Medical and Psychosocial Problems in the Classroom

The Teacher's Role in Diagnosis and Management

Fifth Edition

Edited by
Robert H. A. Haslam
and
Peter J. Valletutti

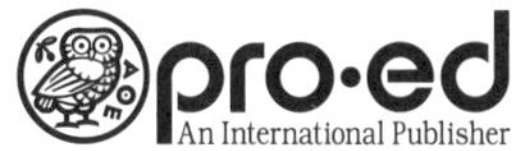

8700 Shoal Creek Boulevard
Austin, TX78757-6897
800/897-3202 Fax 800/397-7633
www.proedinc.com

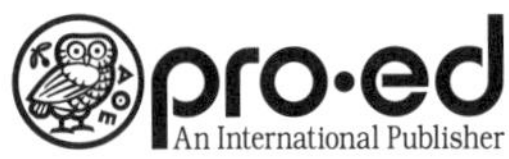

© 2016, 2004, 1996, 1985, 1975 by PRO-ED, Inc.
8700 Shoal Creek Boulevard
Austin, Texas 78757-6897
800/897-3202 Fax 800/397-7633
www.proedinc.com

All rights reserved. No part of the material protected by this copyright notice may be reproduced or used in any form or by any means, electronic or mechanical, including photocopying, recording, or by any information storage and retrieval system, without prior written permission of the copyright owner.

Library of Congress Cataloging-in-Publication Data

Medical and psychosocial problems in the classroom : the teacher's role in diagnosis and management / edited by Robert H. A. Haslam and Peter J. Valletutti. —Fifth edition.
pages cm
Includes bibliographical references and index.
ISBN 978-1-4164-0677-8
1. School health services—United States. 2. School children—Health and hygiene—United States. 3. Children with disabilities—Health and hygiene—United States. 4. Children—Diseases—Diagnosis. I. Haslam, Robert H. A., 1936–II. Valletutti, Peter J.
LB3409.U5M43 2016
371.7'10973—dc23
2015000550

Art director: Jason Crosier
Designer: Tina Brackins
This book was designed in Horley Old Style and Avenir

Printed in the United States of America

1 2 3 4 5 6 7 8 9 10 24 23 22 21 20 19 18 17 16 15

MEDICAL AND PSYCHOSOCIAL PROBLEMS IN THE CLASSROOM

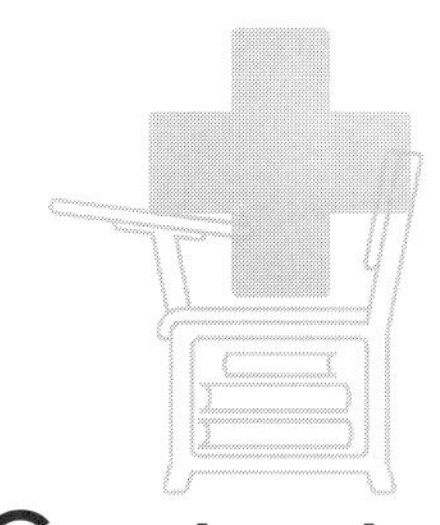

Contents

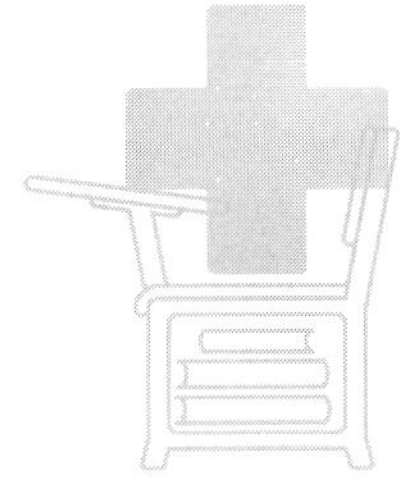

To my wife, Barbara Haslam, BA, MEd, who has been a remarkable inspiration to me since we first met, when she was a special education teacher for children with physical and cognitive disabilities, many years ago. Barb has a knack for teaching students how to think, including our three sons, and a quiet but supportive manner in engaging students in the learning process. Most of all, Barb has supported me in my academic career with advice and ongoing support, which has made the journey together tremendously fulfilling.

—Robert Haslam

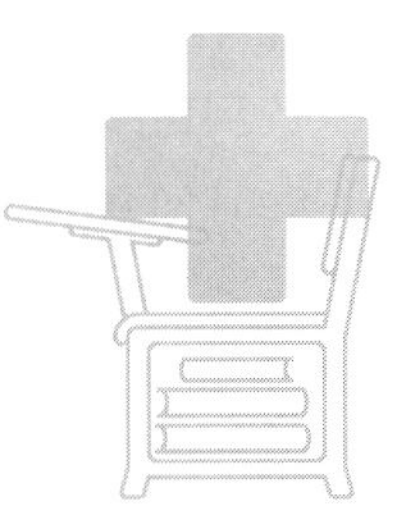

Preface

The role of teachers in the diagnosis and management of students is a multifaceted one that requires a broad range of knowledge and skills. Diagnostic skills may not be sufficiently addressed in some teacher preparation programs, especially when such programs explore their application to the specialized requirements of working with children who have medical and psychosocial problems. The mainstreaming of children with medical and psychosocial problems has markedly expanded the role and professional tasks of teachers, who are now teaching a more diverse population of students. Moreover, because of significant advances in medical care and technology, more children with medical problems are now in school programs and need or are receiving medical attention than there were in former years, when advanced medical procedures were not available.

Teachers can play a significant role in the early identification of students with medical and psychosocial problems, especially when the manifested problems are minor or even moderate. Obviously, a child with severe and profound disabilities most likely will be identified by physicians and parents or other caregivers early in the life of the child. Teachers' professional responsibility to be alert to the existence of medical and psychosocial problems may require an additional task, that is, the need to refer a student for in-depth diagnosis and possible treatment. To expedite such referrals, teachers, consequently, must know whether or not a procedure has been established in the particular school or school system. Teachers must also be knowledgeable about existing school-system-based therapeutic and counseling services as well as those resources available in the community.

WORKING WITH PHYSICIANS AND RELATED PROFESSIONALS

Key Questions to Be Addressed by Teachers

1. What behaviors has the student demonstrated that suggest that he or she may have an undiagnosed medical problem? Are these

behaviors within normal limits, or should a referral be made to a designated staff member, to a primary or medical specialist, to a related service provider (e.g., a physical, occupational, music, or art therapist), or to a speech pathologist?

2. What are the objectives and goals of the specific therapeutic modality, and what are the techniques and materials employed by that specific profession?
3. What medications has the physician prescribed? What are their side effects? What is to be done in a medical emergency?

In addition to working with physicians and related professional service providers, teachers must be knowledgeable and skillful in working with parents or other caregivers of students with medical and psychosocial problems. Many parents of children with disabilities will experience more severe interpersonal, financial, and social problems than will parents without children with disabilities. These parents more likely have many more problems in dealing with their child, with their non-disabled siblings, and with each other. Communicating and collaborating with parents or other caregivers of children with medical and psychosocial problems requires much more effort on the part of teachers.

WORKING WITH PARENTS AND OTHER CAREGIVERS

Key Questions to Be Addressed by Teachers

1. What are the learning and behavioral objectives and goals that parents and caregivers have identified that they believe should be assigned a high educational priority, to better facilitate the improved functioning of their child?
2. What skills is the child demonstrating on a partial or regular basis?
3. What activities, toys, and other items does the child enjoy playing with or using in a functional manner?
4. What particular skills and behaviors are the parents, teachers, and caregivers encouraging and working on? What materials are they using when they engage in these selected teaching activities?
5. What techniques and materials do they use in rewarding their child when he or she shows progress or engages in appropriate behavior?
6. What techniques and materials do they use to modify the child's inappropriate or destructive behavior?

7. What recommendations or suggestions have they made both in informal meeting and during the Individualized Education Program (IEP) process regarding education planning and teaching and behavioral management?
8. What are the best ways for teachers to communicate with parents and caregivers so that they can assist in helping the child acquire needed skills, with special attention to fundamental life skills, and most important, how can parents and caregivers assist teachers in developing functional skills in the real-life setting of home and community?
9. Will parents and caregivers be willing to assist the teacher in helping the child by working with him or her in completing home assignments? Will they also be willing to assist by practicing and reinforcing the work that is ongoing in the classroom?

Finally, in their instructional experiences, teachers must devote sufficient time and effort to addressing the individual needs of all students, a task that is difficult when teaching in a group setting, especially when the group is too large and/or too diverse. Students with medical and psychosocial problems, by their very nature, will have atypical problems that must be addressed. When these students are being taught in a mainstream setting, the challenge is a great one because of larger classes and the greater diversity of the student population.

Furthermore, teachers must direct their attention to meeting the needs of the whole child in terms of the type and severity of the particular treatment and the specific educational and treatment plan. Obviously, when teaching a student with medical and psychosocial problems, a holistic emphasis is more difficult. Teachers, however, need to be aware of the possibility that too great a focus on the disability may result in forgetting the other qualities and needs of the child.

Peter Valletutti

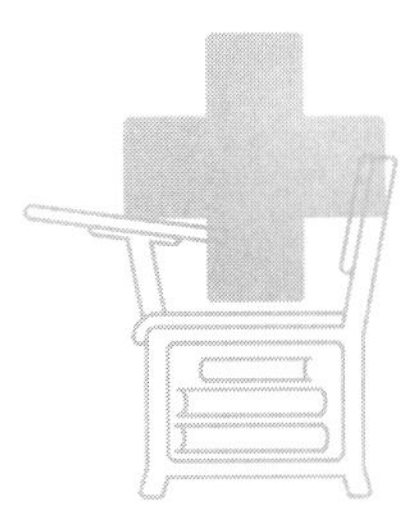

Introduction

Robert H. A. Haslam

> The first edition of *Medical Problems in the Classroom: The Teacher's Role in Diagnosis and Management* was published in 1975. The book was intended for all teachers, both in regular and in special classes. It was also designed for teacher educators as they provided preservice and in-service education for the novice as well as the experienced teacher. In addition, it was developed for school administrators as they sought to better serve the students in their care. It was anticipated that the book would alert readers to the possible existence of various medical problems that may be discovered in the classroom, especially those conditions affecting learning and behavior and the real possibility that the educator might significantly participate in the diagnosis and/or management of the student.

The purpose of this book has not changed over the succeeding 40 years. What has changed are the significantly complex and new medical and social challenges that teachers encounter. Who would have predicted the escalating incidence and various forms of autism, adolescent suicide, bullying, childhood and adolescent obesity, or the seriousness of concussion in the elementary school or adolescent student? For these reasons, the fifth edition of the book has been retitled *Medical and Psychosocial Problems in the Classroom: The Teacher's Role in Diagnosis and Management*, which more accurately reflects what every teacher will encounter during the course of her or his career.

Each chapter in the current edition highlights the important role that the teacher might play in interacting with the health-care team in identifying students with potential serious disorders or working with those professionals to enhance the affected pupil's learning in the classroom. For example, what role might the teacher and school administration play in working with an obese student and family to deal with the problem? What facts should the educator know about a pupil with epilepsy? Is it possible that the child's declining academic performance is due to the medication used to prevent seizures, or are there associated behavioral issues that are interfering with concentration and alertness? What role can the teacher and coach assume in the management of an athlete with significant memory and related symptoms following a concussion during football practice? What steps can the classroom teacher take in assisting the hard-of-hearing student or the child with diabetes mellitus? And what measures might the teacher and school administrators take to prevent school violence and bullying, which unfortunately have become national "epidemics" with frightening consequences?

I am most grateful to each of the authors, all of whom have contributed significantly to the book. Their sharing of experience and knowledge is unparalleled. I am confident that their input will provide the teacher with a valuable resource when encountering a student with one of the disorders covered in this edition.

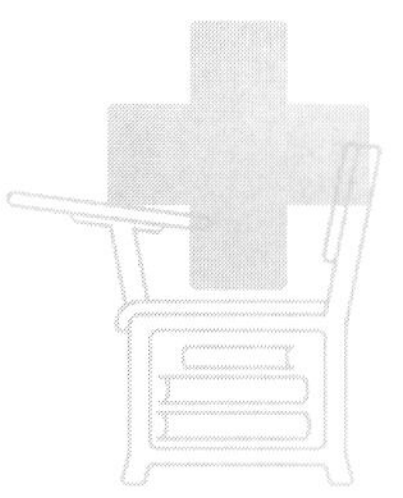

Chapter 1
Infectious Diseases in the Classroom

David B. Haslam and Heidi Andersen

Infectious diseases are exceptionally common among school-age children and are a major cause of school absenteeism. Fortunately, most infections during childhood are brief and resolve either spontaneously or following a short course of antibiotic therapy. Young children may have up to six infections per year, each typically lasting two to four days. Infection of the upper respiratory tract, including the ears, nose, and throat, is most common, followed by viral infections of the lower respiratory tract (bronchiolitis or "bronchitis") and the gastrointestinal tract (gastroenteritis). Most infections during childhood are viral and resolve without the need for antibiotics. However, prolonged infection or severe local symptoms might suggest a bacterial infection that would benefit from antibiotics. Rarely, infections may be life threatening or persist throughout life. Such infections require recognition and effective management, which will include the participation of the child's educator and physician. By definition, an infectious disease can be transmitted from one person to another, and the infected child may pose a risk to his or her classmates or other school attendees. For this reason, children with acute, short-term infections are generally excluded from regular classroom activities while ill and presumed to be contagious. School exclusion is less practical or acceptable during chronic or lifelong infections, especially when the risk of transmission from the infected child to others is low. In those circumstances, an Individualized

Educational Program (IEP) that provides the most appropriate educational environment while ensuring the safety of all school attendees should be developed. Vaccines have been developed against the most severe childhood illnesses and have markedly improved life span and quality of life across the globe. Yet the practice of childhood vaccination has detractors. The failure to vaccinate susceptible individuals and the fact that vaccines are not 100% effective means that some nearly eliminated infectious diseases such as measles still persist in North America. Finally, there is evidence that the seasonal pattern and geographic distribution of some infectious diseases may be changing, at least in part because of alterations in the global climate. This chapter discusses many of the infection-related issues that teachers and administrators will encounter, including life-threatening emergencies, disruptive but short-lived viral infections, lifelong infections, and global changes in infectious disease prevalence.

CLASSROOM INFECTIOUS DISEASE EMERGENCIES

The ABCs of Infectious Disease Emergencies

There are a few infectious diseases that may be life threatening and require prompt medical treatment to ensure the child's survival. Community members, including teachers, are often the first people to recognize such infections and guide those who are affected to emergent care. These infections are life threatening because they involve vital structures or parts of the body that allow for the rapid spread of the virulent organism, a harmful toxin produced by the pathogen, or chemicals released by the body.

Vital structures (ABCs) include the airway, brain, and circulation (heart). Some organisms can infect the epiglottis, located at the top of the airway, where it is responsible for protecting food from entering into and blocking the airways. When infected, the epiglottis swells and can obstruct the airway, resulting in rapid respiratory failure that may be fatal. Children with epiglottitis are classically described as having excessive drooling, making squeaking noises, and refusing to lie down. Epiglottitis is now understood to have been the cause of George

Washington's death. Keeping the child alive requires maintaining an open airway in children with epiglottitis. Ways to help keep the airway open involve keeping the child calm and still, not opening the child's mouth, and refraining from forcing the child to lie down. Essentially, a calm and still child is a calm and still epiglottis. The child with epiglottitis needs to be kept quiet until emergency medical providers can safely protect the child's airway. Other infections can affect the airway and look similar to epiglottitis. Croup is a common viral infection that also affects the upper airways, causing raspy breathing with increased effort required to breathe. Unlike epiglottitis, croup is associated with cough and runny nose, and it is much less likely to be severe or life threatening.

Infections of the brain or surrounding spinal fluid are also life-threatening emergencies. The brain lies in close proximity to the face and sinuses and has a rich blood supply. The eyes, sinuses, nose, mouth, ears, and skin covering the face are all common places for infections. Infection can reach the brain or spinal fluid from any one of these routes. When an infection reaches the brain or spinal fluid, it causes inflammation and swelling of the brain and surrounding tissues. Initially, brain inflammation may be evident as a generalized headache, and as it progresses, it may cause changes in brain activity such as drowsiness, seizures, double vision (diplopia), or inability to move one or more arms or legs. When left untreated, the child with brain infection may go into coma and lose the ability to breathe without help. It is imperative that the child receive medical attention early on in the course of the preceding symptoms.

Some infectious disease emergencies involve the heart and subsequently the circulatory system. When a bacterial infection involves the space between the chest cavity and heart (the pericardium), fluid can accumulate in this space, resulting in increased pressure on the heart. Eventually the pressure can overcome the ability of the heart to pump blood, causing reduced blood flow, low blood pressure, and eventually acute heart failure. A child with acute bacterial pericarditis will complain of chest pain that worsens with breathing but improves with standing rather than lying down, may cough, may have fever, and will become very sweaty, as the heart is struggling to work. In addition to other medical treatment, this child may require emergent drainage of the fluid around the heart to survive.

Sepsis

A special infection of the circulatory system is sepsis, defined as infection of the bloodstream. Organisms may enter the bloodstream from a localized primary site of infection. A common example of this type of sepsis is caused by *Staphylococcus aureus* ("Staph"), the most common cause of boils and skin infections. However, some organisms are notable for living quietly on the body until they get a chance to invade the bloodstream, and without prior warning they result in a rapid progression to sepsis and possibly death. An example of this type of infection is meningococcemia, caused by *Neisseria meningitidis*. Within the bloodstream, infectious organisms cause a marked inflammatory response, leakiness of the blood vessels, and poor blood supply to vital organs, including the brain, heart, lungs, and kidneys. A sustained decrease in blood pressure will result in shock, followed by failure of multiple organs. Replacement of volume to restore the blood pressure and prompt antibiotic treatment is essential for survival.

Toxic Shock Syndrome

Some bacteria produce and release toxins that can also cause shock. The two most common pathogens, *Staphylococcus aureus* and *Streptococcus pyogenes*, are bacteria that are typically found on skin or in the nares and pharynx, respectively. Their toxins are able to cause uncontrolled stimulation of the immune system with release of substantial chemicals causing an overwhelming inflammatory response that appears similar to septic shock. Typically, toxic shock syndrome is described in adolescent females with retained tampon use, because this can lead to colonization by *Staphylococcus aureus*, which is capable of releasing the toxic shock toxin. However, toxic shock is now most often not associated with tampon use and can result simply from carriage of Staphylococcus or Streptococcus on the skin or in the nose. Although toxic shock syndrome typically occurs in healthy persons without a primary infection, shock from *Streptococcus pyogenes* (the bacteria also responsible for strep throat) usually follows a skin infection. The symptoms of toxic shock syndrome include a bright red rash (often similar to a skin burn) and symptoms resulting from low blood pressure and poor blood flow, such as dizziness, rapid and shallow breathing, confusion with difficulty following simple commands, and changes in skin color to a blotchy purplish color. As with other causes of shock, volume replacement with intravenous fluids is essential. Other necessary therapies for children with toxic shock include removing the nidus of an infection (such as the tampon), prompt antibiotic therapy, and consideration of an antitoxin agent. While waiting for emergent medical care, it is prudent in this case to lay the child down and elevate his or her feet to optimize fluid return to the heart for restoration of blood pressure. In addition, it is helpful to cover the child with a blanket to help maintain body temperature while he or she is in shock.

Necrotizing Fasciitis (Flesh-Eating Disease)

There are other ways besides the bloodstream that infections can rapidly spread within the body and cause life-threatening infection. In particular, there is a layer of tissue known as the fascia that lies just above the muscles as a contiguous plane. This plane of tissue can allow for rapid spreading of an infection that can progress significantly before being physically visible as it is covered by the upper skin layers. This type of infection is usually preceded by a traumatic injury or surgical procedure. The first symptoms are often fever, rapid heart rate, and pain that is out of proportion to the injury or appearance of the injury. As the infection spreads, the pain worsens, as does the swelling of the affected areas as a result of the immune system's inflammatory response to the infection. As the swelling continues, it often results in apparent blistering of the visible outer skin layer, along with weeping fluid on the surface. In addition, as the bacteria traveling along the fascia spread, they produce gas, which can be felt on the skin surface, creating a crackly sensation when touched. However, touching the skin will result in excruciating pain. Necrotizing fasciitis is often caused by *Streptococcus pyogenes,* which can also cause toxic shock syndrome, as discussed above, but more commonly causes throat infections (strep throat) or milder skin infections. Bacteria causing this type of infection are often referred to as "flesh-eating bacteria" and are notable for their production of toxins and other factors that break down tissues. Necrotizing fasciitis impairs blood flow to the affected area, making it difficult for antibiotics to reach the infected region. For this reason, antibiotics alone may be unsuccessful, and emergent surgical cleaning of the infected tissue is often required to save the child's life.

COMMON ACUTE INFECTIOUS DISEASES

Below we discuss the most common infections that occur in school-age children. Out of necessity, this is an abbreviated list, but it describes the infections that account for the vast majority of illness-associated absenteeism and visits to the doctor's office. Among these, upper respiratory tract infections, which can take several forms, account for most such illnesses.

Upper Respiratory Tract Infections

Upper respiratory tract infections (URIs) include the common cold, ear infections, sinusitis, and sore throat, and they are by a large margin the most common infections in school-age children. URIs are usually caused by viruses and generally resolve on their own after a few days without treatment. The most common viral causes of URI are rhinovirus, enterovirus, adenovirus, and coronavirus. At the time of this writing, an outbreak of enterovirus D68 had been reported in several states and provinces. In addition to a URI, some of the children in that outbreak developed weakness of an extremity (similar to the pattern of paralysis observed in poliomyelitis). The association of the enterovirus D68 infection and extremity involvement is not clear and is under further study; these things are a reminder that poliovirus is a member of the enterovirus family. The viruses that cause URIs are most readily transmitted by direct contact with infected secretions and are less well transmitted in the air (such as after a child coughs or sneezes). Symptoms begin when the virus comes into contact with the lining of the mouth or nose. There, the virus begins to replicate and cause an injury and immune response. Depending on where the virus was inoculated and where it is best able to establish infection, symptoms will be predominantly in the nose, ears, throat, or sinuses. These sites are all connected at the back of the throat, and it is common for infection in one site to spread to others. Symptoms that begin in the nose or throat often progress to involve the ears or sinuses within a few hours or days. Some viruses also infect the lining of the eyes, causing conjunctivitis, which generally occurs at the same time as infection of the nose or throat. During an acute URI, the child may have fever, nasal congestion, cough, and sore throat. Nasal drainage will initially be clear but will turn yellow or green within one to two days. Green nasal drainage is common in viral URIs and is not alone a sign of bacterial infection or the need for antibiotics. Red, injected eyes with clear drainage are signs of viral conjunctivitis, whereas thick white or green drainage from the eye may indicate bacterial infection. Examination of the child with URI will demonstrate nasal discharge, reddened and inflamed linings of the nose and throat, red and injected eardrums, and often some enlargement of the tonsils and lymph glands in the neck. The child with an uncomplicated URI may be irritable and appear miserable but will generally still interact with her or his surroundings and maintain adequate intake of fluids. Symptoms and fever generally peak on the second or third day of illness, then begin to resolve. During the symptomatic period, the child is contagious and recusal from school is recommended. The virus may be present in secretions for several days afterward, and careful hand washing will prevent further spread.

Bacterial URIs are less common but generally more serious. "Strep throat," caused by the bacterium *Streptococcus pyogenes*, can mimic viral sore throat, but when untreated, it can occasionally cause serious complications, such as infection that spreads into the neck or occasionally into the bloodstream. Rheumatic fever is a rare but very serious complication of strep throat that can damage the heart but has all but disappeared from North America since antibiotics were discovered. Clues to a diagnosis of strep infection are sore throat in the absence of nasal congestion or cough. The tonsils may be quite enlarged and covered with whitish material and lymph nodes in the neck are often swollen and tender. These findings can also be seen in viral infections, however, and the accurate diagnosis of strep throat requires laboratory testing. Treatment is generally highly effective, though reinfection can occur.

Infection of the middle ear (otitis media) and sinuses often begins as a viral infection. During viral infection the tubes that connect the middle ear and sinuses can be blocked by mucus and inflammation-induced swelling of the tissues. Mucus and inflammatory cells become trapped in the middle ear or sinuses, causing sensations of fullness, congestion, pressure, and ultimately pain. These may all occur as a result of viral infection alone. However, when certain bacteria are present in the middle ear or sinuses when blockage occurs, the bacteria may replicate to high numbers and cause a severe inflammatory response. This is usually associated with increased fever and considerable pain. Since this process generally takes a few days to develop, bacterial otitis media or sinusitis may be suspected when ear or sinus pain develop after day 3 to 4 of a URI or when the symptoms are more severe than expected for a typical viral infection. In school-age children it is now generally recommended that antibiotics not be prescribed unless symptoms fail to improve by three to four days or there are severe local symptoms of ear pain or sinus tenderness. Antibiotics can help speed resolution of symptoms when the infection is caused by bacteria and can prevent complications, such as extension of infection into the brain, spinal fluid, or space behind the eyes. However, excessive use of antibiotics in the treatment of a URI, such as during a viral infection, drives the residing bacteria to become resistant and therefore less effective in treating a proven bacterial infection with a specific antibiotic. Decongestants are often used during acute URI but have not conclusively been shown to have any benefit. Since decongestants can have side effects, they are generally not recommended, especially in young children.

Laryngitis is an infection of the lower throat and vocal cords and is almost always viral. In young children laryngitis often causes a barky cough and an upper-pitched noise while taking a breath known as croup. Noise on inspiration is called stridor and is distinguished from wheeze, which is noise when breathing out and is usually seen in lower respiratory tract infections or asthma. Inflammation of the vocal cords and lower throat can make it difficult to take a breath, and the child may have increased work of breathing, manifested by drawing in of the soft spaces above and below the rib cage (often called "retractions"). School-age children with laryngitis are less likely to have classic croup but may still have a barky cough, raspy voice, and mild increased work of breathing. Croup can occasionally be severe and require medical attention in young children, but it is rarely serious in school-age children.

Whooping cough (pertussis) is a bacterial infection that had become rare after introduction of the pertussis vaccine. However, the number of pertussis cases has increased dramatically in the past several years in certain populations of children. In school-age children, whooping cough has symptoms very similar to laryngitis, including a persistent barking cough and occasionally increased work of breathing. Pertussis lasts much longer than laryngitis and is now one of the most common causes of cough lasting more than two weeks. Antibiotic treatment can help shorten the duration and prevent spread of the infection if started within the first few days of infection.

Lower Respiratory Tract Infections

Lower respiratory tract infections (LRIs) involve the lungs and may predominantly involve the airways, the connecting tissue that keeps the air spaces open, or the air spaces themselves. Infections of the airways, often called bronchiolitis, tend to cause cough, wheezing, and increased work of breathing, which is evident as retractions of the spaces between the ribs while the child takes a breath. Infections of the connecting tissue causes increased rate of breathing and cough but does not usually interfere with oxygen uptake. Airway infections are usually viral and generally resolve within four to five days without antibiotic therapy. However, severe cases may compromise the ability to obtain sufficient oxygen and may require medical attention. Viral LRIs can appear similar to an asthma attack, and indeed, asthma is often triggered by an LRI in children.

Bacterial pneumonia is a serious LRI that involves the air spaces and may interfere with oxygen exchange, ultimately leading to respiratory failure. Bacterial pneumonia may follow a viral respiratory tract infection and should be suspected in the child who fails to improve or worsens after the day 3 or 4 of illness. Bacterial pneumonia generally causes fever greater than 39° C (102.2° F), increased rate of breathing, cough, and decreased appetite and energy level. Bacterial pneumonia generally responds to oral antibiotics when treated in early stages but may require hospitalization when more advanced.

Influenza

Influenza viruses cause combined upper and lower respiratory tract infections and are generally more severe than other respiratory viruses. The flu begins with upper respiratory symptoms, often in association with headache, fever, and body aches. Within a couple of days, the infection usually progresses to involve the lung airways and connecting tissues, causing cough, wheeze, and increased rate and work of breathing. Influenza infection can interfere with the lungs' defenses against bacterial infection, and a dreaded complication of the flu is secondary bacterial pneumonia. The influenza virus can occasionally spread to other locations, such as the brain, heart, or muscles, in which case the infection can cause long-term injury. The influenza viruses mutate every year so that immunity to one flu virus does not provide protection in following years. Each year vaccines are developed against the most common strains circulating in the population. The vaccines do not protect against all strains, and for that reason the vaccine is not 100% protective. Nevertheless, widespread use of influenza vaccines results in many fewer cases of the flu, as well as fewer hospitalizations and deaths due to complications of influenza. Antiviral medications have been developed with activity against influenza viruses. These shorten the course of illness and may prevent serious complications if started within the first two days of illness.

Mononucleosis

Classic mononucleosis, caused by the Epstein-Barr virus (EBV), is most common in teenage children and presents with fever, sore throat, and swollen lymph glands. The tonsils are often markedly enlarged and can be covered with whitish material, and together these findings often suggest strep throat. Tonsil swelling can be so severe as to cause difficulty swallowing, and patients can become dehydrated. Physical examination will also reveal an enlarged spleen and enlarged glands under the arm and in the groin. The enlarged spleen may rupture if subjected to blunt trauma, and for that reason students with mononucleosis are usually excluded from contact sports and bicycle riding until the spleen size begins to return to normal. Mononucleosis has an unusual propensity to cause a feeling of tiredness or fatigue that can last for weeks after infection. The virus was once thought to cause chronic fatigue syndrome, but research did not support this idea, and the fatigue from EBV infection usually resolves within weeks to a few months. In rare circumstances, EBV infection has been associated with cancers of the lymph nodes, but this is very rare in people with normal immunity. Younger children can become infected with EBV, but the findings are less typical of mononucleosis, as the pharyngitis is usually mild. Usually young children have fevers that persist for more than one week, swollen lymph glands, and an enlarged spleen. The virus is transmitted in saliva and is often known as the "kissing disease," but contaminated glasses, sports water bottles, and other sites may be the source of infection. After the initial infection the EBV virus becomes dormant in lymphatic cells, and as mentioned later, the infection persists throughout life. There is no effective treatment for EBV infection, but fortunately, in the child with normal immunity, EBV does not tend to cause long-term illness or recur.

Gastroenteritis

Infection of the gastrointestinal tract can be caused by either bacteria or viruses and is the second most common site of infection in school-age children after the respiratory tract. As with respiratory infections, most gastrointestinal infections are caused by viruses. In the well-nourished child with normal immunity, viral gastroenteritis typically causes nausea, vomiting, diarrhea, and low-grade fever. Abdominal pain may be present but is generally mild. Stools can be watery, greenish, and contain mucus but should not contain blood. Nausea and vomiting interfere with food and liquid intake, and the most common serious complication of viral gastroenteritis is dehydration. Young children should urinate every four to six hours, while older school-age children should be able to void at least 500 ml (one pint) of urine every 12 hours. Less urine output can be a sign of dehydration and should prompt medical assessment in the child with gastroenteritis. Until recently, the most common and most severe form of viral gastroenteritis was caused by rotavirus, which infected almost all children by the time they entered school. Effective rotavirus vaccines now exist, and the infection has become much less common. There are as yet no other vaccines available to prevent viral gastroenteritis, and there are no effective antiviral medications for it. Fortunately, these infections are short lived and very rarely cause lasting injury as long as fluid intake is maintained.

Gastroenteritis can also be caused by bacteria such as Salmonella, Shigella, Campylobacter, and Yersinia. These infections are usually acquired from unwashed or undercooked foods, including eggs, chicken, salads, and other vegetables. Distinct from viral gastroenteritis, bacterial infections tend to cause fever greater than 38.5° C (101.3° F) and more severe abdominal pain, and they can cause bloody stools. Bacterial gastroenteritis often resolves without antibiotic therapy, but in certain circumstances it should be treated, and for that reason the student suspected of having bacterial infection should be referred for medical evaluation. A notable form of bacterial gastroenteritis is caused by a type of *E. coli* that produces a toxin and can cause kidney failure and other serious complications. Outbreaks of this infection, called hemolytic uremic syndrome (HUS), are often attributed to contaminated foods (particularly ground beef and unwashed vegetables). HUS may begin as mild diarrhea that suddenly progresses to severe abdominal pain and bloody stools. Fever is usually absent or mild. The kidney injury starts soon after development of abdominal pain. Students suspected of having HUS should always be brought to medical attention.

Head, Body, and Pubic Lice

Infestation with lice, also known as pediculosis, is a common but underreported problem as infestation carries a social stigma. Not a true infection per se, pediculosis has afflicted humans from the earliest recorded times and is caused by small insects approximately the size of sesame seeds that survive by feeding on blood obtained through tiny bites. Different louse species tend to take up residence on different parts of the human body, accounting for distinct infestations of the scalp, the pubic area, and the body. Scalp infection is most common in children and typically manifests as itching of the back of the scalp and behind the ears. Itching is most severe at night, when lice feed, but may persist throughout the day, causing considerable discomfort and distraction. Female insects lay eggs on hair shafts adjacent to the scalp, where the small whitish eggs, called "nits," are often more readily apparent than the adult insects. Visualization with a magnifying glass is often helpful in confirming the diagnosis of head lice. The insects are readily transmitted from person to person by direct contact or through sharing of a contaminated object or article of clothing. For this reason, louse infestation is commonly seen in overcrowded or impoverished settings, but it can occur among students from any socioeconomic background. School children can transmit lice among themselves (and rarely to their educators), and therefore many schools have a "no nit" policy by which children with head lice are excluded from school until they receive effective treatment. Several medications are effective at killing adult lice when applied to the scalp, but most do not kill unhatched nits so a second application approximately 7–10 days later is required to eradicate the infestation. Nit removal using a fine-toothed comb, often assisted by direct visualization and "nit picking" with a pair of tweezers, can be a useful additional measure. Permethrin is usually chosen as the first-line treatment for head lice. Recently, resistance to this drug has been observed, and other agents, such as malathione or ivermectin, may find increased use in the future. Treatment of household and other close contacts is important, as is decontamination of bed linens and other potentially contaminated items. These can be washed and heated at high temperature, or if that is not possible and the item cannot be discarded, sealing the item in a plastic bag for several weeks will kill lice, as they require a blood meal approximately every two weeks to survive.

CHILDREN WITH CHRONIC AND POTENTIALLY TRANSMISSIBLE INFECTIONS

While most infections in childhood are of relatively short duration, some infections persist for life. Such infections include human immunodeficiency virus (HIV), hepatitis B, hepatitis C, herpes simplex virus 1 and 2 (HSV1 and HSV2), and cytomegalovirus (CMV). Each of these is a viral infection that remains in the body through the rest of the infected child's life. In many cases the infection is dormant and, assuming the child has a normal immune system, poses little risk to the child or caretakers. However, even when the student is without symptoms, chronic viral infections can be transmitted by blood or sometimes other body fluids. Universal precautions, as well as the careful handling of any material expelled by a child, should be practiced at all times, regardless of whether the child is known to harbor an infectious agent.

The educator's goal is to provide all children, including those with chronic infection, with the best possible education while also providing protection to all other school attendees. Federal and state courts have ruled that all children with chronic illness have a right to free education in the least restrictive environment possible. The Americans With Disabilities Act and the Canadian Human Rights Act bar schools, colleges, and other organizations from discriminating against children with disabilities. Chronic viral infections are generally covered by these acts, even if the child is without symptoms of infection. State, provincial, and local laws are often in place to further protect the child's right to education in whatever environment is deemed the most appropriate for the child and the protection of other school attendees. The school board should be responsible for developing procedures to manage children with chronic illness, and these are implemented at individual schools, often with the assistance of a specialized task force that includes the school's medical adviser and nurse. With such procedures in place, schools are able to make individual decisions regarding the appropriate educational environment of a child with chronic illness on a case-by-case basis. Most children with chronic infections should be allowed to participate in regular classroom activities. In rare situations, either because of the nature of the illness or factors that could make transmission more likely, alternative arrangements should be made for the child's education, as we describe below.

Students known to have a chronic infectious disease should be individually evaluated to determine whether their condition poses a health risk to others. The school health advisers should work with the child's teacher, parents, physician, and regional or state health officials to establish the most appropriate educational environment for a chronically infected child. While protecting the child's right to an appropriate education, it is necessary to ensure the safety of other school attendees. Although rare, certain features of the student's health condition may require temporary removal from regular classroom activities. For example, a student with chronic infection may place others at risk if the student lacks toilet training, has exposed open sores, or has biting or other behaviors that might pose a risk of disease transmission. In those circumstances, the school nurse, the student's physician, and occasionally local public health authorities should assist in evaluating the level of risk and whether an alternate educational program should be arranged. The school district should have standing policies to guide decisions regarding health-related school removal. In almost all cases, removal from the regular classroom should be considered a temporary adaptation to the child's condition, and plans should be in place for return to the classroom when the advisers deem it safe for the child to do so. School exclusion is not the only feasible approach to a child who might pose a health risk to others. Schools are encouraged to have some flexibility in appropriately educating such a child. In some cases, this might include recusal from individual classes or activities. In each case the school district should attempt to use the least restrictive approach that is able to effectively protect other students and educators. When a child is removed from the school, effort should be made to reassess the educational program on an ongoing basis. A student who is removed from the classroom should be provided with a continuing education program until it is determined that he or she can safely return. The question of when it is safe for a child to return to school must be answered on an individual basis and will involve discussions between the school nurse and health adviser and the child's parents and physician. Occasionally local public health officials should be included in such decisions.

In all the situations described above, the school should respect the privacy of every child. Regional and federal governments have statutes in place to protect the confidentiality of children with HIV or other chronic infections. Such laws typically outline who can be informed of the identity of an infected child. Further, provisions are made regarding which persons should be made aware that an infected child is enrolled at that school, without revealing the child's identity. Only people with a direct need to know (e.g., principal, superintendent, school nurse, the student's teacher) should be informed of the child's identity. Those individuals should be informed by the school board or an infectious diseases task force of any necessary precautions and of confidentiality requirements. It should be noted that some states have laws enabling legal action against a person who willfully discloses confidential information for non-health-related purposes.

Human Immunodeficiency Virus (HIV)

The human immunodeficiency virus (HIV) infects cells of the immune system and, ultimately, leads to profound defects in defense against infection with other organisms. As a consequence, patients with advanced HIV infection are prone to infections with organisms that rarely cause disease in individuals with normal immunity. Such "opportunistic" infections result in poor quality of life and shortened life span in individuals with untreated HIV infection. HIV is transmitted in blood and body fluids and is most often acquired by sexual exposure, intravenous drug use, or transmission from an infected mother to child by passage across the placenta during pregnancy. There is a lag phase between acquisition of the virus and development of immune dysfunction that can range from several months to several years. Infants who acquire the infection during pregnancy tend to have the shortest lag phase if untreated, often presenting with complications of HIV infection in the first two years of life. Prior to the advent of effective medications, up to one-third of babies born to HIV-infected mothers would themselves be infected. One of the major medical advances in recent years was the development of antiviral drugs with potent activity against HIV. With proper identification and treatment, the risk of HIV transmission from an infected mother to her infant has approached zero. As a consequence, the number of young school-age children with HIV infection has dropped precipitously. Occasionally, HIV infection goes unrecognized in a pregnant woman, or she does not receive an effective treatment course, meaning that HIV infections rarely still do occur in young children. Unfortunately, transmission by sexual contact or intravenous drug use has continued unabated, and teenage children represent a significant proportion of new HIV infections annually. Education about safe-sex practices and risks of drug use are important functions of the school in preventing HIV infection.

Treatment of HIV infection is complex but highly effective. Whereas initial therapies were able to delay progression of HIV disease for variable periods of time, new combination therapies effectively prevent progression and result in dramatically prolonged disease-free survival. Indeed, HIV infection is now managed as a chronic disease, much like asthma or diabetes. Regular physician visits and adherence to therapy can prevent immune dysfunction and opportunistic infections, allowing infected individuals to lead essentially normal lives. Most HIV-infected children should have few infection-related school absentee days, aside from intermittent clinic visits. HIV infection still carries some stigma, and its diagnosis can be associated with psychological stress. Additionally, the child with HIV may live in a social environment that is less than optimal for educational achievement. A diagnosis of HIV infection may be an indicator for the need of additional social support structures, perhaps through the utilization of an IEP, somewhat similar to those provided for children with attention-deficit/hyperactivity disorder (ADHD) or other noninfectious behavioral diagnoses.

The HIV virus is transmitted inefficiently. Very sensitive methods can sometimes detect virus particles in saliva or other body fluids from an infected individual, but the risk of transmission from such fluids is extremely low. Even exposure to blood infrequently results in HIV transmission. For example, needle-stick injuries involving blood from an HIV-infected person have approximately 0.3% risk of transmitting the virus. HIV-infected blood splashed on mucus membranes such as the eyes or mouth carries a 0.1% risk of transmission (1 in 1,000). When intact skin comes in contact with blood or other body fluids from an HIV-infected person, the risk of infection approaches zero. Nevertheless, universal precautions, including donning of gloves and other protective equipment when appropriate, is advised for all educators who must come in contact with blood and body fluids such as vomit, stool, urine, or saliva from any child. In the event of a potential contact with infected material, such as a needle-stick injury or bite, an educator or student should be evaluated by local school health representatives, such as the school nurse, regarding the next appropriate course of action. In the case of needle-stick injuries involving blood known to be or at risk of being from an HIV-infected individual, early testing of the exposed individual and a course of antiviral medication may be prescribed to prevent the virus from establishing infection.

Development of a vaccine against HIV has been hampered by the virus's ability to rapidly mutate and escape immune defenses. Recent advances have been made in identifying regions of the virus that are less able to avoid detection by the immune system, and it is hoped that an effective vaccine might be developed in the next several years. In the meantime, educating teens about prevention, early diagnosis, and adherence to therapy are the most effective means of battling HIV infection.

Hepatitis B and Hepatitis C Infection

Both hepatitis B virus (HBV) and hepatitis C virus (HCV) can be acquired at birth from an infected mother and can cause prolonged infections in children. The infections are often silent throughout the school-age years but may cause liver inflammation and injury (hepatitis) that occasionally leads to liver failure or cirrhosis during childhood. Fortunately, the incidence of HBV transmission to newborns has fallen to very low levels in North America since the 1990s, when universal newborn immunization was instituted. As with HIV, most HBV infections among school-age children are the result of sexual exposure or drug use. However, unlike HIV, routine childhood vaccination against HBV has dramatically decreased the incidence of new HBV infections in the teenage years. HBV infection, including transmission from mother to newborn infant, remains a significant problem in much of the world. Children born overseas have a higher likelihood of infection and should be screened by their physician for HBV infection. HBV is transmitted in blood and other body fluids (except stool) and is up to 100 times more contagious than HIV. The risk of transmission is up to 30% following a needle stick involving blood from an HBV infected person. Occupational exposure to HBV is an important mode of transmission, and in many cases, infected workers do not recall explicit contact with infected blood. Therefore, universal precautions and vaccination for all individuals at risk is the safest means of preventing acquisition of the virus. School districts are mandated to provide the hepatitis vaccine to educators who are at increased risk of exposure. Such individuals include school nurses, health assistants, athletic trainers, physical education and special education teachers, first-aid providers, coaches of contact sports, and playground assistants. The vaccine series is not effective in all persons, and blood testing should be done after vaccination to ensure protective antibody levels, particularly in persons with increased risk of exposure. As with HIV exposure, individuals exposed to potentially infectious material should contact the school health adviser for the next appropriate step. If the exposed person is unvaccinated or has not been tested for a protective response, "passive immunization" may be given, which consists of the administration of pooled antibodies from blood donors. Furthermore, the hepatitis vaccine series is initiated or completed in those lacking full immunity. A number of medications have been developed with activity against the HBV virus, but their effectiveness is variable, and they are often associated with intolerable side effects.

Hepatitis C infection presents similar problems to HIV and HBV in that children may acquire the infection at birth and be infected for very prolonged periods. Like hepatitis B, HCV infection often causes no symptoms during childhood but may present with liver injury or failure several years later. Occasionally children will show signs of hepatitis such as jaundice (yellowish discoloration of the eyes or skin), nausea, decreased appetite, and weight loss. HCV is less transmissible than HBV. Indeed, only approximately 5% of mothers transmit the virus to their babies, though co-infection with HIV or sexually transmitted diseases increases the risk. While infant infections with HCV are rare, the infection remains prevalent across North America given its long course and previously high infection rates. Approximately 2% of the U.S. population is chronically infected. Overseas the rate of infection may be considerably higher. Intravenous drug use is the most common means of transmission beyond the newborn period. The virus may be transmitted sexually but much less efficiently than HBV. Unlike with HBV, there is no effective vaccine against HCV, and it is not currently recommended to administer pooled antibody to prevent transmission to an exposed individual. However, recent years have seen remarkable advances in medical therapy for HCV infection. Antiviral medicines with excellent activity against HCV now exist. Patients with advanced liver injury may show dramatic improvement after initiating therapy. Antiviral therapy of infected mothers will likely further reduce the likelihood of transmission and rates of childhood infection. Whether antiviral medication is safe and effective when administered to an uninfected person after exposure to infected blood is an unanswered question. In high-risk situations, such as direct injection with infected blood, a discussion with an infectious diseases specialist regarding preventative therapy might be warranted. Furthermore, these recommendations might change as experience with new antivirals grows.

Herpes Simplex Virus Infection

The herpes virus family includes herpes simplex virus 1 (HSV1), the most common cause of cold sores or "fever blisters," and herpes virus 2 (HSV2), which is associated with genital herpes, as well as viruses not commonly thought of as herpes viruses, such as varicella virus (VZV), the cause of chickenpox and shingles; cytomegalovirus (CMV); and Epstein-Barr virus (EBV), the cause of mononucleosis. These viruses all cause lifelong infection once acquired. Unlike HIV, HBV, and HCV—which have long quiescent periods despite active viral replication—the herpes viruses have a true latent state. They may lie dormant inside the body without active production of infectious virus. With the exception of EBV, which is not thought to reactivate in people with normal immunity, each of the other viruses can reactivate and cause disease at intervals that range from months to many years.

Despite the fact that HSV1 tends to cause oral lesions and HSV2 is associated with genital infections, their behavior is quite similar, and the viruses are often considered together. Either virus may be transmitted to newborn infants, either at the time of birth or shortly thereafter. In that setting HSV1 or HSV2 can cause severe and life-threatening infection. The newborn immune system is ineffective against these viruses, and they may spread to vital organs, including the brain, lungs, and liver. Untreated, newborn infection with either HSV1 or HSV2 is often fatal or severely debilitating. Even in infants diagnosed quickly and treated appropriately, injury may occur. Furthermore, infection can reactivate and in infants younger than 6 months of age there is evidence that reactivation can also involve the brain and cause neurologic injury. For that reason it is now recommended that infants infected in the first month of life be treated with antiviral medication until the age of 6 months, when recurrences become less frequent and it is felt that the risk of injury to the infant brain has subsided. HSV1 and HSV2 are remarkable in that past the newborn period they rarely cause severe or life-threatening infections in individuals with normal immunity. They do, however, cause remitting infections that can interfere with school attendance and quality of life.

HSV1 acquired beyond the newborn period often begins as a clustered eruption of vesicles and scabbed lesions around the mouth, termed "gingivostomatitis." The primary infection can be extensive, involving the lips, inner mouth, and sometimes the back of the throat. Children may refuse to eat or drink because of pain on swallowing and can become dehydrated. Without treatment the eruption lasts 5–7 days before lesions begin to heal and the child is more comfortable swallowing. Early initiation of acyclovir (an antiviral medication), either by mouth or in severe cases by intravenous administration, shortens the course of infection. After initial infection the child develops an immune response that suppresses but does not completely eradicate the virus. Reactivation can occur in intervals ranging from weeks to years, but symptoms are generally much less pronounced. HSV1 can occasionally cause infection at the site of skin breakdown, most commonly on the hand, where it is called "herpetic whitlow." Whitlow is generally not severe, but it may be confused with bacterial cellulitis, which is normally responsive to antibiotic therapy. HSV1 infection will fail such therapy. Very rarely, HSV1 can migrate from the oral location and cause encephalitis, infection of the brain. HSV1 encephalitis is life threatening and may cause significant brain injury. It is generally unknown why the virus attacks the brain in people who otherwise appear to have normal immunity, but recent research has revealed subtle genetic conditions that make HSV1 encephalitis more likely.

HSV1 is transmitted by direct contact with lesions or infected material, such as saliva. Even when the child does not have obvious oral lesions, the virus may be shed in saliva and be transmitted to susceptible individuals, including classmates and teachers. Prevention includes careful hand washing after exposure to saliva and donning of gloves when contact with active lesions is inevitable. Fortunately, the risk to caretakers or classmates is relatively low. Many persons have been infected with HSV1 without their knowledge, as the infection can be completely without symptoms. In North America, approximately half of adults are infected with HSV1.

HSV2 is generally associated with genital herpes. The virus can be acquired by newborn infants during delivery as described above. When the infection involves the skin or mucus membranes, it can reactivate on the skin or mucus membranes and, therefore, does pose some risk of transmission to school attendees if they are in direct contact with infected lesions or saliva. Reactivation is rare after the first year of life and is expected to be very rare in school-age children. Therefore, HSV2 infection will rarely be a concern among school-age children until the teenage years, when it may be acquired by sexual contact. In the event an educator must come into contact with reactivated infection in a young child, universal precautions, including donning of gloves when contacting open lesions and hand washing after exposure to potentially infected saliva, should effectively prevent transmission.

Cytomegalovirus Infection

Cytomegalovirus, like other herpes viruses, causes lifelong infection once acquired. Unlike the other herpes viruses, CMV infection is often completely without symptoms or may present with a mild flu- or mononucleosis-like illness in individuals with normal immunity. CMV infection is common. Greater than 50% of adults in North America are infected, in most cases without individuals having knowledge of infection. However, the virus is notable for causing severe complications in two settings: unborn children and individuals with severely compromised immune defenses. Educators should be aware of the risks of CMV infection to the unborn child. When a pregnant individual who has not previously been infected with CMV becomes infected, there is a significant risk the virus will infect the developing infant. In severe cases CMV infection of the developing infant can lead to brain injury, hearing loss, vision loss, and heart defects. Since CMV infection is common even among young children and the virus can be shed for prolonged periods in saliva and urine, educators are likely to encounter the virus. The infection is generally spread by oral ingestion, such as by touching infected body fluid and then transmitting the virus to the mouth, such as through eating with contaminated hands. Careful attention to hand washing after contact with urine, saliva, or other body fluids effectively prevents transmission and when universal precautions are practiced, the risk of transmission is low. For that reason, pregnant educators or health-care workers are no longer excluded from the care of CMV-infected children but are reminded to be cautious in handling potentially infectious material.

SEXUALLY TRANSMITTED DISEASES

Sexually transmitted diseases (STDs) constitute those infections that are primarily or solely transmitted by sexual contact. The most prevalent infections include chlamydia, syphilis, gonorrhea, and genital warts. HIV, genital herpes (HSV2), hepatitis B (HBV), and hepatitis C (HCV) are often transmitted by sexual contact and are discussed in the prior section regarding chronic infections. Except where discussed in the section on chronic infections in children, an STD will rarely affect a child's ability to participate normally in school activities. However, educators should be aware of the symptoms and implications of sexually transmitted infections, as they may be in a position to advise the student with an STD. As with all medical information, confidentiality of the child with an STD is protected by law and should be closely guarded. A notable exception is that health-care workers must report certain STDs to state health authorities and are mandated to track sexual partners of infected individuals. In those instances where a sexual partner is contacted by a health-care worker, the identity of the infected individual is not disclosed.

The prevalence of sexually transmitted diseases has consistently increased over the past several decades, with chlamydia infection being the most common and accounting for most of the increase. This is somewhat surprising, as teen pregnancy rates have progressively declined since the early 1990s. Declining teen pregnancy rates are thought to be due to a number of factors, including later age at first sexual contact and more frequent condom use. The reason STD infections continue to increase are not completely understood. Each of the STDs is most common in the age range of 20–24, with the next highest rates seen in those aged 15–19 years, who account for approximately one-quarter of cases. Consequently, high school and middle school students account for a large fraction of annual STD diagnoses. Rates are generally higher in females than males, perhaps partly because the infections are more likely to be symptomatic in infected females. Young infants are sometimes affected by a sexually transmitted disease, as they can be acquired from the mother either before or at the time of birth. Most notable among the STDs transmitted to newborns are HIV, syphilis, and HSV2, as described here and in other sections in this chapter.

Chlamydia Infection

Chlamydia trachomatis, the causative agent of genital chlamydia, is the most common STD, infecting approximately 3% of teenage girls and 1% of teenage boys. The infection often causes no symptoms, which may explain why infection rates are so high, but this also likely results in underreporting and missed diagnoses. The organism is readily transmitted by vaginal, oral, or anal intercourse and may have a prolonged incubation period from the time of exposure to development of symptoms. When chlamydia infection does cause symptoms, they are usually confined to the urethra, causing a clear discharge and pain upon urination. However, prolonged untreated chlamydia infection can lead to persistent pelvic pain in women. Infertility is the most serious complication of chlamydia infection, and this can occur even if the infection causes no symptoms. Chlamydia can contribute to pelvic inflammatory disease, a mixed infection that can cause fever, intense pelvic pain, and damage to the fallopian tubes resulting in infertility or ectopic pregnancy. An infected woman may transmit chlamydia to her infant during childbirth. After an incubation period of two to four weeks, the infection may become evident as eye infection (conjunctivitis) or pneumonia, which manifests as increased rate and work of breathing and wheezing. Treatment of chlamydia infection is generally highly effective. A single dose of azithromycin or one week of doxycycline are equally effective and generally safe except in pregnant women, in which case other antibiotics are prescribed. Importantly, sexual contacts should also be treated, and the failure to do so is the most common reason for recurrence of chlamydia infection. The outcomes for persons who complete a course of therapy are otherwise excellent. However, it is prudent to test such individuals for other sexually transmitted infections, as they require alternative treatment approaches.

Gonorrhea Infection

Infection with *Neisseria gonorrhea* is the second most common STD among school-age individuals. Approximately 3 per 1,000 teenagers are diagnosed with gonorrhea annually, with rates approximately twice as high in girls as compared to boys. Like chlamydia, gonorrhea causes urethral irritation but is more likely to cause cloudy urethral discharge and pain on urination. The infection tends to be more aggressive than chlamydia and is more likely to cause pelvic inflammatory disease and intramenstrual bleeding. In boys the infection can extend from the urethra to the epididymis, causing severe testicular pain. Gonorrhea can be transmitted by oral and anal intercourse, and it may present with rectal infection or pharyngitis that is difficult to distinguish from strep throat without specifically identifying the organism in the laboratory. Occasionally gonorrhea infection can disseminate from the genital tract and cause bloodstream infection that can settle in the joints, causing infectious arthritis. In women, gonorrhea can infect the liver, which can be life threatening if not treated aggressively. Like chlamydia, gonorrhea can infect newborns as they transit the birth canal and can cause severe conjunctivitis. Treatment of gonorrhea has become more complicated, as a fraction of gonorrhea strains have become resistant to antibiotics. Recommended treatment currently consists of an intramuscular dose of antibiotic, followed by either a single dose of azithromycin or one week of doxycycline. The oral antibiotic provides two functions: treatment for chlamydia, which often coinfects persons with gonorrhea infection, and backup for the injection, in case the organism is resistant to the antibiotic, which is still rare in North America but seen at much higher rates in other parts of the world. Additionally, azithromycin or doxycycline provides treatment for chlamydia.

Syphilis Infection

Infection with *Treponema pallidum*, the causative agent of syphilis, is found at lower rates in North America than the other STDs described here, affecting approximately 5 per 100,000 adults. Its importance lies in the propensity for syphilis to progress through distinct stages as it causes infection throughout the body and causes severe disease if untreated. Primary syphilis causes a painless ulcerated lesion called a chancre at the site of inoculation. Because the chancre is painless, infected individuals may not seek treatment. Secondary syphilis occurs approximately one month later and results from spread of the organism to the bloodstream. Symptoms of secondary syphilis include fever, body aches, swollen glands, and a distinctive rash often seen on the palms, soles, and lining of the mouth. If untreated at this stage, syphilis may be latent for several months to years, when it may recur with symptoms most prominent in the brain, heart, or essentially any organ. Syphilis may be transmitted during pregnancy from the infected mother to the developing child. Depending on the timing of transmission, syphilis may cause stillbirth, organ damage, or disseminated infection similar to severe secondary syphilis. Recognition of syphilis is therefore important to prevent severe complications both in the infected individual and, if pregnant, to the woman's unborn child. Fortunately, *Treponema pallidum* remains susceptible to penicillin, which remains the treatment of choice. The type of penicillin treatment varies depending on the stage of infection. As with the other STDs described here, reinfection can occur, particularly if sexual partners do not also receive treatment.

Genital Warts and Cervical Cancer

Human papilloma virus (HPV) infection of the genital, anal, or tracheal regions can cause wartlike lesions known as condyloma. There are dozens of HPV strains, many of which can cause genital condyloma. However, serotypes 16 and 18 are most notable, as infection with these strains is associated with a significant risk of developing cancer of the cervix. Overall, HPV infection is common and globally HPV infection is the most common STD. Not all infected individuals have genital warts, however, and their incidence is approximately 1 in 1,000 adults. The true incidence of HPV infection and genital warts is difficult to discern, as there is no system for reporting of the infection. The lesions are almost exclusively transmitted by sexual contact, and it is estimated that up to 75% of persons who have intercourse with an infected partner will eventually develop genital warts. The period from initial HPV infection to development of condyloma is often prolonged, with incubation periods lasting months to years. Condyloma are generally painless but are considered unsightly and therefore may cause considerable anxiety. Treatment is aimed predominantly at removal of the condyloma via laser, cryotherapy, or surgery. Most concerning is the propensity for HPV 16 and 18 to cause abnormalities in infected tissues that progress from relatively benign changes to invasive cancer. HPV is thought to cause essentially all cases of cervical cancer and many cases of vaginal, anal, and penile cancers. Therefore, effective prevention of HPV infection by safe-sex practices and vaccination should markedly reduce the incidence of this devastating cancer. Vaccination against HPV is now recommended for boys and girls at 11–12 years of age. As of 2013, uptake of the vaccine was suboptimal, with only approximately 60% of eligible girls and 30% of eligible boys having received the vaccine. Some of the reluctance to vaccinate young teens apparently arises from parental concern about vaccinating specifically against a sexually transmitted infection. Educational efforts are aimed at alleviating the concern that vaccination condones or leads to earlier sexual activity.

INFECTIOUS DISEASE EXPOSURES ASSOCIATED WITH FIELD TRIPS OR CLASSROOM ACTIVITIES

School field trips can be tremendous experiences to supplement an educational topic being discussed in the classroom, but they may involve exposures to animals or other potential sources of infection. Potential infectious diseases from field trips or camping trips include Lyme disease, Rocky Mountain spotted fever, toxocariasis, encephalitis, rabies, Baylisascaris, acute diarrheal illnesses including hemolytic uremic syndrome, mycobacteriosis, psittacosis, and Q fever. Unfortunately, animals are sources of numerous pathogens. In many cases, animal-associated infections are transmitted by ticks.

Tick-Borne Infections

An adventure in the woods or tall grass may expose the adventurers to ticks, which can harbor the spirochete pathogen responsible for Lyme disease. *Borrelia burgdorferi* is responsible for Lyme disease. A few tips to help prevent contraction of tick-borne illnesses include applying DEET-containing insect spray while outdoors, wearing long-sleeved shirts and pants, and checking adventurers for ticks upon their return. Common sites of tick attachment include the scalp and groin. Lyme disease occurs after a tick has had sufficient attached time to the skin for transmission of the pathogen, which is usually estimated to require more than 24 hours. Fortunately, Lyme disease is neither an emergency nor a life-threatening illness, and it is easily treatable. The characteristic features include a bull's-eye-type rash at the site of tick feeding and occasionally low-grade fever, headache, and muscle aches. If untreated, Lyme disease can cause more serious complications, such as arthritis and infection of the heart or brain. In areas where Lyme disease is common, it is important to observe tick-exposed children for the characteristic features of early disease. Rocky Mountain spotted fever (RMSF) is also transmitted by ticks and is generally more serious. The infection often starts with fever, headache, and muscle pains, but soon it presents with a spotted rash, most prevalent on the palms, soles, or wrists. As the infection progresses, the child may develop a rapid heart rate, stomach pain, and later confusion, low blood pressure, and shock. Early treatment of the child with RMSF will prevent these complications, so any child with tick exposure in the previous 2–3 weeks who develops fever and headache should be evaluated by a medical professional.

Mosquitos are another potential source of infectious diseases in the child. The type of infection transmitted depends upon the environment and the type of mosquito involved. In other parts of the world, malaria, caused by *Plasmodium falciparium*, is responsible for most mosquito-borne infections. In North America mosquitoes are most notable for transmitting viruses that cause encephalitis, an inflammatory infection of the brain. West Nile virus is the most common such infection, although others are also well described. Viral encephalitis usually causes fever, headache, confusion, and occasionally seizures and hallucinations. There are no effective treatments for mosquito-transmitted encephalitis viruses, but fortunately the infections usually resolve without permanent injury. Finally, field trips or classroom pets can expose children to lizards and turtles, each of which can transmit infections. Most notable in this regard is salmonella, a form of bacterial gastroenteritis. The symptoms of salmonella are similar to other causes of bacterial gastroenteritis discussed previously. In the child with normal immunity, treatment is generally not necessary, as the infection will resolve on its own.

CLASSROOM INFECTIONS AFFECTED BY CHANGES IN VACCINATION AND GLOBAL CLIMATE

A number of infectious diseases that were never prevalent or almost eliminated in North America have become increasingly common. Furthermore, infections that were previously localized to distinct geographic areas appear to be expanding their distribution. This stems from a number of factors, including failure to vaccinate susceptible children, problems with vaccine effectiveness, increased international travel, and climate change.

Among vaccine-preventable infections, pertussis (whooping cough) has seen the greatest increase in prevalence. In North America, vaccination had almost completely eradicated whooping cough among school-age children. However, there has been a steady increase in prevalence among children. Although still low by historical standards, recent years have seen the most cases in school-age children since the vaccine was first introduced decades ago. The increase in whooping cough cases has been particularly notable among children aged 7–18, although infant infections are also increasingly common. Some of the increase in whooping cough prevalence may be related to incomplete vaccination, but there is concern that the new "acellular" vaccine, which has fewer side effects than the older "whole cell" vaccine, may be less effective.

Overall, measles and mumps infections are at historically low levels; however, sporadic outbreaks continue to occur. College campuses are often the epicenters for such outbreaks, because it is in college dormitories that students are often first exposed in close quarters to a large number of other individuals. In recent years most infections have surprisingly occurred among fully vaccinated students. Waning immunity might play a role, as might exposure to unvaccinated (or incompletely vaccinated) individuals who shed mumps or measles viruses at a high level and readily transmit the infections.

International travel can be the source of sporadic or epidemic infections. For example, the West Nile virus epidemic that swept across North America is thought to have originated from a mosquito carried by airplane from Europe to New York. Sudden acute respiratory syndrome (SARS) and epidemic influenza outbreaks have occurred on a smaller scale but are reminders that an epidemic may be ignited by a single plane trip. At the time of this writing, the first cases of Ebola infection in North America had been reported, all in travelers or health-care workers returning from overseas. An awareness of outbreaks occurring worldwide will prepare the teacher for unexpected illnesses closer to home.

At the individual level, it is important to remember that a student returning from overseas may present with infections rarely seen in North America. In some cases these illnesses may mimic locally acquired and generally less serious infections. Gastrointestinal infections acquired overseas are more likely to be bacterial and require medical attention than is gastroenteritis acquired in North America. Parasitic infections are also fairly common, particularly after travel to Asia, Africa, or Latin America. Infected students may not have obvious gastrointestinal symptoms, but they may develop weight loss, decreased appetite, or anemia, all of which can interfere with school performance. Similarly, respiratory illness may be due to a novel influenza or coronavirus, to which the student may lack immunity. Tuberculosis is uncommon, especially after brief overseas trips, but it should be considered in a returned traveler with persistent fever, cough, and decreased energy. Malaria is among the more common infections seen in returned travelers and may manifest with "flu-like symptoms," such as fever, headache, sore muscles, and chills. A heightened awareness for atypical infections and a lower threshold for suggesting medical attention are warranted among students recently returned from international travel.

Illnesses formerly acquired only overseas are moving closer to home. Urbanization, human migration, and climate change are associated with expanded habitats of several insects that transmit disease. For example, the mosquitos that carry relatively severe viral infections known as dengue fever and chikungunya virus have expanded their reach into the Caribbean and will likely soon establish themselves in North America. Dengue and chikungunya are already seen with increasing frequency in the United States, and there is concern that these infections may continue to migrate across the continent. Similar forces appear to be at play with Lyme disease. Ticks that carry the Lyme organism (*Borrelia burgdorferi*) are expanding their reach, and the disease is being seen in a broader geographic region than was typically observed. Classrooms also will be affected by the evolving distribution of local and international diseases as temperatures and rainfall patterns continue to change.

PREVENTION OF INFECTIOUS DISEASES BY IMMUNIZATION

In the 1790s Edward Jenner performed the first recorded vaccine trial. Realizing that milkmaids infected with cowpox were subsequently immune to smallpox, Jenner injected pus from a milkmaid's cowpox lesion into the arms of his gardener's son, who was subsequently protected from smallpox challenge. Since then, vaccines have been developed against most of the formerly devastating childhood illnesses. No other advance has saved more lives and prevented more suffering than immunization. Indeed, vaccines may be a victim of their own tremendous success. Whereas smallpox, polio, measles, and other vaccine-preventable diseases were in aggregate the most common cause of childhood deaths in the United States a century ago, they have now been eliminated, or nearly so. The dramatic decline in natural infection has shifted the balance between risks and benefits of vaccination. As a consequence, some parents have concluded that the potential for discomfort, inconvenience, or harm from vaccination outweighs potential benefits. It has been demonstrated that these decisions are often based on incomplete or incorrect information regarding risks of vaccination.

Vaccination consists of administering killed, inactivated, or mutated infectious agents to stimulate a strong immune response against that particular agent. Vaccines are inactivated toxins, killed bacteria or viruses, or live organisms that have been attenuated (mutated) so that they no longer cause disease in children with normal immunity. Most vaccines are given by injection, although some live attenuated vaccines can be administered by mouth or nasal spray. Because the goal is to induce an immune response, some degree of inflammation is expected and can manifest a few days after immunization with mild pain at the inoculation site or low-grade fever. Vaccines vary in their propensity to cause inflammation. Prior to 1991, the whole-cell pertussis vaccine was a notable cause of fever and inoculation site pain. Young children are predisposed to developing seizures when they have fever from any cause, and there was an association between whole-cell pertussis vaccination and subsequent febrile seizures. While seizures are frightening to observe, simple febrile seizures are not associated with any long-term risk of epilepsy and do not have any effect on brain development or cognitive ability. Nevertheless, the clear association between vaccination and febrile seizures contributed to heightened awareness about potential vaccine complications. Confusing the issue, true brain disorders such as infantile spasms, epilepsy, and developmental delays from genetic causes tend to become evident during years when children receive numerous vaccinations. Because vaccination is essentially universal, there is almost always a recent history of vaccine administration to the child recently diagnosed with one of these unrelated brain disorders. Similarly, autism-spectrum disorders often first become evident during the second to third year of life, which follows vaccination with the measles-mumps-rubella (MMR) vaccine at age 12–18 months. Untangling whether vaccination could be a cause of developmental delay, epilepsy, or autism required very large studies to find enough children who had *not* been vaccinated and to determine whether those children have similar rates of illness or to compare rates of serious illness before and after vaccines were introduced. To summarize a vast amount of literature, no carefully controlled, methodologically sound study has demonstrated a causal link between vaccination and any long-term brain disorder. A recent comprehensive review of all vaccine-related injury studies did find an association between MMR vaccination and febrile seizures. The same review was also able to demonstrate strong evidence that MMR is not associated with autism. Further, the review confirms that varicella vaccine can cause infection in children with compromised immunity. Finally, the review finds support for a rare association between rotavirus vaccination and intussusception, a condition in which the bowel inverts upon itself and may become blocked. It is also notable that children may have allergy to components of vaccines, including egg proteins and antibiotics, such as neomycin. To summarize these extensive studies; side effects do occurs with vaccines, but there is no evidence of serious or permanent injury in children with normal immunity. Aside from the concerns discussed above, parents may object to the sheer number of vaccines administered to their children. Indeed, a fully vaccinated child may have received at least 60 vaccine doses and 14 different vaccines by 18 years of age. Concerns about cost, discomfort, and inconvenience are reasonable but must be balanced by the overwhelming evidence that vaccination protects against devastating infections. There are strong individual and societal reasons to undergo vaccination. A trend away from vaccination will increase prevalence of preventable infections in the community and of course put the unvaccinated children at unnecessary risk. It is undeniable that current vaccines prevent vastly more disease and suffering than they cause. Educators and physicians both play important roles in providing accurate information to parents as they make informed decisions about their child's health.

REFERENCES AND FURTHER READING

American Academy of Pediatrics, Committee on Infectious Disease. (2013). *Red book report of the Committee on Infectious Diseases.* Elk Grove Village, IL: Author.

Centers for Disease Control and Prevention. (2010). Sexually transmitted diseases treatment guidelines, 2010. *Morbidity and Mortality Weekly Report, 59*(RR12), 1–109.

Long, S. S., Pickering, L. K., & Prober, C. A. (Eds.) (2012). *Principals and practice of pediatric infectious diseases.* St. Louis, MO: Elsevier.

Maglione M. A., Das, L., Raaen, L., Smith, A., Chari, R., Newberry, S., . . . Gidengil, C. (2014). Safety of vaccines used for routine immunization of US children: A systematic review. *Pediatrics, 134*(2), 325–337.

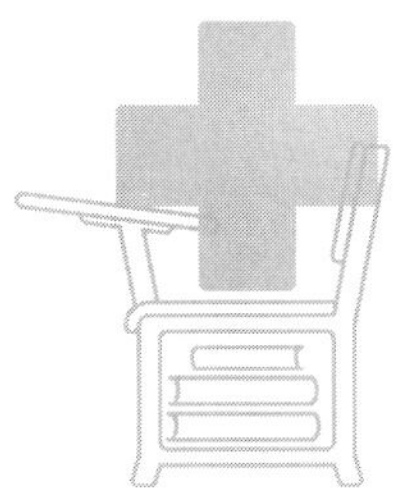

Chapter 2
The Role of Genetic Mechanisms in Childhood Disabilities

Dimitrios Ioannou, Thaddeus E. Kelly, and Helen G. Tempest[1]

Genetic disorders often involve conditions that result in childhood disabilities; thus, an understanding of these conditions is of major importance in the development of educational programs that seek to minimize the impact of a disability on a child. The functional consequences of these disabilities may be any combination of physical, emotional, social, or educational disability. There are literally thousands of genetic conditions, each with its specific consequences. However, it is possible to consider them from their functional consequence in such a way as to allow teachers and allied educational professionals to deal with each child individually and knowledgeably. Because the educational setting is such an important part of any child's life, a full understanding of the social, psychological, physical, and educational limitations imposed on a child by a genetic disorder is crucial for proper placement and support.

Genetic disorders can be considered by the nature of the genetic alteration responsible for the disability or by the nature of the

[1]I wish to acknowledge the late Dr. Thaddeus Kelly's previous contributions as a geneticist to *Medical Problems in the Classroom*, beginning with the first edition of the book published in 1975, when we were colleagues at Johns Hopkins Hospital. Over the successive three editions of the book, he helped countless educators understand the burgeoning field of genetics and its important role in so many disorders affecting children and adolescents. —*R.H.*

functional consequence that they impose. This chapter attempts to provide insight into genetic disorders from both perspectives.

STRUCTURE AND INHERITANCE OF GENETIC MATERIAL

Deoxyribonucleic acid (DNA) is the basis of genetic material that is required for the structure and function of organisms and is essential for transmission of genetic information to the next generation. DNA is a double-stranded helix that is composed of four different nucleotides (adenine, A; thymine, T; cytosine, C; and guanine, G), which are arranged in a specific sequence and code for our genes (see Figure 2.1).

Nucleotides are organized in units of three (codons); each codon specifies the amino acid sequence of a protein. The DNA double-stranded helix is composed of two complementary chains of nucleotides that are intricately coiled and condensed to form chromosomes. The human genome contains approximately 22,500 genes distributed across 46 chromosomes. Chromosomes occur in pairs, with each parent contributing one chromosome of each pair, or 23, to each of his or her children. There are 22 pairs of autosomes and one pair

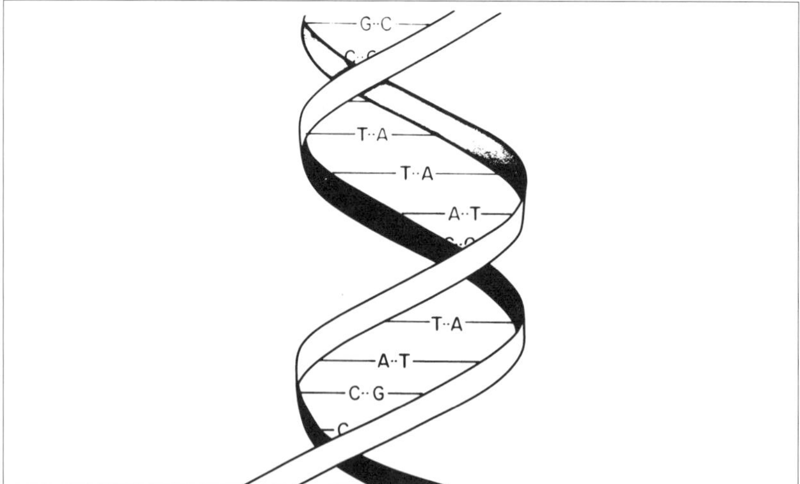

Figure 2.1. The DNA double-stranded helix, with two strands of the DNA helix and the individual nucleotides adenine, guanine, cytosine, and thymine, represented as A, G, C, and T, respectively. The two strands of DNA are held together by hydrogen bonds (represented as two dots) between complementary nucleotides. In the normal situation, A and T as well as C and G always pair with each other. Nucleotides are organized in units of three (codons), with each codon specifying the amino acid sequence of a protein.

of sex chromosomes (X and Y) (see Figure 2.2[A]). A female, whose chromosome constitution is 46,XX, produces eggs with 23 chromosomes, one of which is an X chromosome. A male, whose chromosome constitution is 46,XY, produces sperm with 23 chromosomes, one of which is either an X or a Y chromosome. A female may give either of her X chromosomes to a son or a daughter. A male gives his X chromosome to all of his daughters and his Y chromosome to all of his sons. At the time of conception, the genetic makeup of the embryo serves as a blueprint, containing all the information necessary for the growth and development of an infant. Any alteration in the genetic blueprint of an embryo has the potential to affect the organization, growth, and development of the resulting child.

IDENTIFICATION OF ALTERATIONS IN THE GENETIC MATERIAL

Identification of the genetic causes of childhood disabilities relies on our ability to identify aberrations within DNA, which can vary in size from a single nucleotide to millions of nucleotides. Aberrations can be caused through various mechanisms (e.g., rearrangement of DNA; changing the nucleotide sequence or copy number variations, resulting in gain or loss of genetic material).

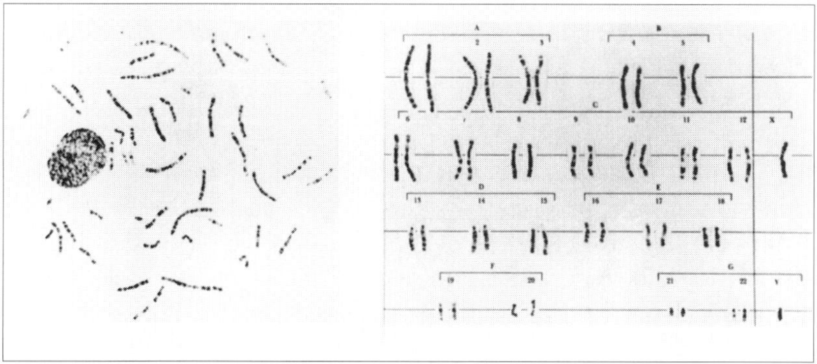

Figure 2.2. (A) Chromosomes of a normal male as viewed under the microscope. These chromosomes are at a specific stage of cell division (metaphase) in which the DNA is at its most condensed. Staining of chromosomes produces a characteristic banding pattern that is used to assist in the identification of each chromosome and to detect chromosome aberrations. (B) Humans have 46 chromosomes (23 pairs), which are numbered from 1 to 22 (the autosomes) and the sex chromosomes (XX female, XY male). Chromosomes are organized in their pairs and studied (karyotyped) based on their size, morphology, and banding patterns. This karyotype is derived from a normal male (46,XY). Karyotyping can detect numerical and structural aberrations (>5Mb) by studying and identifying changes in number, size, morphology, and banding patterns.

Traditionally, chromosomes have been studied by karyotyping (Figure 2.2[B]), or through the identification of chromosomal regions harboring affected genes though family linkage studies. Karyotyping can identify both structural and numerical aberrations, including translocations, inversions, deletions, and duplications involving parts of chromosomes or entire chromosomes. However, this technique has a relatively low resolution, capable only of detecting aberrations that are at least 5 Mb in size (involving more than 5 million nucleotides). Despite the relatively low resolution of karyotyping, it still remains the gold-standard diagnostic test for many genetic conditions.

Family linkage studies have been invaluable in identifying the chromosomal regions harboring genes that contribute to numerous genetic disorders. This approach relies on identifying relatively large families with both affected and unaffected individuals. DNA collected from both unaffected and affected individuals is examined to determine which chromosomal regions are found in affected individuals but not in unaffected family members. This hones in on the region harboring the gene(s) involved, providing areas of the genome to focus the search for the gene causing the condition.

Both karyotyping and linkage studies are genome-wide approaches that have a relatively low resolution; they are time consuming and provide not the gene involved per se, but rather the chromosomal regions to study to identify the genes involved. Once the gene and mutation(s) have been identified, various direct testing methods can be utilized to identify mutations in patients. Despite their drawbacks, these methods remain valuable research and clinical tools. However, the past decade has seen tremendous advances in high-resolution, genome-wide approaches, namely array-comparative genomic hybridization (aCGH) and genome sequencing.

The aCGH approach can detect copy-number changes (gains and losses) and works, in essence, by comparing patient DNA with DNA from a healthy subject (reference DNA). DNA is compared utilizing a microarray slide onto which hundreds of thousands of small pieces of DNA sequence from across the genome are spotted. The patient and reference DNA are both labeled with a different fluorescent dye (red and green), then mixed and hybridized onto the microarray slide. If the entire patient DNA is present, we would expect an equal amount (1:1) of red- and green-labeled DNA to hybridize to each of the spotted DNA sequences on the microarray slide, producing a yellow color. Gains or losses in the patient DNA are detected when there is a shift in this 1:1 ratio showing either a deletion or a duplication of specific regions of DNA.

The advent of the Human Genome Project has significantly advanced our identification and understanding of the genetic causes of disease. The first human genome sequenced cost more than $3 billion and took more than 10 years to complete. However, technological advances have catapulted this technology into clinical diagnostics with the ability to sequence the exome (regions encoding for the genes, ~2% of the DNA sequence) for less than $1,000, or the entire sequence for between $5,000 and $10,000, and a turnaround time of days to weeks. Sequencing of DNA allows us to identify changes in the nucleotide sequence (mutations).

Both aCGH and genome sequencing have dramatically increased our ability to identify the genes involved and are able to provide a molecular diagnosis that, previously, in many cases was not possible. Furthermore, all the methods discussed have led to identification of the genes and pathways involved in disease and will undoubtedly translate to improved diagnosis, prognosis, and eventually treatment therapies.

CHROMOSOMES AND CHROMOSOMAL ABNORMALITIES

Chromosomal abnormalities are common at the time of conception. It is estimated that up to 50% of all conceptions have a chromosomal abnormality. Most of the time, the resultant effect on growth and development of the embryo is so severe that an early spontaneous abortion occurs, often prior to a clinically recognized pregnancy. Only chromosomal abnormalities that have a less severe consequence allow for fetal development and delivery of a live-born infant.

Chromosomal abnormalities include (1) change in the number of chromosomes (aneuploidy), (2) loss or gain of part of a chromosome, and (3) structural chromosome rearrangement. Typically, gain of genetic material is more tolerable than loss of material.

Autosomal Aneuploidies

When a numerical or structural change involves an autosome (see Figure 2.2[B]), there will be three predictable consequences: abnormal growth (short stature), abnormal physical development (birth defects), and abnormal mental development (intellectual disability). For example, Down syndrome results from a chromosomal aneuploidy in which there are three copies of chromosome 21 (trisomy 21) rather than the typical two. Children with Down syndrome have mildly short stature, numerous minor physical birth defects that result in a characteristic appearance, and intellectual disability in the moderate range (see Figure 2.3). Down syndrome occurs in about 1 in 691 liveborn infants in the United States. Of all viable numerical abnormalities of autosomes, Down syndrome is generally the least severe. The presence of a single copy of chromosome 21 at conception is incompatible with fetal life.

Two other viable autosomal aneuploidies include trisomy 13 (Patau syndrome) and trisomy 18 (Edward syndrome). These involve chromosomes larger than chromosome 21 and produce more severe birth defects. Most infants with trisomy 13 or 18 die in the first year of life, but occasionally survival will continue into childhood. Such children have severe intellectual impairment and disabilities from their birth defects, including severe congenital heart disease.

Aneuploidies as a Result of Chromosomal Translocations

In rare cases, chromosome aneuploidies may be a familial disorder if the aneuploidy is the result of a structural chromosome aberration such as a chromosome translocation (see Figure 2.4[A]). Structural abnormalities of chromosomes are defined as balanced if all the genetic material is present but the material is rearranged in a different order, and as unbalanced if there is loss or gain of genetic material. In this

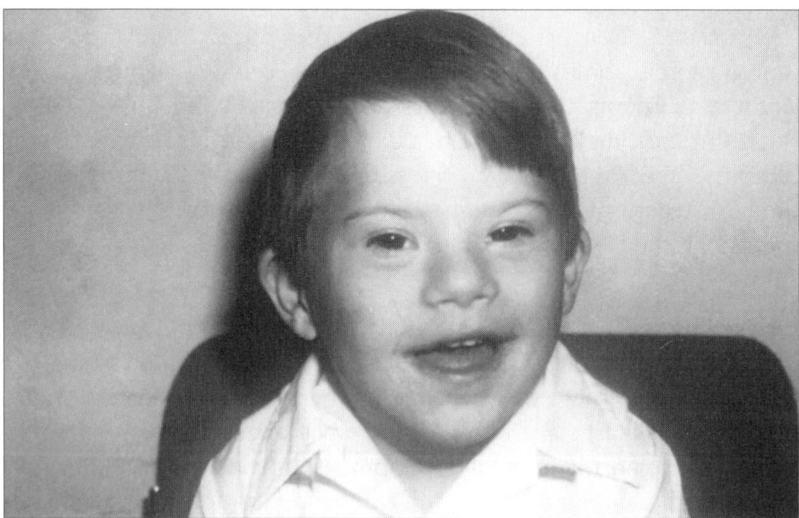

Figure 2.3. A 5-year-old boy with Down syndrome. Down syndrome is associated with a number of physical characteristics (that may or may not be present in all individuals). Note the following in this individual: flat facial features, upward slant to the eyes, and the enlarged tongue with a tendency to stick out.

instance many family members are balanced carriers and are usually phenotypically normal. However, problems arise for future offspring. All chromosomes, including those involved in the translocation, have to undergo cell division to produce either egg or sperm cells with 23 chromosomes. As a balanced translocation progresses through cell division, there are several possible outcomes: (1) normal (inheritance of the normal copies of the chromosomes), (2) balanced (inheritance of the balanced translocation), and (3) unbalanced (aneuploid, inheritance of extra or missing copies of the chromosomes involved in the translocation). In the first two scenarios the offspring will be normal, although balanced offspring will be at risk of having chromosomally aneuploid offspring. Unbalanced conceptions may result in early spontaneous abortions or be live-born with major birth defects, growth retardation, and mental disabilities (depending on the chromosomes involved in the translocation). Figure 2.4(B) provides an example of familial Down syndrome as the result of a balanced translocation between chromosomes 14 and 21. Each normal carrier of a t(14;21) translocation has approximately a 33% chance of having a child with a normal or balanced karyotype, a 57% chance of a spontaneous abortion, and a 10% chance of having a child with Down syndrome with each pregnancy. For these reasons, it is prudent to determine the specific chromosomal change responsible for Down syndrome in all affected children. The consequences for a child with translocation Down syndrome are not different from those for a child with trisomy 21.

Sex Chromosome Aneuploidies

Sex chromosome aneuploidies are different from autosomal aneuploidies in that these conditions have a different pattern of consequences. Several syndromes are discussed in the following sections.

Turner Syndrome

Turner syndrome affects females with a single X chromosome (45,X karyotype). The features of the syndrome include the following:

1. *Short stature.* The average height of an untreated woman with Turner syndrome is about 55 to 58 inches (139 to 147 cm). Currently, various combinations of hormone therapy usually result in an adult height of around 60 inches (152 cm).
2. *Gonadal dysgenesis.* The oocytes, or developing eggs, in the Turner syndrome ovary are unable to properly enter meiotic cell division, which occurs in the germ cells. As a result, the oocytes are rapidly lost in late fetal and early infant life. At puberty, with no ovarian function, there is no secondary sexual development or adolescent

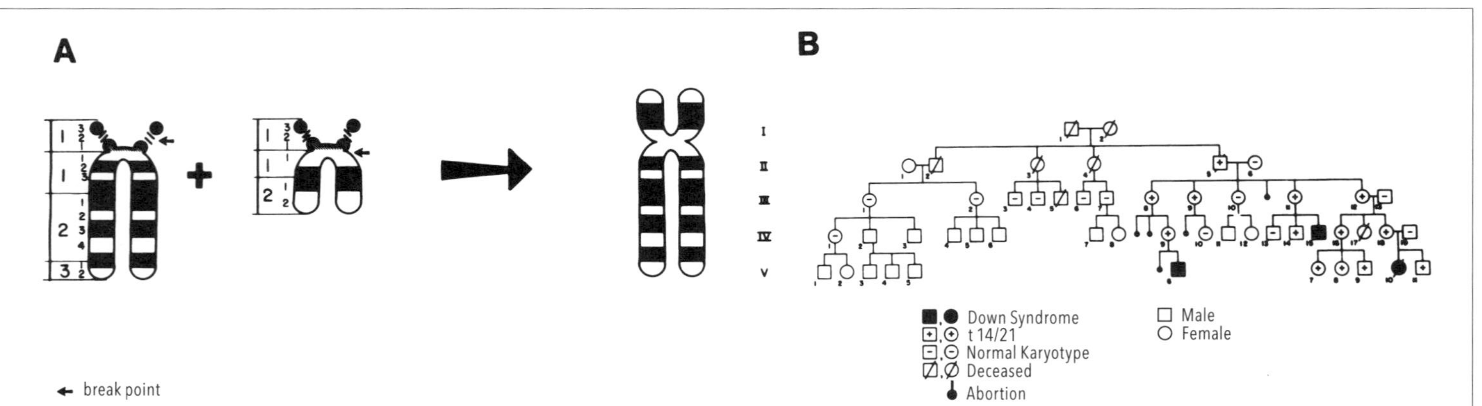

Figure 2.4. (A) Breakage and fusion of chromosome 14 and chromosome 21 to form a chromosome translocation t(14;21). The carrier of such a translocation has 45 chromosomes (instead of the normal 46, due to the fusion of two chromosomes). Typically, an individual with this balanced translocation would be phenotypically normal (the genetic material is rearranged, but there is no loss or gain of material). (B) This shows a pedigree in a family with a t(14;21) chromosome translocation. In this family pedigree there are three Down syndrome offspring (higher incidence rate than would be expected if due to trisomy alone). Also note the incidence of normal karyotypes, balanced karyotypes t(14;21), and the relatively high frequency of spontaneous abortions observed in this family. The high frequency of abortions in this family is most likely due to unbalanced segregation of the chromosome translocation during cell division.

growth spurt. Cyclic hormone replacement therapy with estrogen and progesterone promotes normal sexual development with regular menses. The lack of oocytes precludes natural conception.

3. *Birth defects.* The pattern of birth defects seen with Turner syndrome is the consequence of generalized edema of the body during fetal development. At birth, these female infants have edema of their hands and feet, redundant tissue about their neck, and puffiness around their eyes and ears. The edema generally resolves by 18 to 24 months of age, leaving minor cosmetic consequences. Coarctation, a constriction, of the aorta represents a common and serious birth defect.
4. *Learning disability.* Intellectual disability is not typically a feature of Turner syndrome, but some degree of developmental delays, nonverbal learning disabilities, and behavioral problems are possible. Most commonly this manifests as difficulty with spatial orientation; mathematics is usually their most difficult subject. It should be emphasized that many of these women have achieved meaningful professional careers in a number of fields and enjoy normal social and family lives.

The diagnosis of Turner syndrome may be made at different ages: (1) before birth, by abnormalities noted on ultrasonography or prenatal chromosome testing; (2) at birth, by the presence of the typical physical features of Turner syndrome; (3) during childhood, because of short stature; and (4) during adolescence or later, because of the lack of secondary sexual development, amenorrhea, and infertility.

Variations on Turner Syndrome

Of females with an X chromosome abnormality and gonadal dysgenesis, about 50% have a 45,X karyotype. The remaining cases are due to a wide range of structural abnormalities involving the X chromosome (e.g., loss of part, but not all, of one X chromosome). Three general phenotypes are observed: gonadal dysgenesis with no other manifestations, gonadal dysgenesis with short stature but not the pattern of birth defects seen in Turner syndrome, and all of the typical Turner syndrome features. Note that the common feature is gonadal dysgenesis.

Triple X Syndrome

About 1 in 1,000 live-born female infants have an additional X chromosome (47,XXX). Most of them will go undetected during their lifetime, as 47,XXX often produces no outward manifestations. However, analysis of a large group of 47,XXX females suggests that, as a group there is a 10–15-point reduction in IQ. 47,XXX females have an increased risk of delayed development of speech, language, and motor skills and may also experience behavioral and emotional problems. There is no gonadal dysgenesis or short stature, and fertility is normal, with no increased risk of a sex chromosomal aneuploidy in offspring.

Klinefelter Syndrome

Klinefelter syndrome occurs as a result of a 47,XXY karyotype and has a frequency of about 1 in 500 to 1,000 live-born, unambiguous males. Usually, these males go undetected until they fail to undergo pubertal sex development along with their peers. Untreated teenage males can develop gynecomastia (male breast development), which is particularly distressing socially. Much like Turner syndrome, 47,XXY produces gonadal dysgenesis that results in failure of sexual development and infertility. These males tend to be taller than their male relatives and have small testes (see Figure 2.5). With proper diagnosis and hormone replacement treatment with testosterone, normal sexual development will proceed. For males with gynecomastia, a simple, cosmetic mastectomy will alleviate the associated psychosocial problems. Not unlike 47,XXX females, these males as a group have a small reduction in IQ, such that Klinefelter syndrome is encountered more often than might be expected otherwise among males with learning disabilities and mild intellectual disability.

47,XYY Syndrome

The aneuploidy 47,XYY has a frequency of around 1 in 1,000 live-born males. Most 47,XYY individuals have normal sexual development and fertility. As with the previously mentioned sex chromosome aneuploidies, there may be an increased risk of learning disabilities in 47,XYY individuals. Also of note is the observation that a small percentage of 47,XYY males have been diagnosed with autism-spectrum disorders, which affect their social and communication skills.

MENDELIAN INHERITED SINGLE-GENE DISORDERS

Frequently disorders are not the result of structural or numerical chromosome aberration but are due to a mutation that affects a single gene. A change in the nucleotide sequence of a gene (mutation) can have several outcomes: (1) it may not alter the amino sequence (pro-

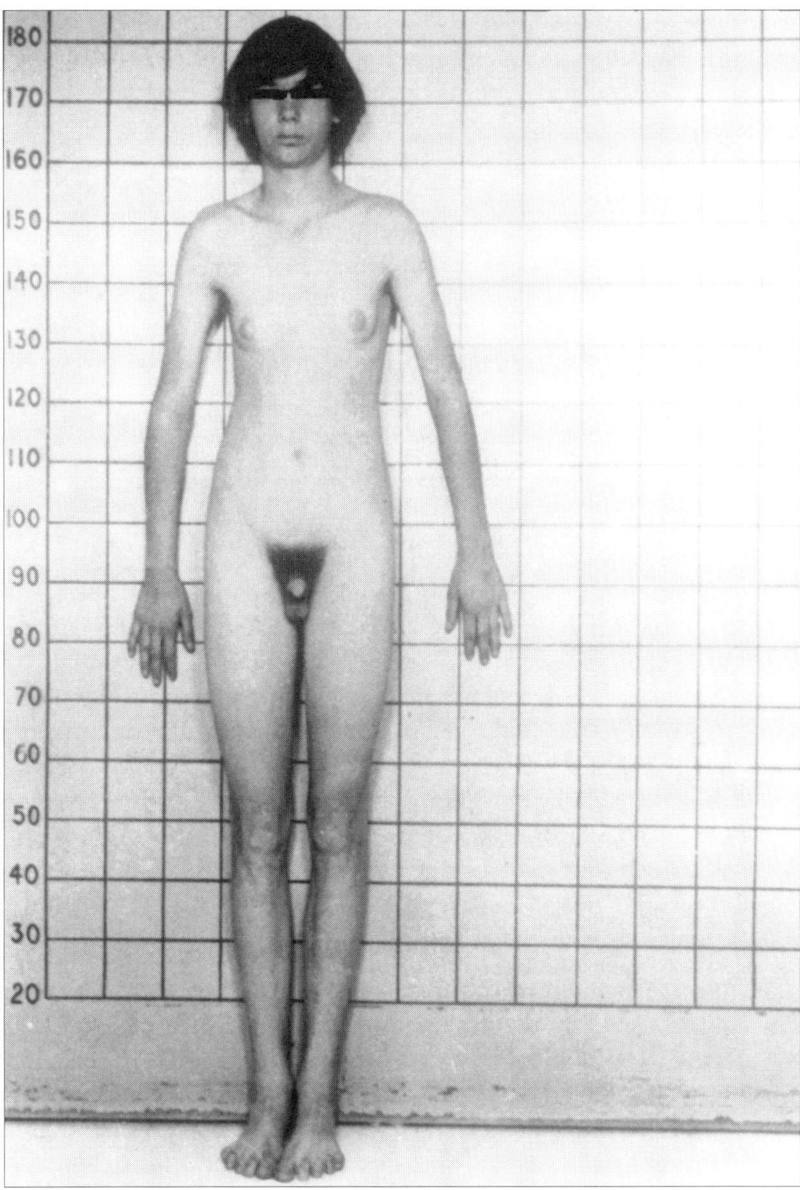

Figure 2.5. An 18-year-old male adolescent with Klinefelter syndrome. Note the relatively tall height, development of gynecomastia, and small testes.

ducing a normal protein with normal function); (2) it may alter the amino acid sequence, resulting in a functionally altered protein; or (3) it may completely eliminate protein production. The manifestations (phenotype) of a single-gene inherited disorder are based on the degree of abnormality in the protein product and its effect on the function normally carried out by that protein. While chromosomal abnormalities have widespread effects on the developing fetus, single-gene abnormalities tend to have more narrow consequences that can be related to the changes in the single gene product. Inherited mutations of single genes have a wide range of functional consequences. These vary from essentially cosmetic concerns to disorders incompatible with life. The patterns of inheritance of single-gene disorders in humans is the same as that described in garden peas by Gregor Mendel in 1866 (i.e., Mendelian inheritance). The various modes of Mendelian inheritance include autosomal dominant, autosomal recessive, and sex-linked inheritance. The hallmarks of these modes of inheritance are highlighted in the following sections, along with examples of disorders that follow these modes of inheritance.

Autosomal Dominant Inheritance

When inheritance of a mutation in only one copy of a pair of genes is required for expression of a trait, that trait is dominantly inherited (see Figure 2.6). There are a large number of dominantly inherited disorders that have important implications for school-age children. In general, the more severe the physical consequences of a dominantly inherited disorder, the more likely it is that an affected child will represent a new mutation. For a dominantly inherited disorder that prevents the individual from being able to reach adulthood and reproduce, all cases must represent a new mutation.

Achondroplasia

This disorder is the most common form of a skeletal dysplasia producing dwarfism. All manifestations of the condition are attributable to defective growth of bones at the site where cartilage is converted to bone in the growth centers of the skeleton. Cell division and growth are typically controlled by the balancing effects of genes that stimulate and inhibit growth. The specific mutation producing achondroplasia results in overexpression of a gene that inhibits skeletal growth. Affected children are quite short (adult height averages 48 inches, or 122 cm) and have a disproportionate shortening of their arms and legs relative to their trunk (see Figure 2.7). Poor growth of the facial bones increases the frequency of ear infections in early childhood and may lead to permanent hearing loss.

Most children with achondroplasia are healthy and bright; their major problem in school years is the psychosocial consequences of their height and appearance. They often have problems getting on

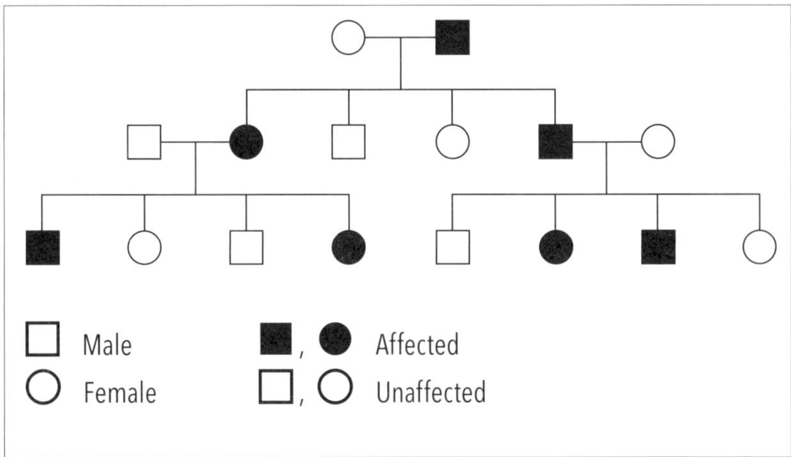

Figure 2.6. Pedigree of a family with an autosomal dominant disorder. In the case of autosomal dominant inheritance, there are several key features: (1) Both males and females have an equal likelihood of expressing the trait; (2) individuals with an autosomal dominant trait have a 50% chance of transmitting the trait to their offspring (male or female). Note the vertical transmission of the trait (every affected individual has an affected parent, unless the mutation has just arisen; see Figure 2.8); and (3) the ratio of affected to unaffected individuals is around 1:1. There are some notable exceptions to the vertical transmission and the ratio of affected to unaffected individuals; these are discussed as part of the exceptions to the rules of Mendelian inheritance.

and off the school bus, reaching a water fountain, using an adult-size toilet, and so on. In addition, there is a tendency to treat such children as though they were younger than their real age. While achondroplasia is an autosomal dominantly inherited disorder, only about 10% to 20% of the time does an affected child have an affected parent (see Figure 2.8).

Neurofibromatosis

Neurofibromatosis type 1 (NF1) typically presents with brown skin spots (café-au-lait spots) and lumpy skin growths (neurofibromas). Mutations in a tumor suppressor gene allow for tumor growth involving tissue of the nervous system. Café-au-lait spots are usually present in early childhood, whereas skin growths commonly appear at puberty. The more serious consequence, however, is the possible development of nerve tumors (neurofibromas) anywhere within the body. These can involve the optic nerve, causing severe visual problems; the acoustic nerve, causing deafness; and nerves along the spine or any part of the brain. Scoliosis (curvature of the spine) occurs commonly in children with neurofibromatosis and is often more difficult to treat than other forms of scoliosis. About 30%–40% of children

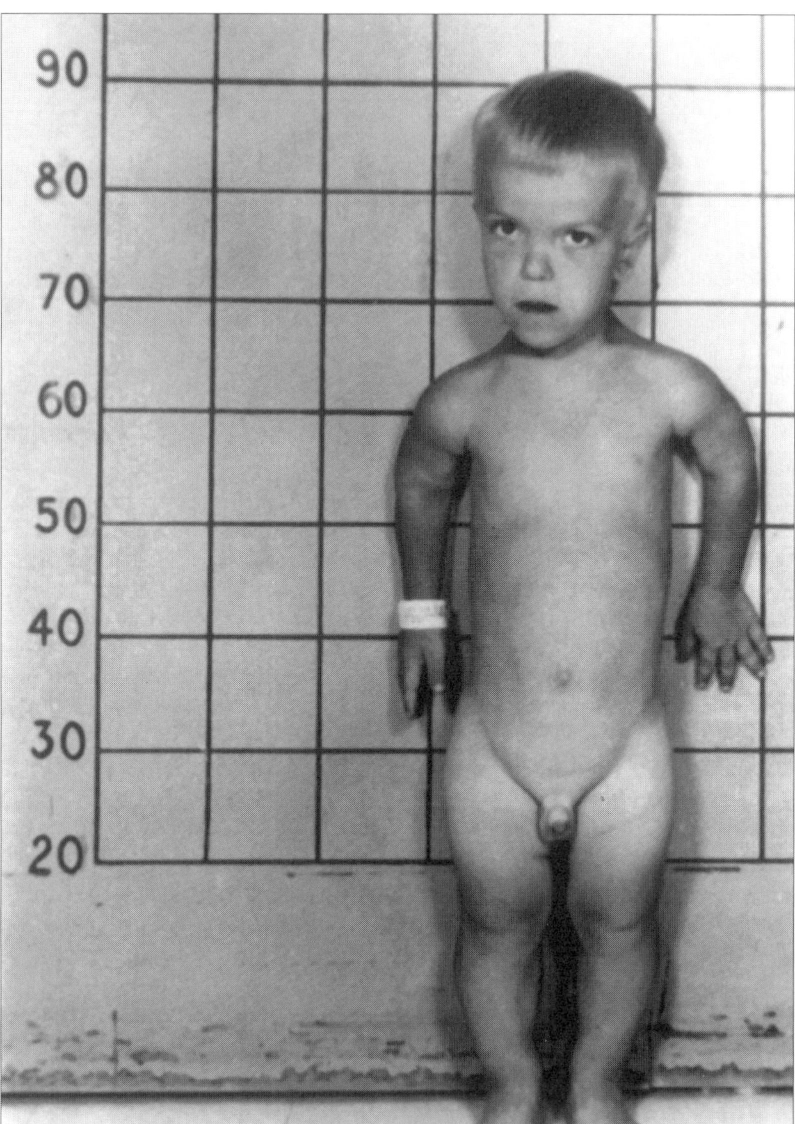

Figure 2.7. A 6-year-old boy with achondroplasia. Note the boy's short stature, poor growth of facial bones, and disproportionate shortening of the limbs relative to his trunk.

with NF1 display a specific pattern of learning disability that is characterized by poor language and reading skills without impaired math skills. They also exhibit deficits in visuospatial and neuromotor skills.

The skin manifestations—spots and lumps—may be the only manifestations of NF1, but they can represent a real emotional concern for a school-age child, depending on the size and location of the

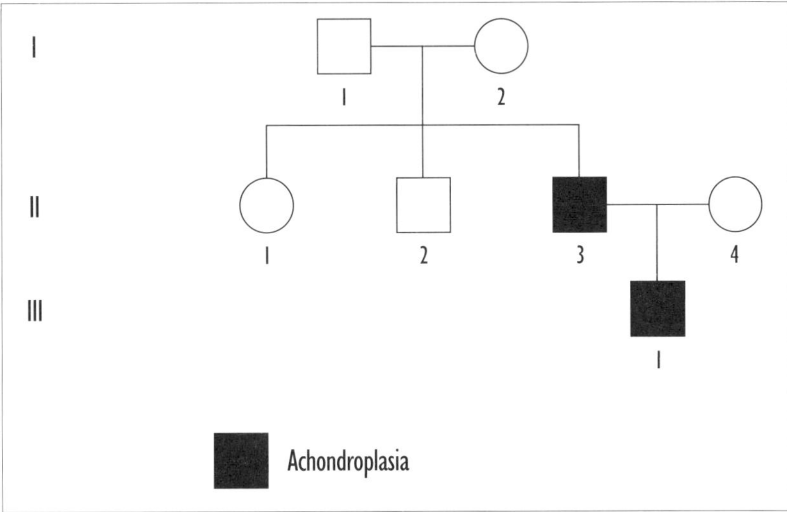

Figure 2.8. Typical family pedigree observed in a family with achondroplasia. Starting from the top of the pedigree, neither of the couple (I-1 and I-2) has achondroplasia. The couple has three children, a girl (II-1) and two sons (II-2 and II-3). II-3 has inherited a new mutation from his parents (either I-1 or I-2) that has arisen in a single sperm or egg cell that gave rise to him; therefore, they do not have an increased risk of having a second affected child. However, the child with achondroplasia (II-3) has the mutation in all his cells, so he has a 50% chance to pass it on to his children; as you can see, he has an affected son (III-1). Note that the de novo achondroplasia mutation preferentially arises during spermatogenesis, and the mutation risk increases with advancing paternal age.

lesions. The size and number may preclude cosmetic surgery for their removal.

Osteogenesis Imperfecta

Osteogenesis imperfecta results from a defect in collagen, which forms the filamentous network upon which bone is mineralized. The most common form of this disorder usually does not result in spontaneous fractures in affected children, but only minimal trauma might be needed to result in a fracture. This form is called osteogenesis imperfecta type 1 (OI1). The fractures heal normally, but recurring fractures may produce skeletal deformity and body asymmetry. Associated features include blue sclerae and joint laxity, with possible early delays in motor milestones. Loss of movement of the bones of the inner ear (otosclerosis) frequently produces a significant hearing loss in young adults. While such children will encounter limitations in their physical activities consistent with the frequency of their fractures, there are no cognitive problems associated with this condition. More severe forms of this condition result in frequent fractures with secondary deformity and poor skeletal growth (OI3). Severely affected children are usually confined to a wheelchair. The most severe forms are incompatible with life and result in stillborn infants or early neonatal death (OI2). The degree of severity is usually consistent within a family but varies widely between families.

Myotonic Dystrophy

Myotonic dystrophy is the most common form of muscular dystrophy among adults. Onset is typically in the twenties, with progression thereafter leading to death in the forties or fifties. The myotonia may be recognized when an individual grasps a door handle and has difficulty releasing his or her grip. Additionally, there is also a congenital form of muscular dystrophy. If the affected infant does not die from respiratory compromise because of the muscle weakness, he or she will later demonstrate intellectual disability and a slowly progressive muscular dystrophy. Increased severity and earlier age of onset of a disorder is referred to as anticipation. Anticipation is covered in more detail in the exceptions to Mendelian inheritance section.

Huntington Disease

Huntington disease (HD) is a progressive form of dementia with involuntary movements usually affecting individuals 45 years of age and older. However, because of anticipation, the disorder may be recognized in young children, as young as 2 to 3 years of age.

Autosomal Recessive Inheritance

Autosomal recessive inheritance is observed when a mutation is required in both copies of the gene (i.e., an individual must receive a mutated copy of the gene from both mother and father) to express the phenotype. Individuals with only one mutation are often phenotypically normal and are known as a carrier. Frequently, having an affected child is the most common means by which carriers for a recessive disorder are recognized (see Figure 2.9). Some autosomal recessive conditions occur more frequently in specific ethnic groups, and carrier testing for these conditions may be available and practical. Consanguinity increases the risk of an autosomal recessive disorder. All states and provinces have a newborn screening program that routinely screens for genetic conditions that can affect childhood health and development for which early detection, diagnosis, and treatment may prevent death or disability. More details regarding carrier testing and newborn screening can be found on the websites of the American

College of Medical Genetics and Genomics and the American Congress of Obstetricians and Gynecologists.

Sickle-Cell Disease

Carriers of a sickle-cell gene mutation possess a biological advantage (sickle-cell trait) that protects them, compared to noncarriers, from contracting malaria but has no adverse medical consequences. This advantage accounts for the high frequency of the disease among

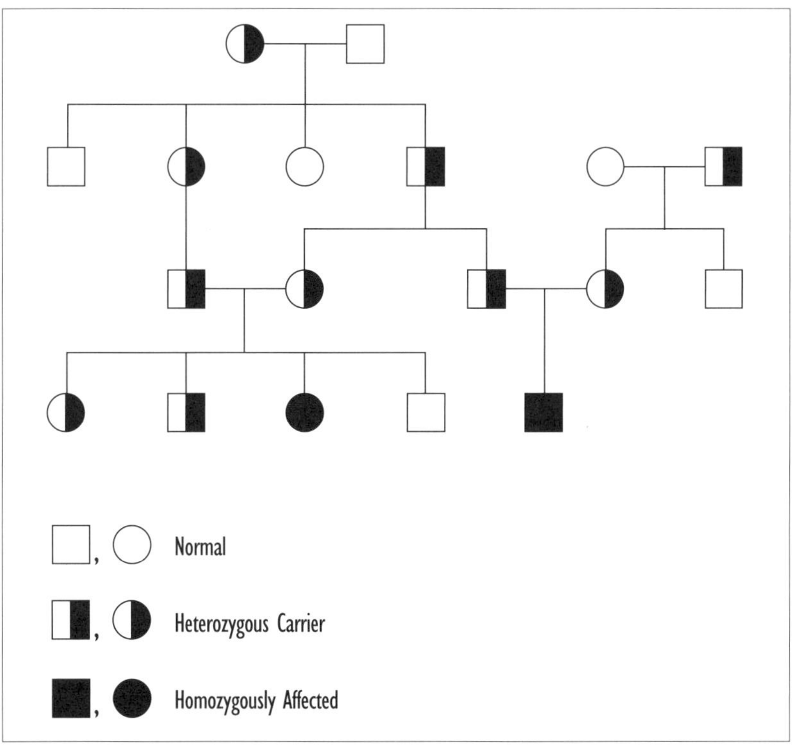

Figure 2.9. An example of a family pedigree with an autosomal recessive trait. The term *heterozygous carrier* refers to the fact that the individual in question has inherited a normal copy of the gene and a mutated copy of the gene (they are often phenotypically normal and unaware that they have the mutation). *Homozygous affected* indicates that the individual has inherited both the mutated copies of the gene and has the disease phenotype. Usually, to be homozygous affected, both parents must be heterozygous carriers. The key features of autosomal recessive inheritance include both males and females being equally affected; the disorder is often expressed in a horizontal pattern (in contrast to the vertical pattern observed with autosomal dominant inheritance; see Figure 2.6); and affected individuals frequently have unaffected parents (heterozygous carriers do not usually express the phenotype). Note that consanguinity, especially with rare disorders, increases the risk for autosomal recessive disorders.

certain populations (e.g., equatorial Africa). However, children who inherit two mutated copies of the sickle-cell gene from their carrier parents have severe consequences. Children with sickle-cell disease display a wide degree of variation in the severity of their disease. In early childhood, overwhelming infections are a major concern. Therefore, many states screen newborn infants for sickle-cell disease. Children are prone to episodes of bone infarction, which produce painful crises. This is the most common cause for a high rate of absenteeism. Chronic anemia results in easy fatigability and the anemia may be sufficiently severe as to require chronic blood transfusion therapy.

Phenylketonuria

Phenylketonuria (PKU) is an inborn error of metabolism, which is screened for in all US states and provinces, because of its frequency and because dietary therapy started in early infancy can prevent the otherwise-inevitable intellectual disability. If untreated, a defect in the metabolism of the amino acid phenylalanine results in severe intellectual disability, without imposing any physical abnormalities. The special diet restricts dietary intake of phenylalanine. Affected children will not be able to participate in the customary eating habits of their peers and will need to bring foods that are low in phenylalanine from home. Without the dietary restrictions, successfully treated children with PKU would not be otherwise recognized as affected in their school.

While dietary therapy is most important in the first two years of life, discontinuance of the diet upon entering school has been shown to result in increased behavioral problems and poorer school performance. Most treatment programs continue children with PKU on some form of dietary therapy throughout their school years. If a female with PKU were successfully treated as a child but went off her diet before starting a family of her own, her PKU essentially places the developing fetus in a PKU environment. Even though the fetus does not have PKU, the result is impaired brain growth and prenatal development. Thus, children born of untreated PKU mothers are severely disabled.

Cystic Fibrosis

Cystic fibrosis (CF) is common among Caucasians of Western European descent, and it results from a defect in the membrane transport of chloride in and out of cells. As a result, the secretions in the respiratory tract are thick and tenacious, which cause repeated pulmonary infections and progressive respiratory failure. The pancreas, which produces enzymes needed for the intestinal digestion of foods, is also affected. Pancreatic enzyme deficiency results in malabsorption of food, creating impaired nutrition. The deficiency can be largely overcome by the use of orally administered enzymes with each meal. School absenteeism is high because of repeated hospitalizations for intensive respiratory therapy. Current therapy requires adherence to a diet, proper use of replacement pancreatic enzymes, frequent antibiotic use, and vigorous chest physical therapy. As each of these aspects of therapy has improved, there has been a continued increase in the life expectancy of individuals with CF. As a result, almost all children with CF are able to participate in school programs from kindergarten through grade 12.

Storage Diseases

Storage diseases result from deficiency of enzymes involved in the degradation of normal, large chemical compounds. Without the necessary catabolism of these large compounds, they accumulate in tissues. The resulting disease depends on the specific tissues in which the involved compounds accumulate. The degree of enzyme deficiency determines the rate of accumulation and, therefore, the rate of progression of the disorder.

Sanfilippo syndrome (mucopolysaccharidosis III) involves defective degradation of large compounds called mucopolysaccharides, or glycosaminoglycans, which accumulate primarily in the brain. Affected children usually are healthy, but delays in their cognitive development become apparent between 2 and 3 years of age. They develop a striking degree of hyperactivity. This form of attention-deficit/hyperactivity disorder (ADHD) is usually not amenable to drug therapy. After about 6 years of age there is slow but unremitting loss of cognitive skills, with a life expectancy into the late teens or twenties.

Two other forms of mucopolysaccharidosis, Morquio syndrome (MPS IV) and Maroteaux-Lamy syndrome (MPS VI), result in severe skeletal problems with dwarfism, but affected children are not cognitively impaired.

Defective Carbohydrate Metabolism

MCAD deficiency (medium chain acyl-carnitine dehydrogenase deficiency) produces a defect in the metabolism of fatty acids. Affected children are prone to hypoglycemia, especially with fasting. Glycogen storage diseases result from an inability of the liver to burn glycogen, the stored form of carbohydrate used for energy production. With both conditions, children require a diet high in complex carbohydrates and low in fat in order to meet their daily energy requirements without recurring episodes of hypoglycemia. With proper diet, most affected children can participate fully in all school activities, and most have normal cognitive function.

X-Linked Inheritance

All chromosomes are present as two copies with the exception of the sex chromosomes; females have two X chromosomes, whereas males have an X and a Y chromosome. Gene dosage is very important; therefore, an elaborate mechanism has evolved to deal with the sex chromosome imbalance between males and females. The Y chromosome contains a small number of genes that are mostly responsible for male sexual development. In females one of the X chromosomes is randomly silenced and hence "inactivated" with the exception of a handful of genes. In essence, this means that genes are expressed only from one X chromosome in females. In general, with the exception of skewed X-chromosome inactivation (discussed in the section on exceptions to Mendelian inheritance), mutations on the X chromosome typically manifest only in males (see Figure 2.10).

Hemophilia

Two forms of X-linked hemophilia can occur: a severe A form (factor VIII deficiency) and a less severe B form (factor IX deficiency). Hemophilia is a result of a deficiency in a factor required for the normal clotting of blood. There is variability in the severity of both forms between different families, ranging from frequent nosebleeds and easy bruising to spontaneous internal hemorrhages. The propensity to bleed with minor trauma leads to restricted activity of affected boys.

Lesch-Nyhan Syndrome

Lesch-Nyhan syndrome is an inborn error of metabolism that affects the part of the brain that controls coordinated speech and muscle activity (the cerebellum). Affected boys are dysarthric (garbled speech) and ataxic (poor sense of balance and coordination). However, they maintain reasonably good receptive language skills, and with communication devices can participate in special education classes. The disorder is progressive; one of the most disturbing complications is the development between the ages of 4 and 6 of self-mutilating behavior. This can be controlled to some extent by a controlled, structured environment, as heightened anxiety tends to set off episodes of finger and tongue biting. Life expectancy is into the late teens or twenties.

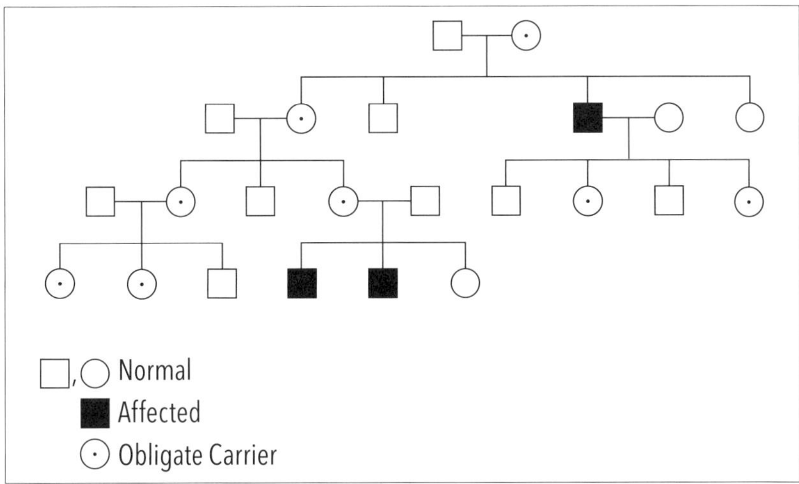

Figure 2.10. An example of a pedigree for an X-linked recessive trait. X-linked recessive conditions display an unusual inheritance pattern due to the phenomenon of X chromosome inactivation and the differences in the sex chromosomes between males and females. The key features of X-linked recessive inheritance include the following: (1) The disease incidence is much higher in males than in females. Males have a single X chromosome, so if the mutation is present it is expressed in all cells, whereas females have two X chromosomes, and typically they do not express the phenotype, as 50% of the protein produced is normal. (2) The allele is passed from an affected male to *all* of his daughters (obligate carrier), and in most cases these daughters will be phenotypically normal. (3) An obligate carrier is heterozygous for the mutation and will have a normal and mutated copy of the X chromosome. In this case she will pass the disease to 50% of her sons, who will express the disease, and 50% of her daughters, who will be carriers. (4) The mutation is never passed from father to son (the father can give only Y chromosome to sons and therefore cannot pass on a mutation on his X chromosome).

Duchenne Muscular Dystrophy

This common, progressive disorder of muscle is usually first apparent at 18 to 24 months by delayed motor skills. A large variety of mutations are known to occur in the dystrophin gene, which results in a wide variability in phenotype. In the most severe forms (e.g., Duchenne muscular dystrophy), the muscle weakness leads to increasing respiratory difficulty, which may be further complicated by cardiac disease and eventually leads to death in the late teens or early twenties. Less severe forms (e.g., Becker muscular dystrophy) may allow for survival well into adult years, with muscle weakness as the only childhood manifestation. Affected boys usually require wheelchairs during their school years.

There are a number of less common forms of progressive muscular dystrophy, most of which are recessively inherited. Cognitive problems are uncommon and the range of disability varies widely in these disorders.

Fragile X Syndrome

Fragile X syndrome is the most common form of intellectual disability caused by a single gene mutation. Its incidence is roughly 1 in 4,000 in males and 1 in 8,000 females, and it accounts for a significant percentage of learning disability in females. Males function in the range of moderate intellectual disability but display no behavioral problems and usually have good social and interpersonal skills. On entering school, they often display a short attention span and immaturity. There are no significant health problems, and life expectancy is not shortened. Males with fragile X syndrome are fully fertile. Originally, the diagnosis of this disorder was based on the cytogenetic appearance of the X chromosome in affected males; it appeared to have a fragile end on the long arm of the X chromosome (see Figure 2.11). Currently, the diagnosis is made by direct DNA analysis of the mutation.

EXCEPTIONS TO THE RULES OF MENDELIAN INHERITANCE

Typically when the same genetic mutation is inherited within the same family, we would expect the affected individuals to have similar disease phenotypes, progression, and age of onset. However, it is becoming increasingly clear that some disorders do not follow the simple rules of Mendelian inheritance and may exhibit patterns of non-Mendelian inheritance. In many cases this can be attributed to the facts that genes are not isolated entities and that many traits are determined and/or influenced by more than one gene and/or the environment. Some examples of these genetic mechanisms are discussed briefly here. It is important to note that in some cases, even though exceptions may alter the disease phenotype, progression, and age of onset, they may still be considered inherited in a Mendelian fashion (autosomal dominant, autosomal recessive, or sex linked).

Incomplete Penetrance

In some cases an autosomal dominant condition may appear to "skip a generation." In the case of dominant conditions, we would expect every affected person to have an affected parent, unless a new mutation has arisen. In some conditions, such as ectrodactyly (absence of one or more of the central digits of the hand or foot), a grandchild may

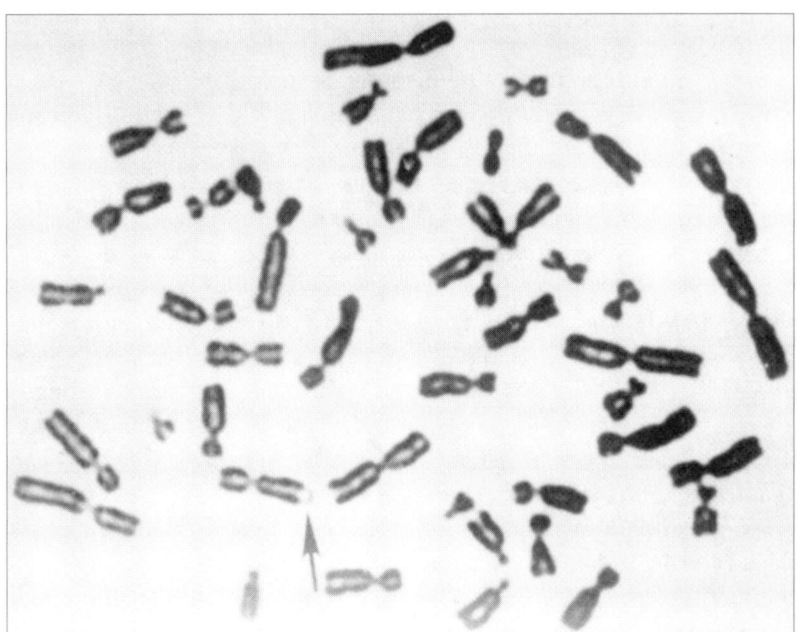

Figure 2.11. A metaphase spread of chromosomes from an individual with fragile X syndrome. The karyotypic manifestation of fragile X syndrome is observed as a fragile site (denoted by the arrow) on the X chromosome.

have an affected grandparent but not an affected parent. This situation is known as incomplete penetrance. Penetrance corresponds to the percentage of individuals who possess the disease mutation and express the phenotype. If an allele has complete penetrance (100%), then everyone who inherits the allele will have the phenotype, which in the case of ectrodactyly penetrance is less than 100%: some individuals will inherit the allele but not express the phenotype, and so can have an affected offspring.

Variable Expressivity

In the case of variable expressivity the allele is 100% penetrant, so every individual who inherits the allele will exhibit a phenotype. However, the severity and expression of the phenotype can vary between individuals within the same family and between families. This is most likely due to which genes are co-inherited with the allele; these may reduce or increase the effect of the allele. Neurofibromatosis type 1 is a good example of variable expressivity, in which some individuals have a handful of café-au-lait spots, whereas others may have neurofibromas.

Anticipation

In some genetic conditions the disorder becomes more severe as it is transmitted over generations within a family, which is known as anticipation. With each generation the disorder starts at a younger age and progresses faster. Examples of conditions in which anticipation occurs include myotonic dystrophy, Huntington disease, and fragile X syndrome. Anticipation is exemplified by a family with myotonic dystrophy (e.g., the grandmother had cataracts but no overt muscle disease, her daughter had typical onset of myotonic dystrophy in her twenties, and the grandchild had congenital myotonic dystrophy). Anticipation arises as the result of dynamic mutations. Littered throughout our genome are regions of highly repetitive segments of DNA; typically, these have little to no effect, and the number of repeats can vary tremendously between individuals. However, it is clear that increased numbers of repeats in and around certain genes can cause phenotypes. To date, more than 20 conditions have been identified that are caused by increased numbers of repeats (typically repeats of three nucleotides, known as trinucleotides). If the number of repeats reaches a critical threshold, then the function of the gene is either lost or altered. If we take fragile X syndrome as an example, unaffected individuals usually have between 10 and 50 copies of a CGG repeat. If this expands to between 50 and 200 repeats, then individuals are said to be premutation carriers, and the repeat is more prone to expand to a full mutation (>200 repeats). Having more than 200 repeats results in affected males and potentially mildly affected females (if skewed X-inactivation occurs). Importantly, in premutation carriers there is often a difference in which trinucleotides are expanded depending on the sex of the transmitting individual. In myotonic dystrophy and fragile X syndrome, the expansion usually occurs in oogenesis (transmitted by mothers), whereas in Huntington disease, the expansion occurs in spermatogenesis (transmitted by fathers).

Skewed X Chromosome Inactivation

As discussed previously, X inactivation can prevent females from manifesting the phenotype of X-linked disorders. In females one of the two X chromosomes is randomly inactivated in early fetal development. Therefore, in a female with a mutation on a single X chromosome, we would expect by random chance 50% of the X chromosome carrying the mutation to be inactivated. Thus, 50% of the normal protein will be expressed, which is usually enough to maintain normal function and therefore not express the phenotype. However, they are carriers of the X-linked condition and can transmit the disease to their offspring. In contrast, a male with a mutation on the X chromosome will not have any normal protein product and hence will display the disease phenotype. In rare instances females can exhibit a milder phenotype when there is skewed X-inactivation (i.e., a deviation from the expected random inactivation). If a higher proportion of unaffected X chromosomes is inactivated, the amount of normal protein produced is reduced. This can result in expression of the phenotype, the severity of which will depend on the proportion of the normal protein produced.

Genomic Imprinting

Initially it was assumed that all genes were biallelically expressed (i.e., the copy received from your mother and father were both expressed). It is now clear that some regions of the genome (around 100 genes) receive genomic imprinting; that is to say, some genes as they are copied in sperm or egg cells are targeted to be "turned off" or silenced. These genes are modified to function differently depending on the sex of the parent. Increasingly, genetic conditions have been identified that involve genes that are imprinted and have arisen either because of aberrant imprinting in the sperm or egg or because of mutations affecting paternally or maternally expressed genes.

Two syndromes, Angelman syndrome and Prader-Willi syndrome, are caused by lack of expression of genes that are normally expressed only on the maternal or paternal chromosome, respectively.

Angelman syndrome is characterized by severe intellectual disability, and affected children are nonverbal. They have a light complexion compared to family members, an unsteady gait, and a seizure disorder. They also appear quite happy, with inappropriate laughter. Angelman syndrome can be caused by a variety of loss-of-function mutations, which all have one thing in common: they all arise on the maternally inherited chromosome. The gene involved is typically silenced on the paternal chromosome and expressed on the maternal chromosome; therefore, loss of function of the maternally expressed gene translates to no expression of the gene. Prader-Willi syndrome involves a neighboring gene, but the converse situation arises: in this case, the gene is paternally expressed and maternally silenced. Therefore, mutations affecting the paternal gene copy cause Prader-Willi syndrome. Prader-Willi syndrome is characterized by striking muscle weakness in infants, and those affected appear quite delayed in all developmental parameters. By age 2, the children have gained considerable muscle strength and made striking motor developmental strides. As older children, they demonstrate mild to moderate intellectual disability, good social and verbal skills, short stature, small hands, and an insatiable appetite. As a result, they develop marked exogenous obesity (see Figure 2.12).

Deletion and Duplication Syndromes

A number of syndromes with several features in common have been described in children. These include short stature, some degree of intellectual disability, and behavioral features and physical findings of a highly specific and diagnostic nature. Affected children are quite similar in their manifestations, and yet the overwhelming majority of cases occur sporadically within families. There have been occasional case reports of an affected parent and child. Therefore, previously it was assumed that while there was the potential for parent-to-child transmission, this was consistent with autosomal dominant inheritance. The disorder was thought to usually arise as a new mutation of a single gene and transmission did not occur largely because the condition greatly reduced the individual's potential for reproduction.

In rare instances a given case has been associated with a visible chromosomal change detected by karyotyping. However, an increasing number of these syndromes occurs as a result of a small, often microscopically invisible deletion or duplication of chromosomal material. Identification of these microdeletions or duplications has advanced as a result of the aCGH, which allows the rapid detection of gains or losses of DNA during transmission of that chromosome from parent to child. These deletions or duplications, though small, can involve a number of contiguous genes. Table 2.1 lists some of the better-known syndromes and chromosomal regions in which deletions have been demonstrated. Figure 2.13 illustrates some chromosomal regions in which recurrent copy-number changes (deletions and duplications) have been identified and associated with intellectual disability and related disorders.

NON-MENDELIAN INHERITANCE

Mitochondrial Inheritance

Mitochondria are organelles within the cytoplasm of cells that function as a cellular furnace, generating and regulating chemical energy production. The mitochondria also contain a small circular chromosome whose DNA codes for some of the proteins involved in

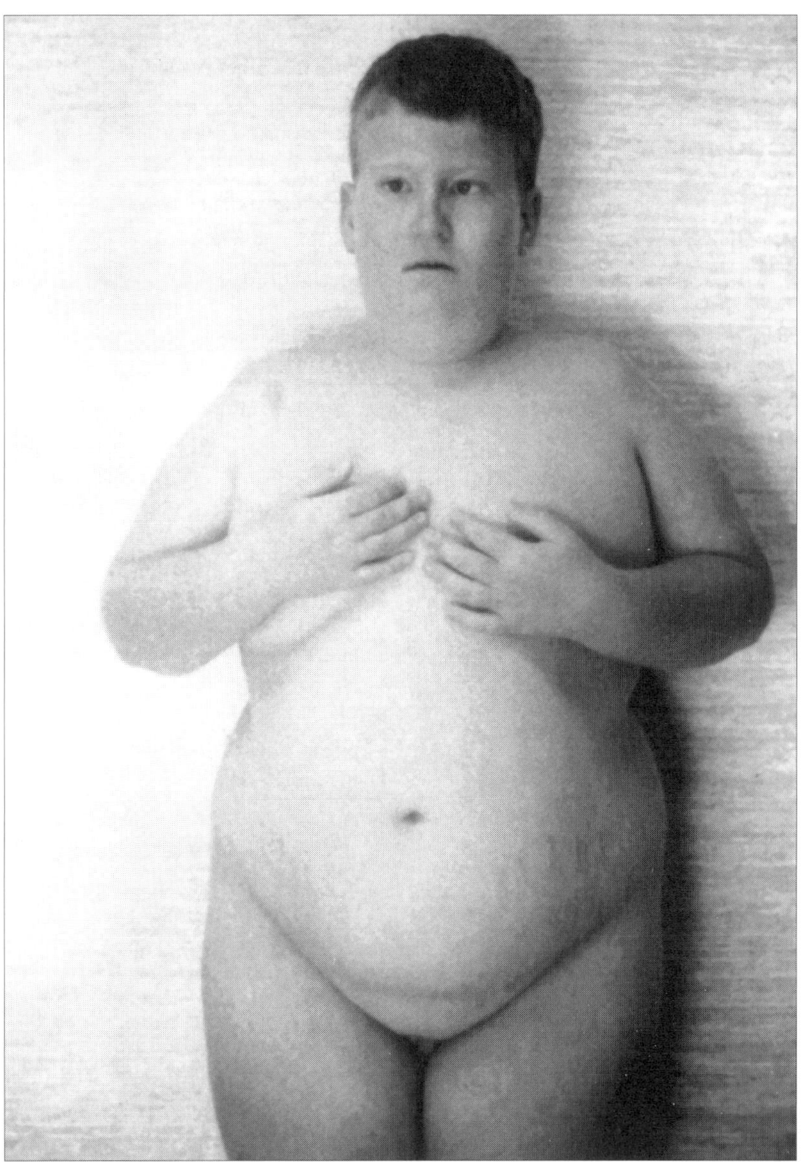

Figure 2.12. A 10-year-old boy with Prader-Willi syndrome. Note the boy's small hands and marked exogenous obesity.

mitochondrial energy production. Genes coding for mitochondrial proteins are also located on the 46 nuclear chromosomes.

Spermatozoa are designed to travel to the site of conception and penetrate the egg in order to transmit the paternal genetic contribution. All the cytoplasm present after fertilization is supplied by the egg, including the mitochondria and the mitochondrial DNA.

Table 2.1

DELETION OR CONTIGUOUS GENE SYNDROMES

Eponym	Chromosomal band deleted	Typical clinical features
Angelman syndrome	15q11-12	Fair complexion, nonverbal, seizures, inappropriate laughter, ataxia
Prader-Willi syndrome	15q11-12	Truncal obesity, insatiable appetite, low muscle tone, fair complexion, small hands
DiGeorge syndrome	22q11.2	Immune deficiency, left-sided congenital heart disease, short stature, cognitive impairment, hypocalcemia
Sprintzen syndrome	22q11.2	Congenital heart disease, elongated mid-face, velo-palatal incompetence, mental illness
Smith-Magenis syndrome	17p11.2	Sleep disorder, hoarse voice, self-destructive behavior, prognathism, puts objects in ears
Williams syndrome	7q11.23	Hyperactivity, good verbal skills, "cocktail party" personality, music skills, poor academic skills
Miller-Dieker syndrome	17p13.3	Lissencephaly (major brain development defect), seizures, forehead furrowing
Beckwith-Wiedemann syndrome	11p.15.5	High birth weight, omphalocele, newborn syndrome hypoglycemia, mild to moderate cognitive impairment, newborn macroglossia

Disorders due to mutations of mitochondrial DNA are transmitted only from the mother to her offspring.

Mitochondrial disorders, whether due to mutations of mitochondrial or to nuclear DNA, are characterized by slowly progressive muscle weakness, often associated with visual impairment, seizures, hearing loss, and some degree of intellectual impairment.

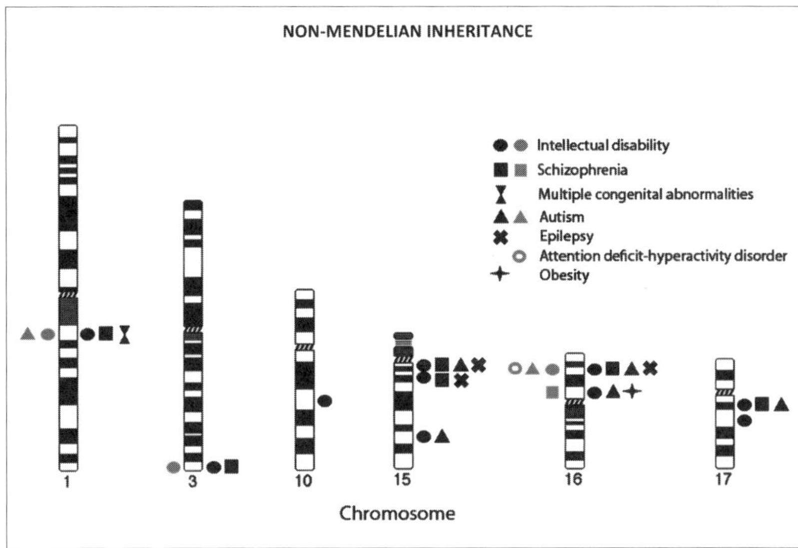

Figure 2.13. Schematic representation of select G-banded human chromosomes (chromosomes 1, 3, 10, 15, 16, and 17). Chromosomal regions associated with recurrent duplications and/or deletions and their associated disorders (indicated by symbols). Black symbols located to the right of each ideogram denote chromosomal deletions, whereas gray symbols to the left of each ideogram denote +D26 chromosomal duplications. Adapted from "Genomics, Intellectual Disability, and Autism," by H. C. Mefford, M. C. Batshaw, and E. P. Hoffman, 2012, *New England Journal of Medicine*, *366*(8), 733–743.

Multifactorial Inheritance

It is readily apparent that many traits are familial. However, it is clear that they are not due to a single gene. These traits are determined by a number of genes acting together and environmental factors that play a role in the expression of many of these traits—thus, the term "multifactorial inheritance." Most common birth defects are caused in this way and, as such, have several characteristics in common:

1. The defects are isolated structural birth defects.
2. The impact on the child results from the physical disabilities imposed by the birth defect.
3. The defect itself is not physically different from that which occurs as part of single-gene or chromosomally inherited syndromes. The distinction is a clinical one; that is, a defect is isolated or part of a wider series of birth defects.
4. The likelihood of recurrence in a family is in the order of 3%–5%, but the risk increases with the severity of the birth defect and the

number of family members affected. Several examples are discussed in the following sections.

Multifactorial inheritance is sometimes referred to as "genetic predisposition" when it is applied to familial adult disorders such as arthritis, coronary artery disease, hypertension, and others.

Cleft Lip and/or Palate

Cleft lip with or without a cleft palate results from a failure of midfacial structures to fuse in the midline during early embryonic life. There are numerous single-gene and chromosomal disorders in which clefting occurs as one of numerous birth defects clustered as a distinct syndrome (e.g., trisomy 13). More commonly, however, clefting occurs as an isolated birth defect. When an infant is born with a cleft, it is important to distinguish between an isolated cleft and one associated with other malformations, as the prognosis for growth and development, as well as the risk for recurrence within the family, is quite different (see also Chapter 10).

Isolated clefting is not associated with growth or cognitive disabilities. The major issue for such children is often the psychosocial problems associated with their appearance and any speech pathology.

Cleft lip and cleft palate requires surgical repair. Clefting may produce feeding problems for the infant, such as regurgitation of milk into the nasopharynx, with associated repeated ear infections. Cleft palate may cause poor closure of the upper airway, giving rise to speech problems that may be aggravated by a hearing loss from repeated infections. Further surgery may be indicated prior to entry into school to achieve a better cosmetic result or to improve the speech of the child. Speech therapy is often required for these children in early school years.

Congenital Heart Disease

Congenital heart disease is also a common component of many single-gene and chromosomal syndromes; only as an isolated defect is it multifactorially caused. Congenital heart disease produces problems for a child by one of three physiological consequences:

1. Blood is rerouted through the heart such that it is not passed adequately through the lungs for oxygenation (e.g., Tetralogy of Fallot).
2. The structure of the heart is such that it cannot work efficiently as a pump, and congestive heart failure results (e.g., ventricular septal defect).

3. There is an obstruction in the pathway by which oxygenated blood from the lungs is delivered to body tissues (e.g., coarctation of the aorta).

Any of these three problems may be partially or completely corrected by heart surgery. Prognosis for a child with congenital heart disease must take into account whether or not the defect is isolated, and if not, what the consequences are of the associated problems. For example, roughly 30% of children with Down syndrome have congenital heart disease.

It is not uncommon for children with functionally insignificant heart disease or surgically corrected heart disease to be unnecessarily restricted resulting in an unnecessary psychological burden.

Neural-Tube Defects

The neural tube consists of the bony encasement of the brain (skull) and the spinal cord (vertebral column). Embryologically, both begin as a flat membrane that folds onto itself and fuses to form a protective tube. At any point, there may be incomplete closure of the tube, ranging from anencephaly (no skull and virtually no brain tissue) to a small skin-covered cyst at the base of the spine that may have no functional consequence. Anencephaly is incompatible with survival beyond a few days after birth. The severity of spina bifida (meningomyelocele) depends on the location along the spine where failure of closure of the neural tube occurs and the degree of damage sustained by the spinal cord. Spina bifida with survival most commonly involves the lower spine with the following consequences:

1. The spinal cord at the site of the open defect is damaged, with resulting paralysis from that point down. The nerves supplying the bladder and lower bowel often are damaged, resulting in incontinence, predisposing individuals to repeated urinary tract infections.
2. The spinal cord is firmly attached to the vertebral column at the site of the defect. As a result, it pulls downward on the brain, creating an obstruction leading to hydrocephalus, which begins to develop before birth and can result in poor intellectual development. Frequently, there is good cognitive development with hydrocephalus as long as infection within the fluid system of the brain (ventricles) is prevented (see Figure 2.14).

A variety of research projects have strongly implicated dietary deficiencies, especially folic acid deficiency, as a causative factor of neural-tube defects. The Centers for Disease Control and Prevention has implemented efforts to increase the folic acid intake of the population as a measure to prevent neural-tube defects.

Diabetes Mellitus

Diabetes mellitus is the most common disorder of carbohydrate (sugar) metabolism. It occurs in two distinct forms: insulin-dependent diabetes and non-insulin-dependent diabetes. Insulin-dependent

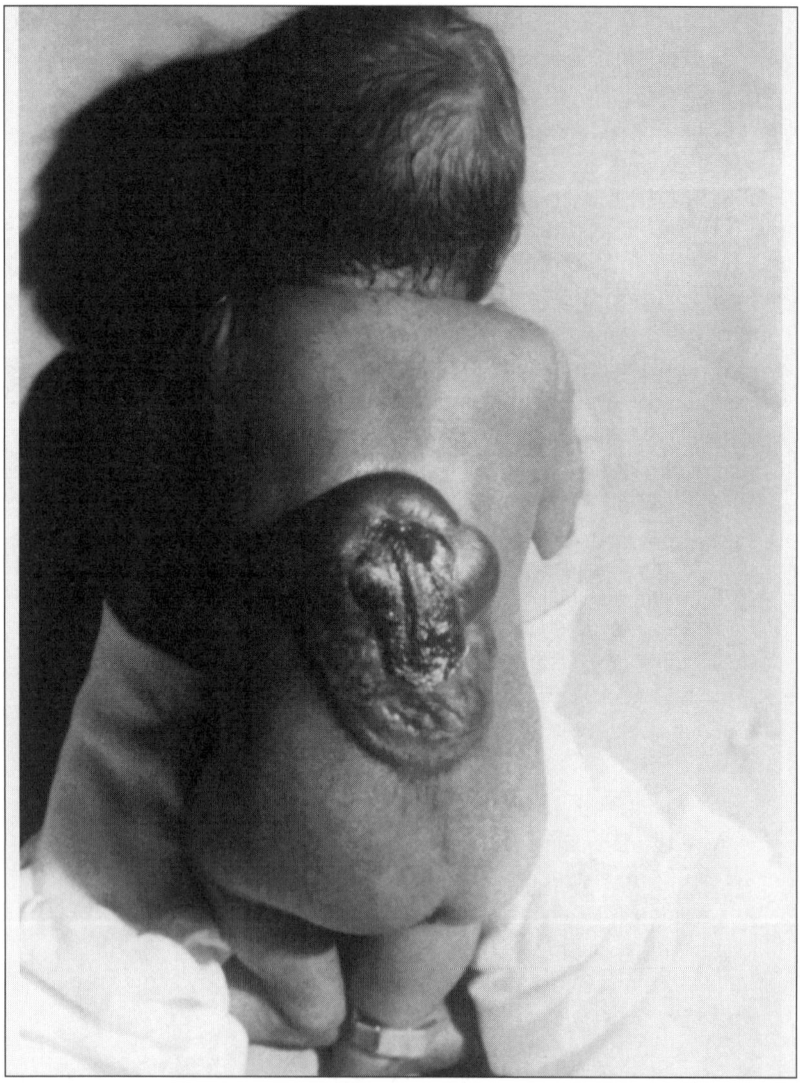

Figure 2.14. Newborn infant with a large thoraco-lumbar meningomyelocele.

diabetes affects younger individuals and produces more severe complications. There is good evidence that it results from a genetic predisposition wherein individuals respond to some viral infections by producing antibodies that destroy the insulin-producing cells of the pancreas. Because of the insulin deficiency, the body attempts to burn fat as a source of energy. Incomplete burning of fats generates compounds (ketones) that lead to excess acids in the body. The combination of impaired sugar metabolism and excess acids (ketoacidosis) chronically results in poor growth, easy fatigability, and increased susceptibility to infection. Acutely, these changes can produce life-threatening chemical imbalances. A combination of proper insulin dosage and diet are required. Insulin administration without proper dietary intake can lead to episodes of confusion and irritability, even coma, because of hypoglycemia (low blood sugar). This can usually be quickly corrected with a sugar snack (see Chapter 8).

Non-insulin-dependent diabetes is a disorder of adults. Proper diet and exercise can usually control it. As the frequency of obesity has increased in children dramatically over recent years, there has been an increased incidence of non-insulin-dependent diabetes in school-age children.

PSYCHOSOCIAL ISSUES

For children, any situation that sets them apart from their peers can produce significant psychosocial problems that often are of greater consequence than physical abnormalities. Genetic disorders set children apart from their peers in many ways that often are unrelated to children's native abilities and skills. Clearly, conditions that result in an obvious and strikingly different physical appearance create considerable emotional stress for children.

BEHAVIORAL CONCERNS

The ability of children with disabilities to take advantage of the educational opportunities open to them is often seriously impeded by associated behavioral problems. While these behavioral problems may have their origin in the inability of the parents or the child to deal with the disability, some genetic disorders have specific behavioral problems as an integral part of the disorder. Table 2.2 shows examples of genetic disorders in which specific and reproducible patterns of behavioral problems arise.

Table 2.2

EDUCATIONAL AND PSYCHOLOGICAL PROBLEMS ASSOCIATED WITH SOME COMMON GENETIC DISORDERS

Disorder	Educational	Psychological
Achondroplasia	None	Dwarfism
Neurofibromatosis	LD	Cosmetic
Fragile X syndrome	Mild to moderate CI	Hyperactivity, immaturity
Lesch-Nyhan syndrome	Ataxia, dysarthria	Self-mutilation
Angelman syndrome	Severe CI	Seizures, inappropriate laughter
Prader-Willi syndrome	Mild to moderate CI	Obesity, pleasant personality
Down syndrome	Moderate CI	Stigmatization
Turner syndrome	Mild LD	Short stature, delayed sexual maturation
Klinefelter syndrome	Mild CI to LD	Social and physical immaturity
Williams syndrome	Moderate CI	Hyperactivity, fearless behavior, gregarious
Osteogenesis imperfecta	None	Limited physical activity
Phenylketonuria	None, if properly treated	Severe dietary restrictions
Sickle-cell disease	None	Pain crises, absenteeism, stroke

Note. CI = cognitive impairment; LD = learning disabilities. Adapted from Mefford, Batshaw, & Hoffman (2012).

SUPPORT GROUPS

Most genetic disorders occur sufficiently infrequently that a primary-care physician may have had no prior experience with a certain disorder. Not only is most medical literature regarding these disorders unintelligible to most laypersons, but also it often does not contain the kinds of information about life experiences and effective management schemes that families seek. Family support groups now exist for virtually all genetic disorders. These support groups provide an invaluable service to families through several mechanisms:

1. The groups usually have prepared pamphlets providing the general kind of information the family seeks about a particular genetic disorder present in their child.
2. They produce a periodic newsletter with updates on research, conferences, and family stories.
3. They sponsor conferences on regional and national levels, which combine research updates with practical information for families and opportunities to meet and socialize with other families.
4. They can provide information about resources needed for the child's care in the family's geographic area. They also can put the family in contact with other families in their geographic area.

It is beyond the scope of this chapter to attempt a listing of all the genetic support groups. Most groups have a website and can be accessed on the Internet by simply typing in the name of the condition in search engines. The Genetic Alliance is able to put families and teachers in contact with specific support groups (www.geneticalliance.org).

REFERENCE

Mefford, H. C., Batshaw, M. L., & Hoffman, E. P. (2012). Genomics and intellectual disability, and autism. *New England Journal of Medicine, 366*(8), 733–743.

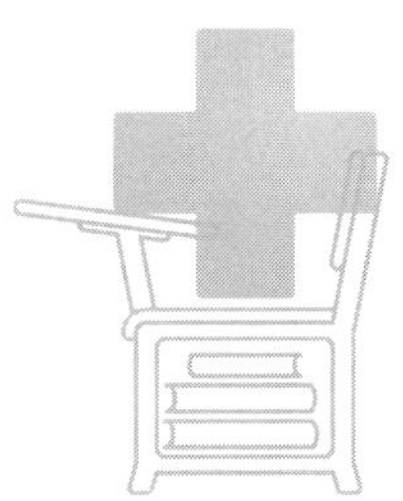

Chapter 3
Growth, Development, and Endocrine Disorders

Denis Daneman

Growth is a complex process that involves the interrelated effects of genetic, environmental, nutritional, hormonal, and psychological factors. Physical growth encompasses changes in the size and function of the organism and begins in utero. Intellectual and emotional growth begin at birth and are dependent on normal neurological and behavioral maturation and on healthy family and peer relationships. From conception to adolescence, growth proceeds in biologically determined cycles that fall into five distinct periods:

1. Intrauterine growth, including organ development and function
2. Early infancy—rapid growth from birth to 2 years of age
3. Childhood—slower growth from 2 years of age to the onset of puberty
4. The rapid pubertal growth spurt up to ages 14 to 16 (earlier in girls than boys)
5. A sharp deceleration to maturity

These periods of physical growth are intertwined with predictable cycles of social and developmental growth in such a way that problems in one may have a profound effect on the other. Figure 3.1 depicts the normal postnatal growth patterns in boys and girls from age 2 to 20.

Problems in growth and development can be a major cause of concern and anxiety to children, adolescents, parents, and teachers. This chapter reviews the normal events of growth and development during each of the five stages described and indicates the common problems

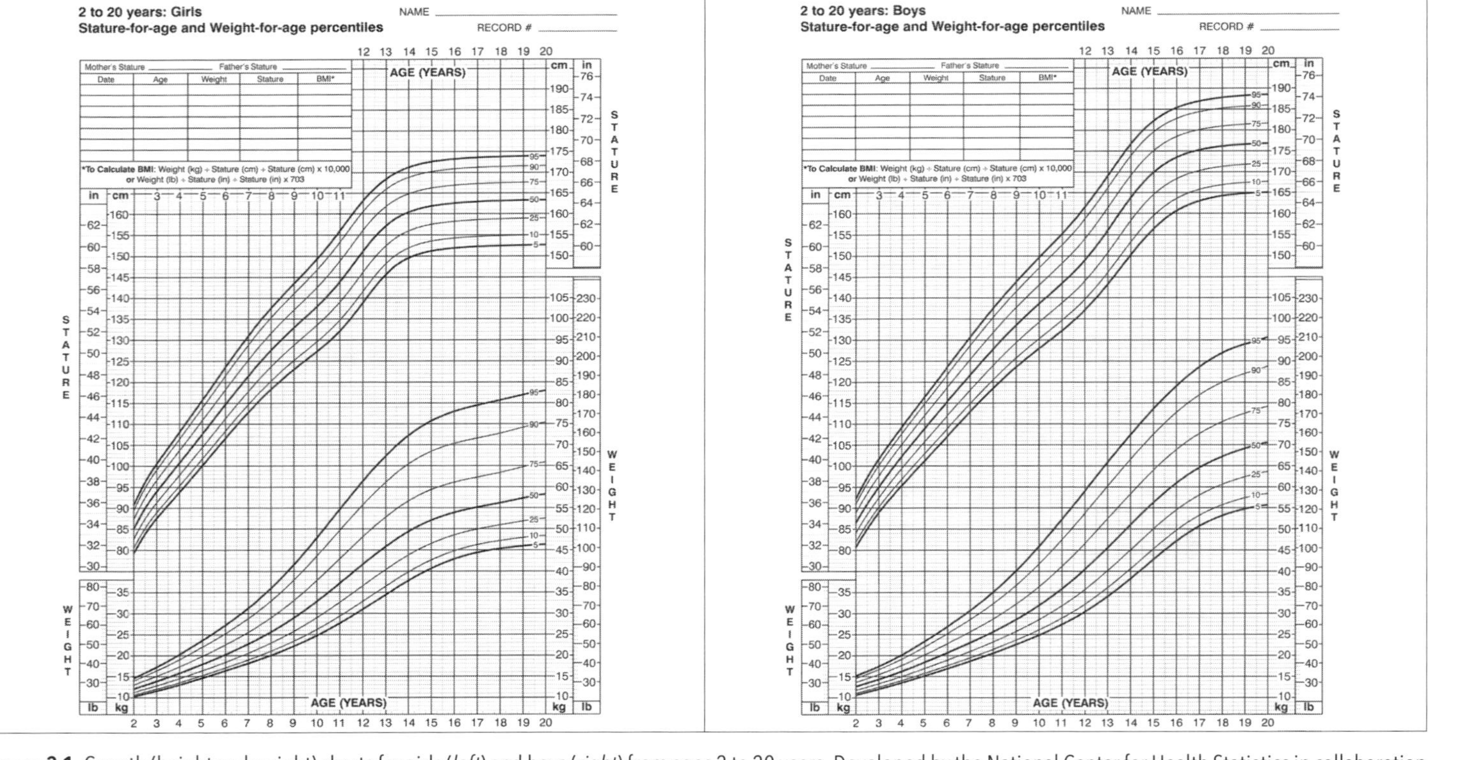

Figure 3.1. Growth (height and weight) charts for girls (*left*) and boys (*right*) from ages 2 to 20 years. Developed by the National Center for Health Statistics in collaboration with the National Center for Chronic Disease Prevention and Health Promotion (2000). Retrieved from http://www.cdc.gov.growthcharts.

that may interfere with these. Other more common disorders of the endocrine system are also discussed.

PHYSICAL GROWTH

The Fetus

Growth begins with the implantation of the fertilized egg in the mother's uterus and subsequent development of the placenta. Normal fetal growth depends on four primary factors:

1. The health and nutrition of the mother
2. The functional integrity of the placenta, the baby's lifeline
3. The size of the mother's uterus and pelvis
4. The potential for normal growth of the fertilized egg

Problems occurring during pregnancy in the mother (e.g., infections, chronic diseases, alcohol or drug abuse), in the placenta (e.g., vascular insufficiency), in the uterus or pelvis (e.g., small size, multiple pregnancies), or in the fetus itself (e.g., chromosomal abnormalities or malformation syndromes) can result in impaired intrauterine growth involving various body tissues and organs, including the brain. This, in turn, can lead to retarded physical, emotional, or intellectual growth both in utero and following birth. Birth injury (e.g., birth trauma, lack of oxygen to the baby's brain) can also result in permanent damage to physical or mental growth.

Just as the hypothalamus and pituitary gland, both located in the brain, act as the master control system in the hormonal regulation of growth in the child and adolescent, so does the placenta control growth in the fetus. Its function is dependent on a healthy nutrient supply from the mother. The placenta secretes a series of messenger hormones, such as placental lactogen, that are capable of stimulating the production of growth-promoting factors in the fetus. These factors, released from organs such as the liver, along with insulin from the fetal pancreas, play a major role in overall fetal cell division and cell growth and differentiation. Interestingly, fetal pituitary growth hormone and thyroid hormone do not exert major influences on intrauterine growth. These hormones, however, become extremely important for normal growth after birth. Disturbances in early pregnancy will interfere with cell division, limiting the number of cells that develop and the potential for catch-up growth after birth. In contrast, problems occurring later in pregnancy may interfere with cell size rather than cell number. These later children, while small at birth, are likely to show catch-up growth after birth once the problem has been removed. What has become clear is that adverse events during pregnancy can seriously affect postnatal outcomes. Many human fetuses have to adapt to a limited supply of nutrients. In doing so, they permanently change their structure and metabolism. These "programmed" changes may be the origins of a number of diseases in later life, including coronary heart disease and the related disorders of stroke, diabetes, and hypertension. This is a process called fetal or intrauterine programming and is accomplished by changes in gene structure and function, called epigenetics.

Extrauterine Growth

Genes

It has long been recognized that growth is closely linked to heredity. This is seen not only in families, where children tend to show patterns of growth similar to their parents, but also in ethnic, tribal, or racial groups, such as in the African Pygmies, whose short stature is genetically determined.

Genes are biological units contained within the chromosomes that have the capacity to direct the synthesis of specific proteins. Thus, certain genes are important in the production of growth-promoting hormones; other genes govern the growth of the receptor tissue to which these hormones are directed. Thus, growth is determined not by a single gene, but rather by many genes working in concert (*polygenic inheritance*).

Both genetic errors that result in abnormal or decreased formation of growth-promoting hormones and those that interfere with receptor tissue growth can cause retarded development. Many types of growth failure, including hormonal disorders such as certain types of hypopituitarism (underactivity of the pituitary gland) and receptor problems such as achondroplasia, are due to genetic errors. Conversely, tall stature may be related to increased production of these hormones either on a genetic basis as occurs in certain races or, rarely, in an abnormal fashion (e.g., a growth-hormone-producing tumor of the pituitary gland).

Hormones

The term *hormone* is derived from the Greek *hormaein,* meaning "to set in motion." Hormones are chemical messengers produced in the endocrine glands of the body (e.g., pituitary gland, thyroid, pancreas, adrenal glands, ovaries, or testes) that are secreted into the bloodstream and exert their influence by altering selected metabolic processes in their specific target organs. Hormones thus are key regulators of cell function.

The master endocrine gland is the pituitary, located in the brain just behind the eyes. It is regulated by the hypothalamus and neural influences and by blood levels of the circulating hormones such as thyroid hormone, estrogen, testosterone, insulin-like growth factor-l (IGF-l), and cortisol. The pituitary secretes hormones that stimulate other endocrine glands such as the thyroid (located at the front of the neck), adrenal glands (which sit on top of each kidney), and ovaries in the female and testes in the male. In response to specific pituitary hormones, the thyroid gland secretes its hormone, thyroxine; the adrenal glands, cortisol; and the ovaries and testes, estrogen and testosterone, respectively. The adrenal glands also produce small amounts of androgens and estrogens. These hormones, in turn, exert their effects on specific target tissues throughout the body. The hormones important for growth include growth hormone; thyroid hormone; and the steroid hormones, including cortisol, androgens (male hormones), and estrogens (female hormones).

Growth hormone produced by the pituitary stimulates the liver and other tissues to produce insulin-like growth factor-I (IGF-I), which stimulates growth of the long bones of the body. The pituitary also produces a hormone, antidiuretic hormone, important in maintaining water balance in the body. Indirectly, this hormone may also influence growth.

Two other endocrine glands are also important in growth: The pancreas, located next to the stomach, secretes insulin, a major regulator of energy metabolism, and the parathyroid glands, embedded in the back part of the thyroid, secrete parathormone, which is essential for calcium metabolism. Insulin is chemically similar to IGF-I and is an essential hormone for fetal growth but also plays a role postnatally. Calcium is critically important in bone growth and strength, factors controlled in part by parathyroid hormone.

Growth occurs by both cell division and cell enlargement. Growth hormone is an important regulator of cell division. Of the other growth-promoting hormones, thyroid hormone increases cell size, insulin increases cytoplasmic growth, and both, in concert with growth hormone and IGF-I, have an effect on cell division.

Long bone growth (e.g., arms and legs) requires cartilage formation and subsequent replacement of cartilage with calcified bone. IGF-I is particularly important in cartilage formation, whereas thyroid hormone is more important in the replacement of cartilage with calcified bone. The sex hormones (androgens and estrogens) exert their influence on both processes.

Growth occurs mainly at the ends of the long bones, although some growth does occur in the spine. The child between the age of 3 and the onset of puberty should grow no less than 2 inches (4 to 5 cm) per year. During puberty, growth rates may increase to 3 to 5 inches (6 to 12 cm) per year. This increased growth rate is due to the combined effects of growth hormone, IGF-I, and the sex hormones.

Puberty

Puberty is the stage of development during which sexual maturation occurs, leading to reproductive capability. Puberty is accompanied by changes in both physical growth and psychological perspective. The terms *puberty* and *adolescence* are used interchangeably.

At puberty, increased production of the hypothalamic hormone, luteinizing hormone-releasing hormone (LHRH), begins. This stimulates production by the anterior pituitary of the two gonadotrophins, luteinizing hormone (LH) and follicle-stimulating hormone (FSH), which together control function of the gonads (ovaries in females, and testes in males). FSH is important in ovulation in the female and sperm production in the male, and LH stimulates estrogen production in the female and testosterone production in the male. Through a feedback mechanism, the hormones produced from the ovaries and testes regulate production of LHRH, LH, and FSH (see Figure 3.2). Small amounts of male hormones, called androgens, are normally produced from the adrenal glands and ovaries in the female, whereas small amounts of the female hormone, estrogen, are produced in the adrenal glands and testes of the male.

In the adolescent female, ovarian estrogens stimulate growth of the uterus, its endometrial lining, and vagina; influence fat deposition; and accelerate linear growth and skeletal maturation. Their secretion is important in reaching menarche (onset of menstrual periods). Androgens stimulate the growth of pubic and axillary hair and contribute to linear growth increase and advanced skeletal maturation. Androgens are also important in the development of the labia majora and clitoris. The mechanism by which adrenal androgens increase at puberty (called adrenarche) is unknown.

In the adolescent male, testosterone and other androgens stimulate growth of the penis and pubic, axillary, and body hair; accelerate growth rate and skeletal maturation; and increase the size and number of muscle cells. Increased amounts of estrogen in the pubertal male may cause transient enlargement and tenderness of the breasts (*gynecomastia*). This occurs to some degree in the majority of pubertal males and generally regresses with time. If the breasts remain large

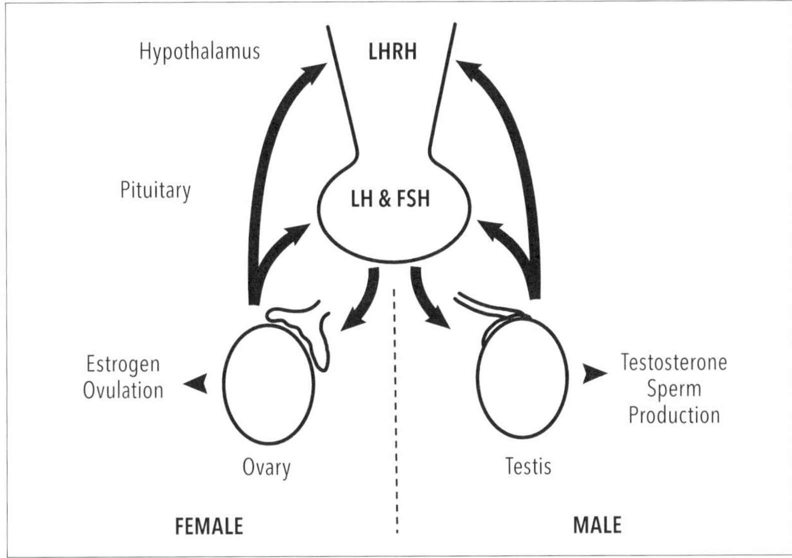

Figure 3.2. Diagrammatic representation of integrated function of the hypothalamic-pituitary-gonadal axis. At puberty, increasing amounts of luteinizing hormone-releasing hormone (LHRH) from the hypothalamus stimulate release from the pituitary of the gonadotrophins, luteinizing hormone (LH), and follicle-stimulating hormone (FSH). These, in turn, lead to release of the sex hormones–estrogen from the ovaries and testosterone from the testes–and production of the ova and sperm, respectively.

or are slow to regress, it may cause considerable embarrassment to the teen, occasionally necessitating surgical reduction.

Androgens appear to exert a permanent organizing influence on the brain both before and during puberty in boys. Males deficient in androgen may have serious defects involving spatial ability and other specific cognitive skills.

The wide age range of the onset and progression of normal pubertal development often arouses fears of abnormality, self-consciousness, and anxiety about body image (see Figure 3.3). In girls, pubertal changes (usually starting with breast development) begin between ages 6 and 13.5, with menarche on average about 2 years later (ages 11 to 15). A recent study in the United States found that the definition of early (precocious) puberty in girls needs to be revised, given that changes are normal in African American girls as young as 6 and in White American girls at 7 years of age. In general, boys start 1 to 2 years after girls, with testicular enlargement beginning at ages 10 to 14. The growth spurt in boys occurs later in the pubertal process than that in girls. The earlier onset of puberty and more rapid growth spurt in girls accounts for their taller stature in early adolescence but shorter adult height than in boys. This leads to an average adult height in males (5 feet 9 inches) 5 inches taller than in females (5 feet 4 inches).

FACTORS AFFECTING GROWTH

Nutrition and Disease

Nutrition has a major influence on both intrauterine and extrauterine growth. Poor nutrition can result in impairments in both physical and mental development. On a worldwide basis, malnutrition is the single most common cause of growth failure and short stature. Malnutrition and, specifically, decreased protein intake may be associated with very low IGF-I levels and high growth hormone levels, which suggests that proper nutrition is an integral component of normal endocrine control. The growth failure associated with many chronic diseases may be the result, at least in part, of poor nutrition.

In females, a determining factor in the onset of puberty and achievement of menarche is the attainment of a critical body weight.

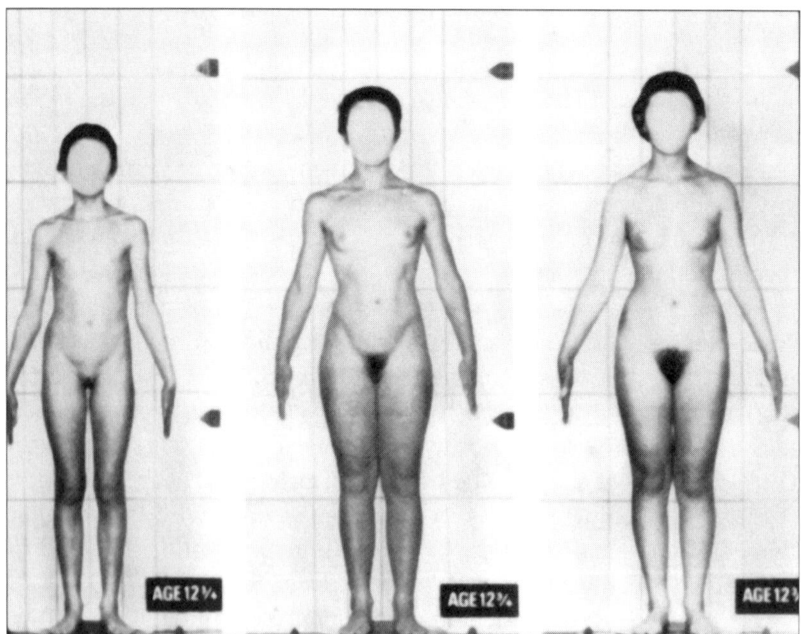

Figure 3.3. Variation in normal sexual development in three girls of the same age (12.75 years). From *Endocrine and Genetic Diseases of Childhood and Adolescence* (2nd ed., p. 28), by L. I. Gardner, 1975, Philadelphia, PA: Saunders. Copyright 1975 by W. B. Saunders Co. Reprinted with permission.

Females who exercise excessively, such as long-distance runners, gymnasts, and ballerinas, may lose body fat and experience a cessation of menstrual function. Such events underscore the importance of good nutrition.

Psychosocial Factors

Growth retardation; disturbances of intellectual, motor, and emotional development; and bizarre behavior have been observed in infants and children living in severely abnormal environments, particularly those devoid of parental love and support. In severe cases, these children may manifest retardation in height, weight, and skeletal maturation comparable to that seen in growth hormone deficiency (hypopituitarism). Motor and intellectual development may also be delayed, and these children may have a range of emotional responses from depressed and withdrawn to inappropriately affectionate. Abnormal feeding behaviors such as rumination, increased thirst, and obtaining food and drink from "bizarre" sources (e.g., garbage cans, drinking from puddles) may also be observed.

The cause of the growth failure is uncertain but may relate to either malnutrition or disturbed growth hormone secretion. With removal from the depriving environment, catch-up growth will be observed. This may require removal of these children from their homes and placement in foster or group homes. This condition, called psychosocial or emotional deprivation, emphasizes the importance of emotional stability in the process of normal growth and development.

Environmental Factors

Socioeconomic factors, such as poverty and poor hygiene, may be associated with poor nutrition and frequent acute or chronic infections, and consequent poor growth. Seasonal variations in growth rates have been observed in certain areas, with the greatest increases in height being seen in the spring and the lowest in the fall. Exercise promotes growth and strength of both muscle and bone. The prolonged use of drugs such as corticosteroids and stimulant medications for attention-deficit/hyperactivity disorder (e.g., methylphenidate, or Ritalin) may also result in growth failure.

CAUSES FOR CONCERN

Linear growth, weight gain, and the onset and progression of puberty are good indicators of the general health and well-being of the child or teenager. All family physicians and pediatricians should maintain growth charts on the children they evaluate in their offices (see Figure 3.1). In this way, they will be able to detect more quickly the subtle changes in growth characteristics that may not otherwise be obvious.

In relation to delayed growth, we should become concerned about the child whose height is

- increasing by less than 1.5 to 2 inches a year (4 to 5 cm)
- more than 2 standard deviations from the mean for age (i.e., below the lowest line on the growth charts)
- "falling off" the percentile the height previously had been following
- considerably shorter than would be expected based on his or her parents' heights

Problems of weight loss, or a weight that is disproportionately lower than height, should also be investigated.

With respect to puberty, girls should be evaluated if breast development occurs before age 6 years in African American girls and age 7 in White American girls (a condition called precocious puberty) or if there is very rapid progression of pubertal development, and if there is no breast development by age 13.5 (delayed adolescence), or if menstrual function has not begun by age 15 (primary amenorrhea). In boys, development of secondary sexual characteristics before age 9–10 or lack of development by age 14 should trigger an evaluation. In general, early puberty is more common in girls than boys, and delayed adolescence is more common in boys.

In all these situations, the presence of other symptoms and signs (e.g., headaches, recent onset of visual disturbance, excessive weight gain with growth failure) in addition to the disorder of growth should alert the physician, parents, and perhaps also school personnel to the possibility of a significant pathological problem.

COMMON CAUSES OF GROWTH DELAY

Normal Variants

Figure 3.4 depicts the numerous factors that may interfere with growth and physical development. The most frequent causes fall into the category of "normal variants":

- *Familial short stature.* In general, short parents tend to have short children, and vice versa.

- *Constitutional delay of growth or adolescence.* Some children, often called "late bloomers," will have a delay in their maturation, reaching their adolescence at a later-than-average age (see Figure 3.5). There is often a family predisposition to this pattern of growth, and it is much more common in boys than in girls.

The two conditions described are quite distinct. Children with familial short stature are healthy in all respects, and puberty is not delayed, leading to a short final adult height. In children who are constitutionally delayed, general health is also normal, but the onset of puberty will be significantly delayed. They will have a normal pubertal growth spurt reaching an adult height well within the normal range. In the prepubertal child, the way to distinguish between these two conditions is by performing a wrist X-ray to determine "bone age." In familial short stature, bony maturation is age appropriate, whereas in the constitutionally delayed, the bone age is less than chronological age (see Figure 3.6). Thus, at any age, the child with constitutional delay will have greater remaining growth potential. These two conditions

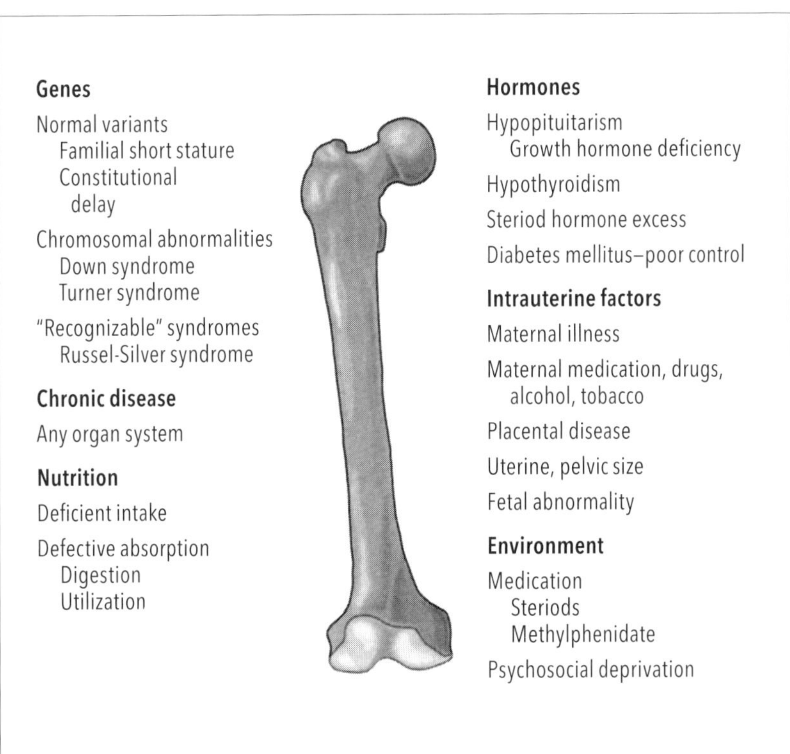

Figure 3.4. Factors responsible for growth failure in children and adolescents.

A

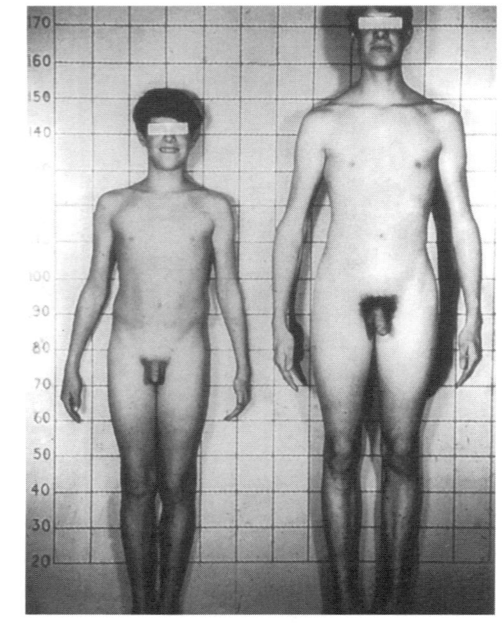

B

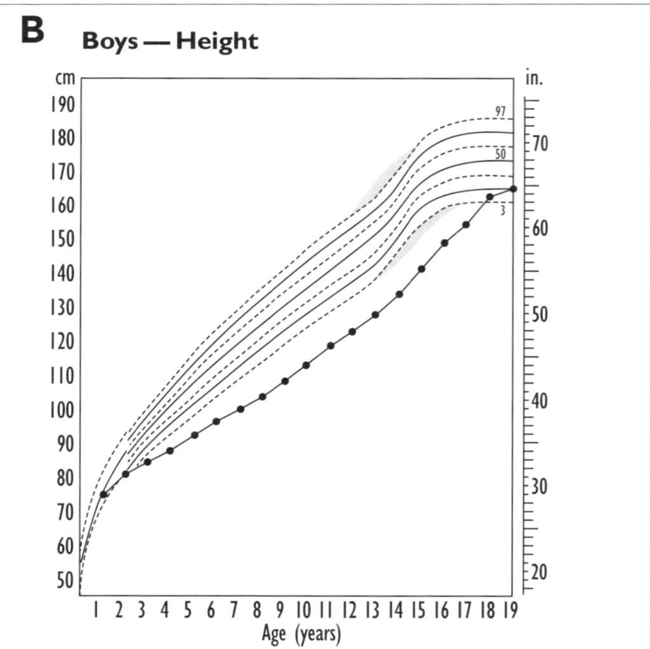

Figure 3.5. Constitutional delay of growth and adolescence in one of a fraternal twin pair. (A) At age 16 years, the brother on the left is shorter and has delayed puberty compared to his twin on the right. (B) Growth change of brother with delayed growth shows falloff in growth before age 3 years, followed by a normal growth rate throughout childhood and a delay in the onset of the pubertal growth spurt until after 16 years. Note that he does achieve a final adult height within the normal percentiles. Growth chart adapted from "Clinical Longitudinal Standards for Height, Weight, Height Velocity, Weight Velocity and Stages of Puberty," by J. M. Tanner and R. H. Whitehouse, 1976, *Archives of Diseases of Children, 51*(3), 170–179. Copyright 1976 by Castlemead Publications. Adapted with permission.

account for more than 80% of cases of short stature presented to the pediatrician or family physician. The remaining 20% or less will fall into one of the other categories described below.

Other Causes of Short Stature

Figure 3.7 illustrates some of the clinical characteristics of the more common "other" causes of short stature. Many of these conditions are distinguished from the normal variants by a growth rate less than normal for age.

Intrauterine Growth Retardation

Any condition that interferes with the well-being of the developing fetus has the potential to limit intrauterine growth and diminish postnatal growth potential. The earlier in pregnancy that the insult occurs, the more likely that the growth will be permanently diminished. Causes of intrauterine growth retardation include the following:

- maternal infection (e.g., toxoplasmosis, syphilis, rubella, cytomegalovirus, HIV, herpes virus)

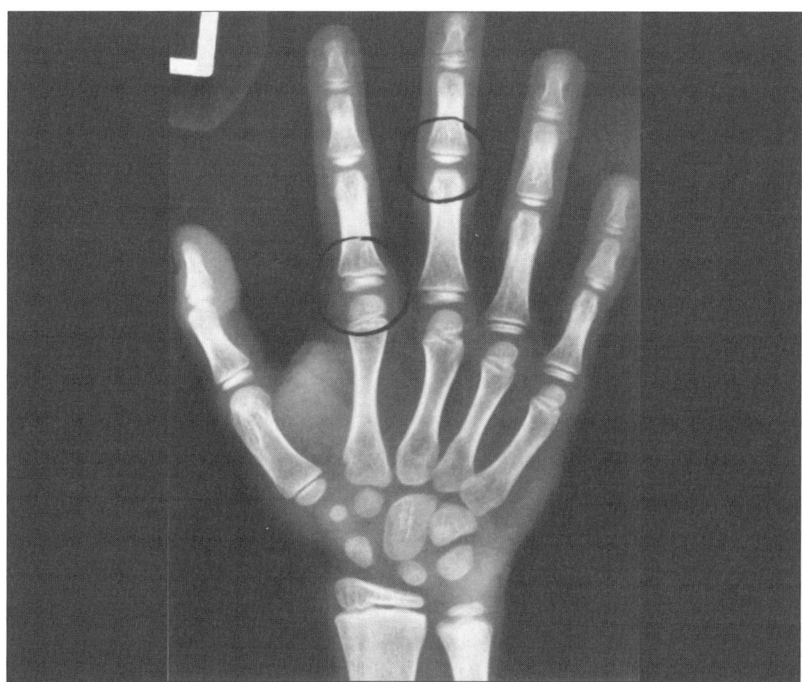

Figure 3.6. X-ray of the right hand. Circles outline growth centers (*epiphyses*), which are studied to determine bone age, here measured to be 7 years in a boy who is 11 years old.

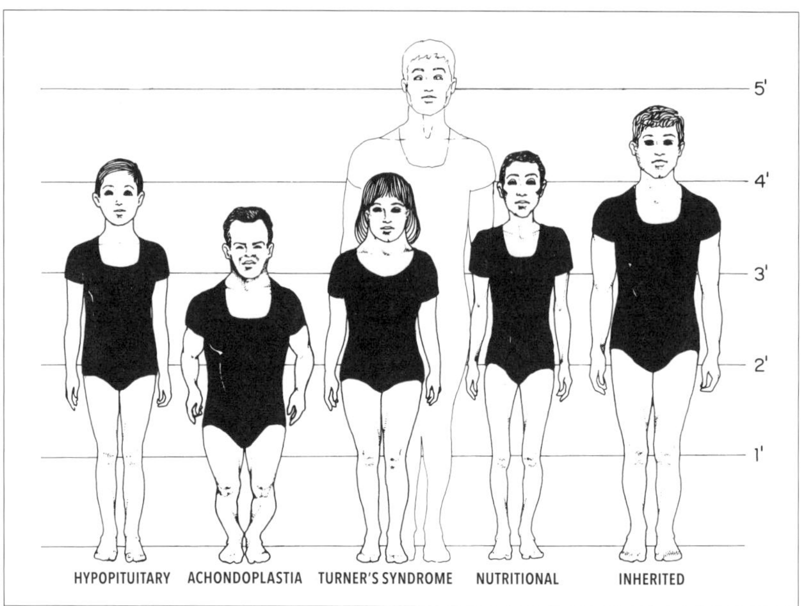

Figure 3.7. Several causes of short stature, illustrating the characteristic features and body proportions associated with each. All children are the same chronological age.

- maternal illness (e.g., cardiac or renal disease, hypertension)
- maternal ingestion of medication that is teratogenic (e.g., phenytoin, Dilantin, thalidomide)
- maternal use of alcohol, tobacco, or illicit drugs during pregnancy
- small uterine or pelvic size
- a chromosomal abnormality (e.g., Down syndrome, Turner's syndrome) or malformation syndrome (e.g., Russell-Silver syndrome)

Children with intrauterine growth retardation are distinguished by a birth weight more than 2 standard deviations below the mean for the gestational age (e.g., less than 2.5 kg at birth in a term infant). By age 2, the infant will usually have caught up to his or her ultimate growth curve. Those who remain low on the percentile charts at age 2 will likely have a permanent decrease in growth potential.

Chromosomal conditions may account for intrauterine growth retardation. Some children are born with either an extra chromosome (a condition called *trisomy,* such as Down syndrome) or a missing chromosome (*monosomy,* such as Turner's syndrome). These are inevitably associated with moderate to severe growth failure of uncertain cause. The growth failure generally starts in utero and is accentuated after birth. In addition to the short stature, these children may exhibit other physical features that clue the physician to their diagnosis (see Chapter 2).

Bony Dysplasias

Conditions that affect the growth of the long bones and spine will lead to disproportionate lack of growth of these bones (bony dysplasias). These conditions are hereditary in nature. One of the most severe forms of bony dysplasia is achondroplasia, but less severe variants also occur. In these conditions, the trunk (chest and abdomen) is often normal in size, but the arms and legs are disproportionately short. In general, children with dysplasias such as achondroplasia do not respond to hormonal therapy. Techniques have been developed to lengthen the long bones and have successfully resulted in marked height increases in some of these children.

Chronic Diseases

Any systemic disease of sufficient severity can interfere with physical growth and development. For example, diseases of the cardiovascular, respiratory, gastrointestinal, genitourinary, and neurological systems all have the potential to have an impact on growth. Most of these disorders will be fairly obvious by the time growth impairment becomes evident. However, a few disorders may be quite "silent" and yet interfere significantly with growth. These include malabsorption conditions of the small bowel, such as celiac disease or inflammatory bowel disease, and kidney conditions, such as undiagnosed kidney infections. Management of the underlying disorder will improve the growth potential, particularly if this occurs before the onset of puberty. In those chronic conditions that cannot be cured, such as chronic renal failure leading to dialysis and/or kidney transplantation, final adult height may be significantly impaired.

Certain medications, such as glucocorticoids, steroids, or stimulant medications used for attention-deficit/hyperactivity disorder (ADHD), may also interfere with growth potential. It is best to maintain these medications at the lowest effective dose to control the underlying condition, in hopes of thereby limiting the growth-retarding side effects.

Malnutrition

Worldwide, malnutrition is far and away the most common cause of short stature. Reversal of malnutrition at an early stage will allow normal growth potential. However, the later the malnourished state is corrected, the less likely the child is to attain genetic height potential. In developed countries, malnutrition is often the result of abuse or neglect, other serious chronic illness, or, occasionally, fad or exclusion diets imposed on these children. Self-imposed malnutrition is an integral part of eating disorders such as anorexia nervosa. If this condition begins before puberty, it has the potential to impair growth (see Chapter 6). Some cases of growth failure have been reported in children, particularly boys, whose restricted caloric intake was due to the fear of obesity.

Psychosocial Deprivation Syndrome

A number of children have been recognized in whom short stature is the result of severe psychosocial deprivation, a serious form of child abuse or neglect. This is an extremely difficult diagnosis to make, as the children often look similar to those with growth hormone deficiency. In fact, their growth hormone levels may be low at the time of initial assessment. They may also exhibit bizarre eating habits and behavior. In fact, many have been noted to drink from toilet bowls, eat dirt, and drink from puddles on the street (Powell, Brasel, & Blizzard, 1967). Removal of these children from the depriving environment usually leads to spectacular catch-up growth.

Endocrine Disorders Leading to Growth Failure

Although hormones such as growth hormone, thyroid hormones, and steroid hormones play an essential role in growth and development, fewer than 10% of children with growth failure have a hormonal deficiency or excess. The more common hormonal conditions that interfere with growth are discussed here.

1. *Growth hormone deficiency.* These children may have isolated growth hormone deficiency or deficiency of multiple pituitary hormones (e.g., those that control the thyroid gland, pubertal development, and the adrenal gland). Although growth hormone deficiency may be an inherited or sporadic (*idiopathic*) disorder, it also may result from damage to the pituitary gland from tumors in this region or from irradiation of the head for treatment of malignant diseases (e.g., leukemia). These conditions require specialized testing and can be managed with replacement of the missing hormones. Growth hormone itself is given as a subcutaneous injection six to seven days a week.

2. *Thyroid hormone deficiency.* Lack of sufficient production of the principal thyroid hormone, thyroxine, will lead to a multitude of symptoms (see the "Other Endocrine Disorders" section), including growth failure.

Hypothyroidism is most commonly a result of chronic thyroid inflammation (Hashimoto's thyroiditis) and can be managed by replacement doses of the missing hormone.

3. *Steroid hormone excess syndromes.* Growth will be impaired if the body is exposed to excessive amounts of the glucocorticoid hormones, either produced by the adrenal glands or used as medications (e.g., hydrocortisone, prednisone, dexamethasone) to control a number of systemic medical conditions (e.g., after organ transplantation to prevent rejection, for lupus erythematosus, and for other arthritides). These steroids may also have an impact on growth, although likely to a lesser degree, when used in the inhaled form for severe asthma or in the topical form for severe skin conditions. In all of these situations, physicians must carefully weigh the benefits of treatment with these agents against their potential side effects.

4. *Very poorly controlled diabetes mellitus.* In children with longstanding, poorly controlled diabetes mellitus, growth impairment may be seen. Improved metabolic control will invariably improve growth velocity.

INVESTIGATION OF THE CHILD WITH SHORT STATURE

All short children deserve evaluation by their physician and referral to a specialist if necessary. The reasons for evaluation are twofold: first, reassurance and counseling for those whose short stature is due to one of the normal variants or genetic syndromes, and, second, management of those conditions amenable to hormonal or other therapy. Investigation will be more urgent in the slow-growing child than in one who is short but showing normal annual height increments (greater than 2 inches a year).

Short stature may have important social implications for children in the classroom. They may be singled out as different and have unpleasant epithets (e.g., "shrimp," "dwarf," "midget") hurled at them by their classmates. In addition, the child who is severely short may face additional difficulties in opening doors, reaching water fountains, and fighting the hustle and bustle around the school. Teachers may inadvertently stigmatize the short child by asking the class to line up according to size or by always choosing these children to do certain tasks or play certain roles (e.g., "the baby") in class activities. Singling out these children may produce emotional disturbance, including withdrawal, aggression, or other acting-out behaviors. While research suggests that short stature is not uniformly damaging emotionally, there may be significant psychological distress in some children.

The strongest source of support for these children will be the guidance and encouragement of their parents, but teachers can also play an important role by encouraging participation in all school activities and avoiding stigmatizing comments or actions. Short children should always be treated according to their mental and chronological age and not according to their size. Occasionally, school personnel may be tempted to hold the short child back a year so that he or she will be with children of more equivalent size in the classroom. This is to be avoided at all costs, unless the child has a learning difficulty that makes holding back appropriate. Special education may be required for certain short children with specific learning disabilities. For example, cognitive impairment is common in Down syndrome, and specific deficits, such as spatial and math deficiencies, are common in Turner syndrome.

These problems also hold true for taller-than-average children, who may be singled out in exactly the opposite way by being expected to perform at an age-inappropriate higher level because of their size.

Treatment of children with disorders of growth and sexual development should not only take into account the obvious medical concerns but also be sensitive to the educational, social, psychological, and vocational needs of these children and adolescents. Medical treatment is not required for all short children. For many, counseling and reassurance with careful follow-up represent the most appropriate therapy.

Some families are willing to "do anything" to enhance the growth potential of their short child. Growth hormone has been approved for use in an increasing number of conditions associated with short stature, including growth hormone deficiency, children born small for gestational age who do not evidence postnatal catch-up, children with idiopathic short stature, and those with chronic renal (kidney) failure or short bowel syndrome, as well as those with Turner, Prader-Willi, and Noonan syndromes. Use of growth hormone should be contemplated only after careful consultation with a pediatric endocrinologist.

OTHER ENDOCRINE DISORDERS

The Thyroid Gland

Thyroxine, the major hormone secreted by the thyroid gland, is one of the most important hormones controlling the metabolic rate of the body. As such, it also affects growth and physical development. The teacher may occasionally face students with either underactivity (*hypothyroidism*) or overactivity (*hyperthyroidism*) of the thyroid gland.

Either condition may have implications for behavior and performance in the classroom.

In the early 1990s, a group of children was identified as having an association between a variant of ADHD and generalized resistance to thyroid hormone action (Hauser et al., 1993). Clinically, these children have nonspecific symptoms and signs of thyroid dysfunction (both hypothyroidism and hyperthyroidism) in addition to the learning disability. However, screening of large groups of children with classical ADHD has failed to reveal an increased incidence of thyroid dysfunction and is likely an unnecessary added investigation in these children.

Hypothyroidism

Thyroid hormone is critically important for early postnatal brain development, and its lack during this period may produce severe cognitive impairment (*cretinism*). Newborn thyroid-screening programs have been developed over the past 35 years to detect the 1 in 3,500–4,000 newborns with congenital hypothyroidism. Treatment in the first week or two of life has been remarkably effective in eliminating any associated intellectual impairment.

Hypothyroidism that develops after the first few years of life will not interfere with intellectual development but may have a major impact in delaying growth and physical development (see Figure 3.8). These children may have a goiter (enlargement of the thyroid gland at the front of the neck); evidence of growth failure; and eventual short stature, weight gain, dry hair and skin, muscle weakness, and poor energy level. They may also become severely constipated and complain of abdominal pains. Even though hypothyroid, they often perform well at school with little distraction from outside activities. The cause of the hypothyroidism is most often Hashimoto's thyroiditis, a chronic inflammatory (autoimmune) condition in which the gland may eventually "burn out." This condition is 10 times more common in girls than boys.

Investigation of hypothyroidism includes measurement of the thyroid hormone levels, with management consisting of replacement treatment with the synthetic hormone, L-thyroxine. This invariably leads to excellent catch-up growth and development and reversal of the symptoms described. However, in the early treatment phase, there may be poor concentration and deteriorating school performance as the body readjusts to a normal thyroid state. Teachers should be informed when one of their students is starting treatment and should be sensitive to changes in the student's performance and attention. Any

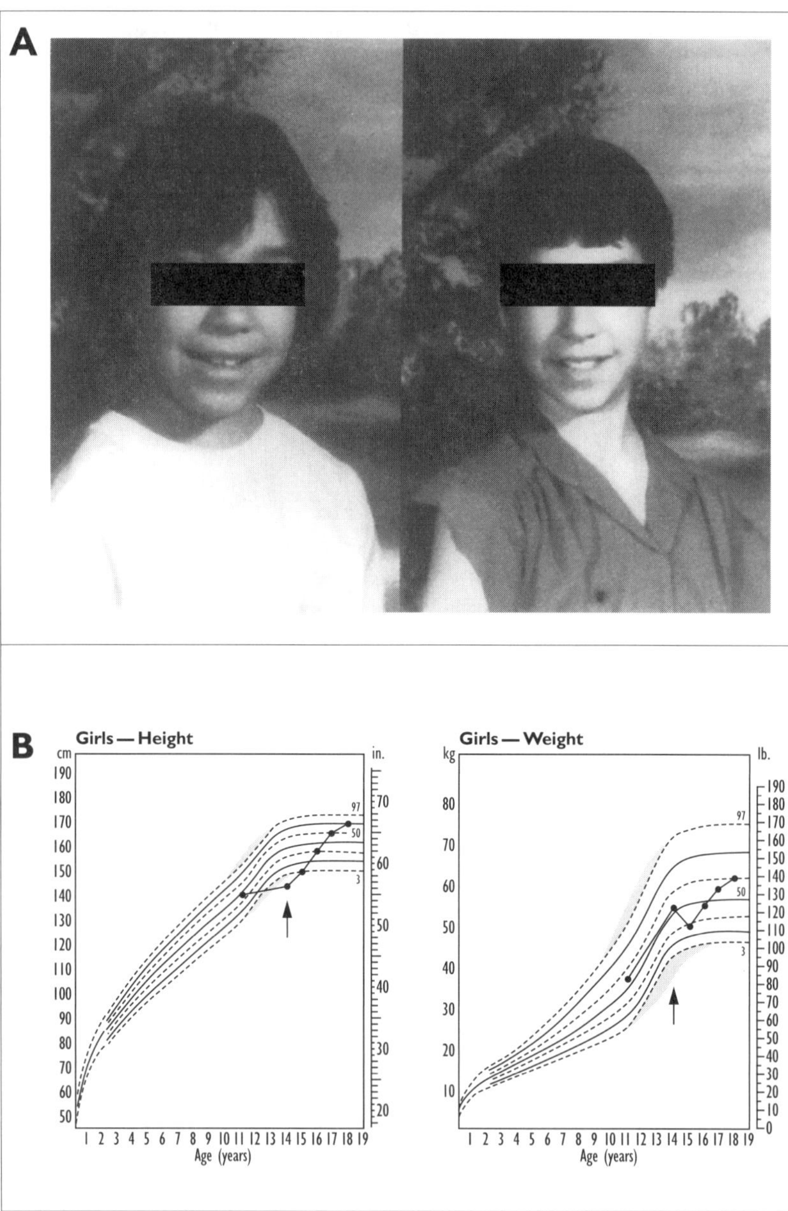

Figure 3.8. Severe acquired hypothyroidism presenting as growth failure in a 14-year-old girl showing (A) facial appearance before (*left*) and one year after (*right*) initiation of thyroid replacement therapy, and (B) growth chart for both height (*left panel*) and weight (*right*). The arrow denotes the time of diagnosis, with a remarkable increase in height and leveling off of weight gain after starting treatment. Growth charts adapted from "Clinical Longitudinal Standards for Height, Weight, Height Velocity, Weight Velocity and Stages of Puberty," by J. M. Tanner and R. H. Whitehouse, 1976, *Archives of Diseases of Children, 51*(3), 170–179. Copyright 1976 by Castlemead Publications. Adapted with permission.

marked changes should be communicated to the parents because the dose of medication may need adjustment.

Hyperthyroidism

This condition, like acquired hypothyroidism, is most frequently the result of chronic inflammation in the thyroid gland (Graves' disease). In some cases, underactivity of the gland ensues; in others, overactivity. While growth is usually not affected by hyperthyroidism, virtually every other system may be involved. In addition to the presence of a goiter, these children may show emotional lability, hyperactivity and short attention span, restlessness and nervousness, increased appetite but weight loss, disturbed sleeping habits, heat intolerance and increased sweating, increased heart rate, tremor of the hands, and diarrhea. These symptoms may lead to deteriorating school performance. In addition, some hyperthyroid children may show prominence of their eyes (*proptosis*).

Diagnosis requires demonstration of elevated levels of thyroid hormones, and treatment consists of thyroid-suppressive medication. In some, failure to respond to oral medications or side effects of these medications may necessitate the use of either radioactive iodine or surgery to ablate the gland. Normal behavior and school performance would be expected to return once the thyroid condition is under control, although noncompliance with medications may lead to a relapse of symptoms and signs. During the period of hyperthyroidism, these students should refrain from vigorous physical activities.

Effects of Excess Cortisone Medication

Cortisone and other glucocorticoid medications may be prescribed for a variety of medical conditions. In addition to impairment of physical growth and development, these medications may cause significant weight gain and change in body habitus, with truncal obesity and thinning of the arms and legs (see Figure 3.9). They may also produce marked acne, face reddening, stretch marks (striae), easy bruising, and a tendency to acquire infections more easily. Because treatment with cortisone diminishes or abolishes the body's ability to secrete more of its own cortisone in response to stress, any intercurrent illness or accident in children receiving these medications may pose a serious threat. Teachers should be aware of this and inform parents immediately should the child develop a serious intercurrent illness at school. Vomiting is particularly dangerous, as it will prevent absorption of the oral medication. Cortisone will then need to be administered by injection.

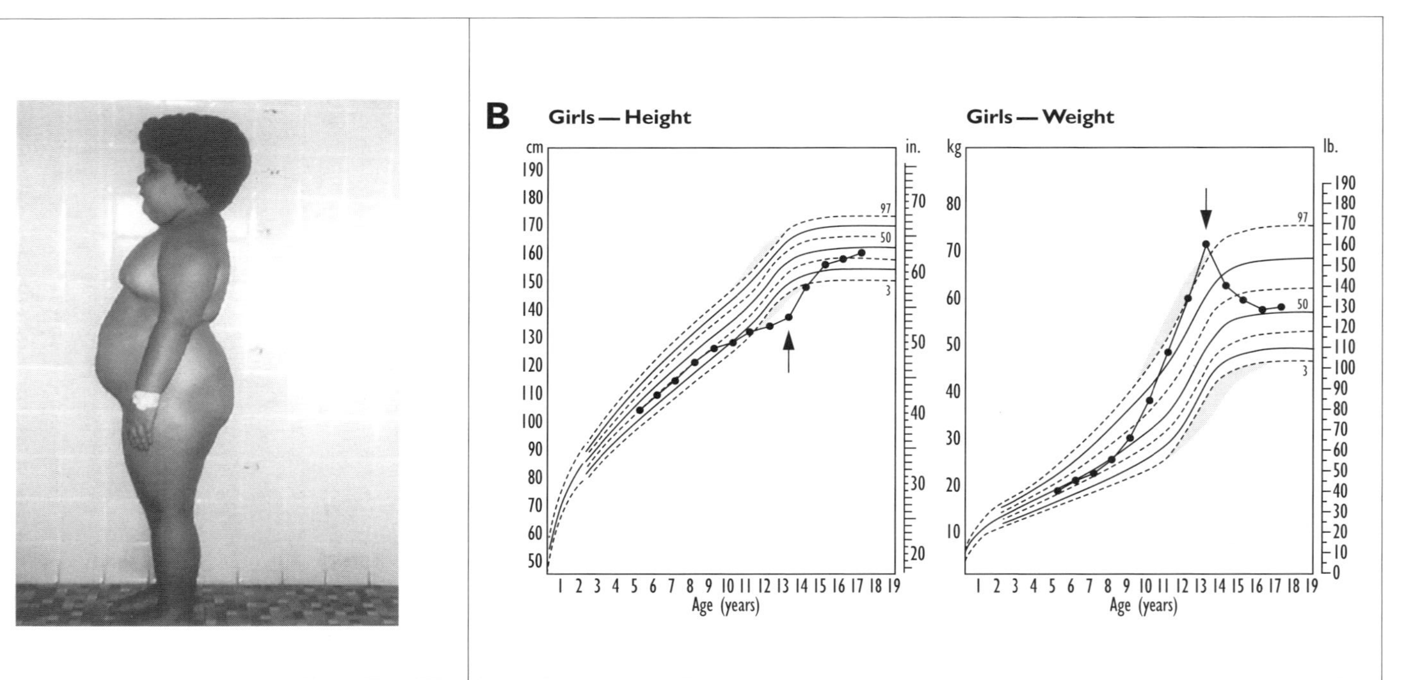

Figure 3.9. Cushing's syndrome (corticosteroid excess) presenting as growth failure and obesity in a 13-year-old girl. (A) The typical truncal obesity and short stature. (B) Height fall-off (*left panel*) and excessive weight gain (*right*) before diagnosis (*arrow*). Removal of her pituitary tumor led to catch-up in height and marked weight loss. Growth charts adapted from "Clinical Longitudinal Standards for Height, Weight, Height Velocity, Weight Velocity and Stages of Puberty," by J. M. Tanner and R. H. Whitehouse, 1976, *Archives of Diseases of Children, 51*(3), 170–179. Copyright 1976 by Castlemead Publications. Adapted with permission.

DISORDERS OF PUBERTY

Any of the conditions that cause short stature may also be associated with a delay in the onset or progression of the secondary sexual characteristics at the time of puberty. This is called delayed adolescence or delayed puberty and can be diagnosed in a girl who has failed to show any breast development by ages 13 to 13.5 or in a boy who shows no enlargement of the testicles by age 14 years. Conversely, early sexual development (before age 6–7 in girls and age 9–10 in boys) is called precocious puberty. Both delayed adolescence and precocious puberty can have serious psychosocial implications for the student.

Delayed Adolescence

This condition is much more common in boys than in girls. In these boys, there is often a family history of late bloomers, and in the absence of obvious chronic disease, it is usually considered a benign condition (normal variant), in that a pathological cause is very rarely found. Treatment will depend on the degree of delay and the psychosocial impact on the particular boy. The most commonly employed therapy is a short course of testosterone injections, which initiate puberty. This may rapidly enhance self-esteem and ego development.

In girls, late onset of puberty is more likely the result of a pathological condition such as anorexia nervosa or other eating disorder or an absence of the ovaries or uterus. Poor ovarian development is a feature of Turner syndrome. In these girls, short stature and characteristic physical features will be associated with the delay. Delayed adolescence in girls, therefore, warrants a more vigorous investigation than it does in boys.

Precocious Puberty

Early sexual development is more common in girls and is almost invariably a benign condition. The earlier the onset and the more rapid the progression of puberty are, the more likely a pathological explanation for the precocity. Conversely, sexual precocity is uncommon in boys, and when it occurs, it warrants full investigation to exclude the possibility of pituitary, testicular, or adrenal conditions that may require therapy.

Treatment of precocious puberty is warranted for one of two reasons: First, early and rapid sexual development will be associated with the pubertal growth spurt. The earlier the growth spurt, the earlier the attainment of final adult height will occur. Thus, children with sexual precocity will show rapid growth and be tall in comparison to other children early in life. However, by reaching final adult height earlier, they may be quite short as adults. Therapy that delays puberty may also increase final height potential. Second, early sexual development may cause significant anxiety and social discomfort among these children and their families. They may be singled out by others and treated as though they were older by teachers, peers, and the population at large. While girls with early development rarely, if ever, show promiscuous sexual behavior, boys with this condition may show aggression, masturbate in public, and generally be disruptive.

The treatment available for precocious puberty consists of monthly injections of a hormone analog called LHRH analog or agonist. This medication overstimulates the pituitary, thereby shutting off its production of the two hormones, LH and FSH, that control ovarian function in the female and testicular function in the male. Discontinuation of these agents at an appropriate age will allow normal progression of pubertal development.

In both delayed adolescence and precocious puberty, the teacher may play an important role in, first, sensitizing the parents to the fact that their child is showing a pattern of development (slow or fast) that differs significantly from their peers. Second, the teacher and other school personnel should remember to treat these students according to their age and not according to their stage of sexual development. In the early-menstruating female, women teachers may be called on to help with the use of tampons at school.

THE TEACHER'S ROLE

Disorders of either growth or other components of the endocrine system may have a wide variety of presentations, including significant implications for healthy personal development and learning. Teachers should be aware of these possibilities and inform parents of students whose growth appears to fall outside of the normal range. Teachers are in a unique position to detect variations in normal growth and pubertal development, since they have a readily available group of classmates as a normal reference. By informing parents of these concerns, teachers will help to initiate appropriate investigation and management, where necessary, earlier rather than later. Furthermore, teachers should deal sensitively with children with disordered growth, preventing their stigmatization by either their classmates or school personnel.

ADDITIONAL RESOURCES

Cheetham, T., & Davies, J. H. (2014). Investigation and management of short stature. *Archives of Diseases of Childhood, 99*, 767–771.

Cohen, L. E. (2014). Idiopathic short stature: A clinical review. *Journal of the American Medical Association, 311*, 1787–1796.

Kaplowitz, P. B. (1999). Reexamination of the age limit for defining when puberty is precocious in girls in the United States: Implications for evaluation and treatment. *Pediatrics, 104*, 936–941.

Kelnar, C. J. H., Savage, M. O., Stirling, H. F., & Saenger, P. (1998). *Growth disorders: Pathophysiology and treatment.* Philadelphia, PA: Chapman and Hall Medical.

Lee, P. A. (1999). Central precocious puberty: An overview of diagnosis, treatment, and outcome. *Endocrinology and Metabolic Clinics of North America, 28*(4), 901–918.

Palmert, M. R., & Dunkel, L. (2012). Clinical practice: Delayed puberty. *New England Journal of Medicine, 366*(5), 443–453.

Rogol, A. D., & Hayden, G. F. (2014). Etiologies and early diagnosis of short stature and growth failure in children and adolescents. *Journal of Pediatrics, 164*(5), S1–14.

Voss, L. D. (2001). Short normal stature and psychosocial disadvantage: A critical review of the evidence. *Journal of Pediatric Endocrinology and Metabolism, 14*(6), 701–711.

REFERENCES

Hauser, P., Zametkin, A. J., Martinez, P., Vitiello, B., Matochik, J. A., Mixson, A. J., & Weintraub, B. D. (1993). Attention deficit-hyperactivity disorder in people with generalized resistance to thyroid hormone. *New England Journal of Medicine, 328*, 997–1001.

Powell, G. F., Brasel, J. A., & Blizzard, R. M. (1967). Emotional deprivation and growth retardation simulating idiopathic hypopituitarism: I. Clinical evaluation of the syndrome. *New England Journal of Medicine, 276*, 1271–1278.

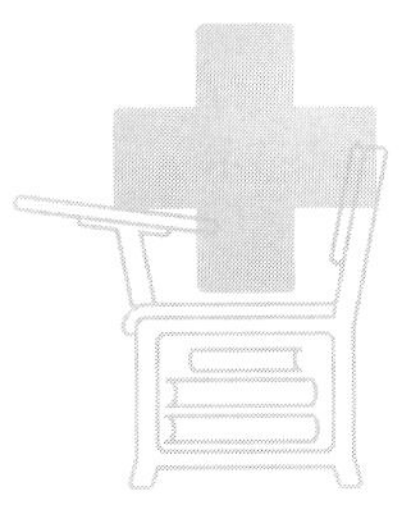

Chapter 4
Intellectual Disability[1]

Pasquale J. Accardo and Jennifer Accardo

The understanding of intellectual disability (or intellectual developmental disorder) has changed dramatically over the past half century. The perceptions that many persons have about what was once called mental retardation are probably still left over from a previous generation rather than informed by recent developments in the understanding of intellectual disability. Thus, the present chapter focuses on some of these major revisions in thought and practice that now characterize the field of intellectual disability. From a medical perspective, most, but not all, of these changes have been for the better, but several offer continuing challenges for optimal interactions between medical and educational professionals.

DEFINITION OF INTELLECTUAL DISABILITY

The classic definition of intellectual disability had three requirements:

1. Significantly below-average intellectual performance, or "failing" a general intelligence test, meaning performing more than 2 standard deviations below the mean for that test. Since most recent tests that generate an intelligence quotient (IQ) have a mean of 100 and a standard deviation of 15, the cutoff for intellectual disability would be an IQ below 70 (the mean of 100 less 30, or twice the standard deviation of 15). It is important that the

[1]The preparation of this chapter was supported in part by Project No. 1 T73 MC 00046 04 from the Maternal and Child Health Bureau (Title V, Social Security Act), Health Resources and Services Administration, Department of Health and Human Services.

intelligence test used measure different aspects of cognition. Earlier editions of the *Stanford-Binet Intelligence Scales* were heavily loaded on verbal items and were therefore more likely to misclassify a child with a significant communication disorder as being intellectually disabled. If using a test with such a bias, it would be important to supplement it with tests that tap other facets of intelligence. Recent revisions of intelligence tests have corrected this bias by assessing a broader range of cognitive skills.

2. In addition to cognitive limitations, the person with intellectual disability needs to exhibit deficits in adaptive functioning; in other words, the intellectual impairment must demonstrate an impact beyond the classroom setting into activities of daily living. This excludes children with severe learning disabilities who might do poorly in all academic areas but who would be able to perform appropriately for age when confronted by the demands of life. In the past, some children with severe learning disabilities were misdiagnosed with intellectual disability. Such confusion was more likely to occur in an era when professional recognition of and diagnostic testing for learning disabilities was still in an early phase.

3. Onset during the developmental period, or before age 18 years. Most intellectual disability is congenital (genetic or related to abnormalities of fetal brain development): it is often present at birth, although it may not be identifiable until years later. Some cases of intellectual disability may result from later childhood "brain damage" due to meningitis, encephalitis, severe head injury, or lead poisoning. Similar severe brain insults causing significant intellectual impairment in persons older than age 18 would be diagnosed as traumatic brain injury rather than intellectual disability.

The most recent American Association on Intellectual and Developmental Disabilities (AAIDD) (Schalock et al., 2009) definition of intellectual disability has maintained these basic criteria for diagnosis of intellectual disability but has notably expanded the requirement for adaptive deficits such that the person with intellectual disability must exhibit significant weaknesses in the conceptual, social, and practical domains. Quantifying the contribution of the adaptive skills criterion is easier with children who are more severely impaired but becomes more subjective in cases of milder severity, which are always more common. A description of the level of needed supports replaces what in the earlier classification was categorized by IQ level alone for the purpose of determining severity of intellectual disability The distinction will be familiar to professionals who participate in the drafting of an Individualized Education Program (IEP): test scores alone do not define the needed classroom supports, but they do provide a rough index of appropriate educational goals for the student:

Mild	50–55 to 65–75
Moderate	35–40 to 50–55
Severe	20–25 to 35–40
Profound	Below 20–25

The American Psychiatric Association and the American Psychological Association still use IQ cutoffs to describe levels of severity. Using IQ levels to characterize levels of severity does allow for more consistent association of degrees of brain impairment with various genetic syndromes and other medical etiologies for intellectual disability. In other words, whatever its utility for the classroom setting, to the physician the IQ remains a neurological marker: it describes the approximate percentage of the child's chronological age that the child's mental age can achieve.

The most important medical statement about intellectual disability is that it is not a medical diagnosis. Rather, it is a term that describes a current functional state. The functional state that intellectual disability describes is, however, most often associated with significant abnormalities of the central nervous system. Although the functional state may change over time, the neurological abnormalities that make up the underlying organic substrate for the functional impairment are most often permanent and will continue to exert a negative and limiting impact on cognition and development into adulthood. The permanence of the "brain damage" that underlies intellectual disability does not, however, mean that a child with intellectual disability will remain at a fixed stage of development. All children, even the most severely impaired, continue to make progress—even if, as in severe and profound intellectual disability, it may be very slow progress. It is the nature of even the most damaged brain to learn and to adapt. Failure to progress and especially regression (the loss of skills) should always be considered indicators of necessary careful medical reevaluation to rule out any complicating, medically treatable conditions. To the physician, intellectual disability is a symptom of neurological dysfunction that needs assessment, monitoring, and sometimes further investigation.

Intellectual disability is classified as a neurodevelopmental disorder, one with a static brain injury that is followed by slower-than-expected developmental progress. This is distinct from a neurocognitive disorder (NCD), in which the brain lesion leads to a loss of function in a person outside the developmental age period. NCDs present with symptoms such as dementia and delirium and are associated with conditions such as Alzheimer's syndrome and Parkinson's disease. In contrast to the course of NCDs, children with neurodevelopmental disorders typically improve over time. Great Britain, Canada, and Australia sometimes employ terms such as "global learning difficulties/disabilities" and "cognitive impairment" (CI). The American Association on Intellectual and Developmental Disabilities (AAIDD) now uses the term "intellectual disability," whereas the International Classification of Diseases (ICD-11) uses "intellectual developmental disorder." Although a diagnosis of intellectual disability might conceivably be made in a fairly young child, there is an increasing tendency for preschool children to be labeled "developmentally delayed" instead of "intellectually disabled." Such terminological substitutions avoid the need to use the emotionally loaded "mental retardation" with families but have no real impact on the nature and course of the developmental disorder. The DSM-V (*Diagnostic and Statistical Manual of Mental Disorders,* 5th ed.; American Psychiatric Association, APA, 2013) recognizes a diagnosis of global developmental delay for children under age 5 who exhibit signs of global delay but are too young to undergo formal testing. If at all possible, this term, along with the nonspecific "developmental delay," should be avoided. Its use represents a failure to adequately assess the child. There will be children and adults at any age who will present with difficulties in the administration and interpretation of test results. One is left with the peculiar situation in which the age level to diagnose autism-spectrum disorders is increasingly lowered while the formal diagnosis of intellectual disability tends to be increasingly delayed. From the physician's perspective, there is a major difference between the medical assessment of a child with mild developmental delay and one with intellectual disability.

OCCURRENCE RATE OF INTELLECTUAL DISABILITY

Intellectual disability occurs in the general population at a rate of just over 1%, with a slight male preponderance. However, this rate varies in different segments of a population. In the more affluent regions of society, the rate may be lower, whereas in poorer areas it might rise above 10%. The reason for this higher rate in lower socioeconomic groups probably reflects a complex interaction among several factors: polygenetic inheritance (a large number of mildly deleterious genes collecting in a population); limited access to prenatal, pediatric well-child, and other preventive health-care services; the long-term impact of poverty; understimulating environments; and substandard schooling. Although the occurrence of intellectual disability seems to have remained relatively constant over the past century, the process of diagnostic substitution is occurring with increasing frequency. Children who previously were diagnosed with intellectual disability are more often being characterized as having autism-spectrum disorders. Good data on the overlap between the two conditions, especially among young children, is not available.

An earlier classification for intellectual disability included the now-defunct category of "borderline intellectual disability," which was used to characterize persons with IQs between 70 and 85. With the inclusion of "borderline" intellectual disability, the incidence of intellectual disability rose to 15%. Such students no longer qualify for the educational and social supports allotted to persons with intellectual disability, but they experience persistent academic difficulties as "slow learners."

DIAGNOSIS OF INTELLECTUAL DISABILITY

The major presenting concern for a child with intellectual disability is developmental delay. The child does not achieve milestones, or do what he or she should be doing at a given age. The child with intellectual disability acts like a much younger child in most or all areas of development. Some children with intellectual disability present at first with behavior problems such as severe tantrums (i.e., when their developmental delay is not recognized), as they become very frustrated when faced with age-appropriate demands that are too difficult for them.

Because motor skills are often least involved in a child with intellectual disability, many such children begin to walk on time and do not exhibit serious motor delays. It is not uncommon to encounter parents and even some professionals who are puzzled as to how a child who walked at 12 months of age could possibly be considered "slow." Later in development, more complex motor planning skills are often impaired.

Language is the most sensitive marker for general cognition, and many children with intellectual disability present first with delayed speech. It is therefore imperative for infants and young children who present with language delay to have their nonverbal intelligence assessed independently of their language skills to differentiate the much more common communication disorder from the less common generalized cognitive impairment. One of the most frequent misdiagnoses places a preschool child with communication delay associated with intellectual disability in an intervention program for young children with speech problems.

The physical examination of the child with intellectual disability includes looking for nonneurological diseases that might negatively affect development and the presence of dysmorphic features that may be indicators of specific genetic syndromes or nonspecifically of early damage to the developing brain. Higher numbers of such "minor malformations" are found in children with intellectual disability, autism, attention-deficit/hyperactivity disorder, learning disabilities, and major psychiatric disorders. The following features are associated with developmental problems:

- electric ("uncombable") hair
- hair-whorl abnormalities (absent, multiple cowlicks, counterclockwise, linear, frontal, widow's peak)
- head circumference: macrocephaly (very large head) and microcephaly (very small head)
- epicanthic folds (prolongation of skin of the upper eyelid in the corner of the eye)
- hypertelorism (wide space between eyes)
- pinna (ear) abnormalities (low set, rotated, rounded, flattened, protuberant, malformed)
- absent ear lobules (adherent earlobes)
- high-arched or steepled palate
- geographic tongue
- clinodactyly (incurving) of the fifth finger
- brachydactyly (shortness) of the fifth finger
- palmar crease abnormality (simian, Sydney, hockey stick)
- sandal-gap deformity of (widened space between) first toes
- syndactyly (decreased space between or partial fusion) of second and third toes
- long middle toe

Abnormalities on the neurological examination may help localize brain damage and identify other deficits associated with the intellectual disability. For example, abnormal gait associated with unilateral weakness of the extremities may imply injury to the cerebral cortex, or incoordination and "staccato"-like speech may indicate a lesion in the cerebellum.

In the presence of significant delays in any major developmental area, a measure of general intellectual functioning should be obtained. If the child's level of intellectual functioning falls into the intellectually disabled range, then a more in-depth interdisciplinary assessment by a team of professionals familiar with the diagnosis of intellectual disability should be carried out. Confirmation of the diagnosis should go side by side with attempts to uncover the reason for the delay. Appropriate parental support, counseling, and educational placement should follow.

With regard to etiology, a detailed medical history should document the presence or absence of a variety of risk factors—with the strong qualification that a risk factor is not the same as a diagnosis. Most children with risk factors exhibit normal development, and many children with developmental diagnoses do not demonstrate common risk factors. Items to be reviewed include family history, infections or exposure to toxins during pregnancy (with alcohol among the most prominent and preventable of these), severe prematurity, perinatal (the time just preceding and following birth) medical complications, severe illnesses in early childhood, meningitis or encephalitis (central nervous system infections), exposure to high levels of lead, general anesthesia, and traumatic brain injury. With regard to the last item, brain injury associated with intellectual disability is much more severe than the usual toddler falls (with scalp lacerations or cuts requiring stitches) that are almost routine in early childhood.

There is no routine biomedical assessment (group of medical tests) for children with intellectual disability (Moeschler, Shevell, & Committee on Genetics, 2014). Selection of which tests and procedures to perform is based on a review of the child's developmental history and functional pattern, physical and neurological findings, and parents' wishes. (Even some so-called noninvasive tests may require general sedation, from which children with intellectual disability are at greater risk for complications.)

Genetic testing technology has made quantum leaps in recent years and continues to advance rapidly. In the not-too-distant past, karyotypes, tests looking at chromosomes for extra materials or deletions, were part of the first line in testing of children with intellectual disability. Now karyotypes are reserved for testing for concerns about specific disorders, primarily Down syndrome. They have been largely replaced by chromosomal microarrays, which screen for small deletions and duplications of genetic material at a higher resolution, with the ability to detect differences of much smaller magnitude affecting specific genes (see Chapter 2). Chromosomal microarrays also supersede the use of specific genetic probes, which often required involvement of a geneticist with expertise in dysmorphology, the study of congenital physical variations that may indicate genetic differences. Even now, more detailed sequencing, capturing even more potential genetic variations, is becoming less expensive and more available. Other potential components of a laboratory assessment for intellectual disability can include the following tests: testing for fragile X syndrome, thyroid function studies (thyroid conditions are potentially treatable), creatine kinase (CK, which can be associated with muscular dystrophies that manifest with low muscle tone and intellectual disability), and plasma amino and urine organic acid levels (markers for disorders of metabolism). In addition, procedures such an electroencephalograms (EEGs), to evaluate patterns of brainwaves, and neuroimaging of the brain (computerized tomography, CT, and magnetic resonance imaging, MRI, scans) can be considered. Neuroimaging generally captures structure, so that a normal MRI should not be taken to imply normal function.

In a large population of children with intellectual disability, five out of six children will have delays in the mild range (IQs above 50), whereas only one out of the six will have moderate to severe delays (with IQs below 50). Detailed biomedical assessments are likely to uncover a specific etiology for intellectual disability in one-third of all cases. That one-third is, however, asymmetrically composed of three-quarters with more severe delay and less than one-quarter with mild delay.

It is of concern to note that a number of children with significant cognitive impairment who have received extensive and repeated interdisciplinary evaluations to determine functional levels may be placed in special education for years without ever having had any other medical assessment than well-child visits. Professionals competent to perform an appropriate medical evaluation of the child with intellectual disability include child neurologists, neurodevelopmental pediatricians, developmental and behavioral pediatricians, and clinical geneticists. The failure to identify a specific genetic etiology may place the family at risk for the recurrence of a condition associated with intellectual disability. Appropriate early identification of such causes allows secondary prevention.

SYNDROME IDENTIFICATION

A quarter of a century ago the scientific literature published papers on different aspects of mild and moderate intellectual disability. Today these are almost completely absent. Medical and other professional journals instead publish research papers on specific conditions such as Down syndrome, fetal alcohol syndrome (FAS), Prader-Willi syndrome (PWS), fragile X syndrome, and the like. The earlier classification by degrees of severity of intellectual impairment (IQ level) no longer makes sense within the current medical understanding of the neurological substrate of intellectual deficiency. Many syndromes are no longer associated with a specific narrow IQ range but are known to occur with a fairly wide range of IQs. For example, FAS and PWS can occur in the presence of normal intelligence. In these latter examples, although the IQ may be in the normal range, a child's learning profile is still affected, so that specific language, learning, behavioral, and often severe attentional problems still characterize these syndromes.

Today there is less concern to identify the IQ range associated with a syndrome than to describe the behavioral and learning profiles (of which IQ is one component) associated with that specific syndrome. This pattern of cognitive strengths and weaknesses associated with specific behavioral markers (behavioral phenotyping) (O'Brien & Yule, 2002) represents one of the frontiers of modern genetics and promises to be of use in the classroom management of children with such syndromes (see Table 4.1).

MEDICAL MANAGEMENT OF INTELLECTUAL DISABILITY

When the human brain is sufficiently impaired to produce global cognitive limitation, there is no traditional medical treatment to "cure" the resulting intellectual disability. The treatment for intellectual disability remains education. There are, however, a number of areas in which the physician can contribute to the well-being of the child with intellectual disability.

Primary Medical Care

A half century ago many children with intellectual disability were placed in institutional settings. Their basic medical care was marginal, and their environment fostered the spread of diseases that would ultimately shorten their life span. Today children with intellectual disability live at home and make use of community health and educational resources. The life span of persons with even severe cognitive impairment more closely approximates the average life span of persons without intellectual disability. Providing primary health care to children with intellectual disability can be challenging because of limitations in the child's ability to communicate. With the increase

Table 4.1

BEHAVIORAL PROFILES FOR SYNDROMES ASSOCIATED WITH SEVERE INTELLECTUAL DISABILITY

Syndrome	Behavioral characteristics
Down syndrome (trisomy 21)	Developmental deceleration, delayed expressive language, sitting down, escape behavior, visual-spatial STM better than auditory STM
Williams syndrome (17q11 deletion)	Fluent expressive language ("cocktail party" speech) without corresponding receptive language strengths; auditory STM better than visual STM
Smith-Magenis syndrome (17p11.2 deletion)	Self-hugging ("spasmodic upper-body squeeze"), onychotillomania (pulling out finger- and toenails), and polyembolokoilamania (insertion of foreign bodies into bodily orifices)
Prader-Willi syndrome (15q11-13 deletion, paternal)	Hyperphagia (overeating, leading to life-threatening obesity if not controlled), obsessive-compulsive traits, skin picking
Angelman syndrome (15q11-13 deletion, maternal)	Unbalanced (marionette-like) gait, paroxysmal laughter
Lesch Nyhan (Xq27-q28 mutation)	Severe self-mutilation
Rett syndrome (MECP2 on Xq28)	Gaze aversion, hand stereotypies (wringing, clapping, tapping, washing, and mouthing), some autistic features
Fragile X syndrome (more than 200 CGG repeats on q27)	Poor eye contact, cluttered speech, hyperactivity, aggressive behavioral outbursts, autistic features

Note. STM = short-term memory.

in knowledge of medical implications of different genetic syndromes, physicians can monitor and anticipate various medical complications as, or even before, they arise (Wilson & Cooley, 2006). Thus, routine thyroid screening is part of the recommended management of children with Down syndrome. The onset of hypothyroidism can explain why a child with Down syndrome becomes more sluggish and apathetic and falls off his or her learning and growth curves; it is also very treatable. The mild diseases of childhood can have a greater impact on the development of a child with intellectual disability than on a typically developing child.

Specialty Medical Care

Children with medical syndromes associated with their intellectual disability are more likely to exhibit various medical problems. On the one hand, such children are less likely to complain about or describe their symptoms; on the other hand, even mild chronic disorders can have a severe impact on the child's development. A higher percentage of children with intellectual disability have seizure disorders than in the general population. In treating epilepsy, it is important to avoid worsening the cognitive impairment or facilitating problem behaviors by judicious use of anticonvulsants, which can have significant side effects.

Behavioral Medications

Although some controversy remains about the use of psychotropic medications to manage challenging behaviors in persons with neurodevelopmental disorders, there is little doubt that the use of such drugs often allows the child with intellectual disability to function in a less restrictive environment and to make better use of various educational and behavioral interventions. Without discussing particular drugs, two major considerations need to be kept in mind:

- If a child is to be maintained for the long term on a drug, resulting behavioral improvements should be dramatic, not marginal.
- The child should exhibit *no* side effects to the drug, including sedation or sometimes not-so-subtle personality changes. *Primum non nocere*: first, do no harm. Medication should facilitate (not force) behavioral improvement in the child.

Over the past several decades, some schools have modified their originally antagonistic attitudes toward use of pharmacotherapeutic agents as not appropriate to an educational program to almost too-eager acceptance of their use to minimize the need for intensive behavioral supports in an educational system with increasingly limited fiscal resources. However, the concern should be with each child's needs rather than policy. Again, with behavioral disorders it is first important to make certain that other appropriate medical factors are not contributing to the problem (e.g., the anticonvulsant levetiracetam can induce or worsen irritability). If functional behavioral analyses (FBAs), with their associated positive behavior improvement plans, were conducted with appropriate diligence, a significant percentage of medication usage might be spared.

Prevention

Intellectual disability from some causes can be prevented. The *Haemophilus influenzae* (HIB) vaccine has virtually eliminated the associated meningitis, a once-common cause of intellectual disability and hearing loss in children. Universal newborn screening allows early preventive treatment of causes of progressive intellectual disability. The disorders routinely identified include hypothyroidism (formerly cretinism), phenylketonuria (PKU), urea cycle defects, and a variety of disorders that involve the metabolism of amino acids, organic acids, fats, sugars, and vitamins.

Again, it is very important to attempt to identify the cause of intellectual disability in young children: genetic etiologies may pose an identifiable recurrence risk for the family, and toxic exposures such as alcohol and lead can also be expected to influence later children in the same family environment.

So-called medical treatments that claim a neurological basis but lack scientific evidence for efficacy in the treatment of intellectual disability have come and gone over the years, preying on hopeful parents. These include patterning, masking (intermittent suffocation to induce CO2 rebreathing), nutritional additives (glutamic acid, megavitamins, trace elements, amino acids), elimination diets, music therapy, nootropics (drugs to increase intelligence, such as piracetam), sicca-cell therapy, osteopathy (craniosacral therapy or skull massage), hormones (in the absence of documented endocrine deficiencies), antioxidants, and antimold (antiyeast or anticandidiasis) drug treatment.

Transition

Since the 1990 amendments to the Individuals With Disabilities Education Act, the school's role in the provision of transition services has been greatly expanded. Transition planning starts at age 14 years and involves the setting of goals for and the determining of activities to achieve the maximum of adult independence for students with intellectual disability. Issues of employment, adult education, independent living, and community integration all need to be addressed (Antosh et al., 2013). Both educational and community resources need to be organized to achieve the goals negotiated with the child and family. For various reasons the successful implementation of transition is often elusive. Some of the problems reside in the school system, whereas other barriers arise from the community. The difficulties that characterize the educational achievement of successful transition to adulthood are dwarfed by the difficulties that occur with regard to the provision of medical care. Persons with intellectual disability require time, patience, and consideration from their primary-care physician; persons with intellectual disability and complex medical problems require even more time, patience, and consideration from their relevant subspecialty care providers. The critical variable here is quite simply that the number of physicians available to provide such care is inadequate to the demand. Measures to address this critical shortage are still in the discussion phase.

THE TEACHER'S ROLE

The teacher is an important member of the team in the medical management of children with intellectual disability. Establishing open communication among teacher, parents, and medical professionals is a priority. The following is a list of ways teachers can contribute to the medical care of children with intellectual disability:

- "Medical home": Encourage families to have a primary care pediatrician who is familiar with the child with intellectual disability. Sporadic emergency room visits are not an acceptable equivalent for such care.
- Do not recommend the use of medications, either specific agents or medications in general. Do encourage parents of children with intellectual disability to make certain that their child's developmental disorder has been adequately medically assessed, with both a careful search for etiologies and an evaluation of possible medical therapies (including medications).
- When children with intellectual disability are diagnosed with specific syndromes, ask for information on both medical and behavioral implications of the diagnosis. The school nurse should be a resource to help the teacher become familiar with these associations.
- When children with intellectual disability are placed on specific drugs, ask for information on both medical and behavioral

implications of such drugs. Again, the school nurse can function as a liaison between the teacher and the prescribing physician.

- When responding to physicians or parents with regard to drug effects, include any changes noted, even if these were not specifically identified as possible effects. Some medication effects are rare or idiosyncratic and may not appear in a list of potential adverse effects.
- When behavior or learning deteriorates, consider a medical reassessment even in the absence of obvious signs of physical illness.

In addition, the following guidelines concern the management of children with intellectual disability in the classroom:

- The special education teacher's classroom role is generally carefully spelled out in those items included in the child's Individualized Educational Program. When that IEP is negotiated (or reviewed), a reasonable point to address is the identification of any unique needs specific to the child's learning profile and any associated medical condition.
- When the child with intellectual disability is mainstreamed into a regular education setting, close communication with the child's special education teacher (and any other specialty service providers) should be maintained.
- Proactive preparatory education to sensitize regular education students for the reception of special needs students is indicated.
- Significant underachievement with regard to reasonable IEP goals may reflect medically treatable complications to the child's condition and not merely lack of motivation.

REFERENCES

American Psychiatric Association. (2013). *Diagnostic and statistical manual of mental disorders* (5th ed.). Washington, DC: Author.

Antosh, A. A., Blair, M., Edwards, K., Goode, T., Hewitt, A., Izzo, D. R., . . . Wehmeyer, M. (2013). *A collaborative interagency, interdisciplinary approach to transition from adolescence to adulthood.* Silver Spring, MD: Association of University Centers on Developmental Disabilities.

Education for All Handicapped Children Act. Amendments of 1990. P.L. 101-476.

Moeschler, J. B., Shevell, M., & Committee on Genetics (2014). Comprehensive evaluation of the child with intellectual disability or global developmental delays. *Pediatrics, 134*(3), e903–e918.

O'Brien, G., & Yule, W. (1995). *Behavioural phenotypes in clinical practice.* London, UK: MacKeith Press, Clinics in Developmental Medicine.

Schalock, R. L., Borthwick-Duffy, S. A., Bradley, V. J., Buntinx, W. H. E., Coulter, D. L., Craig, E. M., . . . Yeager, M. H. (2009). *Intellectual disability: Definition, classification, and systems of supports* (11th ed.). Washington, DC: American Association on Intellectual and Developmental Disabilities.

Wilson, G. N., & Cooley, W. C. (2006). *Preventive health care for children with genetic disorders: Providing a primary care medical home.* New York, NY: Cambridge University Press.

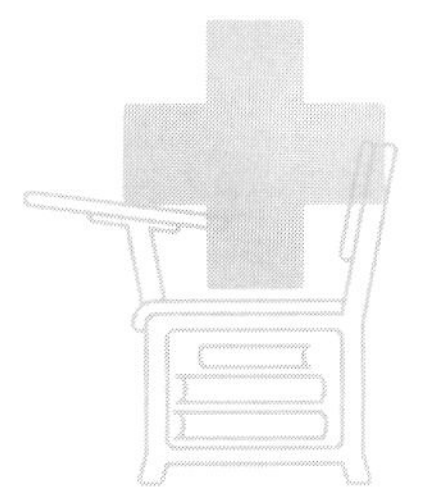

Chapter 5
Attention-Deficit/ Hyperactivity Disorder

Dilip J. Karnik[1]

Attention-deficit/hyperactivity disorder (ADHD) is a common condition that affects a child's education and behavior. If untreated, ADHD may lead to profound and long-term consequences. With proper management, most children with ADHD improve and become happier, better-adjusted individuals. Although many benefit from medication, the use of medication alone has not been shown to facilitate the best outcomes. A multimodality approach that incorporates the use of classroom adaptations, behavior modification strategies, counseling, parent training, tutoring, and therapies, in addition to the use of medication, when appropriate, is the most effective treatment approach for ADHD. Parents, teachers, and clinicians all play important roles in assisting these children to achieve the best outcomes. However, without a doubt, teachers who work with ADHD children can make the greatest impact on the ability of these children to learn, achieve, and feel better about themselves. The classroom teacher has a vital role in the diagnosis and therapeutic process.

DEFINITION AND INCIDENCE

ADHD is one of the most common neurobiological conditions that affect children. In May 2013, the *Diagnostic and Statistical Manual of*

[1]The author would like to thank Dr. Emily Gutierrez, DNP, C-PNP, chief of neuronutrition, Karnik Institute, for providing assistance in the nutrition therapy section and for editing of this chapter.

Mental Disorders, Fifth Edition (DSM-5) issued a revised definition and criteria for ADHD (American Psychiatric Association, APA, 2013). Revisions highlighted changes to the age of onset of ADHD and the manifestations seen in older children.

Persons affected with ADHD typically have problems paying attention to tasks and being impulsive, and often display hyperactivity not appropriate for their age or chronological neurodevelopment. These issues are severe enough to affect at least two different settings and are present in a child's life for at least six months. Most often symptoms affect school-age children in academic settings and social environments. Some children with ADHD may have only inattentive symptoms, and others may have additional symptoms of impulsivity and hyperactivity. The severity and frequency of symptoms have individual variations. For example, a child may show interest in sports or video games. It is not uncommon for a teacher to be concerned about ADHD symptoms in a child but for a parent not to share those concerns.

The DSM-5 states that ADHD occurs in 5% of children (APA, 2013); however, some studies have shown it to be much higher (Barkley, Fischer, Smallish, & Fletcher, 2002). The Centers for Disease Control and Prevention (CDC) have reported that incidences of ADHD vary from state to state. For example, the incidence of ADHD in Nevada is 5.6%, in contrast to Kentucky, where it has been reported as high as 18.7%. ADHD is more common in boys (13.2%) than in girls (5.6%). Approximately 11% of children are diagnosed with ADHD between the ages of 4 and 17 years. Approximately 6.1% of those diagnosed with ADHD in 2011 were put on medications (CDC, 2001).

CHARACTERISTICS

Children affected with ADHD display increased motor activity, impulsiveness, and inattention, with a considerable variation in the degree and frequency of these symptoms. When severe, ADHD can affect a child's learning, social skill development, and self-esteem. ADHD can have a significant and lifelong impact on an individual.

Learning

Children with ADHD have a greater likelihood of having emotional, cognitive, developmental, and academic problems (Cuffe, Moore, & McKeown, 2005; Flory, Milich, Lynam, Leukefeld, & Clayton, 2003). These coexisting conditions can vary in severity and significantly affect a child's school performance, social-emotional development, and future vocational success. Not all children with ADHD display all of these problems, but many experience at least some of these conditions to an extent that they are greater than seen in children without ADHD.

Children with ADHD may be delayed in intellectual development. Research has shown that children with ADHD score an average of 7 to 15 points below control groups on standardized intelligence tests (Jepsen, Fagerlund, & Mortensen, 2009). However, these children are likely to represent the entire spectrum of intelligence, from superior to mild cognitive impairment.

Learning disabilities can coexist with ADHD (Dyck & Piek, 2014). Studies have shown that about 8%–39% of children with ADHD have a reading disability, 12%–30% have a mathematical disability, and 12%–27% have a spelling disorder (Biederman & Faraone, 2005).

Studies have shown that children with ADHD tend to perform below average on various language evaluations, including tests of simple verbal fluency, complex language fluency, and discourse organization (Mathers, 2006). In addition, children with ADHD appear to produce less speech in response to confrontational questioning and are sometimes less competent at verbal problem-solving tasks. Their narrative stories tend to produce less information and are less organized in presentation (Scott & Windsor, 2000).

Some children with ADHD demonstrate deficits in the processing of auditory input in the absence of an intellectual or hearing impairment (Sawyer, 2001). This condition is known as a central auditory processing disorder (CAPD).

Children with ADHD may exhibit deficits in executive brain functions, including decreased nonverbal and verbal working memory, impaired planning ability, impaired sense of time, and possibly impaired behavioral and verbal creativity. These cognitive problems can affect the learning abilities of children with ADHD (Barkley, 1998).

Neurological "soft signs" related to fine motor coordination problems and delayed motor development are found more frequently in children with ADHD (Halperin et al., 2013). Tests of fine motor coordination, including balance tasks, paper-and-pencil mazes, and tracking activities, reveal that children with ADHD tend to be less coordinated than children without ADHD. As a result of delays in fine motor coordination, children with ADHD often have difficulties with handwriting. Their drawings are often sluggish and sloppy. They are frequently characterized by inconsistent letter formation, excessive errors, poor page organization, poor hand movement fluency, and incorrect pencil grasps. Other deficits in written language may include problems with spelling, punctuation, and capitalization. All these characteristics of dysgraphia indicate that children with ADHD experience problems with motor planning, motor control, and motor memory (Mariani & Barkley, 1997).

Behavior

Children with ADHD have a higher risk for developing other psychiatric disorders, including anxiety disorder, depression, bipolar disorder, conduct disorder, and oppositional–defiant disorder (Ghanizadeh, Mohammadi, & Moini, 2008). Children with any of these disorders may experience behavioral problems and difficulties in their relationships with peers, teachers, and family members.

Having additional psychiatric disorders can compound ADHD symptoms and challenges. Children with conduct disorder may display deceitful characteristics and show aggression toward people, animals, and property. Oppositional–defiant disorder occurs in approximately 14% of children with ADHD. They may be less compliant with parent and teacher requests and be moody, aggressive, negative, or hostile. The primary identifying symptoms of these conditions include anxiety, defiance, excessive mood swings, aggressive behavior, and depression (APA, 2013).

Anxiety disorders are more common in children with ADHD than in the general population (Ghanizadeh et al., 2008). Anxiety is a normal emotional experience for stressful situations. Children with anxiety disorders experience emotions in greater severity and frequency. These children may have unrealistic worries about events, school performance, and social interactions. They may look for constant reassurance from teachers or parents. They may have phobias to things such as dark places, bathrooms, elevators, being separated from a parent, or speaking in front of a class. When a coexisting anxiety disorder is present, this condition should be appropriately managed for the best outcomes.

Many children with ADHD have coexisting sleep disorders or disturbances. This can include difficulties falling asleep or maintaining sleep. It can also include restless-leg syndrome, which is characterized by disruptive body or leg twitching that occurs during sleep. In addition, some children have breathing difficulties while asleep, such as those with sleep apnea.

Children with ADHD have an increased incidence of tics, which is characterized by eye blinking, facial grimacing, and/or nonpurposeful sounds.

Appropriate evaluation and management of children with neuropsychiatric symptoms is of paramount importance. Children with psychiatric disorders require special attention, and involved personnel should proceed with caution when identifying these disorders. Conversely, a child who exhibits symptoms of a behavioral disorder and/or inattention, hyperactivity, and impulsiveness may not necessarily have ADHD but rather a psychiatric disorder with symptoms mimicking ADHD. For example, a child with absence seizures (petit mal epilepsy) manifested in frequent staring episodes may not pay attention in class. Likewise, a child with bipolar disorder may initially present with inattention and hyperactivity. Disorders such as pervasive developmental disorder, mild cognitive impairment, and learning disabilities can also be mistaken for ADHD.

CAUSES OF ADHD

Despite extensive research, the exact cause of ADHD is not known. Most children with ADHD have no evidence of a brain injury. Studies suggest the following contributory factors:

- Genetic factors (Barkley, 1998; Faraone et al., 1993)
- Molecular genetic factors (Banaschewski, Becker, Scherag, Franke, & Coghill, 2010)
- Developmental factors (Bennett, Wolin, & Reiss, 1988; Hartsough & Lambert, 1985; Mick, Biederman, & Faraone, 1996; Nichols & Chen, 1981).
- Neurological factors (Adisetiyo et al., 2014; Arnsten, Steere, & Hunt, 1996; Barkley, 1997, 2013; Benton, 1991; Cortese, Angriman, Lecendreux, & Konofal, 2012; Cortese, Azoulay et al., 2012; Heilman, Voeller, & Nadeau, 1991; Hynd et al., 1993; Konofal et al., 2008; Matles, 1980).
- Neurotransmitter factors (Owens et al., 2013)
- Factors related to diet and food additives (Bloch & Qawasmi, 2011; DiGirolamo & Ramirez-Zea, 2009; McCann et al., 2007; Mousain-Bose et al., 2005; National Institutes of Health, NIH, 2014; Perlmutter, 2013)

DIAGNOSIS OF ADHD

When a child is identified as having significant symptoms of inattention, impulsiveness, or hyperactivity, a comprehensive evaluation for ADHD is warranted. Because of the complex nature of ADHD, diagnosis can be difficult, especially when a child manifests symptoms in only one setting. Behavioral observations and teacher concerns may be the only clue that a child has a problem. Frequently, parents, teachers, and clinicians struggle to separate typical from atypical behavior.

The clinician should obtain a detailed history from the child and the parent. A history should also be acquired from the child's teacher through a personal interview or a questionnaire. Open and candid communication between the child's teacher and the clinician is critical to the evaluation of this disorder. Behavioral questionnaires, such as those developed by Conners, Goldstein, Kendall, Braswell, or Gilliam, can be useful in the evaluation for ADHD (Conners, 2008; Goldstein & Goldstein, 1990; Kendall & Braswell, 1985; Gilliam, 2015).

According to the American Academy of Child and Adolescent Psychiatry, there are many useful rating scales for ADHD. The most commonly used scales are the following:

- Parent-completed Child Behavior Checklist
- Teacher Report Form (TRF) of the Child Behavior Checklist
- ADD-H: Comprehensive Teacher Rating Scale (ACTeRS)
- Barkley Home Situation Questionnaire (HSQ)
- Barkley School Situation Questionnaire (SSQ)

Another commonly used and free questionnaire that teacher and parents can use is the National Institute for Children's Health Equality (NICHQ) Vanderbilt Assessment Scales (Wolraich, 2002). These can be found at the websites of the American Academy of Pediatrics (http://www.aacap.org) and Children and Adults with Attention-Deficit/Hyperactivity (CHADD) (http://www.chadd.org).

The Abbreviated Conners' Teacher Questionnaire (see Figure 5.1) can be of help in the evaluation process.

In addition to obtaining the child's history, the physician should perform a complete physical and neurological examination. Tests of visual and hearing acuity should also be performed to rule out any sensory disorders affecting vision or hearing.

The diagnosis of attention-deficit/hyperactivity disorder is essentially made through a subjective clinical diagnosis. To date there are no laboratory tests or neurological scans that can identify the disorder with certainty. Physical examination of ADHD children is generally normal and does not necessarily help identify the condition except to rule out other physical or medical conditions that could be causing symptoms. It is important to ascertain whether the child has any associated conditions. For this reason, the clinician should evaluate

ABBREVIATED CONNERS' TEACHER QUESTIONNAIRE

Child's Name ______________________

Today's date ____/____/____
Month Day Year

Parent's Name ______________________

Teacher's Name ______________________

Instructions: Listed below are items concerning children's behavior or the problems they sometimes have. Read each item carefully and decide how much you think this child has been displaying this behavior at this time. (Check only one box for each row.)

	Frequency			
Observation	**Not at all**	**Just a little**	**Often**	**Almost always**
1. Has difficulty sitting still; is excessively fidgety, restless.	☐	☐	☐	☐
2. Has difficulty staying seated; is often on the go.	☐	☐	☐	☐
3. Starts things without finishing them; does not complete tasks.	☐	☐	☐	☐
4. Does not seem to listen attentively when spoken to.	☐	☐	☐	☐
5. Has difficulty following oral directions.	☐	☐	☐	☐
6. Is easily distracted; has difficulty concentrating.	☐	☐	☐	☐
7. Has difficulty staying with a play activity.	☐	☐	☐	☐
8. Acts before thinking.	☐	☐	☐	☐
9. Has difficulty organizing work.	☐	☐	☐	☐
10. Needs a lot of supervision.	☐	☐	☐	☐
11. Interacts poorly with other children.	☐	☐	☐	☐
12. Expects demands to be met immediately; is easily frustrated.	☐	☐	☐	☐
13. Changes mood quickly; cries; has temper outbursts.	☐	☐	☐	☐

Comments ______________________

____

____

Figure 5.1. Abbreviated Conners' Teacher Questionnaire. Adapted from "Revision and Restandardization of the Conners' Teacher Rating Scale (CTRS-R): Factor Structure, Reliability, and Criterion Validity," by C. K. Conners, G. Sitarenios, J. D. Parker, and N. Epstein, 1998, *Journal of Abnormal Child Psychology, 26*(4), 279–291.

for motor coordination problems by checking for "soft neurological" signs. These signs are normally present in very young children up to age 6 years; but as the brain matures, they generally disappear. Persistence of these signs suggests immaturity of the central nervous system and may be present in children with ADHD or motor dyscoordination disorder. In addition, if learning disabilities are suspected, the child should be referred for a comprehensive evaluation. Educational diagnosticians or school psychologists can administer these tests.

MANAGEMENT OF ADHD

Research has demonstrated that the use of multiple modalities, including academic support, behavioral counseling, parent training, and pharmacotherapy, is the most successful approach in the treatment of ADHD. Not all children diagnosed with ADHD require medication. Mild cases may respond to educational and or behavioral modalities and may not need medications. More severe cases may warrant immediate introduction of drugs in the therapy. Some clinicians may use medications only after a trial of nutritional, behavioral, and educational modalities. Regardless of these different individual views, current research suggests that when compared with the use of nonmedication modalities alone, treatment with psychotropic drugs is statistically more effective in improving ADHD symptoms (Karanges, Stephenson, & McGregor, 2014).

A prominent research study known as the Multimodal Treatment of Attention Deficit Hyperactivity Disorder (MTA) was a major multisite trial that compared outcomes by utilizing medications alone, psychosocial or behavioral therapy alone, or a combination of both therapies in 579 children with ADHD. Researchers initially showed that intensive medication management alone or in combination with behavior therapy made the best impact. The follow-up study published in 2007 showed that this advantage waned after 14 months (NIH, 2009).

The American Academy of Pediatrics (AAP, 2011) recommends the following strategies:

- Children aged 4–5 years: Evidence-based parent- and/or teacher-administered behavioral therapy as the first line of management. If this does not improve ADHD symptoms, methylphenidate should be considered.
- Children aged 6–11 years: Approved medications and/or evidence-based parent- and/or teacher-administered therapy should be considered. There is stronger evidence that stimulants are more

effective for ADHD than drugs such as atomoxetine, the extended form of guanfacine, or clonidine.

- Adolescents aged 12–18 years: Approved medication and consideration of behavioral therapy.

COUNSELING

Once the diagnosis of ADHD is made, the clinician should discuss with the parents the nature of treatment options available. Every effort should be made to give parents a clear picture of this condition and help them accept the diagnosis and prepare for long-term management. Through counseling, the clinician may be able to help remove incorrect ideas and misinformation, guilt, or denial parents may be experiencing. Ineffective or counterproductive parenting patterns should be identified and discouraged. High parent expectations of the child and/or the school system should also be discussed and measures suggested for management.

Counseling by a psychologist or a social worker may be warranted, especially if the child has significant associated conditions, such as depression, anxiety, aggression, and/or antisocial behavior. Counselors can develop behavioral programs that teachers and parents can follow. Such counseling may consist of individual parent sessions to promote realistic and effective parenting strategies (Barkley, 1990; Chacko et al., 2008; Wender, 1987). The child may be given specific instruction in the area of socialization, communication, organization, and better study habits (Furman, 1980; McConnell & Ryser, 2005).

ACADEMIC INTERVENTIONS

Helping a child manage ADHD can become an overwhelming task for a teacher. Monitoring, recording, and implementing behavioral management strategies can be time consuming and at times impractical. The following guidelines are essential to the successful treatment of ADHD in the classroom:

- Professionals who work with ADHD children should understand ADHD as a condition. It is important that educators keep up to date with the current literature as well as attend appropriate seminars and conferences. Misunderstanding the disorder can lead to undue stress and adverse relationships.
- Teachers should be aware that children with ADHD are highly inconsistent in the manifestation of symptoms. A child with

ADHD may perform well one day and poorly on another. In addition, he or she may seem behaviorally normal in some situations and "out of control" in others.

- Professionals should be sensitive to situations in which a child with ADHD might be extremely anxious so as to avoid embarrassing the child, especially in front of his or her peers.

Teacher's Personality

Understanding of the following characteristics is important to the successful treatment of children with ADHD and should be considered when assigning a teacher to take on the management of these children. Teachers need to be the following:

- *Flexible:* Teachers who are open to adjustments will have more success. Flexibility helps both the teacher and the child experience more success.
- *Creative:* Teachers who are creative and innovative in the development and implementation of teaching strategies are more likely to find what works for students with ADHD.
- *Sensitive:* Many children with ADHD have low self-esteem. Keeping communications about their grades, behavior, or medical condition private can certainly help. In addition, if a child must take medication at school, being discreet in assisting with the administration of the drug can lessen any stigma for the child.

Teaching Style

Children with ADHD perform better when teachers do the following:

- Present lessons that are organized
- Are vibrant and energetic
- Allow plenty of time for presenting material
- Emphasize key or important points
- Maintain eye contact with each student to gauge student attention
- Use a variety of teaching aids, such as pictures, hands-on demonstration and manipulatives, videos, role-play, and other audiovisual techniques
- Are interactive
- Demonstrate mutual respect

Management Strategies

Effective management strategies may be primarily related to the classroom setting, the child, or the teacher. Following are some recommended strategies for these three areas. Classroom accommodations include the following:

- Allowing the student to sit near the teacher.
- Seating the student near a model student.
- Seating the student away from noisy equipment, such as the air conditioner or heating unit.
- Allowing the student to sit away from high-traffic or distracting areas.
- Keeping the student in small groups if at all possible.
- Keeping the student away from students who may engage in bullying.
- Keeping visual and auditory distractions to a minimum when students are working independently.
- Reducing the disturbance caused by extraneous noise through the use of calming background music or white noise.
- Installing FM system and headphones especially for children with a central auditory processing disorder.
- Engaging in close supervision so teachers are aware of particular difficulties and challenging subjects—it may be necessary to provide additional time and assistance in instruction of some subjects.
- Considering tutoring from an independent source—when possible, teachers should pursue tutoring for students who are falling behind in academic development.
- Facilitating a preview of the material before it is presented in the classroom, such as notes, a copy of the chapter, or books about the subject to read ahead of time, so the child becomes somewhat familiar with the topic and to enhance comprehension and learning.

Child-centered approaches (Barkley, 1985) include the following:

- Rehearsing the instructions and having the student review and repeat the instructions before starting the task. This can prevent the child from an impulsive and poorly organized start.
- Facilitating planning and organization before the student begins the task. Once a teacher is sure that the student has understood

the instructions, he or she can help the child plan and organize a response by breaking the task down into steps and prioritizing these steps.

- Helping students explore other ways of accomplishing a task, and assisting the child in choosing the best option for achieving the desired outcome when necessary.
- Teaching and demonstrating organizational strategies, such as how a large and complex assignment can be divided into a series of small assignments that lead to an accurate and timely completion of the task. Teachers can also show students how to use assignment books and time management strategies to help meet deadlines.
- Teaching appropriate communication strategies that are respectful yet assertive. Students can be encouraged to talk about the effectiveness of various strategies and teaching techniques. This kind of exchange can go a long way in empowering and motivating children with ADHD.
- Monitoring behavior. Discuss with a student what signals he or she feels can be helpful in lessening inappropriate behavior. Strategies such as standing next to the student, making eye contact, and tapping him or her on the shoulder might help in redirecting a student and preventing the escalation of inappropriate behavior.

Teacher-Centered Approaches

Teachers should do the following:

- Follow a consistent routine.
- Avoid information overload. Children vary in their ability to attend and concentrate. They also differ in speed of processing. Children with ADHD are particularly vulnerable to problems with processing information. Periodically check to see whether a student with ADHD comprehends instructions and information and that he or she is not becoming overwhelmed by the amount of material being presented.
- Consider which are the primary problems affecting the child with ADHD and concentrate on helping him or her work on those issues. To the extent possible, ignore the problems that do not interfere with learning, such as restlessness, hyperactivity, fidgeting, unusual postures, and noise-making or tapping.
- If noise is a problem in the classroom, the teacher may wish to use a noise meter. The teacher can reward the class for keeping noise below a certain level.

Behavior Management

The teacher can identify problem behaviors and work on reducing those behaviors by establishing a reward system for appropriate substitute behaviors. Examples of behaviors that could be targeted include the following:

- Working independently without disturbing others
- Completing assignments
- Remaining seated at desk or workstation
- Taking appropriate notes
- Improving grades

Some rewards could be any of the following:

- Reduced homework
- Verbal praise
- Computer access
- Additional recess
- Class job or responsibility (e.g., class monitor)
- Field trip
- Lunch with parent or teacher
- Points or tokens
- Prize, food, or toy
- Being first in line (leader)
- Show-and-tell

Target the behaviors that are critical to the child's ability to learn and make sure the rewards are meaningful to the child. Parents should be involved in the identification of the target behaviors and rewards to the extent possible. It is important to establish positive rewards and avoid negative consequences such as criticism, insults, and humiliation.

The first step in developing a point or token system for behavior modification is to identify the behaviors that most frequently interfere with the child's ability to learn and function in the classroom. It may be helpful to fill out a behavioral questionnaire such as the follow-up sheet for ADHD Behavior Score. Figure 5.2 shows a simple questionnaire that teachers and parents can use to help identify problems and assist them in monitoring progress.

Planned Ignoring

There are undesirable behaviors that are best addressed by ignoring them when they occur. This technique can be a viable method

FOLLOW-UP SHEET
FOR ADHD BEHAVIOR SCORE

Child's Name ______________________________

Parent's Name ______________________________

Teacher's Name ______________________________

Dates: From ____/____/____ To ____/____/____

Instructions: Identify the behaviors that need to be extinguished. For each negative behavior, suggest an appropriate or target behavior the child should exhibit instead. Grade the child's behavior by using the following point system. Reward the child if improvement is shown. Counsel the child if no improvement is seen on weekly basis.

0–no problem	2–moderate problem
1–mild problem	3–severe problem

Observation	Points 0	1	2	3	Suggested behavior	Points 0	1	2	3
Gets off task	☐	☐	☐	☐	Stays on task	☐	☐	☐	☐
Interrrupts	☐	☐	☐	☐	Raises hand/ waits for turn	☐	☐	☐	☐
Overactive/ fidgety	☐	☐	☐	☐	Remains calm	☐	☐	☐	☐
Forgets assignment	☐	☐	☐	☐	Writes down assignment	☐	☐	☐	☐
Ignores instructions	☐	☐	☐	☐	Listens and repeats instructions	☐	☐	☐	☐
Acts before thinking	☐	☐	☐	☐	Thinks before acting	☐	☐	☐	☐
Talks back	☐	☐	☐	☐	Is respectful	☐	☐	☐	☐
Gets angry	☐	☐	☐	☐	Controls anger	☐	☐	☐	☐
Has difficulty playing	☐	☐	☐	☐	Shares/ cooperates	☐	☐	☐	☐
Is not organizied	☐	☐	☐	☐	Organizies	☐	☐	☐	☐
Loses things	☐	☐	☐	☐	Does not lose things	☐	☐	☐	☐

Instructions:

Child is making progress at the end of 4 weeks: ☐ Yes ☐ No

If yes, progress is: ☐ Mild ☐ Moderate ☐ Significant

Figure 5.2. Questionnaire for identifying ADHD problems and monitoring progress.

for weakening and extinguishing behaviors such as whining, pouting, throwing temper tantrums, demanding, complaining, making inappropriate noises, using foul language, and crying. In general, ignoring these behaviors and not reacting to them will gradually weaken them over a period of time.

Proximity Control

Some undesirable behaviors may be curtailed by simply standing next to the student and assuming a firm body posture and facial expression. Such proximity control techniques can be useful in controlling mild, nonaggressive behaviors.

The Premack Principle

Having the child do unpleasant and difficult work first can help the child complete assignments efficiently. Teachers and parents may consider assigning more difficult tasks at the beginning of the class or homework period.

Signal System

Teachers or parents, together with the child, can develop a signal system to reduce undesirable behavior. For example, using a specific hand signal, calling the child in a different tone of voice, standing near the child's desk, or putting a finger over lips when the child is talking out of turn.

Negative Consequences

Negative consequences can be aversive, such as evoking pain or discomfort, or deprivation events, such as taking away a pleasurable object or activity from the child. Research and experience has shown that the aversion method is generally ineffective, as there are many short- and long-term undesirable effects (Kaplan, in press).

Children respond best to a behavior modification system when the teacher

- is specific about the behavior to improve, and suggests the appropriate substitute behavior in language the student understands
- rewards appropriate behavior, and punishes only the inappropriate ones that can't be ignored
- pays minimal attention to minor behavior problems
- is consistent with rewards and punishment
- rewards and punishes immediately when possible
- rewards with social praise or with privileges that are meaningful to the child

- avoids the use of physical punishment
- does not expect big changes in behavior immediately

NEUROPHARMACOLOGICAL APPROACHES

Some children with ADHD, especially those who have not improved with the use of educational and behavioral modification strategies, may benefit from medications. Research data has clearly demonstrated that appropriate use of medication can significantly benefit children with ADHD (Karanges et al., 2014).

Given the diverse population associated with ADHD and the numerous medications available to treat the condition, clinicians face significant challenges. Medications choices include the following (Kaplan, Sadock, & Sadock, 2014):

- stimulants
- nonstimulants
- antidepressants
- anticonvulsants
- antihypertensives
- neuroleptics

Stimulants are widely used to improve attention, alertness, and wakefulness in children and adults. Although the exact mechanism is unknown, research suggests they influence the availability of norepinephrine and/or dopamine neurotransmitters in the brain. Stimulants improve ADHD symptoms in about 70% of children and adults.

Stimulant medications have been shown to improve selective attention, reduce impulsiveness, and increase self-control. These drugs can also help enhance social skills by improving the ability to perceive and integrate social cues (Hunt, Paguin, & Payton, 2001).

Common side effects of stimulants include headaches, abdominal pain and discomfort, nausea, loss of appetite, and insomnia. Some children will also experience a rebound effect as the drug level tapers off. During this phase, children become irritable and more impulsive. Use of longer-acting preparations may prevent this problem. Stimulants may exacerbate preexisting tics, and concerns have been raised about growth suppression.

When stimulants are contraindicated or not tolerated in a person with ADHD, nonstimulants should be considered next to improve symptoms. Nonstimulant medications work by improving norepinephrine modulation in the attention area of the brain.

Various antidepressants have been used to treat children with ADHD, especially when anxiety or depression are present. Although there is an improvement in task performance, they are generally less effective than stimulants in improving overall behavior.

Anticonvulsants have been used in special situations, such as with children with ADHD and an associated mood disorder, bipolar disorder, or aggression.

All these medications must be prescribed and monitored by an experienced physician.

UNPROVEN THERAPIES

A number of therapies that have been proposed over the years to help children with ADHD do not have scientific evidence to support their claims. Unproven alternative therapies can be expensive and should be discouraged. A few examples of such therapies include megavitamins (Haslam, Dalby, & Rademaker, 1984), optometric training (AAP, 1998), and various herbs, including Pycnogenol (Heimann, 1999). Most studies show that at least 40% of the parents of children initially presenting for medical evaluation with the diagnosis of ADHD will not share the fact that their child is on some form of alternative or complementary treatment unless asked during the history taking. Furthermore, some alternative therapies may cause a serious adverse reaction when taken along with a drug prescribed by the physician. It is important for the clinician to address the parents in a supportive and informative manner and to point out the importance of using evidence-based therapies in the management of children with ADHD. Educators should be aware of scientifically proven therapies and encourage parents to discuss these with their physician.

REFERENCES

Adisetiyo, V., Jensen, J. H., Tabesh, A., Deardorff, R. L., Fieremans, E., Di Martino, A., . . . Helpern, J. A. (2014). Multimodal MR imaging of brain iron in attention deficit hyperactivity disorder: A noninvasive biomarker that responds to psychostimulant treatment. *Radiology, 272*(2), 524–532.

American Academy of Pediatrics, Committee on Childhood Disabilities. (1998). Learning disabilities, dyslexia, and vision: A subject review. *Pediatrics, 102*(9), 124.

American Academy of Pediatrics. (2011). ADHD: *Clinical practice guideline for the diagnosis, evaluation and treatment of attention-deficit/hyperactivity disorder in children and adolescents.* Elk Grove Village, IL: Author.

American Psychiatric Association. (2013). *Diagnostic and statistical manual of mental disorders* (5th ed.). Washington, DC: Author.

Arnsten, A. F. T., Steere, J. C., & Hunt, R. D. (1996). The contribution of alpha-2-noradrenergic mechanism of prefrontal cortical cognitive function. *Archives of General Psychiatry, 53,* 448–455.

Banaschewski, T., Becker, K., Scherag, S., Franke, B., & Coghill, D. (2010). Molecular genetics of attention deficit/hyperactivity disorder: An overview. *European Child and Adolescent Psychiatry, 19,* 237–257.

Barkley, R. A. (1985). *Defiant children: A clinician's manual for parent training.* New York, NY: Guilford Press.

Barkley, R. A. (1990). *Attention-deficit hyperactivity disorder.* New York, NY: Guilford Press.

Barkley, R. A. (1997). *ADHD and the nature of self-control.* New York, NY: Guilford Press.

Barkley, R. A. (1998). *Attention deficit hyperactivity disorder: A handbook for diagnosis and treatment.* New York, NY: Guilford Press.

Barkley, R. A. (2013). *Taking charge of ADHD: The complete, authoritative guide for parents* (3rd ed.). New York, NY: Guilford Press.

Barkley, R. A., Fischer, M., Smallish, L., & Fletcher, K. (2002). The persistence of attention deficit/hyperactivity disorder into young adulthood as a function of reporting source and definition of disorder. *Journal of Abnormal Psychology, 111,* 279–289.

Bennett, L. A., Wolin, S. J., & Reiss, D. (1988). Cognitive behavioral and emotional problems among school-aged children of alcoholic parents. *American Journal of Psychiatry, 145,* 185–190.

Benton, A. (1991). Prefrontal injury and behavior in children. *Developmental Neuropsychology, 7,* 275–282.

Biederman, J., & Faraone, S. V. (2005). Attention deficit hyperactivity disorder. *Lancet, 366,* 237–248.

Bloch, M. H., & Qawasmi, A. (2011). Omega-3 fatty acid supplementation for the treatment of children with attention-deficit/hyperactivity disorder symptomatology: systematic review and meta-analysis. *Journal of American Academy of Child and Adolescent Psychiatry, 50*(10), 991–1000.

Centers for Disease Control and Prevention. (2001). *Attention deficit/hyperactivity disorder: A public health perspective.* Retrieved from http://www.cdc.gov/ncbddd/adhd/research.html

Chacko, A., Wymbs, B. T., Flammer-Rivera, L. M., Pelham, W. E., Walker, K. S., Arnold, F. W., & Herbst, L. (2008). A pilot study of the feasibility and efficacy of the strategies to enhance positive parenting (STEPP) program for single mothers of children with ADHD. *Journal of Attention Disorders, 2,* 270–280.

Conners, C. K. (2008). Conners-3: *Conners, third edition continuous performance test.* North Tonawanda, NY: MultiHealth Systems.

Cortese, S., Angriman, M., Lecendreux, M., & Konofal, E. (2012). Iron and attention deficit/hyperactivity disorder: What is empirical evidence so far? A systemic review of the literature. *Expert Review of Neurotherapy, 12*(10): 1227–1240.

Cortese, S., Azoulay, R., Castellanos, F. X., Chalard, F., Lecendreux, M., Chechin, D., . . . Mouren, M. C. (2012). Brain iron levels in attention deficit/hyperactivity disorder: A pilot MRI study. *World Journal of Biological Chemistry, 13*(3), 223–231.

Cuffe, S. P., Moore, C. G., & McKeown, R. E. (2005). Prevalence and correlates of ADHD symptoms in the national health interview survey. *Journal of Attention Disorders, 9*, 392.

DiGirolamo, A., & Ramirez-Zea, M. (2009). Role of zinc in maternal and child mental health. *American Journal of Clinical Nutrition, 89*(3), 940S–945S.

Dyck, M. J., & Piek, J. P. (2014). Developmental delays in children with ADHD. *Journal of Attention Disorders, 18*, 466.

Faraone, S. V., Biederman, J., Lehman, B., Keenan, K. I., Norman, D., Seidman, L. J., . . . Chen, W. (1993). Evidence for the independent familial transmission of attention deficit hyperactivity disorder and learning disabilities: Result of a familial genetic study. *American Journal of Psychiatry, 150*, 891–895.

Flory, K., Milich, R., Lynam, D. R., Leukefeld, C., & Clayton, R. (2003). Relation between childhood disruptive behavior disorders and substance use and dependence symptoms in young adulthood: Individuals with symptoms of attention-deficit/hyperactivity disorder and conduct disorder are uniquely at risk. *Psychology of Addictive Behaviors, 17*(2), 151–158.

Furman, W. (1980). Promoting social development: Developmental implications for treatment. In B. Lahey & A. Kazden (Eds.), *Advances in clinical child psychology* (pp. 1–40). New York, NY: Plenum.

Ghanizadeh, A., Mohammadi, M. R., & Moini, R. (2008). Comorbidity of psychiatric disorders and parental psychiatric disorders in a sample of Iranian children with ADHD. *Journal of Attention Disorders, 12*, 149–155.

Gilliam, J. E. (2015). ADHDT-2: *Attention-deficit/hyperactivity disorder test* (2nd ed.). Austin, TX: PRO-ED.

Goldstein, S., & Goldstein, M. (1990). *Managing attention disorder in children*. New York, NY: Wiley.

Halperin, J. M., Marks, D. J., Bedard, A. V., Chacko, A., Curchack, J. T., Yoon, C. A., & Healey, D. M. (2013). Training executive, attention, and motor skills: A proof-of-concept study in preschool children with ADHD. *Journal of Attention Disorders, 17*, 711–721.

Hartsough, C. S., & Lambert, N. M. (1985). Medical factors in hyperactivity and normal children: Prenatal development and health history findings. *American Journal of Orthopsychiatry, 55*, 190–210.

Haslam R. H. A., Dalby, J. T., & Rademaker, A. W. (1984). The effects of megavitamin therapy on children with attention deficit disorder. *Pediatrics, 74*, 103–111.

Heilman, K. M., Voeller, K. K. S., & Nadeau, S. E., (1991). A possible pathophysiological substrate of attention deficit hyperactivity disorder. *Journal of Child Neurology, 6*, 74–79.

Heimann, S. W., (1999). Pycnogenol for ADHD? *Journal of the American Academy of Child and Adolescent Psychiatry, 38*(4), 357–358.

Hunt, R. D., Paguin, A., & Payton, K. (2001). An update on assessment and treatment of complex attention-deficit hyperactivity disorder. *Pediatric Annals, 30*, 162–172.

Hynd, G. W., Hern, K. L., Novey, E. S., Eliopuous, D., Marshall, R., Gonzalez, J. J., & Voeller, K. K. (1993) Attention deficit hyperactivity disorder and asymmetry of caudate nucleus. *Journal of Child Neurology, 8*, 339–347.

Jepsen, J. R. M., Fagerlund, B., & Mortensen, E. L. (2009). Do attention deficits influence IQ assessment in children and adolescents with ADHD? *Journal of Attention Disorders, 12*, 551–562.

Kaplan, H. I., Sadock, B. J., & Sadock, V. (2014). *Synopsis of psychiatry* (11th ed., pp. 1193–1200). Riverwoods, IL: Lippincott Williams and Wilkins.

Kaplan, J. S. (in press). *Beyond behavior modification: A cognitive-behavioral approach to behavior management in the school* (4th ed.). Austin, TX: PRO-ED.

Karanges, E. A., Stephenson, C. P., & McGregor, I. S. (2014). Longitudinal trends in the dispensing of psychotropic medications in Australia from 2009–2012: Focus on children, adolescents and prescriber specialty. *Australian & New Zealand Journal of Psychiatry, 48*, 917–931.

Kendall, T. C., & Braswell, L. (1985). *Cognitive behavioral therapy for impulsive children.* New York, NY: Guilford Press.

Konofal, E., Lecendreux, M., Deron, J., Marchand, M., Corlese, S., Zaim, M., . . . Arnult, I. (2008). Effects of iron supplement on attention deficit/hyperactivity disorder in children. *Pediatric Neurology, 38*, 20–26.

Mariani, M., & Barkley, R. A. (1997). Neuropsychological and academic functioning in preschool children with attention deficit disorder. *Developmental Neuropsychology, 13*, 111–129.

Mathers, M. E. (2006). Aspects of language in children with ADHD: Applying functional analyses to explore language use. *Journal of Attention Disorders, 9*, 523–533.

Matles, J. A. (1980). The role of frontal lobe dysfunctions in childhood hyperkinesis. *Comprehensive Psychiatry, 21*, 358–369.

McCann, D., Barrett, A., Cooper, A., Crumpler, D., Dalen, L., Grimshaw, K., . . . Stevenson, J. (2007). Food additives and hyperactive behaviour in 3-year-old and 8/9-year-old children in the community: A randomised, double-blinded, placebo-controlled trial. *Lancet, 370*, 1560–1567.

McConnell, K., & Ryser, G. (2005). *Practical ideas that really work for students with ADHD* (2nd ed.). Austin, TX: PRO-ED.

Mick, E., Biederman, J., & Faroane, S. V. (1996). Is season of birth a risk factor for attention deficit hyperactivity disorder? *Journal of the American Academy of Child and Adolescent Psychiatry, 35*, 1470–1476.

Mousain-Bose, M., Roche, M., Polge, A., Pradal-Prat, D., Rapin, J., & Bali, J. P. (2005). *Improvement of neurobehavioral disorders in children supplemented with magnesium-vitamin B6.* Poster presentation at Gordon Research Conference on Magnesium in Biochemical Processes and Medicine, Ventura, CA.

National Institutes of Health. (2014). *Who is at risk for iron deficiency anemia?* Retrieved from http://www.nhlbi.nih.gov/health/health-topics/topics/ida/atrisk.html

Nichols, P. L., & Chen, T. C. (1981). *Minimal brain dysfunction: A prospective study.* Hillsdale, NJ: Erlbaum.

Owens, J., Gruber, R., Brown, T., Corkum, P., Cortese, S., O'Brien, L., . . . Weiss, M. (2013). Future research directions in sleep and ADHD: Report of a consensus working group. *Journal of Attention Disorders, 17*, 550–564.

Perlmutter, D. (2013). *The grain brain.* New York, NY: Little, Brown.

Sawyer, J. (2001). Short bits. *Word of Mouth, 13,* 15–16.

Scott, C., & Windsor, J. (2000). General language performance measures in spoken and written narrative and expository discourse of school-age children with language learning disabilities. *Journal of Speech, Language, and Hearing Research, 43,* 324–339.

Wender, P. H. (1987). *The hyperactive child, adolescent, and adult: Attention deficit disorder through the lifespan.* New York, NY: Oxford University Press.

Wolraich, M. L. (2002). NICHQ *Vanderbilt assessment scale.* Retrieved from http://www.nichq.org/childrens-health/adhd/resources/vanderbilt-assessment-scales

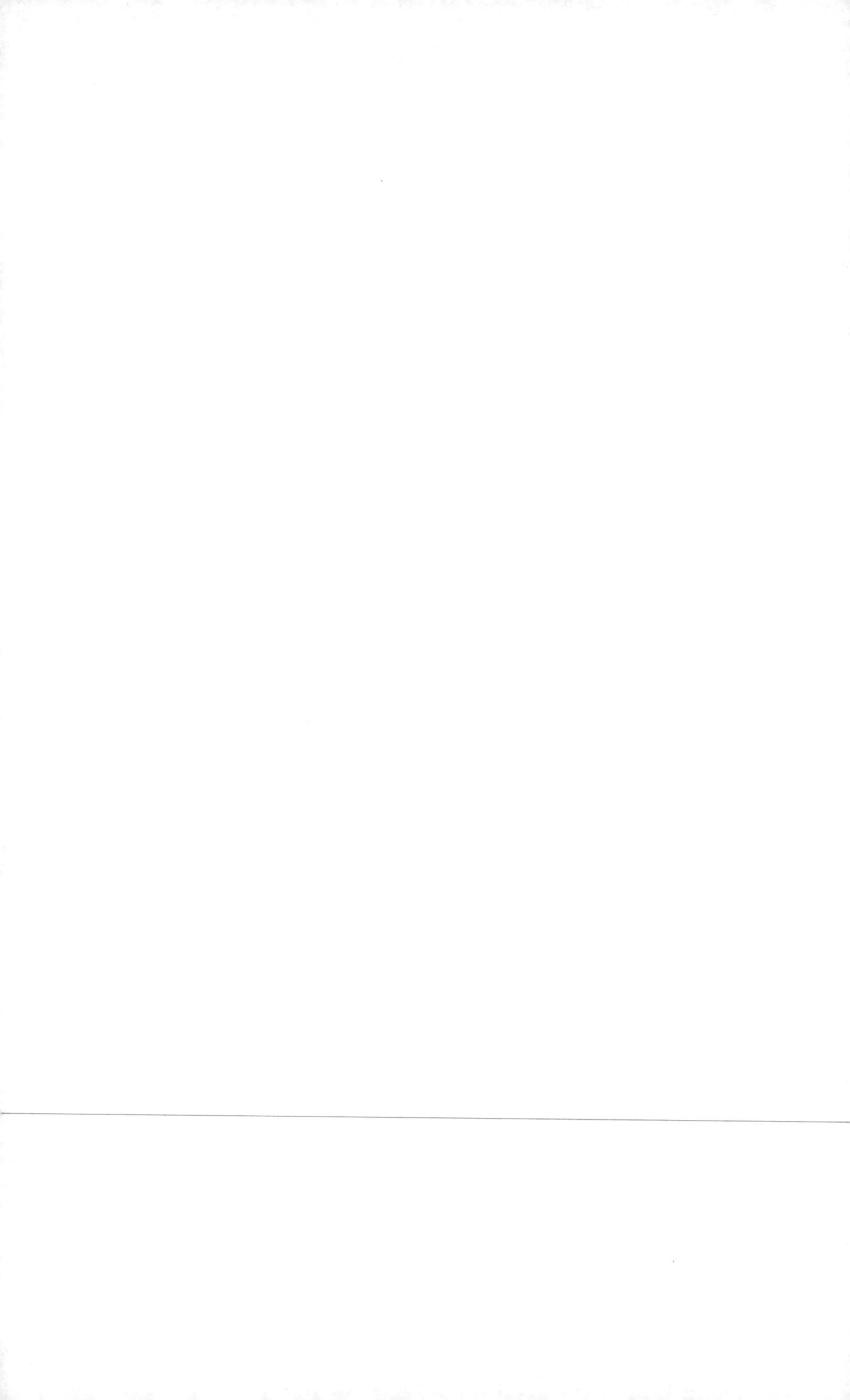

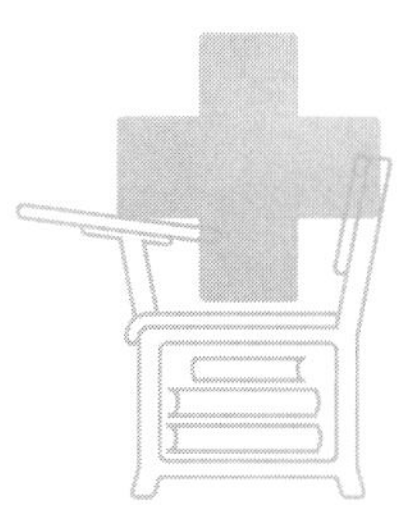

Chapter 6
Adolescent Eating Disorders

Ashley Vandermorris and Debra K. Katzman

Eating disorders are complex illnesses that are affecting adolescents with increasing frequency. Given this rising incidence, people who work with children and adolescents need to become familiar with these disorders. Schools provide a natural place to teach young people about health issues, specifically nutrition and exercise. Teachers working with adolescents probably will encounter students or parents of students who are experiencing problems in regard to food, diet, and weight. Teachers can play an important role in imparting cultural values and cultivating healthy attitudes toward the body and the self. They thus can have a strong impact on the prevention of eating disorders and growing preoccupation with weight. They are in an excellent position to soften the impact of the sociocultural factors causing food and weight problems and to help in their early detection and treatment.

This chapter is a summary of current aspects of eating disorders in the adolescent, paying particular attention to the teacher's role. It describes the clinical presentation, medical and developmental issues, and kinds of treatment specific to adolescents. It is our hope that the information presented here will increase the teacher's knowledge about adolescent eating disorders and facilitate prevention, early detection, and referral.

DIAGNOSIS

The fifth edition of the *Diagnostic and Statistical Manual of Mental Disorders* (standard criteria for the classification of mental disorders) includes a new section on feeding and eating disorders (American Psychiatric Association, APA, 2013). This section includes several changes to better represent the symptoms and behaviors of children and adolescents with these conditions. This chapter discusses the characteristics of the most common eating disorders observed in children and adolescents, including anorexia nervosa, bulimia nervosa, binge-eating disorder, and avoidant/restrictive food intake disorder, also commonly referred to as ARFID. However, at this time very little data exist on binge-eating disorder and ARFID in children and adolescents, and thus the remainder of this chapter focuses primarily on anorexia nervosa and bulimia nervosa.

Anorexia Nervosa

Anorexia nervosa is characterized by emaciation, a relentless pursuit of thinness and inability to maintain a normal or healthy weight, a distortion of body image, and intense fear of gaining weight or persistent behaviors that interfere with weight gain. Adolescents with anorexia nervosa will often control their weight by restricting both the quantity and type of food and by exercising strenuously to eliminate calories.

Commonly, the adolescent begins a weight-reducing diet in response to comments made by friends or family. At first, the young person wants to lose a few pounds, and so eliminates sweets and desserts. Gradually, the choice of food becomes more restricted, as the adolescent begins skipping meals and eating only high-protein, low-carbohydrate, no-fat foods that are low in calories. The young person may consume as little as one-quarter of the typically required number of calories per day (Marzola, Nasser, Hashim, Shih, & Kaye, 2013). As the adolescent's weight gets lower and lower, she or he develops a sense of accomplishment and begins to psychologically feel better. This period of dieting and weight loss often wins praise from others, which encourages the young person to continue the same practices.

Dieting is accompanied by changing weight goals, social isolation, and (in some) increased physical activity. Most of these young people become preoccupied with food and eating. They often entertain magical beliefs about their routines and food, consider many foods forbidden, and eat the same foods at the same time every day. If the caloric allotment is exceeded or a prohibited food eaten, the adolescent may become overwhelmed with guilt and reduce the caloric intake yet further. The adolescent with anorexia nervosa often likes to cook for other family members but refuses to eat any of the food. She or he typically avoids meals with other family members and offers numerous excuses: "I've already eaten," "I have the flu," or "I'm going out for dinner." If these young people sit down to a meal with others, they often cut their food into tiny pieces, rearrange it around their plate, or chew food and spit it out. They often weigh themselves several times a day.

Bulimia Nervosa

Bulimia nervosa is characterized by recurrent episodes of binge eating and inappropriate compensatory behaviors, such as self-induced vomiting, laxative and diuretic abuse, fasting, and excessive exercise to prevent weight gain. Like individuals with anorexia nervosa, teenagers with bulimia nervosa are overly concerned with their body shape and weight; however, bulimia nervosa is more prevalent among those who have been previously obese. Typically, bulimia nervosa begins with unwanted weight gain during or following puberty. Research studies indicate that the onset of bulimic symptoms is often followed by periods of prolonged caloric deprivation (Herpertz-Dahlmann, Holtkamp, & Konrad, 2012; Kaye, 2008). Binges may occur regularly or as a result of an unpleasant feeling, and they are marked by the rapid and out-of-control consumption of a large amount of high-calorie food in a short period of time. At the start of a binge the young person typically feels a surge of euphoria, but as the behavior continues, the individual experiences fear, self-disgust, guilt, or anxiety about impending weight gain. The patient may consume as many as 5,000 calories during a binge.

The binge eating and inappropriate compensatory behaviors both occur at least once a week for three months in patients with bulimia nervosa. These behaviors are often followed by efforts to prevent weight gain, such as self-inducing vomiting, misusing laxatives or diuretics, taking syrup of ipecac, using complementary and alternative medications, exercising, or starving between episodes. A variety of methods are used to induce vomiting; the most common is sticking a finger or toothbrush down the throat. Some patients can vomit spontaneously. Purging produces another episode of euphoria. Several hours after the binge–purge behavior, patients often feel depressed and hopeless. Occasionally, they get desperate enough to hoard or steal food or steal money to buy food. Initially, the binge–purge activity is infrequent, but its frequency may increase to daily or even to many times a day. Both bingeing and purging behaviors are often secretive.

Binge-Eating Disorder

Binge-eating disorder is defined by recurrent episodes of binge eating (like those found in bulimia nervosa) that are not followed by compensatory behaviors. An adolescent with binge-eating disorder may eat too quickly, even when he or she is not hungry, or may have feelings of guilt, embarrassment, or disgust, and may binge eat alone to hide the behavior. This disorder is associated with marked distress and occurs at least once a week over three months. Binge-eating disorder is distinguished from overeating in that it is far more severe and is associated with significant physical and psychological problems (APA, 2013).

Avoidant/Restrictive Food Intake Disorder

Avoidant/restrictive food intake disorder (ARFID) is a new diagnostic category. These children and adolescents are unable to take in adequate calories or nutrition through their diet and experience significant associated physiological or psychosocial problems. Because children and adolescents are not able to get nutrition through their diet, they may end up losing weight or may not gain weight or grow as expected. There are many types of eating problems that might warrant an ARFID diagnosis, including children who avoid foods of certain colors or textures or children who are afraid to eat after a frightening episode of choking or vomiting (APA, 2013).

The DSM-5 includes the full diagnostic criteria for anorexia nervosa, bulimia nervosa, binge-eating disorder, and ARFID (APA, 2013).

The diagnosis of an eating disorder requires ruling out other medical and psychiatric conditions: malignancy, brain tumors, seizures, inflammatory bowel disease, endocrine and metabolic diseases, infection, and pregnancy. Patients with one of these conditions do not pursue thinness or distort their body image. Weight loss may also occur with psychiatric disorders such as schizophrenia, depression, conversion disorder, and obsessive–compulsive disorders. However, it is important to keep in mind that an eating disorder can occur simultaneously with another medical or psychiatric disorder. Determining an accurate diagnosis is the first step for clinicians to establish a treatment plan.

EPIDEMIOLOGY

Over the past 20 years, major changes have occurred in the epidemiology of eating disorders in adolescents. Between 13% and 27% of adolescent girls and 7% and 20% of adolescent boys report disordered eating attitudes or behaviors (Domine, Berchtold, Akre, Michaud, & Suris,

2009; Jones, Bennett, Olmsted, Lawson, & Rodin, 2001; Neumark-Sztainer & Hannan, 2000). Anorexia nervosa, bulimia nervosa, and binge-eating disorder are considered serious public health problems. Teachers and others who work with teenagers are encountering increasing numbers of adolescents with eating disorders.

The prevalence of anorexia nervosa among girls ages 15–19 years ranges from 0.4% to 1% (APA, 2013; Smink, van Hoeken, & Hoek, 2012). It is the third most common chronic illness among adolescent girls, after obesity and asthma (Golden et al., 2003; Yeo & Hughes, 2011). The age range of highest risk is between 12 and 25 years; females aged 15–19 account for 40% of all cases of anorexia nervosa (Halmi, Casper, Eckert, Goldberg, & Davis, 1979; Smink et al., 2012). Girls and women were historically thought to account for 90% to 95% of all reported cases. More recently, studies have suggested that significantly more males are affected. While the DSM-5 continues to report a male-to-female ratio of 1:10 for the overall population, a recent Canadian study found a male-to-female ratio of 1:6 among children less than 13 years old presenting with a restrictive eating disorder (APA, 2013; Pinhas, Morris, Crosby, & Katzman, 2011). This increasing recognition of the frequency of anorexia nervosa among younger boys is important when considering which adolescents are at potential risk.

Bulimia nervosa tends to strike in middle adolescence, either as a result of anorexia nervosa or as an isolated occurrence. The prevalence of bulimia nervosa is up to 3% of adolescent and young adult women (Swanson, Crow, Le Grange, Swendsen, & Merikangas, 2011). It is much less common in males than in females. It is rare in children younger than 14 years of age (Peebles, Wilson, & Lock, 2006; Walker et al., 2014).

Although it was previously thought that eating disorders were more prevalent among certain ethnicities, cultural backgrounds, and socioeconomic groups, it is now recognized that eating disorders affect all groups in society. The incidence of eating disorders is not significantly associated with parental education or household income (Swanson et al., 2011). Eating disorders affect North Americans of all race/ethnicities (Franko, 2007). Eating disorders are reported worldwide, including in the Middle East, Brazil, the Caribbean, and Asia (Becker, 2007; Makino, Tsuboi, & Dennerstein, 2004; Rosen, 2010). It is thought that the detection and diagnosis of eating disorders in minority groups in the United States may be influenced by cultural differences in the experience and expression of body dissatisfaction, differential access to care, and lack of adequate research among minority populations (Becker, 2007).

RISK FACTORS

Although the exact causes of anorexia nervosa and bulimia nervosa are unknown, the causes of these disorders are known to be multifactorial. Biological, psychological, and societal factors all have been implicated. Studies of twins suggested that identical twins have a higher concordance rate for anorexia nervosa than fraternal twins, which supports the view that genetic factors play a role in the causation of anorexia nervosa (Bulik, Sullivan, Wade, & Kendler, 2000; Holland, Sicotte, & Treasure, 1988). Heritability is as high as 50%–70% at puberty, whereas before puberty it is nearly zero (Bulik et al., 2010; Klump et al., 2012). This suggests a biologic vulnerability that may be "turned on" by puberty. The rate of bulimia nervosa is higher among twins of patients with this disorder, and identical twins have a higher concordance than fraternal twins (Kendler et al., 1991). Relatives of an individual with anorexia nervosa are 11.3 and 12.3 times more likely to develop anorexia nervosa than the general population (Strober, Freeman, Lampert, Diamond, & Kaye, 2000), whereas relatives of an individual with bulimia nervosa are 4.4%–9.6% more likely to develop bulimia nervosa (Thornton, Mazzeo, & Bulik, 2011). Although these studies indicate a clear genetic component, the development of eating disorders is also influenced by environment and experiences, as evidenced by the less-than-100% concordance among identical twins. In eating disorders, nonshared environmental factors, which are experiences that are unique to an individual within his or her family (e.g., differential parental treatment or peer group characteristics), have been found to contribute more significantly to the variance in development of an eating disorder than shared environmental factors, such as socioeconomic status (Klump, Wonderlich, Lehoux, Lilenfeld, & Bulik, 2002; Thornton et al., 2011). Studies examining how environmental factors may affect genes that in turn may influence the development of eating disorders in genetically vulnerable individuals, a field known as epigenetics, further emphasize that the causes of eating disorders are multifactorial (Clarke, Weiss, & Berrettini, 2012).

Adolescents with eating disorders have extremely low self-esteem and a sense of ineffectiveness (Cervera et al., 2003; Jacobi, Paul, de Zwaan, Nutzinger, & Dahme, 2004). Typically, adolescents with eating disorders put pressure on themselves to please others and do nothing to please themselves. Patients with eating disorders do not experience pleasure from their bodies. They often believe that they have little control over their world: eating and losing weight become the methods they choose to exert control. During adolescence, young people begin to experience a sense of personal identity. Those who are vulnerable to an eating disorder have difficulty with autonomy and feel ineffectual when they are in situations that place new and different demands on them (Bruch, 1973; Jacobi et al., 2004). They fear the inevitability of maturity and independence.

Cultural trends may contribute to the increased frequency of eating disorders, especially in adolescent girls. Society gives them the message that looking attractive is the most important achievement. The media perpetuates this message: Teen role models are usually portrayed as attractive, self-disciplined, in control—and always slender.

Puberty, which usually occurs at age 11 years in girls and 13 years in boys, is associated with numerous physical and emotional changes. Pubertal development as a cause of eating disorders is supported by studies showing that dieting and disordered eating increase with both menarche and breast development and appear to be independent of chronological age (Killen et al., 1992). Another report suggested that the early onset of puberty (Klump et al., 2012) and a tendency to being overweight (Calzo et al., 2012) may predispose a young person to developing an eating disorder.

Some adolescents have a documented medical illness that places them at a high risk for developing an eating disorder. Studies have suggested relationships between insulin-dependent diabetes mellitus and bulimia (Jones, Lawson, Daneman, Olmsted, & Rodin, 2000; Rodin & Daneman, 1992; Smith, Latchford, Hall, & Dickson, 2008) and between Turner's syndrome and anorexia nervosa (Muhs & Lieberz, 1993). One study found that eating disorders occurred in 20% of diabetics (Rodin, Johnson, Garfinkel, Daneman, & Kenshole, 1986), representing a sixfold increase in anorexia nervosa and a twofold increase in bulimia nervosa over the expected prevalences in similar nondiabetic individuals.

CLINICAL CHARACTERISTICS

Patients with anorexia nervosa display distinct clinical characteristics. They often look much younger than their chronological age and are often perceived as active, energetic, and therefore physically well. Patients who are quite ill, in contrast, may be lethargic and irritable. Their skin is often yellow, they lose scalp or pubic hair and subcutaneous fat, they develop lanugo (fine downy hair) on the body, their hands and feet are usually cold and mottled, and they may experience sleep disturbances, cold intolerance, and constipation. Young patients may appear sad, depressed, and socially isolated, and they show a decline in school performance. Patients with anorexia nervosa frequently deny their physical and psychological symptoms.

Patients with bulimia nervosa can hide their illness more successfully than can those with anorexia nervosa. They may show signs of weakness, muscle aches, stomach bloating or pain, and a puffy face. In addition, calluses may develop over the back of the hand or knuckles, known as Russell's sign, caused by the repeated trauma of their teeth (the central incisors) striking the skin of the hand they use to stimulate the gag reflex. Other clues to bulimia nervosa include painless swelling of the parotid gland, dental enamel erosion, and tooth decay. These patients may complain of swelling of the hands and feet, chest pain, and fatigue. Patients with both anorexia and bulimia nervosa may exhibit features of both disorders.

Patients with binge-eating disorder may not have any obvious physical signs or symptoms. These patients may be overweight or obese, or may be normal weight. The most prominent sign of binge eating is weight gain. Patients with binge-eating disorder have a higher incidence of depression, anxiety, and substance abuse.

ARFID usually presents in infancy or childhood, but it can also present or persist into adulthood. The course of ARFID is unknown. In children or adolescents, the eating issues may be related to emotional difficulties. An example of a young person with ARFID includes an individual who likes only foods of a certain color or texture, and who therefore has great difficulty consuming enough energy to sustain normal growth and development. Another example includes an adolescent who is unwilling to eat any solid foods as a result of choking and therefore has decreased intake that affects his or her growth/weight gain.

MEDICAL ASPECTS

Physical complications involving nearly every organ system in the body have been described (Palla & Litt, 1988). However, many of these young people are so embarrassed about their illness that they rarely disclose their physical symptoms.

Cardiovascular abnormalities are frequent in adolescents with eating disorders and cause significant morbidity and mortality. Electrocardiographic changes occur in up to 75% of hospitalized patients. These include bradycardia (slow heart rate) and other abnormalities, and they are probably a result of malnutrition or electrolyte depletion. Postural changes in both blood pressure and pulse are common, but these are reversible with hydration and nutritional rehabilitation. Approximately 17% of patients with bulimia induce vomiting with syrup of ipecac, an over-the-counter product used as first aid in cases of accidental poisoning (Steffen, Mitchell, Roerig, & Lancaster, 2007). Ipecac contains a cardiotoxic substance, emetine, which is a muscle poison and can, with repeated use, lead to irreversible cardiomyopathy (primary myocardial disease, with sudden death) or peripheral muscle weakness (Ho, Dweik, & Cohen, 1998; Mitchell, Seim, Colon, & Pomeroy, 1987). Changes in cardiac dimensions, including reduction in chamber size, have been described in emaciated patients (Isner, Roberts, Heymsfield, & Yager, 1985; Mont et al., 2003; Oflaz et al., 2013; Ulger et al., 2006). Refeeding of these patients may cause congestive heart failure as a result of an increase in cardiac output, expansion of plasma volume, and increase in metabolic rate. An association between eating disorders and mitral valve prolapse has been reported (Johnson, Humphries, Shirley, Mazzoleni, & Noonan, 1986; Oflaz et al., 2013). Abnormalities are typically reversible with refeeding (Mont et al., 2003; Ulger et al., 2006).

Abnormalities of fluids and electrolytes can also occur, as the result of starvation, vomiting, laxative or diuretic abuse, and/or water loading. Low potassium levels, called *hypokalemia*, have been reported to be the most common electrolyte abnormality (Fisher, Simpser, & Schneider, 2000; O'Connor & Nicholls, 2013; Ornstein, Golden, Jacobson, & Shenker, 2003; Palla & Litt, 1988). Hypokalemia is associated with abnormal cardiac rhythms, muscular weakness, constipation, and cramping. The patient may present with dehydration or abnormal serum levels of sodium, potassium, chloride, carbon dioxide, and blood urea nitrogen. Several renal abnormalities may also be observed (Bouquegneau, Dubois, Krzesinski, & Delanaye, 2012; Kanbur & Katzman, 2011).

Growth retardation and short stature, both known complications of anorexia nervosa, can be very severe when the disorder develops before the growth spurt (Lantzouni, Frank, Golden, & Shenker, 2002; Modan-Moses et al., 2012; Nussbaum, Baird, Sonnenblick, Cowan, & Shenker, 1985; Pfeiffer, Lucas, & Ilstrup, 1986; Root & Powers, 1983; Weiner, 1989). During early adolescence, there is marked acceleration in weight and modest acceleration in linear growth in both girls and boys, averaging 4 kg and 6 to 7 cm and 6 kg and 6 to 7 cm, respectively (Carswell & Stafford, 2008). Development of an eating disorder during this period can adversely affect adult height for both genders (Lantzouni et al., 2002; Nussbaum et al., 1985), particularly among boys (Misra, 2008; Modan-Moses et al., 2003).

Menstrual dysfunction is common with eating disorders. Amenorrhea can occur in patients with anorexia nervosa. Reports have indicated that 20%–50% of female patients with anorexia nervosa lose their menstrual period even before they lose a significant amount of weight (Katz & Vollenhoven, 2000; Kaye, Gwirtsman, & George, 1989; Poyastro Pinheiro et al., 2007). Up to half of female patients with bulimia nervosa may experience irregular menstrual function, and up to 40% can have absent periods (Gendall, Bulik, Joyce, McIntosh, & Carter, 2000; Newman & Halmi, 1988; Poyastro Pinheiro et al., 2007). Many factors may contribute to the amenorrhea, including loss of body fat, excessive exercising, emotional disturbances, and alterations in the regulation of the hypothalmic–pituitary function (Golden & Shenker, 1992). Moreover, adolescents with anorexia nervosa have delayed sexual maturation. Weight loss not only interferes with the onset of menarche but also inhibits normal pubertal development in the premenarchal girl and causes secondary amenorrhea in the postmenarchal girl. With the onset of an eating disorder during puberty, there is delay of breast and testicular development, depletion of auxiliary and pubic hair, and loss of growth of pelvic contours in girls.

Bone-mineral density is a measure reflecting the strength of bones. Low bone-mineral density is an established complication of anorexia nervosa in adolescents. The reduction in bone-mineral density may be severe enough to cause painful and disabling bone fractures. The extent to which low bone-mineral density in anorexia nervosa is reversible remains uncertain. To date, current recommendations for the treatment for low bone-mineral density includes sustainable weight restoration via nutritional rehabilitation, resumption of menstrual function, and optimal calcium (1,300 mg/day of elemental calcium) and vitamin D (600–1,000 IU units/day) intake. High-impact physical activity should be discouraged during active disease, especially in those adolescents with low bone-mineral density (Katzman & Misra, 2013).

Clinical evidence of mild hypothyroidism is evident in patients with anorexia nervosa. Features include constipation, cold intolerance, bradycardia, dry skin, and relaxation of reflexes. Thyroid function, as determined by the serum levels of thyroxine and thyrotropin, is usually in the low-normal to normal range. Some patients have difficulty concentrating their urine in response to water deprivation, possibly because of defective osmoregulation of the secretion of the hormone vasopressin.

The structural abnormalities found in the brains of adolescents with anorexia nervosa are among the earliest and most striking physical consequences. Using a neuroimaging technique called magnetic resonance imaging (MRI), studies have demonstrated that acutely ill adolescents with anorexia nervosa have significant deficits in both gray- and white-matter volumes (Katzman et al., 1996; Kohn et al., 1997; Lambe, Katzman, Mikulis, Kennedy, & Zipursky, 1997). Studies of weight-recovered patients have shown that young people may have persisting deficits in gray-matter volumes (Katzman et al., 1996; Lambe et al., 1997). Very little is known about the functional significance of these brain abnormalities. Patients who had adolescent-onset anorexia nervosa and remain amenorrheic or have irregular menstrual periods have significant cognitive deficits across a broad range of domains. It appears that resumption of menstrual function and therefore increasing levels of the hormone estrogen have a positive impact on cognitive function in girls with anorexia nervosa.

In addition, patients with anorexia nervosa have been found to have cognitive rigidity, difficulties with set shifting (the ability to switch or alternate between tasks) (Tchanturia et al., 2012; Tchanturia et al., 2011), and extreme attention to detail. Current research is looking at new models of treatment to address these cognitive characteristics. It is essential that teachers be aware of the cognitive characteristics of adolescents with anorexia nervosa and attend to these known deficits.

Hematologic disturbances in anorexia nervosa include leukopenia (reduction of the number of leukocytes in the blood), anemia (decreased red blood cells in the blood), and thrombocytopenia (reduction of the number of platelets in the blood) (Hutter, Ganepola, & Hofmann, 2009; Misra et al., 2004; Sabel, Gaudiani, Statland, & Mehler, 2013). However, it does not appear that these patients are more susceptible to infection (Nova, Samartin, Gomez, Morande, & Marcos, 2002).

Gastrointestinal complications occur frequently as a result of starvation, bingeing, vomiting, or purging. Constipation and abdominal pain may result from delayed gastric emptying and slowed intestinal motility. Complaints of bloating after a meal are often reported in this patient group, even after snacks or small meals. Acute dilatation of the stomach (clinically defined as abdominal pain, nausea, distended abdomen, constipation, absence of bowel sounds, and rebound tenderness) is a life-threatening event. Other serious gastrointestinal disorders that have occurred in the course of anorexia nervosa include gastric perforation, trichobezoar (a ball of swallowed hair), and acute pancreatitis. As a result of starvation, liver function test results and cholesterol levels are mildly elevated, a condition that seems reversible with refeeding.

Patients with bulimia nervosa expose their teeth to a steady immersion in acid from stomach contents, resulting in enamel erosion and tooth decay. They may also have associated esophagitis,

Mallory-Weiss tears (mucosal tears and bleeding where the esophagus joins the stomach), and even esophageal erosion and rupture. Some patients with bulimia nervosa may develop a nonpainful enlargement of the parotid glands.

Young people with eating disorders may develop dermatologic complications as a result of malnutrition, vomiting, or drugs used to lose weight. For example, those with anorexia nervosa may have dry skin, brittle hair and nails, an orange discoloration to the skin, edema, and loss of subcutaneous skin (Tyler, Wiseman, Crawford, & Birmingham, 2002).

TREATMENT

The successful management of adolescents with eating disorders involves early restoration of a normal nutritional and physiologic state, establishment of trust, involvement of the family in the treatment program, and a team approach. Professionals generally accept that a multidisciplinary team approach is most effective in the treatment of adolescent eating disorders (Kreipe & Uphoff, 1992). All healthcare providers must have a clear understanding of adolescent health: psychosocial, cognitive and physical growth and development, educational achievement, family and peer interaction, substance use, and sexual behaviors.

Adolescents with eating disorders should be treated at a facility with staff members who understand these problems and have experience in treating young people. Treatment may be carried out in an outpatient, inpatient, residential, or day-hospital setting. The goals of treatment are to diagnose the disorder rapidly and restore the patient's physical and psychological health. Initial goals are medical stabilization and nutritional rehabilitation; they must be achieved before any psychological therapy can be beneficial. Some adolescents with these disorders are admitted to hospital because of cardiovascular or metabolic instability, profound weight loss, inability to gain weight as an outpatient over an extended period, delayed growth and development, or suicidal behavior. Special consideration should be given to younger adolescents, who lose a higher percentage of body weight sooner and experience delays in growth and sexual development.

The treatment modality with the strongest evidence base for anorexia nervosa and bulimia nervosa in adolescents is family-based treatment (FBT), sometimes known as the "Maudsley" method (Lock & Le Grange, 2005). This is an intensive outpatient treatment that recognizes that the adolescent is part of a family system. As such, the initial focus of FBT is to empower the parents (as primary caregivers) to renourish their child to get him or her back to health. Once the adolescent is well nourished, he or she begins to take on more responsibility for eating. Later in the course of treatment, issues such as autonomy, expression of individual feelings, and conflict resolution may be explored. Adolescents should be closely monitored by their physician during FBT. The physician follows the adolescent's growth and development, menstrual irregularities, bone-mineral density, and biochemical indices (Katzman, Peebles, Sawyer, Lock, & Le Grange, 2013).

Day-treatment programs provide an alternative approach to the management of eating disorders. The patient participates in the therapeutic setting and meals are supervised. Most of these programs function five days a week; patients go home for the night and on weekends. Treatment may be provided in groups, on an individual basis, or with the family. This approach encourages autonomy, fosters the ability to test newly acquired skills in regulating eating behavior, and avoids a lengthy separation of the adolescent from his or her family.

For those adolescents whose eating disorders have persisted despite intensive inpatient, outpatient, or day-hospital interventions, residential programs may be available. These programs involve a longer-term intensive and structured treatment program outside of the hospital setting (Brewerton & Costin, 2011). Short-term outcomes in adolescents seem to be promising; however, there are limited data on long-term outcomes for adolescents treated in the residential setting (McHugh, 2007).

Cognitive behavioral therapy (CBT) in older adolescents and adults with bulimia nervosa is effective in the majority of patients (Mitchell, Raymond, & Specker, 1993). A study that used an adapted adult CBT program for youth with bulimia nervosa found results similar to those in adults (Lock, 2005). However, there is only one study to date comparing CBT to FBT for adolescents with bulimia nervosa. This study found no differences in outcomes between those two interventions (Schmidt et al., 2007). More research in this area is warranted.

There are few studies exploring the role of pharmacologic treatment in children and adolescents with eating disorders. It is not clear whether selective serotonin reuptake inhibitors (SSRIs) provide improvement in eating disorder psychopathology or symptoms (Holtkamp et al., 2005) or prevent relapse (Kaye et al., 2001; Walsh et al., 2006). SSRIs may be a consideration in the treatment of bulimia nervosa in adolescents given the evidence in the adult population and in one study in adolescents with bulimia nervosa (Kotler, Devlin, Davies, & Walsh, 2003). Atypical antipsychotics may prove helpful for adolescents with anorexia nervosa (Hagman et al., 2011). At present, medication is not recommended as primary treatment for adolescents with eating disorders; however, there may be a role for medications in patients who have coexisting mental health disorders, such as anxiety or depression (Couturier, Kimber, & Szatmari, 2013).

THE TEACHER'S ROLE

Although teachers cannot be expected to identify or diagnose psychiatric illness, they should be able to recognize the adolescent who is experiencing emotional, psychological, and social difficulties. Teachers are in an advantageous position to identify a student with an eating disorder early and may be the first to observe changes in behavior or appearance. Table 6.1 lists the warning signs of anorexia nervosa and bulimia nervosa. Teachers who suspect that a student has an eating problem should have the opportunity to discuss their concerns with other school professionals, such as an educational psychologist, school nurse, or counselor. These discussions may help teachers present their concerns to the student and his or her parents. The teacher's initial approach to the student should take the form of a compassionate and honest conversation rather than a diagnostic interview. School staff need to be respectful and supportive while recognizing the difference between constructive assistance and overinvolvement. The teacher should be informed about the steps in the referral process, and school officials should know about the services available for the diagnosis and treatment of adolescent eating disorders.

For the most part, adolescents with eating disorders do not come to the school's attention, since their academic performance is high, their attendance excellent, and their behavior compliant and polite. When the teacher looks more closely, however, it becomes apparent that these adolescents do have problems. Their struggles with peer and adult relationships are manifested at school in social withdrawal and isolation. The teacher and school resource staff can assist with issues of self-esteem, social interaction, peer relations, and education about healthy and appropriate nutrition and exercise.

Adolescents with eating disorders often deny their illness or its symptoms. They may continue to participate in regular school activities. School staff should therefore be well informed about the medical and psychological complications of these patients so that they can meet their needs. Often the school can adjust a student's schedule, offer a restricted physical education program if weight remains a concern, and help compensate for absence from school because of medical appointments or prolonged hospitalization. The school's involvement

Table 6.1
WARNING SIGNS OF ANOREXIA NERVOSA AND BULIMIA NERVOSA

Anorexia nervosa
Significant weight loss in the absence of related illness
Extremely thin appearance
Signs of starvation: thinning hair; hair loss; the appearance of fine, raised white hair (lanugo) on the cheeks, neck, forearms, and thighs; repeated gastrointestinal problems; yellowish appearance of the palms or soles of the feet
Significant reduction in eating coupled with a denial of hunger
Strenuous dieting when not overweight
Amenorrhea in women
Unusual eating habits: preference for foods of a certain texture or color, compulsively arranging food, unusual mixtures of food
Obsessive and prolonged exercising despite weakness, fatigue, illness
Complaints of feeling bloated or nauseated after eating a small or normal amount
Bulimia nervosa
Evidence of binge eating: actual observation, verbal reports, large amounts of food missing, stealing money or food
Habitual overeating in response to stress
Frequent weight fluctuations of 10 pounds or more
Eating (not sampling) foods such as dough, canned frostings, or maple syrup without preparing them
Evidence of purging by vomiting, laxative or diuretic use, emetics (e.g., syrup of ipecac), frequent fasting, excessive exercising
Swelling of the glands under the jaw (caused by frequent vomiting), causing a "chipmunk" appearance

and support may help alleviate the patient's anxiety about missing classes.

Students with a serious eating disorder who remain in school should be participating in a suitable treatment program and their general medical safety monitored by clinicians. The school can work with clinicians to determine a student's ability to participate in athletic and other extracurricular activities. Students with a serious eating disorder may be advised to take a leave of absence if they are seriously ill.

Teachers and coaches can play a vital role in strengthening self-acceptance and promoting positive attitudes toward body size and shape and the enjoyment of physical activity (Levine, 1987). They should encourage healthy adolescents to participate in physical activity regardless of their body shape, size, or weight, and foster healthy attitudes toward the body and nutrition. Teachers and coaches working with adolescent athletes participating in at-risk sports (e.g., gymnastics, ballet, or figure skating for girls; bodybuilding and wrestling for boys) need to be aware of early symptoms of eating disorders. Coaches should be discouraged from performing weekly weigh-ins, announcing body weights, or determining changes in body fat in their students. Even the seemingly benign act of weighing a young person as part of a sports evaluation can be a much more serious psychological experience than one might think. School-based approaches to preventing eating disorders that focus on positive self-esteem, resiliency, and healthy engagement in physical activity have been found to have significantly better results than previous models that emphasized calorie counting, categorizing food as good or bad, and the dangers of weight-loss techniques. These more negative, problem-oriented approaches run the risk of suggesting techniques for weight loss and of inadvertently triggering or even glamorizing eating disorders among youth (McVey, 2005).

Teachers should be aware of the impact of the mass media on young people. Television, films, videos, magazines, newspapers, and books continue to glamorize thin, beautiful women and sculpted, attractive men, projecting unrealistic images and false symbols of success, self-control, competence, and strength. The role of the school in counteracting these influences is particularly important. In addition, teachers should examine their own views about body size, attitudes to food, and eating behaviors so they can have a positive influence on young people. Their beliefs can unintentionally affect the body images their adolescent students are in the process of forming.

Health-care professionals can serve as trainers, coordinators, and professional supports for peer-counseling efforts at school and dormitories (residential schools). School health services and school-based health clinics must be alert to identifying early signs and symptoms of eating disorders.

Finally, teachers, school administrators, school nurses, and guidance counselors need to be prepared for an emergency. Students with eating disorders may demonstrate acute medical symptoms (e.g., fainting, vomiting blood, abdominal pain, seizures) as a result of starvation, bingeing, or purging. In some cases they may be suicidal.

PROGNOSIS AND OUTCOME

Research studies of the outcome and prognosis of patients with eating disorders have differed so widely in methodology (e.g., number of patients studied, populations studied, standardization of diagnostic and recovery criteria, differences in duration of illness at time of diagnosis) that generalizations are difficult. However, factors that frequently predict a positive outcome in patients with anorexia nervosa include earlier age of onset, good parent–child relationship, and brief duration of illness (Steinhausen, Rauss-Mason, & Seidel, 1991). The literature on prognosis and outcome in patients with bulimia nervosa is inconclusive and contradictory. Bulimic patients often continue the same pattern of behavior, marked by frequent relapses (Herzog & Sacks, 1993). Studies have found that psychiatric symptoms, including alcohol abuse (Lacey, 1983), suicide attempts (Abraham, Mira, & Llewellyn-Jones, 1983), increased depression at follow-up (Swift, Kalin, Wamboldt, Kaslow, & Ritholz, 1985), association of vomiting and other purging behaviors, and association with anorexia nervosa may predict a poor outcome in patients with bulimia nervosa.

The course of anorexia nervosa is typically protracted. Outcome studies show that approximately 50% of patients will have complete resolution of the illness, whereas 30% will have residual features that come and go in severity well into adulthood. The disease will follow a chronic course in 10% of patients, and another 10% will die from the disorder (Strober, Freeman, & Morrell, 1997). Although less is known about the long-term prognosis for patients with bulimia nervosa, 50% recover and 20% continue to meet full criteria anywhere from 5 to 10 years after their initial presentation

CONCLUSION

People who work with children and adolescents should all become familiar with eating disorders. Parents, teachers, guidance counselors, and health professionals can help identify and prevent these disorders by understanding the risk factors thought to contribute to their development. Early detection of abnormal adolescent eating behaviors may also help reduce morbidity and mortality. Teachers, other school staff members, and parents can help the adolescent by promoting self-esteem, self-acceptance, and a healthy lifestyle. Concerned, sensitive, and well-informed school staff are in a position to help make a difference in how adolescents feel and think about themselves.

REFERENCES

Abraham, S. F., Mira, M., & Llewellyn-Jones, D. (1983). Bulimia: A study of outcome. *International Journal of Eating Disorders, 2*, 175–180.

American Psychiatric Association. (2013). *Diagnostic and statistical manual of mental disorders* (5th ed.). Arlington, VA: Author.

Becker, A. E. (2007). Culture and eating disorders classification. [Review]. *International Journal of Eating Disorders, 40*, S111–S116. doi:10.1002/eat.20435

Bouquegneau, A., Dubois, B. E., Krzesinski, J. M., & Delanaye, P. (2012). Anorexia nervosa and the kidney. [Review]. *American Journal of Kidney Diseases, 60*(2), 299–307. doi:10.1053/j.ajkd.2012.03.019

Brewerton, T. D., & Costin, C. (2011). Long-term outcome of residential treatment for anorexia nervosa and bulimia nervosa. *Eating Disorders, 19*(2), 132–144. doi:10.1080/10640266.2011.551632

Bruch, H. (1973). *Eating disorders.* New York, NY: Basic Books.

Bulik, C. M., Sullivan, P. F., Wade, T. D., & Kendler, K. S. (2000). Twin studies of eating disorders: A review. [Review]. *International Journal of Eating Disorders, 27*(1), 1–20.

Bulik, C. M., Thornton, L. M., Root, T. L., Pisetsky, E. M., Lichtenstein, P., & Pedersen, N. L. (2010). Understanding the relation between anorexia nervosa and bulimia nervosa in a Swedish national twin sample. *Biological Psychiatry, 67*(1), 71–77. doi:10.1016/j.biopsych.2009.08.010

Calzo, J. P., Sonneville, K. R., Haines, J., Blood, E. A., Field, A. E., & Austin, S. B. (2012). The development of associations among body mass index, body dissatisfaction, and weight and shape concern in adolescent boys and girls. *J Adolescent Health, 51*(5), 517–523. doi:10.1016/j.jadohealth.2012.02.021

Carswell, J. M., & Stafford, D. E. J. (2008). Normal physical growth and development. In L. S. Neinetein, C. M. Gordon, D. K. Katzman, D. S. Rosen & E. R. Woods (Eds.), *Adolescent health care: A practical guide* (5th ed.). Philadelphia, PA: Lippincott Williams & Wilkins.

Cervera, S., Lahortiga, F., Martinez-Gonzalez, M. A., Gual, P., de Irala-Estevez, J., & Alonso, Y. (2003). Neuroticism and low self-esteem as risk factors for incident eating disorders in a prospective cohort study. *International Journal of Eating Disorders, 33*(3), 271–280. doi:10.1002/eat.10147

Clarke, T. K., Weiss, A. R., & Berrettini, W. H. (2012). The genetics of anorexia nervosa. *Clinical Pharmacology and Therapeutics, 91*(2), 181–188. doi:10.1038/clpt.2011.253

Couturier, J., Kimber, M., & Szatmari, P. (2013). Efficacy of family-based treatment for adolescents with eating disorders: A systematic review and meta-analysis. *International Journal of Eating Disorders, 46*(1), 3–11. doi:10.1002/eat.22042

Domine, F., Berchtold, A., Akre, C., Michaud, P. A., & Suris, J. C. (2009). Disordered eating behaviors: What about boys? *Journal of Adolescent Health, 44*(2), 111–117. doi:10.1016/j.jadohealth.2008.07.019

Fisher, M., Simpser, E., & Schneider, M. (2000). Hypophosphatemia secondary to oral refeeding in anorexia nervosa. [Case Reports]. *International Journal of Eating Disorders, 28*(2), 181–187.

Franko, D. L. (2007). Race, ethnicity, and eating disorders: Considerations for DSM-V. [Comment]. *International Journal of Eating Disorders, 40*, S31–S34. doi:10.1002/eat.20455

Gendall, K. A., Bulik, C. M., Joyce, P. R., McIntosh, V. V., & Carter, F. A. (2000). Menstrual cycle irregularity in bulimia nervosa. Associated factors and changes with treatment. *Journal of Psychosomatic Research, 49*(6), 409–415.

Golden, N. H., Katzman, D. K., Kreipe, R. E., Stevens, S. L., Sawyer, S. M., Rees, J., . . . Rome, E. S. (2003). Eating disorders in adolescents: Position paper of the Society for Adolescent Medicine. *Journal of Adolescent Health, 33*(6), 496–503.

Golden, N. H., & Shenker, I. R. (1992). Amenorrhea in anorexia nervosa: Etiology and implications. *Adolescent Medicine, 3*(3), 503–518.

Hagman, J., Gralla, J., Sigel, E., Ellert, S., Dodge, M., Gardner, R., . . . Wamboldt, M. Z. (2011). A double-blind, placebo-controlled study of risperidone for the treatment of adolescents and young adults with anorexia nervosa: A pilot study. *Journal of American Academy of Child & Adolescent Psychiatry, 50*(9), 915–924. doi:10.1016/j.jaac.2011.06.009

Halmi, K. A., Casper, R. C., Eckert, E. D., Goldberg, S. C., & Davis, J. M. (1979). Unique features associated with age of onset of anorexia nervosa. *Psychiatry Research, 1*(2), 209–215.

Herpertz-Dahlmann, B., Holtkamp, K., & Konrad, K. (2012). Eating disorders: Anorexia and bulimia nervosa. [Review]. *Handbook of Clinical Neurology, 106*, 447–462. doi:10.1016/B978-0-444-52002-9.00026-7

Herzog, D. B., & Sacks, N. R. (1993). Bulimia nervosa: Comparison of treatment responders vs. nonresponders. *Psychopharmacological Bulletin, 29*(1), 121–125.

Ho, P. C., Dweik, R., & Cohen, M. C. (1998). Rapidly reversible cardiomyopathy associated with chronic ipecac ingestion. [Case Reports]. *Clinical Cardiology, 21*(10), 780–783.

Holland, A. J., Sicotte, N., & Treasure, J. (1988). Anorexia nervosa: Evidence for a genetic basis. *Journal of Psychosomatic Research, 32*(6), 561–571.

Holtkamp, K., Konrad, K., Kaiser, N., Ploenes, Y., Heussen, N., Grzella, I., & Herpertz-Dahlmann, B. (2005). A retrospective study of SSRI treatment in adolescent anorexia nervosa: Insufficient evidence for efficacy. *Journal of Psychiatric Research, 39*(3), 303–310. doi:10.1016/j.jpsychires.2004.08.001

Hutter, G., Ganepola, S., & Hofmann, W. K. (2009). The hematology of anorexia nervosa. [Review]. *International Journal of Eating Disorders, 42*(4), 293–300. doi:10.1002/eat.20610

Isner, J. M., Roberts, W. C., Heymsfield, S. B., & Yager, J. (1985). Anorexia nervosa and sudden death. [Case Reports]. *Annals of Internal Medicine, 102*(1), 49–52.

Jacobi, C., Paul, T., de Zwaan, M., Nutzinger, D. O., & Dahme, B. (2004). Specificity of self-concept disturbances in eating disorders. *International Journal of Eating Disorders, 35*(2), 204–210. doi:10.1002/eat.10240

Johnson, G. L., Humphries, L. L., Shirley, P. B., Mazzoleni, A., & Noonan, J. A. (1986). Mitral valve prolapse in patients with anorexia nervosa and bulimia. *Archives of Internal Medicine, 146*(8), 1525–1529.

Jones, J. M., Bennett, S., Olmsted, M. P., Lawson, M. L., & Rodin, G. (2001). Disordered eating attitudes and behaviours in teenaged girls: A school-based study. *Canadian Medical Association Journal, 165*(5), 547–552.

Jones, J. M., Lawson, M. L., Daneman, D., Olmsted, M. P., & Rodin, G. (2000). Eating disorders in adolescent females with and without type 1 diabetes: Cross sectional study. *British Medical Journal, 320*(7249), 1563–1566.

Kanbur, N., & Katzman, D. K. (2011). Impaired osmoregulation in anorexia nervosa: review of the literature. [Review]. *Pediatric Endocrinology Review, 8*(3), 218–221.

Katz, M. G., & Vollenhoven, B. (2000). The reproductive endocrine consequences of anorexia nervosa. [Review]. *British Journal of Obstetrics & Gynecology, 107*(6), 707–713.

Katzman, D. K., Lambe, E. K., Mikulis, D. J., Ridgley, J. N., Goldbloom, D. S., & Zipursky, R. B. (1996). Cerebral gray matter and white matter volume deficits in adolescent girls with anorexia nervosa. *Journal of Pediatrics, 129*(6), 794–803.

Katzman, D. K., & Misra, M. (2013). Bone health in adolescent females with anorexia nervosa: What is a clinician to do? [Case Reports]. *International Journal of Eating Disorders, 46*(5), 456–460. doi:10.1002/eat.22102

Katzman, D. K., Peebles, R., Sawyer, S. M., Lock, J., & Le Grange, D. (2013). The role of the pediatrician in family-based treatment for adolescent eating disorders: Opportunities and challenges. *Journal of Adolescent Health, 53*(4), 433–440. doi:10.1016/j.jadohealth.2013.07.011

Kaye, W. (2008). Neurobiology of anorexia and bulimia nervosa. [Review]. *Physiology & Behavior, 94*(1), 121–135. doi:10.1016/j.physbeh.2007.11.037

Kaye, W. H., Gwirtsman, H. E., & George, D. T. (1989). The effect of bingeing and vomiting on hormonal secretion. *Biological Psychiatry, 25*(6), 768–780.

Kaye, W. H., Nagata, T., Weltzin, T. E., Hsu, L. K., Sokol, M. S., McConaha, C., . . . Deep, D. (2001). Double-blind placebo-controlled administration of fluoxetine in restricting- and restricting-purging-type anorexia nervosa. *Biological Psychiatry, 49*(7), 644–652.

Kendler, K. S., MacLean, C., Neale, M., Kessler, R., Heath, A., & Eaves, L. (1991). The genetic epidemiology of bulimia nervosa. *American Journal of Psychiatry, 148*(12), 1627–1637.

Killen, J. D., Hayward, C., Litt, I., Hammer, L. D., Wilson, D. M., Miner, B., . . . Shisslak, C. (1992). Is puberty a risk factor for eating disorders? *American Journal of Diseases of Children, 146*(3), 323–325.

Klump, K. L., Culbert, K. M., Slane, J. D., Burt, S. A., Sisk, C. L., & Nigg, J. T. (2012). The effects of puberty on genetic risk for disordered eating: Evidence for a sex difference. *Psychology Medicine, 42*(3), 627–637. doi:10.1017/S0033291711001541

Klump, K. L., Wonderlich, S., Lehoux, P., Lilenfeld, L. R., & Bulik, C. M. (2002). Does environment matter? A review of nonshared environment and eating disorders. [Review]. *International Journal of Eating Disorders, 31*(2), 118–135.

Kohn, M. R., Ashtari, M., Golden, N. H., Schebendach, J., Patel, M., Jacobson, M. S., & Shenker, I. R. (1997). Structural brain changes and malnutrition in anorexia nervosa. *Annals of New York Academy of Science, 817*, 398–399.

Kotler, L. A., Devlin, M. J., Davies, M., & Walsh, B. T. (2003). An open trial of fluoxetine for adolescents with bulimia nervosa. *Journal of Child & Adolescent Psychopharmacology, 13*(3), 329–335. doi:10.1089/104454603322572660

Kreipe, R. E., & Uphoff, M. (1992). Treatment and outcome of adolescents with anorexia nervosa. *Adolescent Medicine: State of the Art Reviews, 3*(3), 519–540.

Lacey, J. H. (1983). Bulimia nervosa, binge eating, and psychogenic vomiting: A controlled treatment study and long term outcome. *British Medical Journal (Clinical Research Edition), 286*(6378), 1609–1613.

Lambe, E. K., Katzman, D. K., Mikulis, D. J., Kennedy, S. H., & Zipursky, R. B. (1997). Cerebral gray matter volume deficits after weight recovery from anorexia nervosa. *Archives of General Psychiatry, 54*(6), 537–542.

Lantzouni, E., Frank, G. R., Golden, N. H., & Shenker, R. I. (2002). Reversibility of growth stunting in early onset anorexia nervosa: A prospective study. *Journal of Adolescent Health, 31*(2), 162–165.

Levine, M. P. (1987). *How schools can help combat student eating disorders: Anorexia nervosa and bulimia.* Washington, DC: National Education Association.

Lock, J. (2005). Adjusting cognitive behavior therapy for adolescents with bulimia nervosa: results of case series. [Clinical Trial]. *American Journal of Psychotherapy, 59*(3), 267–281.

Lock, J., & le Grange, D. (2005). Family-based treatment of eating disorders. [Review]. *International Journal of Eating Disorders, 37*, S64–S67 (discussion S87–69). doi:10.1002/eat.20122

Makino, M., Tsuboi, K., & Dennerstein, L. (2004). Prevalence of eating disorders: A comparison of Western and non-Western countries. [Comparative Study Review]. *Medscape General Medicine, 6*(3), 49.

Marzola, E., Nasser, J. A., Hashim, S. A., Shih, P. A., & Kaye, W. H. (2013). Nutritional rehabilitation in anorexia nervosa: Review of the literature and implications for treatment. *Biomedical Central Psychiatry, 13*, 290. doi:10.1186/1471-244X-13-290

McHugh, M. D. (2007). Readiness for change and short-term outcomes of female adolescents in residential treatment for anorexia nervosa. *International Journal of Eating Disorders, 40*(7), 602–612. doi:10.1002/eat.20425

McVey, G. L. (2005). Preventing eating disorders by educating teachers, coaches and counselors. In D. K. Katzman & L. Pinhas (Eds.), *Help for eating disorders: A parent's guide to symptoms, causes and treatments.* Toronto, ON: Robert Rose.

Misra, M. (2008). Long-term skeletal effects of eating disorders with onset in adolescence. [Review]. *Annals of the New York Academy of Science, 1135*, 212–218. doi:10.1196/annals.1429.002

Misra, M., Aggarwal, A., Miller, K. K., Almazan, C., Worley, M., Soyka, L. A., . . . Klibanski, A. (2004). Effects of anorexia nervosa on clinical, hematologic, biochemical, and bone density parameters in community-dwelling adolescent girls. *Pediatrics, 114*(6), 1574–1583. doi:10.1542/peds.2004-0540

Mitchell, J. E., Raymond, N., & Specker, S. (1993). A review of the controlled trials of pharmacotherapy and psychotherapy in the treatment of bulimia nervosa. [Comparative Study Review]. *International Journal of Eating Disorders, 14*(3), 229–247.

Mitchell, J. E., Seim, H. C., Colon, E., & Pomeroy, C. (1987). Medical complications and medical management of bulimia. [Review]. *Annals of Internal Medicine, 107*(1), 71–77.

Modan-Moses, D., Yaroslavsky, A., Kochavi, B., Toledano, A., Segev, S., Balawi, F., . . . Stein, D. (2012). Linear growth and final height characteristics in adolescent females with anorexia nervosa. *PLoS One, 7*(9), e45504. doi:10.1371/journal.pone.0045504

Modan-Moses, D., Yaroslavsky, A., Novikov, I., Segev, S., Toledano, A., Miterany, E., & Stein, D. (2003). Stunting of growth as a major feature of anorexia nervosa in male adolescents. [Comparative Study]. *Pediatrics, 111*(2), 270–276.

Mont, L., Castro, J., Herreros, B., Pare, C., Azqueta, M., Magrina, J., . . . Brugada, J. (2003). Reversibility of cardiac abnormalities in adolescents with anorexia nervosa after weight recovery. *Journal of the American Academy of Child & Adolescent Psychiatry, 42*(7), 808–813. doi:10.1097/01.CHI.0000046867.56865.EB

Muhs, A., & Lieberz, K. (1993). Anorexia nervosa and Turner's syndrome. [Case Reports Review]. *Psychopathology, 26*(1), 29–40.

Neumark-Sztainer, D., & Hannan, P. J. (2000). Weight-related behaviors among adolescent girls and boys: Results from a national survey. *Archives of Pediatric and Adolescent Medicine, 154*(6), 569–577.

Newman, M. M., & Halmi, K. A. (1988). The endocrinology of anorexia nervosa and bulimia nervosa. [Review]. *Endocrinology and Metabolism Clinics of North America, 17*(1), 195–212.

Nova, E., Samartin, S., Gomez, S., Morande, G., & Marcos, A. (2002). The adaptive response of the immune system to the particular malnutrition of eating disorders. [Review]. *European Journal of Clinical Nutrition, 56*, S34–S37. doi:10.1038/sj.ejcn.1601

Nussbaum, M., Baird, D., Sonnenblick, M., Cowan, K., & Shenker, I. R. (1985). Short stature in anorexia nervosa patients. *Journal of Adolescent Health Care, 6*(6), 453–455.

O'Connor, G., & Nicholls, D. (2013). Refeeding hypophosphatemia in adolescents with anorexia nervosa: A systematic review. [Review]. *Nutrition and Clinical Practice, 28*(3), 358–364. doi:10.1177/0884533613476892

Oflaz, S., Yucel, B., Oz, F., Sahin, D., Ozturk, N., Yaci, O., . . . Oflaz, H. (2013). Assessment of myocardial damage by cardiac MRI in patients with anorexia nervosa. *International Journal of Eating Disorders, 46*(8), 862–866. doi:10.1002/eat.22170

Ornstein, R. M., Golden, N. H., Jacobson, M. S., & Shenker, I. R. (2003). Hypophosphatemia during nutritional rehabilitation in anorexia nervosa: Implications for refeeding and monitoring. *Journal of Adolescent Health, 32*(1), 83–88.

Palla, B., & Litt, I. F. (1988). Medical complications of eating disorders in adolescents. *Pediatrics, 81*(5), 613–623.

Peebles, R., Wilson, J. L., & Lock, J. D. (2006). How do children with eating disorders differ from adolescents with eating disorders at initial evaluation? [Comparative Study Research Support]. *Journal of Adolescent Health, 39*(6), 800–805. doi:10.1016/j.jadohealth.2006.05.013

Pfeiffer, R. J., Lucas, A. R., & Ilstrup, D. M. (1986). Effect of anorexia nervosa on linear growth. *Clinical Pediatrics (Phila), 25*(1), 7–12.

Pinhas, L., Morris, A., Crosby, R. D., & Katzman, D. K. (2011). Incidence and age-specific presentation of restrictive eating disorders in children: A Canadian Paediatric Surveillance Program study. *Archives of Pediatric & Adolescent Medicine, 165*(10), 895–899. doi:10.1001/archpediatrics.2011.145

Poyastro Pinheiro, A., Thornton, L. M., Plotonicov, K. H., Tozzi, F., Klump, K. L., Berrettini, W. H., . . . Bulik, C. M. (2007). Patterns of menstrual disturbance in eating disorders. *International Journal of Eating Disorders, 40*(5), 424–434. doi:10.1002/eat.20388

Rodin, G. M., & Daneman, D. (1992). Eating disorders and IDDM. A problematic association. *Diabetes Care, 15*(10), 1402–1412.

Rodin, G. M., Johnson, L. E., Garfinkel, P. E., Daneman, D., & Kenshole, A. B. (1986). Eating disorders in female adolescents with insulin dependent diabetes mellitus. *International Journal of Psychiatry & Medicine, 16*(1), 49–57.

Root, A. W., & Powers, P. S. (1983). Anorexia nervosa presenting as growth retardation in adolescents. *Journal of Adolescent Health Care, 4*(1), 25–30.

Rosen, D. S. (2010). Identification and management of eating disorders in children and adolescents. [Review]. *Pediatrics, 126*(6), 1240–1253. doi:10.1542/peds.2010-2821

Sabel, A. L., Gaudiani, J. L., Statland, B., & Mehler, P. S. (2013). Hematological abnormalities in severe anorexia nervosa. *Annals of Hematology, 92(*5), 605–613. doi:10.1007/s00277-013-1672-x

Schmidt, U., Lee, S., Beecham, J., Perkins, S., Treasure, J., Yi, I., & Eisler, I. (2007). A randomized controlled trial of family therapy and cognitive behavior therapy guided self-care for adolescents with bulimia nervosa and related disorders. *American Journal of Psychiatry, 164*(4), 591–598. doi:10.1176/appi.ajp.164.4.591

Smink, F. R., van Hoeken, D., & Hoek, H. W. (2012). Epidemiology of eating disorders: Incidence, prevalence and mortality rates. [Review]. *Current Psychiatry Report, 14*(4), 406–414. doi:10.1007/s11920-012-0282-y

Smith, F. M., Latchford, G. J., Hall, R. M., & Dickson, R. A. (2008). Do chronic medical conditions increase the risk of eating disorder? A cross-sectional investigation of eating pathology in adolescent females with scoliosis and diabetes. *Journal of Adolescent Health, 42*(1), 58–63. doi:10.1016/j.jadohealth.2007.08.008

Steffen, K. J., Mitchell, J. E., Roerig, J. L., & Lancaster, K. L. (2007). The eating disorders medicine cabinet revisited: A clinician's guide to ipecac and laxatives. *International Journal of Eating Disorders, 40*(4), 360–368. doi:10.1002/eat.20365

Steinhausen, H. C., Rauss-Mason, C., & Seidel, R. (1991). Follow-up studies of anorexia nervosa: A review of four decades of outcome research. [Review]. *Psychological Medicine*, 21(2), 447–454.

Strober, M., Freeman, R., Lampert, C., Diamond, J., & Kaye, W. (2000). Controlled family study of anorexia nervosa and bulimia nervosa: Evidence of shared liability and transmission of partial syndromes. *American Journal of Psychiatry, 157*(3), 393–401.

Strober, M., Freeman, R., & Morrell, W. (1997). The long-term course of severe anorexia nervosa in adolescents: Survival analysis of recovery, relapse, and outcome predictors over 10–15 years in a prospective study. *International Journal of Eating Disorders, 22*(4), 339–360.

Swanson, S. A., Crow, S. J., Le Grange, D., Swendsen, J., & Merikangas, K. R. (2011). Prevalence and correlates of eating disorders in adolescents. Results from the national comorbidity survey replication adolescent supplement. *Archives of General Psychiatry, 68*(7), 714–723. doi:10.1001/archgenpsychiatry.2011.22

Swift, W. J., Kalin, N. H., Wamboldt, F. S., Kaslow, N., & Ritholz, M. (1985). Depression in bulimia at 2- to 5-year follow-up. *Psychiatry Research, 16*(2), 111–122.

Tchanturia, K., Davies, H., Roberts, M., Harrison, A., Nakazato, M., Schmidt, U., . . . Morris, R. (2012). Poor cognitive flexibility in eating disorders: Examining the evidence using the Wisconsin Card Sorting Task. *PLoS One, 7*(1), e28331. doi:10.1371/journal.pone.0028331

Tchanturia, K., Harrison, A., Davies, H., Roberts, M., Oldershaw, A., Nakazato, M., . . . Treasure, J. (2011). Cognitive flexibility and clinical severity in eating disorders. *PLoS One, 6*(6), e20462. doi:10.1371/journal.pone.0020462

Thornton, L. M., Mazzeo, S. E., & Bulik, C. M. (2011). The heritability of eating disorders: Methods and current findings. [Review]. *Current Topics of Behavioral Neuroscience, 6*, 141–156. doi:10.1007/7854_2010_91

Tyler, I., Wiseman, M. C., Crawford, R. I., & Birmingham, C. L. (2002). Cutaneous manifestations of eating disorders. [Review]. *Journal of Cutaneous Medical Surgery, 6*(4), 345–353. doi:10.1007/s10227-001-0054-5

Ulger, Z., Gurses, D., Ozyurek, A. R., Arikan, C., Levent, E., & Aydogdu, S. (2006). Follow-up of cardiac abnormalities in female adolescents with anorexia nervosa after refeeding. *Acta Cardiologica, 61*(1), 43–49.

Walker, T., Watson, H. J., Leach, D. J., McCormack, J., Tobias, K., Hamilton, M. J., & Forbes, D. A. (2014). Comparative study of children and adolescents referred for eating disorder treatment at a specialist tertiary setting. *International Journal of Eating Disorders, 47*(1), 47–53. doi:10.1002/eat.22201

Walsh, B. T., Kaplan, A. S., Attia, E., Olmsted, M., Parides, M., Carter, J. C., . . . Rockert, W. (2006). Fluoxetine after weight restoration in anorexia nervosa: A randomized controlled trial. *Journal of the American Medical Association, 295*(22), 2605–2612. doi:10.1001/jama.295.22.2605

Weiner, H. (1989). Psychoendocrinology of anorexia nervosa. *Psychiatric Clinics of North America, 12*(1), 187–206.

Yeo, M., & Hughes, E. (2011). Eating disorders: Early identification in general practice. [Review]. *Australian Family Physician, 40*(3), 108–111.

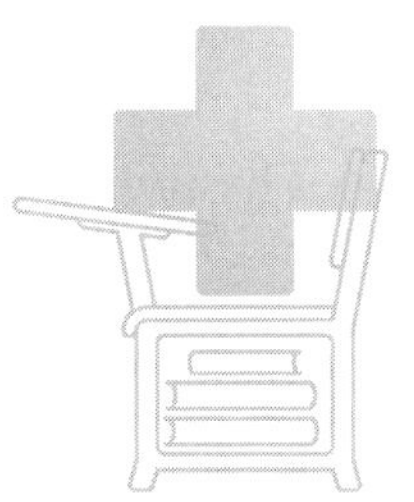

Chapter 7
Sports Medicine

Kate Berz and Robert H. A. Haslam

Pediatricians are often asked to evaluate a child's health status as it relates to his or her ability to participate in sport. This is especially important for children with certain medical conditions, either short term (acute) or long standing (chronic). For example, a child with a fever of 100.4 °F or higher should not participate in athletic activity because of the increased demands placed on the cardiovascular system. A child with a congenital heart condition or one that he or she acquired may or may not be cleared to play sports based on the type of sport and the type of heart problem. In some cases, modifications to sport or the addition of special equipment can make it safer for children with specific medical conditions to participate. An important part of this process is to educate the athlete and parents on the risk of injury given the child's medical condition.

The American Academy of Pediatrics' (AAP) Council on Sports Medicine and Fitness (COSMF) has outlined common medical conditions along with a recommendation for whether it is appropriate for a child with specific medical conditions to participate. Many times the pediatrician makes a clinical judgment call on whether to clear the child for participation.

In most cases, children are cleared to play sports. The conditions that are an absolute contraindication to sport participation are: fever (100.4° F or above), infectious mononucleosis, and carditis (inflammation of the heart). Common conditions that when well controlled do not affect sport participation include asthma, a seizure disorder, and diabetes. The teacher can play an important role by being aware of the child's condition and making sure that the environment is safe for the child to participate in sport activity if appropriate (Rice, 2008).

The pre-participation physical examination is a tool that physicians use to screen children in middle and high school for certain medical conditions. The ultimate objective is to discover previously undiagnosed cardiovascular abnormalities that can lead to sudden cardiac death (SCD). The exam includes a thorough history; certain elements of the physical examination can give clues to cardiac diseases. One difficulty with this method of screening is that the number of eligible young athletes to be screened falls in the range of 10–12 million, and the cardiac diseases that can lead to SCD are rare; the prevalence is estimated at less than or equal to 0.3%. Once the disease is identified, recommendations on sports participation for those with cardiovascular abnormalities are based on the strenuousness of the sport (Maron, Douglas, Graham, Nishimura, & Thompson, 2005).

School personnel should consult a pediatrician or the AAP (national, state, or local chapter) for the most up-to-date practices in their area regarding the pre-participation physical and medical conditions affecting sport.

SPORTS INJURIES

Concussion

Concussion is the most frequent closed-head injury in youth and adolescents. Sports injuries among boys and girls account for a significant proportion of these injuries. It has been estimated that approximately 1.5 million cases of recreational and sports-related concussions occur annually in the United States (Faul, Xu, & Coronado, 2010; Langlois, Rutland-Brown, & Wald, 2006). As most of these individuals are students in junior and senior high school, it is imperative that school administrators and teachers have a good working knowledge of the symptoms and sequelae of concussions and sound advice as to how they may assist in their rehabilitation.

Definition

A consensus statement on concussion in 2013 defined concussion as a "complex pathophysiological process affecting the brain, induced by traumatic biological forces" with the following defining components:

- Concussion is caused by a forceful strike to the head, face, or neck.
- The immediate aftermath is followed by a brief but reversible period of neurological impairment.

- The symptoms associated with concussion are the result of physiological disturbances of the brain rather than structural damage.
- Concussion results in a series of clinical symptoms that may be associated with loss of consciousness.
- Routine imaging studies by computerized tomography (CT scan) and magnetic resonance imaging (MRI) are typically normal (McCrory et al., 2012). Recently, studies using specialized MRI techniques (e.g., diffusion tensor imaging) may show changes in the myelin due to swelling or demyelination in certain areas of the brain, especially the corpus callosum, following concussion. Follow-up studies have been variable; some show complete recovery and others loss of volume of the brain (Dr. A. Rauscher, personal communication, 2013).

The precise biological and physiological mechanisms following concussion in the human brain is not known. Clearly, a significant blow to the head causes the brain to undergo rotational forces resulting in shearing or stretching of axons and their multiple connections. Studies in animals post-concussion have shown abnormal flux of sodium, potassium, and calcium ions across the various ion channels within the brain. Following such experiments, it has been noted that recovery of the ion channels may take up to seven days. This may explain in part why the symptoms following concussion in the human, especially in the adolescent, may take up to several weeks or longer to resolve.

Symptoms of Concussion

Headache is the most common symptom of concussion. There is no particular pattern of the headache except that it can be overwhelming and interfere with cognitive function. Vomiting often occurs acutely, but if prolonged or intense, the pupil should be immediately examined in a hospital. The injured individual should be questioned for both retrograde and anterograde amnesia. Retrograde amnesia refers to the ability to recall events leading up to the insult and anterograde amnesia refers to the accuracy in recalling the timing of events following the trauma. Generally speaking, the longer the period of amnesia, the greater the injury to the brain. The following list highlights the common symptoms associated with concussion, dividing them into four categories: physical, cognitive, emotional, and sleep (US Department of Health & Human Services, Centers for Disease Control and Prevention, "Heads-Up," 2013):

Physical	Cognitive	Emotional	Sleep
Headache	Feeling mentally "foggy"	Irritability	Drowsiness
Nausea	Feeling slowed down	Sadness	Sleepy
Vomiting	Difficulty concentrating	More emotional	Insomnia
Poor balance	Difficulty remembering	Repeats questions	
Visual complaints	Forgetful of recent information		
Fatigue	Confused about recent events		
Light sensitivity	Answers questions slowly		
Noise sensitivity			
Dazed			
Stunned			

Although the majority of youth and adolescents recover from a concussion in two to four weeks, it is not uncommon for the symptoms to persist. These symptoms are variable but most often interfere with concentration and learning. In this case the pupil and family may be provided with a post-concussion symptom-scoring scale. Several post-concussion symptom-scoring scales are available that are used by the student and parents to monitor the progress of symptoms over time. The scoring scale developed by Alia, Sullivan, Hale, and McCrory (2009) lists most of these symptoms. The student is asked to grade each symptom from 0 (*asymptomatic*) to 6 (*severe*) using the Likert sliding scale over time. As the scores in each of the categories move from 6 to 0, the student is assured that significant progress is being made.

Medical and Psychological Evaluation of Concussion

It is imperative that any student who has had a head injury while playing a sport be immediately removed from the game and prohibited to return to play that day. In the immediate period following a head injury, it is important to examine the injured student, looking for abnormal neurological signs and cognitive dysfunction. Loss of consciousness is a medical emergency and demands transfer to a hospital with precautions to stabilize the cervical spine as a spinal cord injury may be present. In addition, if localizing signs are uncovered, such as weakness of the extremities, pain on neck movement, sensory changes in the extremities, or persistent unawareness such as the inability to answer the correct day or place, then transfer to a hospital is essential. As mentioned above, imaging studies are not necessary in an uncomplicated concussion but are certainly warranted if any of the previously mentioned signs are present. Generally, psychological testing in the acute phase is not helpful and should be reserved for those individuals with persistent post-concussion symptoms.

Treatment of Concussion

The initial most important step by the physician in the treatment of concussion is to reassure the pupil and parents that a thorough neurological examination and other diagnostic tests are normal and a complete recovery is to be expected. This is also the time to inform parents and the youth that full recovery may be slow and that it is imperative not to rush to resume pre-concussion activities, as this may exacerbate the problem and cause the return of various symptoms. It is essential that a parent or caregiver be provided with instructions to carefully monitor the athlete at home for 24–48 hours following the injury and be made aware of danger signs that necessitate transfer to a hospital. Analgesics for the treatment of headache have not proved effective in most cases. If drugs such as acetaminophen, aspirin, and ibuprofen (a nonsteroidal anti-inflammatory agent) are overused, they may promote bleeding in the recently traumatized brain. Melatonin has been advocated by some clinicians for the treatment of significant sleep disturbances in post-concussion patients. The use of melatonin awaits evidence-based clinical trials. Patients with significant anxiety and depression may be treated in the short term with an antidepressant agent.

The most important therapy protocol may be "mind or brain rest." This is the part of the therapy in which the teacher may play a primary role in treatment. As outlined in the symptom list earlier, symptoms such as fatigue, sensitivity to light and loud noises, confusion, and memory loss, as well as irritability and drowsiness, may be prominent in the pupil. It may be impossible for the student to attend school in this state. As the symptoms lessen and return to school is possible, perhaps beginning with a half day or even less, placement of the student in a surrounding with non-fluorescent lighting or the temporary use of sunglasses may be beneficial if bright lights aggravate the symptoms. Decreasing noise may be helpful by using headphones when loud noises may interfere with the student's concentration. Watching television, texting, or excessive reading may provoke the symptoms. In addition, consideration should be given to initially lessening the homework assignments and withholding tests, as the results will be unreliable in the early stages of recovery and almost certainly will increase the stress already affecting the student. Typically, the experienced teacher will discover that each of the affected students requires an individualized program. In contrast, the teacher should not encourage the student to take time off or receive special license when it is clear that the recovery process is proceeding satisfactorily (Halstead, McAvoy, Devore, Carl, & Lee, 2013).

Another important component in the treatment of concussion is appropriate physical or "body" rest. This means that even minor physical activity should not be resumed until the individual has no symptoms during rest for two to three weeks. When exercise is resumed, activities such as bicycle riding, skateboarding, skiing, weight lifting, and so on should be delayed until graded activities such as walking and swimming are symptom-free. Progressive physical exercise is guided by at least a 24-hour symptom-free period since that previous set of planned exercises.

Unfortunately, depression is a common sequelae of concussion. The pupil may require a neuropsychological evaluation and benefit by a referral to a mental health team of professionals. Many methods of treatment have been proposed, including various exercises, rotational devices that spin the subject, and a series of medications. None of these methods have undergone strict scientific study.

The educator is in a unique position to inform colleagues in the educational system about the symptoms of concussion, the behaviors associated with the condition, and early recognition of the various complications of concussion. Furthermore, the teacher who has experience working in the classroom with a concussed youth will have valuable insight into assisting in the recovery of the subject that he or she may share with colleagues.

An excellent resource for teachers and parents is provided by the Centers for Disease Control (CDC) website Heads Up, which focuses on students who have suffered from an athletic head injury (Halstead & Walter, 2010).

How Many Concussions Are Too Many?

Precise data and research information is unknown, and the answer likely depends in part on the force of the initial blow to the head and the duration between concussive episodes, as well as the time to complete recovery from previous concussions. Several studies have shown that two concussions, particularly if occurring close together, can have a detrimental effect on school performance. Other studies have shown that three or more concussions in school-age youth may cause long-term cognitive defects. If two concussions are very close together, the brain may undergo marked swelling that may result in severe and persistent cognitive impairment and memory loss.

Role of the Teacher

The physical education teacher and school coaches must learn the early symptoms of concussion and take every blow to the head seriously. They must not accept a student's assertion such as "I saw stars after that ding to my head coach—but I am OK and ready to get back out onto the field." It is imperative that no student who has suffered a concussion or even a possible concussion be allowed to return to play the same day. Rather, coaches and physical education teachers should follow a stepwise "back to play" protocol following a concussion. Each step should last not less than 24 hours and proceed as follows:

1. Complete "body and mind" rest following a concussion until symptom-free
2. Minimal physical activity such as walking at a moderate pace or swimming
3. Moderate physical activity such as training exercises but no head impact
4. Training protocols used in regular and routine team exercises
5. Full-contact practice and examination, and approval by a physician
6. Return to play

If symptoms recur at any stage during the stepwise program, the pupil returns to the previous step and proceeds following a minimum of 24 hours symptom-free. The above "back to play" protocol should not be implemented until the athlete has been symptom-free for two to three weeks.

It is important that school administrators, physical education teachers, and coaches ensure that equipment used in the gymnasium and playground, as well as protective headgear, including correct-fitting helmets, meet current standards. It is important that all school trainers and coaches are knowledgeable in the diagnosis, risks, and management of concussion. In addition, many schools have benefited from using coaches and trainers in the establishment of concussion protocols that have focused on preventing and recognizing a head injury. Finally, it is incumbent upon a coach to contact the parents after suspected concussed student occurrences and provide them with a list of symptoms to be on the lookout for, with instructions as to when to contact the hospital for further observation.

OVERUSE INJURIES

Children and adolescents are especially vulnerable to overuse injuries. Since all of their bones are not completely developed until the teenage years, the growth centers are a site of frequent injury. Growth plates, or epiphyses, are located at the ends of long bones. The epiphysis is a part of the bone that is composed of cartilage, and it is replaced by solid bone when the child is fully grown, which occurs sometime during adolescence. Until the growth plates are closed or fused, this is an area of frequent injury because of either accident (acute injury) or overuse.

Overuse injuries occur as a result of repetitive activity, which leads to microtrauma to a bone, muscle, or tendon. The painful area has been subjected to stress without time to heal. There are four stages of overuse injuries: pain after activity, pain during activity, pain during activity that affects performance, and pain during activity and at rest. A teacher can look out for these signs of overuse injury and encourage the child or adolescent to rest and recommend to the family that the child see his or her pediatrician (Brenner, 2007).

Upper Extremity

In the upper extremity, there are growth plates at each end of the humerus (upper arm) and the two bones in the forearm (radius and ulna). Common overuse injuries in the upper extremity include the following (Brenner, 2007; DiFiori et al., 2014):

- Wrist pain or gymnast's wrist: This results from repeated backward bending of the wrist at the radial growth plate. The injury is usually seen in gymnasts who spend time "walking" on their hands. The child will have pain at the wrist after no known injury or trauma and a history of gymnastics or other activity that puts a repetitive load on the wrist.
- Little League elbow or shoulder. This overuse injury occurs most often in a young baseball pitcher. The child will complain of pain at the shoulder or the elbow, and it is caused by improper throwing technique or too much time spent throwing with not enough rest.
- Swimmer's shoulder. This is seen in an athlete who repeatedly performs overhead activity like a swimming stroke or volleyball serve. Unlike Little League shoulder, this overuse injury may be seen in a child whose growth plates are closed.
- Common acute injuries in the upper extremity include fractures, sprains, and contusions. Any child with a suspected fracture should be removed from the activity and seen by his or her pediatrician.

Baseball and Softball

Injuries to the upper extremity are commonly seen in baseball and softball, although baseball and softball are among the safest sports in which youth participate. Common injuries include head injuries, finger, wrist, and hand injuries, and knee and ankle injuries. Baseball and softball players are subjected to overuse injuries because of the repetitive nature of throwing on an unprepared or immature musculoskeletal system.

Injuries are often age related. Younger children are more likely to be injured before or after games and practices during warm-ups or unsupervised play. In addition, young pitchers are more likely to be hit by a ball. Young catchers are also at risk for being hit by a pitch. Adolescents are more likely to be injured in a collision with another player, be hit by a foul tip, or sustain an overuse injury.

Overuse Injuries Commonly Seen in Throwing Athletes

Baseball pitchers are the players that are most commonly affected by overuse injuries, although any throwing athlete may be affected. An understanding of the anatomy and biomechanics of throwing is helpful for coaches and teachers who may be the first to hear about arm pain in these athletes.

The shoulder is a highly mobile joint that can become unstable when the muscles are fatigued. The shoulder is made up of the following:

- clavicle (collarbone)
- scapula (shoulder blade)
- humerus (upper arm)
- muscle attachments
- ligamentous attachments

The strength and endurance of the muscles and ligaments around the scapula are essential to safe throwing, especially for the repetitive demands of baseball pitching. The source of power of a throw goes beyond the arm and shoulder and includes the muscles of the legs, pelvis, back, and abdomen. This is often referred to as the "core." For softball pitchers the core is especially important. The lower body serves to support the upper body during the windmill motion of softball pitching.

Little League shoulder presents as shoulder pain in throwing, most often a baseball pitcher. This is an overuse injury that occurs when the player throws too many pitches or maximum-effort throws without sufficient rest. It is also seen in throwing athletes using improper technique. The treatment is rest until pain-free, correct the improper throwing mechanics, and build the muscles needed to support proper throwing. If left untreated, this can lead to chronic shoulder pain.

Little League elbow is pain at the medial or middle side of the elbow in throwing athletes. This is caused by the traction of the tendon on the growing bone at the elbow that occurs during throwing. The traction can cause separation of the tendon from the bone and lead to chronic elbow pain and instability. The treatment involves rest until pain free, correction of poor throwing mechanics or muscle deficits, and gradual return to sport (Rice & Congeni, 2012).

Any athlete who participates in a throwing activity, whether or not he or she is a pitcher, should see his or her pediatrician when shoulder or arm pain develops and does not resolve with rest.

Prevention of Upper Extremity Overuse Injuries

For prevention of upper extremity overuse injuries, baseball organizations have set pitch limits based on age. The AAP recommendations are as follows:

- Pitchers should not pitch on multiple teams.
- Players should have three months of rest per year from competitive pitching.
- The pitcher should not also catch for the team because catchers throw more frequently than pitchers.
- Preparation for the season should include exercises focusing on core strength, shoulder stabilization, and proper throwing mechanics (Rice & Congeni, 2012).

Catastrophic Injuries in Baseball and Softball

The rate of catastrophic injury in baseball and softball is very low, at one injury per one million participants annually. These injuries are caused by direct trauma, illness, or a complication of an injury (Rice & Congeni, 2012).

A direct ball impact to the area of the chest right over the heart can cause cardiac arrest in children. This phenomenon is called *commotio cordis* and is the second-highest cause of death in pediatric athletes. Children are thought to be more vulnerable to this injury because of their elastic chest wall. Baseball and softball are considered high-risk sports because the player is often in the direct path of a thrown or batted ball. Commotio cordis causes cardiac arrest secondary to a lethal heart arrhythmia. The treatment involves activation of the emergency response system and immediate use of cardiopulmonary resuscitation (CPR) or an automated external defibrillator (AED). Prevention of commotio cordis involves protective gear, lighter-weight balls, limits on the composition of metal bats, teaching batters to turn away from an inside pitch, and fielders' proper body position.

Equipment for acute injury prevention in baseball and softball includes the following:

- proper weight and compressibility of ball according to age and according to the manufacturer
- proper bat, which includes length, size, and composition of metal bat
- for Little League, the maximum bat length is 33 inches and a diameter of 2.25 inches; the bat performance factor may not exceed 1.15, which is a comparison to the wood bat
- breakaway bases to prevent foot and ankle injuries when sliding
- rubber spikes, not metal spikes
- a runner's base to prevent collisions at first base
- equipment that fits properly and is properly maintained and cleaned to prevent the spread of infection
- padded sliding pants to protect against bruises and abrasions from sliding
- gloves to protect against abrasions when sliding headfirst
- batting gloves to protect against bat blisters
- chest protectors for catchers for prevention of blunt injuries from missed or foul balls
- helmets for base runners
- face and eye shields for batters and infield players
- players who wear eyeglasses or sunglasses should use a lens that will not shatter if hit by a ball or another player
- hard plastic athletic cup to protect the testicles of male players
- knee savers for catchers
- shin guard for batters
- elbow guard for batters (Rice & Congeni, 2012)

Lower Extremity

In the lower extremity, there are growth plates at the ends of each of the long bones, at different sites on the pelvis, in the knees, and in the heels. These are sites of muscle attachments that can put a strain on the growth plates when subjected to repetitive stress and not enough rest time.

Common Lower-Extremity Overuse Injuries

Hip pain is common in athletes who rely on lower-body strength for their sports. High-risk sports include dance, track, and gymnastics. Overuse injuries of the hip may begin as generalized pain in the area of the hip or groin, which progresses to include mechanical symptoms such as a "snapping hip." This condition starts out without any pain and includes a "snapping" or "popping" feel and sound in the hip. It can progress to include painful snapping or popping in the side or front of the hip. A snapping hip is the result of weakness or imbalances in the core muscles.

Thigh pain can sometimes start out as the feeling of a pulled muscle either in the front or back of the upper leg. A fracture from repeated stress on the thigh (stress fracture) can start out just hurting with strenuous activity, but then progress to pain both during activities of daily living and at rest. A stress fracture can be a sign of poor nutrition or other underlying health problems.

Anterior knee pain or pain in the front of the knee is a common occurrence, especially in female athletes. One study of female basketball players showed a prevalence of 34% for high school girls (Barber Foss, Myer, Chen, & Hewett, 2012). Causes of anterior knee pain include the following growth plate problems:

- *Osgood Schlatter's disease (OSD)* occurs when the tendon that connects the kneecap or patella to the shin bone or tibia becomes painful or inflamed at the site of the tibial attachment. It is sometimes possible to feel or see a bump over the site of the tibial growth plate or tibial tubercle.
- *Sinding-Larsen-Johansson (SLJ) syndrome* manifests with pain at the site of the attachment of the patellar tendon, but on the kneecap or patellar side of the tendon. The cause of SLJ and OSD is repeated jumping, cutting, and running, which put stress across the growth plates on either side of the patellar tendon.
- *Shin splints or tibial stress fracture.* Lower-leg pain is common in all sports. Medial tibial stress syndrome or shin splints occur when there is inflammation around the muscles that attach to the tibia or shin. The child may first feel pain in the front of the leg only when running. This pain may progress to pain even when walking. If this is the case, then concern should be raised for a stress fracture. Cause of shin splints and stress fractures is multifactorial, including hard or inappropriate training surfaces, poor running mechanics, poor nutrition, or a quick or accelerated increase in activity over a short period of time.

- *Heel pain or Sever disease.* The heel is the site of the growth plate where the Achilles' tendon attaches the foot to the calf muscle. Repeated flexion and extension (pointing and flexing) of the foot plus pounding of the heel on any kind of surface like a court or field may cause irritation at the site of this growth plate.

Prevention of overuse injuries is important and involves parents, teachers, and coaches. In general, when starting out a sport or training program, children should avoid intense and excessive jumps. Coaches should provide appropriate days off from training. Time should be spent to review proper technique and children should be supervised to make sure they are using good mechanics. For example, when throwing a ball, the child should use his or her entire body, which utilizes core muscles, and avoid using just the arm. Supervising adults should have a working knowledge of the demands of the sport or activity and watch out for signs of overuse.

Common acute injuries in the lower extremities include the following:

- *Knee ligament tear.* The anterior cruciate ligament (ACL) is a structure inside the knee that provides stability. It is often abruptly injured during cutting, jumping, and pivoting sports such as basketball, soccer, and football. Females are 4–10 times more likely to tear the ACL for a variety of reasons (Hewett, Myer, & Ford, 2006). The common story is that the child plants the foot, pivots, and feels a "pop," followed by pain, swelling, and instability. The treatment for an ACL tear for a child who would like to return to sport is surgical repair and intensive rehabilitation to build up the muscles surrounding the hip and knee (Hewett et al., 2006).
- *Ankle sprain.* The ankle is often injured during sport or daily activity. A common mechanism is to invert or turn the ankle, injuring the ligaments on the lateral side or outside of the ankle. In a skeletally immature child or adolescent, this injury can involve the growth plate. The ankle will often be swollen and painful and may have bruising.
- *Fractures of the bones of the lower leg, the tibia, and fibula.* Common in children and adolescents. A child suspected of having a fracture should see his or her pediatrician.

Soccer

Soccer is a popular team sport throughout the world. The sport requires very little equipment and can be played in a variety of settings.

The injury rate in soccer is relatively high when compared to other team sports. Soccer is classified as a high to moderate intensity contact or collision sport. Soccer injuries occur mostly from player to player contact when two players are challenging each other for the ball. Noncontact injuries are also common in soccer. These occur when a player is running, cutting, jumping, and twisting with or without the ball. Injuries to the lower extremity, including ankle and knee sprains and strains, are the most common injury in soccer. Players are more likely to be injured during games than practices (Koutures & Gregory, 2010).

The concussion rate in soccer is similar to that of American football and ice hockey and results more often from player-to-player collision and less often from heading the soccer ball or contact with the goal post. Although heading the soccer ball has not been proven to cause concussions either through one event or through repeated heading, it is worthwhile to learn the proper technique and children should not head the soccer ball until they can demonstrate head, neck, and trunk control sufficient for heading. The use of soft helmets in soccer has not been shown to prevent head injury.

Catastrophic Injuries in Soccer

Soccer-related injuries involving collision with the goalpost have been reported, and, since 1979, 28 fatalities from falling goalposts have been reported (Koutures & Gregory, 2010). Grounding of the goalposts and padding of the goalposts is recommended to prevent fatalities.

Equipment for injury prevention in soccer include the following:

- The field should be free of holes and uneven playing surfaces to prevent lower extremity landing, tripping, or twisting injuries.
- Participants should wear proper shoes to avoid slipping or the alternative, too much gripping.
- Hard fields and ill-fitting shoes with insufficient support can lead to overuse injuries like Sever disease.
- Participants should wear shin guards to prevent bruises to the lower leg during kicking or defending.
- Goalposts should be secured to the ground.
- Participants should learn proper heading technique.
- Protective eyewear is strongly recommended by the AAP and the American Academy of Ophthalmology and should be mandatory for participants with only one functional eye.

TREATMENT OF OVERUSE OR ACUTE INJURIES

Overuse injuries are treated with rest of the affected area. Ice for inflammation and over-the-counter analgesics such as ibuprofen or acetaminophen may be used for pain control. Crutches, braces, or casting is sometimes used to completely rest the area.

For acute injuries like fractures or sprains, it is important to protect the area that has been injured with a splint or a brace until the injury can be evaluated by medical personnel. In addition, ice may be applied for pain relief.

Specific exercises recommended by a doctor or a physical therapist are often part of the treatment program for overuse or acute injuries and can also help prevent future injuries. For more information on sports injuries: www.stopsportsinjuries.org.

Sports Drinks and Energy Drinks

Sports drinks and *energy drinks* are terms that are often used interchangeably, but they are different products. Both are marketed to children and adolescents, and in most cases their use by children and adolescents is inappropriate.

Sports Drinks

Sports drinks are flavored beverages that contain mostly electrolytes and carbohydrates for use before, during, and after a period of strenuous exercise. Often marketed to increase athletic performance, they are intended to replenish water and electrolytes that may be lost through sweating during exercise. Sports drinks may be beneficial to the child or adolescent athlete participating in an hour or more of high-level exercise; however, they are not meant for routine physical activity or for consumption during meals or snacks.

Energy Drinks

Studies have shown that approximately 30% of teenagers report regular use of energy drinks (Seifert, Schaechter, Hershorin, & Lipshultz, 2011). Marketed to boost energy, decrease tiredness, and increase concentration, these beverages contain mainly stimulants, such as caffeine and guarana, in addition to carbohydrates. Even though energy drinks contain carbohydrates, a major energy source, the main ingredient is caffeine, a central-nervous-system stimulant. Guarana is another common ingredient. It is a plant extract that contains caffeine. Since energy drinks are considered supplements by the Food and Drug Administration (FDA), the contents are not regulated, and there is no limit on the amount of caffeine. In contrast, soft drinks are considered a food and have a limit of 32.4 mg of caffeine per 6 oz. In addition, it is difficult to determine the caffeine content of energy drinks because the amount is not always prominently displayed on the packaging.

In body tissues, caffeine blocks a chemical called adenosine, which then affects many organs (Babu, Church, & Lewander, 2008).

Effects of caffeine include increases in heart rate, blood pressure, attention, rate of speech, stomach secretions, urination, and body temperature.

In adults, caffeine has been shown to increase aerobic endurance, strength, and reaction time, and to decrease fatigue. These effects have not been studied in children and adolescents, and there is concern regarding the effects of caffeine on the developing neurologic and cardiovascular system.

Other ingredients in energy drinks include electrolytes, amino acids, vitamins, and minerals, which can all easily be consumed through a healthy diet and are unnecessary to drink. The best method for a child or adolescent to increase energy levels is through a balanced diet.

Hydration is necessary for maintaining the body's physiologic function. In general, water is the appropriate beverage for use on the sports field or at school. The daily amount of water each child needs is determined by a number of factors, including his or her size, medication use, diet, and the presence of illness. Daily water losses occur through sweating, breathing, urinating, and bowel movements. During exercise the body's need for water increases. Environmental conditions such as heat and humidity, the child's level of conditioning, and the amount that the child sweats all factor into the amount of water that the child needs.

Carbohydrate-containing beverages are usually unnecessary. One exception is prolonged vigorous activity, during which muscle glycogen stores are depleted. This is the most appropriate use of a carbohydrate-containing sports drink. Carbohydrate-containing drinks at mealtime should not be a replacement for water or milk and may result in excessive caloric intake (AAP, 2011).

For most children and adolescents, water is adequate to meet the body's daily needs, and the routine use of water should be encouraged. Children should be able to drink as much water as they want during school hours and should have free access to water before, during, and after exercise.

Nutrition Standards for Foods in School, published by the Institute of Medicine in 2007, makes specific recommendations that are relevant to sport and energy drink use. The report recommends limits on sugar, restriction of carbonated, fortified, or flavored beverages, as well as the restriction of sports drink use to children participating in vigorous and prolonged physical activities, and it prohibits the use of energy drinks and the sale of caffeinated beverages at school (Stallings & Yaktinee, 2007).

Strength Training

It has previously been considered that children could not make gains in strength training and that strength training was harmful to a growing skeleton (Lloyd et al., 2014). This is no longer the case and children and adolescents may choose to participate in strength training for a variety of reasons, including injury prevention or rehabilitation and improved sports performance. In addition, school-sponsored sport and physical fitness programs may involve a strength-training component.

The benefits of strength training include cardiovascular fitness and improvements in body composition and bone-mineral density. The blood lipid profile and a child's mental health may also be positively affected by strength training. Focusing on core strength, or strength of the muscles that support the body's trunk (abdominals, gluteals, thigh muscles, and pelvic muscles) can be good for sport specific skill acquisition and also for balance. Strength training, coupled with plyometrics or specific jumping activities, has been related to a decrease in ACL injuries in adolescent females (McCambridge & Sticker, 2008).

Is Strength Training Safe?

Injuries do occur during strength training, but most have been related to the unsafe use of the equipment, the use of home equipment, or an unsupervised setting. Common injuries include muscle strains, and the most common body parts injured are the hand, lower back, and upper trunk. Lower injury rates are seen in settings where there is supervision and when children are taught the proper technique.

Medically speaking, strength training is safe and has no effects on linear growth, growth plates, or the child's cardiovascular system as long as the child is healthy. The following chronic conditions may exclude children from weight lifting because of potential adverse effects (McCambridge & Sticker, 2008):

- hypertension (high blood pressure)
- history of chemotherapy

- certain heart problems, cardiomyopathy, pulmonary hypertension
- Marfan syndrome, with dilated aortic root
- uncontrolled seizure disorder

Which Skills and Equipment Are Required for Strength Training?

Although no minimum age exists for a child to participate in strength training, he or she should be able to accept and follow directions and should appreciate the benefits of training. For maximum benefit and safety, the child should have balance and postural control, which are skills usually attained by age 7 or 8 years.

Children should be strictly supervised by an adult with an appropriate level of certification or knowledge in strength training. The adult-to-child ratio should not exceed 1:10. The adult should be able to provide feedback on proper technique. Children should gain the motor skill competency first and acquire proper form for weight lifting prior to adding any weight or resistance. For general health benefits, strength training should be combined with aerobic training programs for general health benefits. Children should practice their sport specific skills in addition to strength training for maximum benefit when strength training is introduced to improve in a sport.

Prior to skeletal maturity or before the growth plates are closed, children should not participate in power lifting or perform explosive lifting during strength training. The proper technique may be difficult to maintain, and the actions of this type of lifting may stress the body tissues too abruptly.

One repetition maximum, or "maxing out," is often used by coaches or trainers to provide appropriate training intensity. Proper supervision is required for this activity and alternatives to assessing strength should be considered (Lloyd et al., 2014).

How to Strength Train

Once a child has been medically cleared, he or she may participate in a strength-training program. For maximum safety and health benefits, the following additional elements are recommended by the AAP Council of Sports Medicine and Fitness (McCambridge & Sticker, 2008):

- use appropriate-sized weights or use the body for resistance
- include all major muscle groups
- perform 8–15 repetitions of the weight that allows the child to demonstrate proper form

- use weights 1–3 times per week for 20–30 minutes
- sessions should include a 10-minute warm-up and cool-down period that incorporates aerobic activity like jogging, biking, or jumping rope and stretching
- add in weight at 10% increments when the child can perform the repetitions with ease and perfect form

REFERENCES

Alia, S., Sullivan, S. J., Hale, L., & McCrory, P. (2009). Self report scales/checklists for the measurement of concussion symptoms: A systematic review. *British Journal of Sports Medicine, 43*(1), i3–i12.

American Academy of Pediatrics, Committee on Nutrition and the Council on Sports Medicine and Fitness. (2011). Sports drinks and energy drinks for children and adolescents: Are they appropriate? *Pediatrics, 127*(6), 1182–1189.

Babu, K. M., Church, R. J., & Lewander, W. (2008). Energy drinks: The new eye-opener for adolescents. *Clinical Pediatric Emergency Medicine, 9*, 35–42.

Barber Foss, K. D., Myer, G. D., Chen, S. S., & Hewett, T. E. (2012). Expected prevalence from the differential diagnosis of anterior knee pain in adolescent female athletes during preparticipation screening. *Journal of Athletic Training, 47*(5), 519–524.

Brenner, J. S. (2007). Overuse injuries, overtraining, and burnout in child and adolescent athletes. *Pediatrics, 119*(6), 1242–1245.

DiFiori, J. P., Benjamin, H. J., Brenner, J., Gregory, J. S., Jayanthi, N., Landry, G. L., & Luke, A. (2014). Overuse injuries and burnout in youth sports: A position statement from the American Medical Society for Sports Medicine. *Clinical Journal of Sport Medicine: Official Journal of the Canadian Academy of Sport Medicine, 24*(1), 3–20.

Faul M., Xu L., & Coronado V. (2010). *Traumatic brain injury in the United States: Emergency department visits, hospitalizations and death.* Atlanta, GA: Centers for Disease Control and Prevention, National Center for Injury Prevention.

Halstead, M.E., McAvoy, K., Devore, C.D., Carl, R., Lee, M. (2013). Returning to learning following a concussion. *Pediatrics, 132*, 948–957.

Halstead, M. E., & Walter, K. D. (2010). Sport-related concussion in children and adolescents. *Pediatrics, 126*, 597–616.

Hewett, T. E., Ford, K. R., & Myer, G. D. (2006). Anterior cruciate ligament injuries in female athletes: Part 2, a meta-analysis of neuromuscular interventions aimed at injury prevention. *American Journal of Sports Medicine, 34*(3), 490–498.

Hewett, T. E., Myer, G. D., & Ford, K. R. (2006). Anterior cruciate ligament injuries in female athletes: Part 1, mechanisms and risk factors. *American Journal of Sports Medicine, 34*(2), 299–311.

Koutures, C. G., & Gregory, A. J. (2010). Injuries in youth soccer. *Pediatrics, 125*(2), 410–414.

Langlois, J. A., Rutland-Brown, W., & Wald, M. M. (2006). The epidemiology and impact of traumatic brain injury: A brief overview. *Journal of Head Trauma & Rehabilitation, 21*(5), 375–378.

Lloyd, R. S., Faigenbaum, A. D., Stone, M. H., Oliver, J. L., Jeffreys, I., Moody, J. A., . . . Myer, G. D. (2014). Position statement on youth resistance training: The 2014 International Consensus. *British Journal of Sports Medicine, 48*(7), 498–505.

Maron, B. J., Douglas, P. S., Graham, T. P., Nishimura, R. A., & Thompson, P. D. (2005). Task Force 1: Preparticipation screening and diagnosis of cardiovascular disease in athletes. *Journal of the American College of Cardiology, 45*(8), 1322–1326.

McCambridge, T. M., & Stricker, P. R. (2008). Strength training by children and adolescents. *Pediatrics, 121*(4), 835–840.

McCrory, P., Meeuwisse, W., Aubrey, M., Cantu, R. C., Dvorak, J., Echemendia, R. J., . . . Turner, M. (2013). Consensus Statement on Concussion in Sport: The 4th International Conference on Concussion in Sport, Zurich, November 2012. *Journal of Athletic Training, 48*(4), 554–575.

Rice, S. G. (2008). Medical conditions affecting sports participation. *Pediatrics, 121*(4), 841–848.

Rice, S. G., & Congeni, J. A. (2012). Baseball and softball. *Pediatrics, 129*(3), e842–e856.

Seifert, S. M., Schaechter, J. L., Hershorin, E. R., & Lipshultz, S. E. (2011). Health effects of energy drinks on children, adolescents, and young adults. *Pediatrics, 127*(3), 511–528.

Stallings, V. A., & Yaktine, A. L. (Eds.) (2007). N*utrition standards for foods in schools: Leading the way toward healthier youth.* Washington, DC: National Academies Press.

U.S. Department of Health & Human Services. (n.d.). *Heads-up.* Retrieved from http://www.cdc.gov

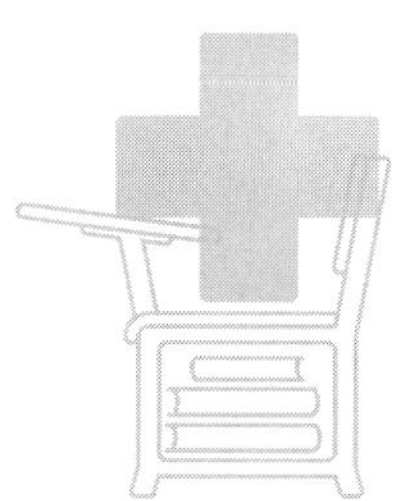

Chapter 8
The Student With Diabetes Mellitus

Denis Daneman

Type 1 diabetes (previously called insulin-dependent diabetes mellitus, IDDM, or juvenile-onset diabetes) is one of the most common chronic disorders of childhood. In fact, it is second in prevalence only to asthma. In Canada and the United States, the incidence of this type of diabetes is 10 to 20 or more new cases per 100,000 youth younger than the age of 20 each year. Incidence has been increasing throughout the world by 2%–5% per year. Although type 1 diabetes can present at any time in childhood, the peaks of incidence are in the early school-age and early adolescent years. By the end of high school, approximately 1 in 400–500 individuals has developed this condition.

Type 2 diabetes (previously called non-insulin-dependent diabetes mellitus or maturity-onset diabetes) has begun to increase rapidly in particular high-risk population groups in North America, including Native American and First Nation individuals, African Americans, and Hispanics. This type of diabetes is often associated with a strong family history of diabetes and a propensity to obesity.

Diabetes cannot be cured. However, children and adolescents with well-controlled diabetes can expect to enjoy healthy school years, participate in the same kinds of activities as their nondiabetic siblings and friends, and look forward to a healthy future. For young people with diabetes, good health over the short and long term is hard work, an achievement resulting from careful attention to a rigorous program of self-management (Daneman, Frank, & Perlman, 1999; Haire-Joshu, 1992). More specifically, these individuals, with the help and support of their families, take multiple (2–5) insulin injections each day or use continuous subcutaneous insulin-infusion pumps, frequently monitor their blood-sugar (glucose) levels, attend to their diet, plan for their activities, and respond to acute emergencies of high and low blood-sugar concentrations. Clearly, the demands of such a regimen cannot help but have an impact on the school life of these children.

Teachers and other school personnel need to be aware of the student with diabetes in the classroom. By understanding the essential features of diabetes management, the teacher can facilitate healthy adjustment of the student to the classroom situation and in peer relationships. Teachers also have an important role in ensuring the ongoing safety of these students in the classroom, on the playground, and on school trips; in alleviating parental anxiety; and in preventing minor crises from getting out of hand.

The teacher's ability to provide the student with the appropriate level of support is contingent on a sound understanding of diabetes and its implications. A number of studies have documented the relatively inadequate knowledge base that most teachers have concerning diabetes (Anderson, Hess, & Hiss, 1989; Pinelli et al., 2011). Given the incredibly large number of disorders teachers may encounter among their students, this is not surprising; health-care providers and parents should not be critical about this seeming lack of preparedness. Furthermore, in a study evaluating the effectiveness of mass education of 244 teachers in the Salt Lake Valley, Utah, Gesteland and Lindsay (1989) concluded that this approach was largely ineffective. The conclusion to be drawn from this and other studies is that diabetes education for teachers should be targeted to those who presently have or will have in the coming year a student with diabetes in their classrooms (Anderson et al., 1989; Bradbury & Smith, 1983; Gesteland & Lindsay, 1989; Henderson, 1993). By virtue of having completed a diabetes education program and having taken care of their child's diabetes at home, the parents should be considered experts in diabetes management and the major source of information for their child's teachers.

In this chapter, we provide teachers with an overview of diabetes and principles of management; describe the impact of diabetes on lifestyle and daily activities; outline expectations for general health, school attendance, and performance; define the teacher's role in relation to that of the student and his or her family; and offer helpful hints in dealing with special situations such as school activities, trips, and party days. Although we focus on type 1 diabetes, many of the same principles apply to the management of type 2 diabetes. Where differences exist, these are highlighted. For additional information, teachers might wish to contact the organizations or refer to the websites listed at the end of this chapter.

OVERVIEW OF DIABETES

Type 1 diabetes is caused by a lack of insulin in the body. Insulin is a hormone produced by the pancreas. More specifically, the beta cells, which are housed in the islets of Langerhans, secrete insulin in response to increasing blood glucose concentrations. Insulin circulates in the blood, binds to its target cells, and stimulates a series of events that lead to glucose uptake by the cell. Without insulin, glucose cannot be used as the energy source of the cells, and life cannot be sustained.

Children with type 1 diabetes develop a complete lack of insulin secretion from the pancreas and, as a result, require insulin replacement, by injection, for life. This situation is quite different from the more common type 2 diabetes, which occurs with increasing prevalence in older individuals and accounts for about 85% of all cases of diabetes. Type 2 diabetes often presents in overweight adults and teens at high risk (as a result of strong family history, obesity, ethnicity); insulin secretion is present but inadequate to meet the demands of the aging and enlarging body. The symptoms are usually much less severe, and the condition can often be managed by either diet alone or diet in combination with pills that increase insulin secretion or action. Because most people know adults with type 2 diabetes, teachers should take care to avoid extrapolating from their experiences with such individuals to the care of their students in the classroom. However, with the increasing prevalence of childhood obesity, type 2 diabetes is being recognized in increasing numbers of teens, particularly those in high-risk groups.

Causes of Diabetes in Children

The cause of type 1 diabetes is not well understood. It is probably the result of a combination of factors leading to chronic inflammation and destruction of the islet cells that produce insulin (Atkinson & Eisenbarth, 2001; Wherrett & Daneman, 2011). That there is a genetic or hereditary component to type 1 diabetes is beyond doubt; however, it is the predisposition to the condition, not the diabetes itself, that appears to be inherited. Unidentified environmental influences appear to be important in converting this predisposition into disease. A few myths need to be exploded for the classmates of the student with newly diagnosed diabetes: (1) Diabetes is *not* an infectious disease, and (2) it is *not* the result of eating too much sugar. Type 2 diabetes tends to have a stronger inherited component and to be closely related to the development of obesity and a sedentary lifestyle in high-risk individuals.

Signs and Symptoms of Untreated or Uncontrolled Diabetes

Without insulin, children are unable to use sugar from the food they eat as a source of energy. Instead, the unused sugar builds up in the blood (*hyperglycemia*) and is "dumped" out in the urine, dragging with it large amounts of water. This increased urination, day and night and often associated with enuresis (bed-wetting), may be the first sign of the onset of diabetes in a previously well child; in someone with diagnosed diabetes, it may signal that the level of control is less than optimal. The increased urination and water loss creates an increase in thirst. Because glucose loss in the urine represents energy loss, there will often also be associated hunger, weight loss, and increasing fatigue or lethargy. Finally, fat breakdown will occur in an effort to replace glucose as the energy source. Eventually this results in a buildup of acid in the blood, severe dehydration, and a potentially life-threatening condition called diabetic ketoacidosis.

These symptoms and signs—increased urination, increased thirst, increased or decreased appetite, weight loss, and poor energy level—will clue the family and physician to the diagnosis of diabetes in an otherwise well child. At school, the teacher may notice that the child leaves the class frequently to urinate, has a poor energy level, and generally appears unwell. These same symptoms and signs may occur after the diagnosis of diabetes during periods of intercurrent illness or if insulin dosages are inadequate or omitted. Well-controlled diabetes should eliminate all these symptoms.

Of note, a study in Italy showed that when teachers and other school personnel were made aware of these symptoms of diabetes, they were often able to facilitate an early diagnosis in students before ketoacidosis developed (Vanelli et al., 1999; Vanelli, Chiari, Lacava, & Iovane, 2007). The awareness of school personnel was accomplished by the strategic placement of colorful posters that reminded teachers of the symptoms of diabetes.

PRINCIPLES OF DIABETES MANAGEMENT

Concept of Balance

In nondiabetic individuals, insulin secretion is so finely regulated that blood glucose concentrations are maintained in an extremely narrow range: 60–110 mg/dl (3.3–6.0 mmol/L) before meals and less than 180 mg/dl (10 mmol/L) after eating. In children with diabetes, the internal regulation of glucose levels is lost. Therefore, diabetes management entails the reestablishment of blood glucose balance through a multicomponent treatment program:

1. Insulin is replaced either by multiple (two to five) daily injections of short- and longer-acting insulin preparations or, increasingly throughout the world, by continuous infusion using a portable pump.
2. Meals and snacks are taken at consistent times and in consistent amounts to provide some predictability to the action of the injected insulin.
3. Regular monitoring of blood glucose (and urine ketones when indicated) provides feedback regarding the effectiveness of the treatment program.

This approach can mimic the functioning of the nondiabetic (normal) pancreas only to a degree. Despite their very best efforts, students with type 1 diabetes and their families will not always be able to achieve perfect blood-sugar control. At times, the blood glucose may be high (hyperglycemia); at other times it may drop precipitously low (hypoglycemia). Achieving the balance can be difficult and frustrating, especially early on after diagnosis. Teachers need to maintain a nonjudgmental attitude as these families adjust to their new reality. The challenge for children and adolescents is to learn as much as possible about their diabetes and to incorporate the treatment measures into their daily lives so as to minimize the risks of both hyperglycemia and hypoglycemia and to maintain good health over both the short and long terms.

Diabetes Education for Families

Successful diabetes management depends on the child's and family's mastery of the necessary cognitive and technical skills, as well as their healthy adjustment to the disorder. From the time of initial diagnosis, children and their families should have the opportunity to participate in a developmentally appropriate program of diabetes care, education, and support. In most centers, this comprehensive program is provided by a multidisciplinary team of health-care providers with expertise in childhood diabetes. Members of such a team include a physician, diabetes nurse, dietitian, and social worker or psychologist (Haire-Joshu, 1992).

In general, parents are highly motivated and quickly learn about the pathophysiology and management of diabetes. They learn to monitor the effectiveness of the treatment program and make the adjustments necessary to maintain good diabetes control. They are taught strategies to detect, treat, and prevent diabetes-related emergencies and are informed about the long-term complications of the disease. The child's level of involvement will depend on his or her age and cognitive maturity. Younger children are not able to comprehend the intricate details of diabetes care, whereas most older children and adolescents can be active participants in the program. Ongoing education of the child and family will serve two purposes: reinforcing present skills and knowledge, and keeping the child's understanding consistent with his or her developmental stage.

Contact between teachers and members of the health-care team should be encouraged for the cooperative dissemination of information and assistance in problem solving (Henderson, 1993). The parents' agreement is obviously required to allow such interchange to occur. In a number of centers, a member of the diabetes team attends the child's school after diagnosis to help school personnel understand the crucial aspects of diabetes care, to answer their questions and those of the student's classmates, and to establish a line of communication between the school and the health-care team. Unfortunately, this is a luxury most diabetes teams cannot easily afford.

Goals of Therapy

Current treatment regimens for type 1 diabetes are based on the need to achieve and maintain blood-sugar levels as close to those in nondiabetic individuals as possible while at the same time minimizing the risks of hypoglycemia (low blood sugar). These goals are determined by the results of the landmark Diabetes Control and Complications Trial (from 1982 to 1993), which demonstrated a close relationship between the level of blood sugar and the risk of the long-term complications of diabetes, such as damage to the eyes, kidneys, and nerves (Diabetes Control and Complications Research Trial Group, 1993). These goals translate into the attempt to achieve premeal blood-sugar levels in the 70–145 mg/dl (4–8 mmol/L) range in teens and older children, 70–180 mg/dl (4–10 mmol/L) range in younger school-age children, and 110–220 mg/dl (6–12 mmol/L) range in infants and toddlers.

INSULIN REPLACEMENT

Insulin was discovered at the University of Toronto in 1921 by the Canadian physician Frederick Banting and his student Charles Best. Prior to the discovery of insulin, children with type 1 diabetes died.

The only way to replace insulin is by injection; taken by mouth, insulin, which is a protein hormone, would be digested in the stomach and rendered ineffective.

Usually a syringe with a short, fine needle or a pen injection device is used to inject the insulin into the subcutaneous tissue (fatty tissue under the skin) of the upper arms, thighs, abdomen, or buttocks. Injected insulin enables the individual with type 1 diabetes to use glucose for his or her energy supply. Its effect is to lower the blood glucose concentration, but unlike naturally secreted insulin, there is no internal regulation. In other words, the effect of the injected insulin does not wear off until it has all been absorbed from the subcutaneous site and used in the body. Thus, injected insulin may lower the blood glucose too much if there is an inadequate supply of glucose from food to balance its action.

At present, most children with type 1 diabetes take insulin injections multiple times each day. Most diabetes experts prescribe three or four injections a day for children and teens with diabetes. There is also a rapidly increasing trend toward the use of insulin pumps in children and teens with type 1 diabetes. These pumps deliver insulin through a rubber tube (catheter) placed under the skin. Insulin is delivered constantly at a low (basal) rate throughout the day and night, with extra doses (boluses) given at each meal (and snack) time. There is no doubt that increasingly intensified approaches to diabetes management place greater demands on the student during the school day. As a result, the role of teachers and other school personnel in supporting these children and teens has also increased.

In general, insulin injections are administered by the parents of young children, with self-administration under supervision being encouraged as the child reaches about age 10. Wide individual differences exist in the age at which children begin self-injection. As parents transfer the technical responsibility of insulin injection to their children, they should supervise the activity closely until the child reaches a high level of maturity and demonstrated skill (Daneman, 1991).

With intensive treatment approaches, teachers and other school personnel are being called on more frequently to participate in the diabetes routines (e.g., supervising or performing injections of blood-sugar tests). Policies differ in various jurisdictions as to the role teachers may or may not play in such management.

Diet

Maintenance of the appropriate balance between food and insulin is essential to good blood glucose (diabetic) control. When the parents or health-care providers decide on an insulin dose for the child with type 1 diabetes, they assume that the food intake will be kept relatively consistent. Although teachers do not need to know all the details of a student's meal plan, they should understand that the diet for people with diabetes is based on the following principles:

1. The child should eat a similar quantity of food each day.
2. The child should eat meals and snacks at the same times each day.
3. The child should avoid foods containing excess amounts of concentrated sugars (e.g., candies, regular soft drinks).

These principles should be followed not only on a regular day-to-day basis at school but also during field trips, other school trips, and even detentions. It is almost always possible to integrate the child's meal plan into the daily school schedule. For example, snacks can be taken at recess or during snack time. Only occasionally will it be necessary for the student to eat his or her snack during class. Every effort should be taken to avoid criticizing or singling out these students. Many students find that low-noise foods, such as cheese or dried fruit, minimize classroom disruption.

Younger children with diabetes will likely require extra supervision in both the classroom and the lunchroom to ensure that they eat most of what has been provided for each meal or snack. Overeating or eating candies will not cause an immediate problem but is cause for concern if done regularly, in which case school personnel should inform parents of such behavior. A far more serious problem may arise if the student misses a meal or snack or has much too little food at such time. Lower food intake may precipitate a medical emergency by causing the blood glucose to drop too low. This condition is called an insulin or hypoglycemic reaction. The appropriate treatment for such a reaction is to have the student ingest a quickly absorbable form of sugar (for details see the "Hypoglycemia" section later in this chapter).

With a little planning, students with diabetes can eat most of the foods that their classmates eat. Parents of younger children should be notified ahead of time of parties, hot dog or pizza days, or other special events involving food. Suitable treats include popcorn, fruit, cookies, potato chips, and pizza.

Increasingly, children and teens with type 1 diabetes are learning to adjust insulin dosages according to the amount of carbohydrate-containing food to be ingested at the next meal or snack, an approach called "carbohydrate counting." However, in most cases, teachers and other school personnel cannot be expected to participate in this process.

Monitoring

To assess the effectiveness of their treatment regimens, and to prevent hypoglycemia and hyperglycemia, every student with diabetes should have a system for monitoring blood glucose concentrations on a regular basis. Blood glucose testing is performed by pricking a finger with a spring-loaded device and then applying a drop of blood to a strip, which is read by a blood glucose meter. In addition, children and teens should use urine-testing strips to detect the presence of ketones, a product of fat breakdown. Usually they are encouraged to test blood-sugar levels four or more times a day, before the main meals and at bedtime, but specific protocols vary with different treatment centers. Urine ketones should be monitored during periods of illness or poor metabolic control.

With older children and adolescents, school personnel usually are not requested to participate in testing routines unless the student is having significant problems with control and requires assistance in performing the test at school. However, with increased efforts to achieve tight glucose control in most treatment centers, teacher involvement in testing routines is often required. Teachers and other school personnel involved in such testing require instruction regarding technique, method of recording, and interpretation of test results. Furthermore, they must observe universal precautions to prevent potential transfer of blood-borne diseases. Also, if teachers are involved in monitoring at school, they should have very clear, and preferably written, guidelines about what actions should be taken in response to the result of the test.

One problem that can occur when students monitor under the guidance of school personnel is the tendency for school staff to become overinvolved in a student's diabetes care and overconcerned that every nuance of behavior is a result of changes in blood glucose. Teachers caught in such a situation should request help from the parents and health-care team to clarify and redefine their role in the child's diabetes care at school.

SPECIAL SITUATIONS

Hypoglycemia

Hypoglycemia, insulin reaction, and insulin shock are different names for the same thing: an emergency situation caused by a low blood-sugar level. Because the normal pancreas is able to turn insulin secretion on and off as required, the risk of low blood glucose levels in individuals without diabetes is essentially nonexistent. In those with type 1 diabetes, however, hypoglycemia is an ever-present risk and can develop within minutes of the child's appearing healthy and normal.

The causes of hypoglycemia include the following:

- too much insulin (this is usually inadvertent, but occasionally intentional)
- not enough food, due to a delayed or missed meal or snack
- too much unplanned, vigorous activity (i.e., inadequate provision of extra food for additional physical activities)

For many episodes of hypoglycemia, however, the cause cannot be determined.

The symptoms of hypoglycemia can be divided into the early warning symptoms, caused by increased secretion of the counterregulatory or stress hormones of the body (glucagon, adrenaline or epinephrine, cortisol, and growth hormone), and those caused by poor glucose supply to the brain, termed *neuroglycopenia*. The early warning symptoms include a feeling of shakiness or jitteriness; hunger; cold, clammy, or sweaty skin; tiredness or drowsiness; blurring of vision; anxiety or nervousness; headache; abdominal pain or nausea; and looking quite pale ("white as a ghost"). In younger children, the main features may be behavioral change, with irritability, hostility, or mood swings. The neuroglycopenia will present as increasing confusion and clumsiness or staggering gait, with progression to a decreasing level of consciousness, coma, and a seizure or convulsion if left untreated. Mild, occasional hypoglycemic episodes that can be easily identified and treated are quite commonplace. Most people with type 1 diabetes report at least one a week. More severe episodes that require outside assistance are quite uncommon in the school setting. Every effort should be made to avoid these by careful planning, regular monitoring, and the establishment of realistic goals for blood glucose control.

Treatment of mild hypoglycemia requires ingestion of simple sugar, such as juice, regular soft drinks, or glucose tablets. At home, children are encouraged to test their blood sugar to confirm the presence of hypoglycemia, then to take a modest amount of simple sugar (e.g., 4 ounces of juice or regular soda, two to four glucose tablets). At school, if the student does not have testing equipment easily available, treatment should be initiated without testing. The student should be treated in the classroom, so sugar should be readily available for emergencies. It may take some encouragement to get these children to drink or eat, but the teacher must insist they do. If there is no noticeable improvement in about 10–15 minutes, the treatment should be repeated. When the condition has improved, the child should have some solid food, usually in the form of the next regular meal or a snack. The child should not be left unsupervised until fully recovered. To facilitate treatment of hypoglycemic episodes, the parents should provide the teacher or other school personnel with a handy supply of juice, soda, or glucose tablets. This should be replenished after each episode.

If the hypoglycemic episode is more severe—that is, confusion or beyond—the school should call the local ambulance service and have the child treated by qualified health professionals. The teacher must not give anything by mouth if the child is unconscious, as the child may aspirate the food into his or her lungs.

For home management of severe hypoglycemia, all families have learned to give glucagon. When injected during severe hypoglycemia, this medication quickly raises the blood glucose level and the child recovers. It is rarely necessary for school personnel to learn how to administer glucagon. If, however, the parents and health-care team consider it appropriate for school personnel to know how to give glucagon, instruction can be accomplished with the help of the parents, school nurse, or health-care team.

Prevention of hypoglycemia is an important component of diabetes management. Careful attention to the total treatment package, with rational adjustment of insulin, an appropriate nutritional plan, regular monitoring, and exercise planning, will help prevent many, but not all, hypoglycemic episodes. Parents should be informed of all hypoglycemic episodes that occur at school, because these may signal a need to alter the treatment regimen and thus prevent further and potentially more severe events from developing.

If the teacher is unsure as to whether the child is having a low-blood-sugar reaction, the safest course of action is to give sugar. A temporary excess of sugar will not harm the child, but a low blood glucose reaction is potentially very serious.

Intercurrent Illness

More myths to be exploded: Students with diabetes do *not* acquire more frequent or more severe illnesses than their nondiabetic peers, and they are *not* poor healers. However, when children with diabetes become ill with the usual fevers and other childhood illnesses, the blood glucose balance is likely to be upset (Daneman & Frank, 1984). Careful monitoring with blood glucose and urine ketone tests, a clear fluid diet, and extra (or less) insulin may be required. This is the responsibility of the parents, not the school personnel.

When a child with diabetes becomes ill at school, the parents should be notified immediately so they can take appropriate steps to prevent the development of either hypoglycemia or ketoacidosis. Vomiting or the inability to retain food or fluids is a potentially serious situation that requires prompt attention. If the child vomits, the teacher should inform the parents immediately; if they cannot be reached, the child should be taken directly to the nearest hospital.

Virtually all episodes of hypoglycemia and ketoacidosis during illness should be preventable. Recurrent episodes of ketoacidosis requiring repeated hospitalization are the result of insulin omission and signal significant family dysfunction and distress in the student.

Exercise and Special Events

Children with diabetes should be encouraged to participate in as many school activities as they choose, and they should be included in school trips. For students who participate in vigorous physical activity, good planning is essential to maintain good diabetes control. Physical activity requires extra energy and thus an increased need for glucose. In a child with diabetes, involvement in physical activities will likely lead to a decrease in blood glucose levels and the possibility of developing hypoglycemia. This may occur during the activity or for several hours afterward. In general, students with diabetes are encouraged to take extra food when embarking on physical activities that are beyond those they do on a daily basis (e.g., gym at school, sports events). Some students will decrease their insulin dose in anticipation of such activities. Teachers should be aware of the particular student's exercise-related food habits and, at least for younger children, provide appropriate supervision. As part of the information provided by the parents (see Figure 8.1), common practices around exercise should be included as special instructions.

Ensuring safety in the classroom and on the playground on a day-to-day basis is the major focus for a teacher who has students with diabetes. However, the teacher must be prepared for special events that might occur during the school year, including day and overnight trips, special sporting events, and classroom celebrations such as birthdays and public or religious holidays. Careful preparation for such events helps to prevent unnecessary problems. Consultation with the family and, where applicable, the health-care team is indicated before taking a child with diabetes on any significant trips away from the school. If the trip involves an overnight stay or absence from the home at the time of an insulin injection or blood glucose test, an individual (teacher, other school personnel, or parent) must be identified who will

PERSONAL INFORMATION TO BE PROVIDED BY PARENTS

Name ________________ Age ______ Grade ______

Parent's name ________________

Address ________________

Home phone ____________ Business phone ____________

Alternate person to call in an emergency ________________

Are there other siblings in school? ________________

Name ________________ Grade ______

Doctor's name ________________ Phone ____________

Health Insurance number ________________

Time of day when low blood glucose is most likely to occur ____________

Symptoms commonly experienced ________________

____

What has been provided to treat hypoglycemia ____________

____

Where is it located? ________________

Alternatives: 4 oz fruit juice / 4 oz pop (not diet)

Type of morning snack ________________

Type of afternoon snack ________________

Suggested treats for school parties ________________

Special instructions ________________

____

____

____

____

PHOTO

Figure 8.1. Example of an information sheet that parents should provide to the school to assist with the management of a child's diabetes. Reprinted with permission of the Canadian Diabetes Association.

take responsibility for either performing or supervising the specific task. Furthermore, the school personnel should have available simple sugars for treating mild hypoglycemia, perhaps glucagon for injection for severe reactions, as well as phone numbers to call in case of an emergency.

Being aware of the child's specific dietary needs and general diabetes routines will provide the teacher with a sense of comfort in dealing with the child without too much fuss or bother. Similarly, when special occasions arise at school, the informed teacher will be able to provide additional food before unplanned extra exercise and assess the likely impact of classroom treats brought in by other students.

THE TEACHER'S ROLE

The general health care of the student with diabetes is the responsibility of the family in conjunction with members of their health-care team. Teachers and other school personnel (excluding the school nurse) are not health-care professionals, but they do have an important role in ensuring the safety and comfort of the student. In addition, they have a unique opportunity to contribute to the healthy adjustment of the child to his or her diabetes and the school situation (American Diabetes Association, 2014). It is unrealistic to expect teachers to maintain adequate knowledge and skills because of the possibility of having a student with diabetes in the classroom at some time. Nevertheless, when such a student is in a class, it becomes essential for that teacher and other select school personnel to exhibit appropriate attitudes and to acquire the necessary know-how (Henderson, 1993). The poorly informed or misinformed teacher who has great anxiety about having a student with diabetes in the classroom can add to the adjustment and management difficulties encountered by these children and their families (Pinelli et al, 2011).

Once the family has informed the school of the child's diabetes, a meeting should be organized that includes the teacher, other key school personnel, parents, and the student to discuss the diabetes and the student's individual needs and characteristics (see Figure 8.1 for the kinds of information to be ascertained at the meeting). Such a meeting should be held soon after diagnosis and at the beginning of each school year. Written information is helpful but does not replace personal contact. When the teacher recognizes the expertise of the parent and student and when the expectations of the teacher match those of the family from the outset, the child has the best possible head start for a healthy, happy, productive school year.

The teacher and other school personnel can contribute enormously to the well-being of the student by developmentally appropriate support of the child's activities at school. The child's age and cognitive maturity, as well as other individual and family issues, will have a major impact on management of the child's diabetes. In younger children, care is parent-oriented, whereas in late childhood and early adolescence, there is a steady transition toward self-care. By late adolescence, the expectation is that the teens will have assumed virtually all the responsibility for the day-to-day management of their diabetes. To achieve a smooth transition from parent- to self-oriented care, management of diabetes requires a developmental approach with expectations for self-care balanced against age, maturity, and demonstrated competence. The expectations of and demands placed on teachers to participate in this care will vary greatly according to the child's age and stage of development, parents' expectations and demands, and the nature of the treatment regimen established for the particular student.

Sometimes problems may arise when the expectations of teachers, parents, and students with diabetes do not balance. For example, parents may expect a high level of independence at a young age, such as expecting a child of 8 years to perform tests, administer insulin, and adjust diet without supervision (Daneman & Frank, 1984). Conversely, the parents may expect school personnel to take responsibility for tasks about which they have inadequate knowledge and skills. As mentioned already, these problems can generally be alleviated by advance planning.

That teachers of students of all ages need to be able to recognize and respond to hypoglycemia (low blood glucose or insulin reactions) is not disputed. However, the role of the teacher in prevention of such episodes is also important. For teachers of older students, this entails awareness of and attention to the special needs of the student at school (e.g., regular meal and snack times, planning for gym classes) so that food, insulin, and monitoring requirements can be incorporated safely and unobtrusively into the school schedule, not only on regular school days but also during examinations and other special events. Younger children, of course, require direct supervision during school activities. Teachers may need to remind young children of snack and meal times, ensure adequate lunchroom and playground supervision, and provide extra food for extra activity as instructed by the parents. In addition, teachers need to collaborate with the parents to develop a sensitive system for handling special occasions involving food.

Also, the teacher should be aware of the symptoms of hyperglycemia (high blood sugar), such as increased urination and thirst and decreased energy level. Rather than criticize the student for frequent trips to the bathroom during class, the teacher should inquire as to the level of metabolic control and inform parents of these types of symptoms. The sudden appearance of these symptoms together with another illness (e.g., influenza), especially if the child is vomiting, should trigger an immediate phone call to the parents to allow them to intervene before more serious problems arise. Because viral illnesses are much more common in younger children than in adolescents, it is the teachers of these children who need to be most alert to changes that may occur during the school day.

An increasing number of parents of students with diabetes, particularly younger children, have been making increased demands on school personnel not only to supervise meals and snacks and treat minor hypoglycemic events but also to perform blood glucose testing and administer insulin and glucagon (the latter for severe hypoglycemic events). Although these medical acts are not the usual responsibility of teachers, many are willing to become proficient in these techniques in an attempt to best integrate the student into everyday activities with minimal risk. In fact, in the United States, Public Law No. 94-142, the Education for All Handicapped Children Act of 1975, entitles all "physically, developmentally, emotionally, and other health-impaired children to free appropriate public education" (as cited in Gray, Golden, & Reiswerg, 1991). Type 1 diabetes is identified in the regulations as an eligible condition, implying that schools, in the United States at least, are obligated to provide for specific health-related needs that would otherwise interfere with normal school participation. This means that all the components of diabetes care should be provided by school personnel where indicated.

The identification of children and adolescents with type 1 diabetes as students with "special needs" ought to be done with the utmost caution. Diabetes should not be seen as a label that accompanies the child throughout his or her school years and into adult life. Educators' continuous efforts should be to help these students function in as normal a manner as possible. Because the stigmatizing effect of labeling may be long lasting, labeling should be used only insofar as it serves to identify children with special needs and allows the particular school system to mobilize the necessary resources on their behalf.

Adequate knowledge of diabetes and its management will allow teachers to integrate their students with diabetes into all school activities without the unnecessary stigmatizing or labeling that may have a serious negative effect on a child's self-esteem and classroom adjustment. A well-informed teacher will be able to offset the negative comments of other students and quickly and efficiently deal with contingencies that may arise. It is also ideal for classmates to have appropriate information about the student's diabetes. However, the teacher should not involve the class in a discussion about diabetes without the student's permission to do so. The student is often the best one to lead such a discussion, even at a relatively young age. Teachers can encourage students to share their expertise with classmates through projects, speeches, and so forth. Not only is the information helpful for other students, but it may also serve to boost the self-esteem of the student with diabetes.

Type 1 Diabetes

Studies have shown that children with chronic diseases have greater school absenteeism than their healthy peers. Although type 1 diabetes is one of the most common chronic disorders of childhood, most children with this condition are otherwise healthy. Research suggests that school performance of children with diabetes is similar to that of their nondiabetic peers. Furthermore, although a pilot study showed that children with diabetes do miss, on average, less than 1 week more of school per year than their nondiabetic siblings, most of the difference can be accounted for by visits to health-care professionals rather than as the result of intercurrent illness (Glaab, Brown, & Daneman, 2005; Vetiska, Glaab, Perlman, & Daneman, 2000). Parental overprotection or lack of trust in the ability or willingness of school personnel to provide appropriate supervision may be reasons for greater absenteeism in some children with chronic disorders.

The teacher should be alerted when the student with diabetes has poor school attendance, frequent hospitalizations, or recurrent diabetes-related events at school. Communication with parents should be escalated at these times, and the advice of the child's health-care team should be sought. These episodes may be related to a poor understanding of diabetes and its management on the part of the child and parents. They may also result from family dysfunction where the diabetes bears the brunt of the fallout. Regardless, interventions are required to restore or maintain the child's health and end the disruption to his or her school experience.

Type 2 Diabetes

Although considerably less common than type 1 diabetes, type 2 diabetes is seen with increasing frequency in teens at high risk (strong family history, obesity, member of high-risk ethnic group). Many can be managed with careful attention to diet and exercise; however, oral hypoglycemic agents, medications that help lower blood-sugar levels, or insulin injections may be required in a significant number. Schools should promote physical fitness and healthy eating as part of their mandate. For teens with type 2 diabetes, school personnel should provide support for their treatment regimen in much the same way as for those with type 1 diabetes.

CONCLUSION

Abraham Lincoln once said, "If I had eight hours to chop down a tree, I'd spend six sharpening my axe," underscoring the need for adequate preparation when embarking on a new and unfamiliar task. Such ought to be the case when teachers are faced with the prospect of having a student with diabetes in their classroom. We believe that it is the primary responsibility of parents to inform the school about their child's diabetes and to provide general literature for key school personnel through personal contact. They should also provide specific information regarding their child's diabetes (e.g., diet issues, testing requirements, specific symptoms when hypoglycemia occurs). Teachers should acknowledge and respect the expertise of the parents and student. Wherever possible, the parents should encourage contact between the school and members of the child's diabetes health-care team. Sometimes a visit to the school by a member of the team or someone from the local branch of the volunteer diabetes organization (e.g., the American or Canadian Diabetes Associations) can be arranged to bring more information for both the school personnel and the other students in the child's classroom.

Despite the fact that diabetes is a serious, lifelong disorder with potentially dangerous acute and chronic complications, our experience is similar to that of many others: the vast majority of students with diabetes adjust well to their disorder and attend and perform normally in school. Teachers have an important role to play in early detection of diabetes, in ensuring the safety of the student, and in promoting a healthy adjustment to diabetes in the school setting.

ADDITIONAL RESOURCES

An excellent listing of diabetes-related materials can be obtained from the following organizations:

National Diabetes Information Clearing House
Information Way
Bethesda, MD 20892-3560

Phone 301-654-3327 or 800-860-8747.
e-mail: ndic@info.niddk.nih.gov
http://www.diabetes.niddk.nih.gov

Support can be obtained through the local branches of the American and Canadian Diabetes Associations. The addresses of the national offices of these two organizations are as follows:

American Diabetes Association

1701 N. Beauregard Street Alexandria, VA 22311
Phone 800-342-2383
http://www.diabetes.org

Canadian Diabetes Association

1400-522 University Avenue, Toronto, ON M5G 2R5
Phone 800.226-8464
http://www.diabetes.ca

The following highly informative website, Children With Diabetes, is available in addition to those of the American and Canadian Diabetes Associations:

http://www.childrenwithdiabetes.com

REFERENCES

American Diabetes Association. (2014). Diabetes care in the school and day care setting. *Diabetes Care, 37*(1), S91–S96.

Anderson, R. M., Hess, G. E., & Hiss, R. G. (1989). The knowledge and attitudes of elementary and high school teachers regarding diabetes. *Diabetes Educator, 15*, 314–318.

Atkinson, M. A., & Eisenbarth, G. S. (2001, July 21). Type 1 diabetes: New perspectives on disease pathogenesis and treatment. *Lancet, 358*, 221–229.

Bradbury, A. J., & Smith, C. S. (1983). An assessment of diabetic knowledge of school-teachers. *Archives of Diseases of Children, 58*, 692–696.

Daneman, D. (1991). When should your child take charge? In *Diabetes Forecast* [pamphlet], 61–66.

Daneman, D., & Frank, M. (1984). Managing intercurrent illness in the child with diabetes. *Clinical Diabetes, 2*, 1–7.

Daneman, D., Frank, M., & Perlman, K. (1999). *When a child has diabetes.* Toronto, ON: Key Porter Books.

Diabetes Control and Complications Trial Research Group. (1993). The effect of intensive treatment of diabetes on the development and progression of long-term complications in insulin-dependent diabetes mellitus. *New England Journal of Medicine, 329*, 977–986.

Gesteland, H. M., & Lindsay, R. N. (1989). Evaluation of two approaches to educating elementary schoolteachers about insulin-dependent diabetes mellitus. *Diabetes Educator, 15*, 510–513.

Glaab, L. A., Brown, R., & Daneman, D. (2005). School attendance in children with type 1 diabetes. *Diabetic Medicine, 22*(4), 421–426.

Gray, D. L., Golden, M. P., & Reiswerg, J. (1991). Diabetes care in schools: Benefits and pitfalls of US Public Law 94-142. *Diabetes Educator, 17*, 33–36.

Haire-Joshu, D. (Ed.) (1992). Management of diabetes mellitus: *Perspectives of care across the life span*. St. Louis, MO: Mosby-Yearbook.

Henderson, G. (1993). A diabetes education service for school personnel: Safety and health for the student with diabetes. *Beta Release, 17*, 20–24.

Pinelli, L., Zaffani, S., Cappa, M., Carboniero, V., Cerutti, F., Cherubini, V., . . . Lorini, R. (2011). The ALBA project: An evaluation of needs, management, fears of Italian young patients with type 1 diabetes in a school setting and an evaluation of parents' and teachers' perceptions. *Pediatric Diabetes, 12*(5), 485–493.

Vanelli, M., Chiari, G., Ghizzoni, L., Costi, G., Giacalone, T., & Chiarelli, F. (1999). Effectiveness of a prevention program for diabetic ketoacidosis in children: An 8-year study in schools and private practices. *Diabetes Care, 22*(1), 7–9.

Vanelli, M., Chiari, G., Lacava, S., & Iovane, B. (2007). Campaign for diabetic ketoacidosis prevention still effective 8 years later. *Diabetes Care, 30*(4), e12.

Vetiska, J., Glaab, L., Perlman, K., & Daneman, D. (2000). School attendance of children with type 1 diabetes. *Diabetes Care, 23*, 1706–1707.

Wherrett, D. K., & Daneman, D. (2011). Prevention of type 1 diabetes. *Pediatric Clinics of North America, 58*(5), 1257–1270.

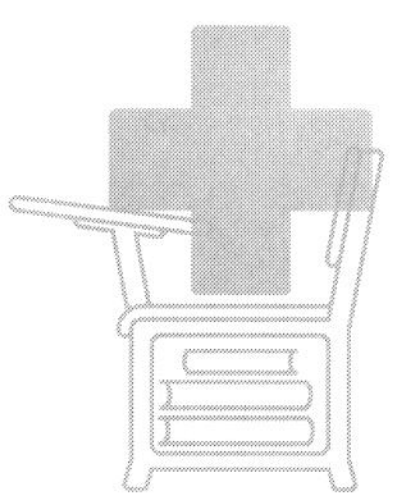

Chapter 9
Hearing Loss and the Classroom Teacher

Vicky Papaioannou

For many years, Deaf and hard-of-hearing children have made up the largest group of students requiring special services in schools (Flexer, Wray, & Ireland, 1989). In addition, most of these students have been mainstreamed into regular classrooms in regular schools. In the past 15 years, universal newborn hearing screening (UNHS) programs have become increasingly common across North America. It is the ultimate intent of these programs to identify children with hearing loss early (usually before 6 months of age) and to allow these children access to the services that will enable them to enter the school system with the same level of communication as their normal-hearing peers. If these goals are realized, it is likely that even more children will be educated in the mainstream. For these children to succeed in this environment, teachers need to be aware of several issues for which a basic understanding of hearing, the consequences of hearing loss, amplification, assistive listening devices, and instructional and classroom management strategies is necessary. What is wonderful about these accommodations is their universal benefit to all students in the classroom and to the teacher as well.

STRUCTURE AND FUNCTION

In describing the structure and function of the auditory system, it is useful to look at the ear in four sections:

1. The *outer ear* includes the ear itself (auricle or pinna) and the ear canal (external auditory canal).

2. The *middle ear* includes the eardrum (tympanic membrane), the three middle-ear bones (ossicles) with their associated muscles and tendons, and the eustachian tube.
3. The *inner ear* contains both the organs of balance and hearing. Only part of the inner ear, the cochlea, belongs to the auditory system.
4. The *central auditory nervous system* includes all the auditory interconnections between, and including, the auditory nerve and the auditory cortex.

OUTER EAR

The external skin flap, the pinna, and the external auditory canal (ear canal) direct sound to the eardrum. There is great variation in terms of pinna shape and size from individual to individual. Functionally, the pinna is important for sound localization, or knowing from where in space a sound originates.

The external auditory canal is an oval tube approximately 2.5 cm or 1 inch in length, ending at the eardrum. The path of the ear canal is generally not straight and varies between individuals. In the canal there are hair follicles and glands that secrete cerumen, commonly referred to as ear wax. The wax helps moisten the skin of the canal and also serves a protective function, which is to keep the ear canal clean. The outer ear structures are illustrated in Figure 9.1.

MIDDLE EAR

This region is a small air-filled cavity within the skull. It begins at the eardrum, the thin, oval-shaped, semitransparent membrane that

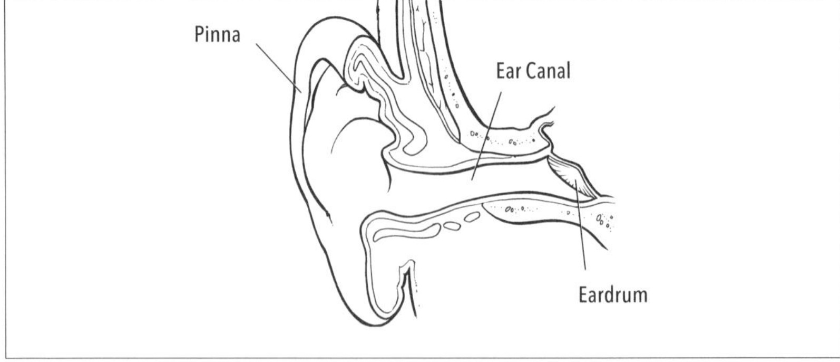

Figure 9.1. The outer ear and tympanic membrane (eardrum).

lies at the end of the ear canal and separates the outer ear from the middle ear.

The middle ear contains the three bones of hearing, the malleus, the incus, and the stapes (more commonly known as the hammer, anvil, and stirrup), which transmit sound from the eardrum to the inner ear. The largest of these bones, the malleus, is attached to the eardrum. The incus is the middle bone and transfers sound vibrations from the malleus to the stapes. The footplate of the stapes, the smallest of the three bones (in fact, the smallest bone in the body), is attached to the cochlea at an area leading to the inner ear known as the oval window.

Two small muscles are found in the middle ear. The tensor tympani is attached to the malleus and functions to tense the eardrum by pulling on the malleus medially. The stapedius muscle is attached to the stapes and serves to prevent excessive movements of this bone by pulling the stapes posteriorly. Together, these muscles provide the ear with some protection from very loud sounds.

The eustachian tube connects the middle ear and the nasopharynx (back of the nose). It functions to equalize pressure on both sides of the eardrum and for drainage of fluid from the middle ear space. Figure 9.2 illustrates the middle ear structures.

INNER EAR

The cochlea is the part of the inner ear that resembles a snail's shell. The cochlea itself is divided into three compartments: the scala vestibuli, scala tympani, and scala media or cochlear duct. The scala vestibuli and scala tympani contain a fluid called perilymph. The

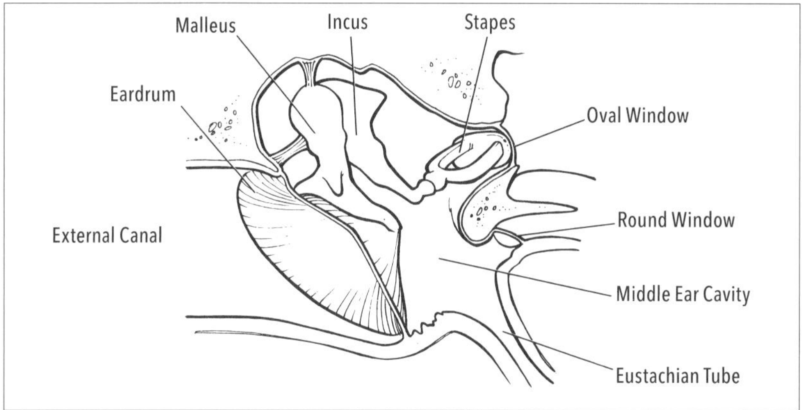

Figure 9.2. The external auditory canal and the middle ear structures.

scala media is found between the two compartments and contains a different fluid called endolymph. Movements of the stapes acting on the oval window transmit sound vibrations from the middle ear to the fluid filled cochlea. A second "window" into the cochlea, the round window, is covered by a thin membrane and allows fluids within the cochlea to move and stimulate the sensory cells of hearing.

The basilar membrane separates the scala media from the scala tympani. Attached to the basilar membrane is the organ of Corti, formed by this group of sensory cells and related supporting structures. This is the actual receptor organ for hearing. The sensory or receptor cells themselves are called hair cells. The structures of the inner ear are shown in Figure 9.3.

CENTRAL AUDITORY NERVOUS SYSTEM

The sensory hair cells connect to nerve fibers that transmit sound information in the form of neural impulses to the central auditory nervous system (CANS). The nerve fibers make up the auditory nerve. Sound information is processed at various levels within the auditory pathway. Our awareness of sound and the recognition of speech is the result of processes at the highest cortical levels. A view of the auditory system up to and including the auditory nerve is illustrated in Figure 9.4.

HOW DOES IT ALL WORK?

To hear, then, the pinna and the ear canal direct the sound to the eardrum. The eardrum vibrates in response to the sound, transferring

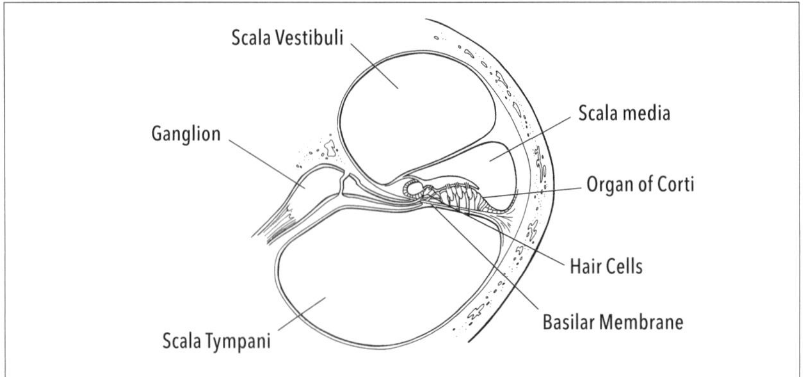

Figure 9.3. The cochlear portion of the inner ear and the auditory nerve.

the sound from the outer ear to the middle ear. In the middle ear, the intensity of the sound is increased as it passes from each middle-ear bone to the next before finally being passed on to the inner ear. These vibrations are changed in the inner ear into nerve impulses, which travel up the auditory nerve to the brain. The brain then translates those impulses into what is perceived as sound.

TYPES OF HEARING LOSS

A hearing loss is present when there is a problem in one or more parts of the auditory system. As described, the system can be divided into different sections. A problem can occur in any one of these areas or in more than one area. This will result in different types of hearing loss as described below.

CONDUCTIVE HEARING LOSS

In a conductive hearing loss, an abnormality exists in the outer or middle ear and causes sound to be reduced in loudness before it reaches the inner ear. This affects the mechanical transfer of sound to the inner ear, which functions normally. This type of loss can often be treated with either medication or surgery. The most common conductive hearing loss seen in young children is caused by otitis media (ear infections causing accumulation of fluid in the middle ear). Other causes include extreme wax buildup, eardrum perforation, small or absent ear canals or pinnas, and ossicular abnormalities. All of these

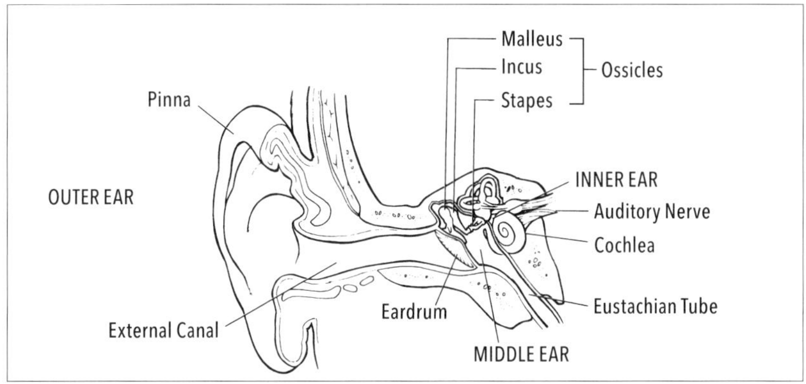

Figure 9.4. The outer, middle, and inner ear structure.

examples hinder the transmission of sound through the external or middle ear and result in a hearing loss. Conductive hearing loss may fluctuate over time and may be temporary (e.g., wax buildup) or may be permanent (e.g., missing ossicles).

SENSORINEURAL HEARING LOSS

In this type of loss, the problem lies in the inner ear or in the transmission of impulses along the auditory nerve. Within the cochlea, the site of damage is often the sensory hair cells. As a result of the hearing loss, not only does the individual notice decreased sensitivity to sound, but there is often a decrease in the clarity of sound as well. Sound may reach the inner ear, but because of damage to the cochlea or auditory nerve, it is not received clearly by the brain, even if it is made sufficiently loud through the use of hearing aids. There is usually no medical or simple surgical treatment for this type of hearing loss and it is, therefore, generally permanent. Potential causes include heredity, exposure to certain drugs, anatomical abnormalities of the cochlea, noise exposure, head injuries, prolonged high fevers, intrauterine cytomegalovirus infection (transplacental infection from mother to fetus), meningitis, mumps, and measles. In many cases, especially when the child is born with the hearing loss, the cause remains unknown.

MIXED HEARING LOSS

A mixed hearing loss is a combination of both a conductive and a sensorineural hearing loss. Often, the conductive component can be treated with medication or surgery, but no treatment is available for the sensorineural component. A child with a sensorineural hearing loss who gets, for example, an ear infection, would have a subsequent mixed hearing loss.

CENTRAL OR CORTICAL HEARING LOSS

Central or cortical hearing loss refers to the inability of the brain to interpret sound information even though the peripheral hearing sensitivity is essentially normal. Hearing aids are not expected to be of benefit in this type hearing loss. Varying degrees of auditory comprehension result. This type of hearing loss is very rare and can be associated with other disease processes, for example, affecting the cortex.

AUDITORY NEUROPATHY SPECTRUM DISORDER

Over the past two decades another disorder has appeared to surface that is often confusing to both parents and professionals. Auditory neuropathy spectrum disorder (ANSD) is not a new disorder, but it has become better defined and recognized with improvements in technology and the increasing prevalence of newborn hearing screening programs worldwide. Children with this disorder present as somewhat of a challenge, as they have some commonly used indicators of normal hearing with some commonly used indicators of hearing loss.

ANSD can occur in isolation or with various other symptoms and conditions (e.g., cerebral palsy), and these can make management even more difficult. In addition, individuals with this disorder often present very differently from one another. For example, there is significant variation in terms of the audiometric thresholds found in individuals with ANSD. Some children have thresholds in the normal hearing range, whereas others fall in the profound hearing loss range. Others have thresholds somewhere in between. Some individuals have hearing thresholds that fluctuate, which make learning language extremely difficult. One relatively consistent finding among these individuals is their difficulty hearing in noisy environments—hence its particular relevance once the child enters school.

ONE EAR OR TWO?

Hearing loss is also referred to as either unilateral or bilateral, depending upon whether one or both ears are affected. In a unilateral hearing loss, there is a hearing loss in one ear and normal hearing in the other. Unlike children with bilateral hearing loss, children with unilateral hearing loss typically hear and respond to conversational-level speech and to environmental sounds and demonstrate relatively normal speech and language development. Before universal newborn hearing screening, the average age at which a child with a unilateral hearing loss was identified was later than that of a child with a bilateral hearing loss. Thus, many of these children were not identified until they were in school. Universal newborn hearing screening has changed this somewhat, but it is still not uncommon for children to be identified with a unilateral hearing loss once they reach school. Individuals with unilateral hearing loss find sound localization extremely difficult. That is, they have problems determining where a sound originates. These children also have difficulty hearing in noisy environments. These are important considerations for a child in the mainstream classroom. Many of the educational implications for children with bilateral hearing loss apply to a child with a unilateral hearing loss as well.

COMMON CAUSES OF HEARING LOSS

As we have discussed, there are many different types of hearing loss caused by all different mechanisms. Hearing loss present from birth is called congenital hearing loss. Many congenital hearing losses are thought to be genetic. With advances in genetic testing, many genes responsible for hearing loss have been identified.

Other hearing losses develop after birth. These are called acquired hearing losses. These too could be genetic, but they could also be caused by different diseases or infections such as meningitis or mumps.

As we age, we know that our vision gets worse and that our hearing does too. Hearing loss due to aging is called presbycusis. Noise exposure can cause hearing loss and is seen more frequently in younger and younger individuals, perhaps in relation to the increased use of personal listening equipment, such as MP3 players.

Even a cold can cause a hearing loss, although this would tend to be temporary. In the classroom environment, even this slight temporary hearing loss can have an impact on student learning.

CLASSIFICATIONS OF HEARING LOSS

There are individuals with a wide range of hearing abilities between those deemed to have "normal hearing" and those who have very little or no ability to hear. The term "culturally Deaf" is usually reserved for individuals who identify with and participate in the language, culture, and community of Deaf people, based on a signed language such as American Sign Language (ASL), regardless of their degree or type of hearing loss. For those children who use their residual hearing to learn speech and language and who use spoken language at least some of the time, the term "hard of hearing" is generally used.

HEARING ASSESSMENT

The sounds that we are able to hear can be measured by pitch (frequency) and loudness (intensity). Humans have the ability to hear sounds as low in frequency as 20 hertz (Hz) and as high in frequency as 20000 Hz. The current practice in audiology is to measure hearing in the range of 250 Hz to 8000 Hz, as most speech sounds are found in this range. Intensity is measured in decibels (dB), which are expressed in reference to normal hearing (dB HL). Sounds can be presented at very quiet levels (0 dB HL) or at very loud levels (120 dB HL). Conversational speech occurs at approximately 50 dB HL.

The audiogram is a graph illustrating the softest sound that an individual can hear (their threshold) at various frequencies. It shows frequency along the horizontal axis and intensity along the vertical axis. Figure 9.5 illustrates an audiogram of an individual with normal hearing. Information below the threshold line is audible, whereas sounds above the line cannot be heard. Because the decibel scale is logarithmic, hearing loss cannot be expressed in terms of a percentage. Instead, hearing loss is described in terms of severity, as listed in Table 9.1.

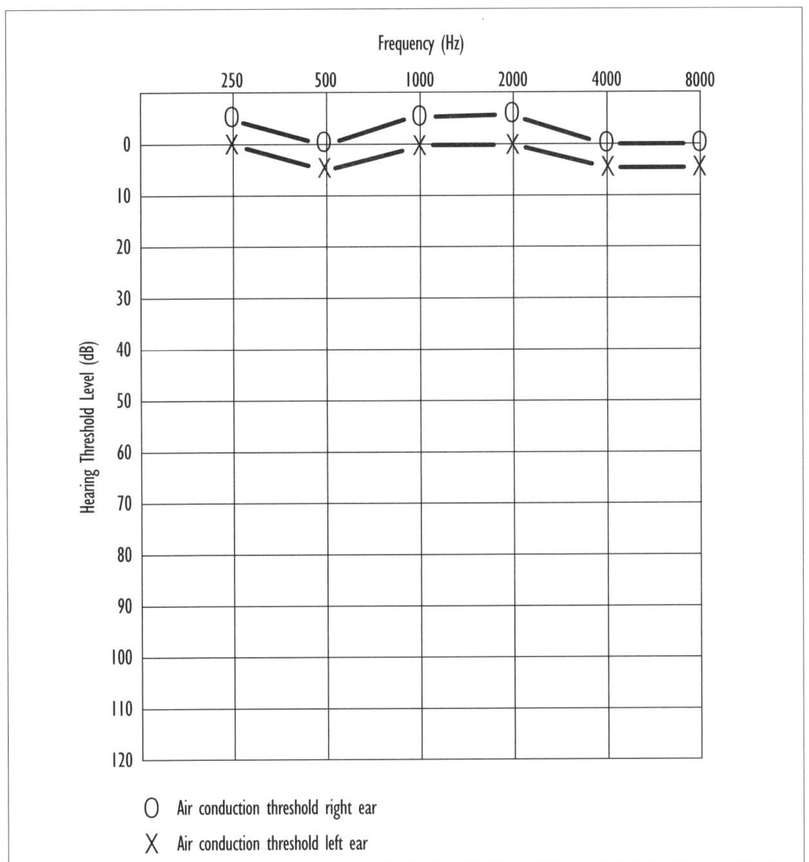

Figure 9.5. Characteristic pure-tone audiogram of an individual with normal hearing.

Table 9.1
CLASSIFICATION AND IMPLICATIONS OF HEARING LOSS

Average hearing threshold in dB HL[a]	Classification	Implications
-10 to 15	Normal hearing	The child is able to detect speech even at very soft levels
16 to 25	Slight or minimal hearing loss	Some children will experience difficulty with quiet or distant speech, especially if the classroom is noisy. Speech and/or language development may be affected.
26 to 40	Mild hearing loss	The child will miss some of the speech signal. Difficulty increases with distance from the teacher and background noise levels. Speech and/or language development will likely be affected. Hearing aids will likely be necessary.
41 to 55	Moderate hearing loss	The child will be able to hear and understand speech only at very close range without amplification. Speech and language development will likely be affected. The child requires hearing aids.
56 to 70	Moderately severe hearing loss	The child will only be able to *detect* speech without hearing aids and only at very close range. Speech and language development will be delayed. The child requires hearing aids.
71 to 90	Severe hearing loss	The child is able to detect loud environmental sounds, but not conversational speech. The child requires hearing aids for speech and language development. Sign language would be an alternative mode of communication.
91+	Profound hearing loss	The child is likely aware of vibrations more than sounds. The child may or may not receive benefit from traditional hearing aids. Hearing aids or a cochlear implant would be required if oral communication is desired. Sign language would be an alternative mode of communication.

[a]The average pure-tone air conduction threshold of 500 Hz, 1000 Hz, and 2000 Hz.

An audiologist administers a variety of tests in a soundproof booth that depend upon the child's age and ability. No child is too young to have his or her hearing tested. Assessment methods vary depending on the child's age or developmental ability.

Hearing loss is ideally detected long before the child reaches school. With universal newborn hearing screening, this should be the norm. Unfortunately, this is not always the case. For a wide variety of reasons, a child may slip through the cracks and a hearing loss may go unnoticed. The child may have acquired the hearing loss later in life or perhaps the child has come from an environment where identification or management of hearing loss is unavailable. Once a child enters the school system, it is the teacher who interacts with that child more than any other professional. Identification of hearing loss may be tricky, as its presentation can vary greatly from child to child. Factors such as type, degree, and duration of the hearing loss, etiology of the hearing loss, and even the child's intelligence may affect how the child responds to his or her hearing difficulty. A list of behaviors a teacher may notice in a child with a hearing problem is found in Table 9.2. If a student exhibits any signs of hearing loss, it is essential to determine whether or not a hearing loss exists. A number of options are available to the teacher, and several are listed in Table 9.3.

AUDIOLOGICAL (RE)HABILITATION

Once a child's hearing difficulty has been identified and it has been determined that nothing can be done medically or surgically to restore the hearing to "normal," the child will likely be fitted with one or two hearing aids depending upon whether one or both ears are equally affected. Hearing aids simply make sound louder at those pitches at which the child cannot hear the sounds at a normal level. An audiologist will usually prescribe the hearing aids and will choose them on the basis of the child's hearing loss, lifestyle, educational environment, and family and personal preferences.

All hearing aids consist of three main components: a microphone, an amplifier, and a receiver. Very basically, the microphone receives the sound into the hearing aid. The amplifier makes it louder, and the receiver directs the sound from the hearing aid into the ear via the earmold or earpiece. Other components that may be found on the hearing aid are an on/off and "T" switch, as well as a volume control, although this varies with the type of hearing aid. The T switch activates the hearing aid's telecoil and may be used when the child uses a compatible

Table 9.2

SIGNS OF HEARING LOSS THAT TEACHERS MAY OBSERVE

Demonstrates signs of inattentiveness
Appears to daydream frequently
Demonstrates signs of frustration
Has frequent colds and earaches
Often fails to respond to his or her name when it is called
Often requests repetition of what was said
Appears confused while the teacher is providing instructions
Engages in inappropriate behaviors, even when given very precise instructions
Watches what other children do and then imitates their actions
Responds inappropriately to questions
Speaks either very quietly or very loudly
Has articulation errors, especially with high-frequency sounds like *s, z, t, k*, and *f*.
Appears fatigued before the day is through
Watches the speaker's facial expressions and lip movements more than other children do
Shows an inability to hear in group situations or in noisy environments
Cannot locate a sound source and struggles to follow the speaker in a group conversation, especially when the child cannot see the speaker
Directs one ear toward the speaker in an attempt to hear better
Withdraws from the group, often preferring to work or play alone
Prefers to interact with younger children, who often accept the child more readily

telephone or an FM system. Hearing aids, of course, need a power source; different types and models use different sizes of batteries.

With increasing advances in technology, hearing-aid choices seem endless. Not all hearing aids are the same, and they need to be perfectly tuned to the hearing levels of the individual child.

Table 9.3

STRATEGIES AVAILABLE TO TEACHERS ONCE A HEARING LOSS IS SUSPECTED

Examine the student's records for previous evidence of hearing loss, including hearing test results.
Consult with the principal, school nurse, speech–language pathologist, or educational audiologist, discussing your concerns and what to do about them.
Contact the child's parents to discuss your observations.
Suggest to the child's parents that the student's hearing be checked, recommending an audiological assessment through the child's physician.
If the student is old enough, discuss the suspected hearing difficulties with him or her.

In general, there are two basic styles of hearing aids:

1. *Custom hearing aids*, which include in-the-ear (ITE), in-the-canal (ITC), and completely-in-the-canal (CIC) hearing aids—these hearing aids are housed entirely within an individual's ear. In general, ITC hearing aids are prescribed for mild to moderately severe hearing losses, whereas ITE and CIC hearing aids are prescribed for mild to severe hearing losses.
2. *Behind-the-ear (BTE) hearing aids*, which include hearing aids like open-fit hearing aids, receiver-in-the-canal (RIC) hearing aids, and receiver-in-the-ear (RITE) hearing aids, as well as the more traditional behind-the-ear (BTE) hearing aid worn with a custom made earmold—these hearing aids have a component that sits behind the pinna and a component that delivers the sound into the ear, which sits in the ear canal. In general, a true open-fit hearing aid could be used for a mild or moderate hearing loss or a high-frequency hearing loss. RIC or RITE hearing aids can be fit to hearing losses ranging in degree from mild to perhaps severe. Traditional behind-the-ear hearing aids with an earmold can be used for any degree of hearing loss. Examples of commonly used hearing aids are illustrated in Figure 9.6.

Behind-the-ear hearing aids are often preferred for children for several reasons. The earmold material prescribed for children should be soft so that during the rough-and-tumble activities of childhood,

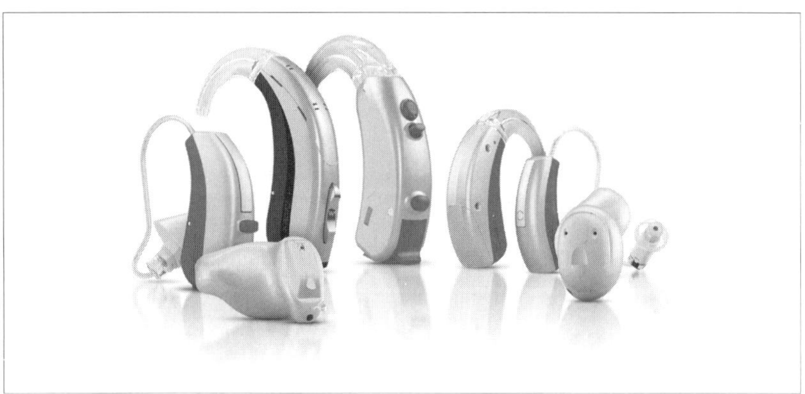

Figure 9.6. Custom and behind-the-ear (BTE) hearing aids, provided by Widex Canada, Burlington, ON.

the child is not hurt by a blow to the head or to the ear. An earmold made of a hard material or a custom hearing aid could cause significant discomfort to the child in such a situation. Retention is also an important factor, and BTE hearing aids with custom earmolds often stay in place better than other hearing devices. Durability is also extremely important for children, as their hearing aids need to be able to withstand much more than the hearing aid of a more sedate adult. Hearing aids that have been knocked off, dropped, or chewed by the family pet are seen much more often for children than for adults. Furthermore, for BTE hearing aids with custom earmolds, the earmolds themselves can be easily replaced as the child grows, much more quickly and easily, and often at a lesser expense, than recasing a custom hearing aid. Growing children may need to have their earmolds replaced as often as every three months. A sign that the child needs a new earmold, or needs his or her custom hearing aid recased, is a squealing noise (called feedback) coming from the hearing aid when the child is wearing the hearing aid at its usual volume.

Another advantage of BTE hearing aids is their compatibility with various assistive listening devices. This compatibility is especially important in an educational environment, and it is discussed later in the chapter.

SURGICAL IMPLANTATION

Today there are more surgically implanted "hearing aids" than ever before. All involve an external sound processor programmed by an audiologist that works with the internal components implanted by the surgeon.

Bone-Anchored Hearing Aid

The internal part of a bone-anchored hearing aid is placed surgically in the bone above and behind the pinna. The external hearing aid or sound processor is worn on the corresponding site on the skin. The hearing aid is attached to the internal component via a small coupling (abutment) that goes through the skin. Newer technology allows for the sound processor to be attached to the head with a magnet. Bone-anchored hearing aids have traditionally been provided to children with conductive hearing loss, although they have more recently been marketed to individuals with single-sided deafness (SSD), which is also known as profound unilateral hearing loss. For children with absent pinnas and/or external auditory canals or children with chronically draining ears due to ear infections, it is often a welcome surgical intervention (see Figure 9.7).

If a child or family is averse to the idea of surgery, the external sound processor can be used on a headband, which allows the child to use the device without having surgery. Alternatively, a more traditional bone conduction hearing aid could be used. This hearing aid delivers sound to a vibrator, usually placed on the mastoid bone behind the ear and held in place either using a headband or double-sided tape. The sound vibrations are transmitted through the skull and to the inner ear, thus allowing the child to hear. Many children who are candidates for bone-anchored hearing aids first undergo a trial with a traditional bone conduction hearing aid or with the external sound processor worn on a headband.

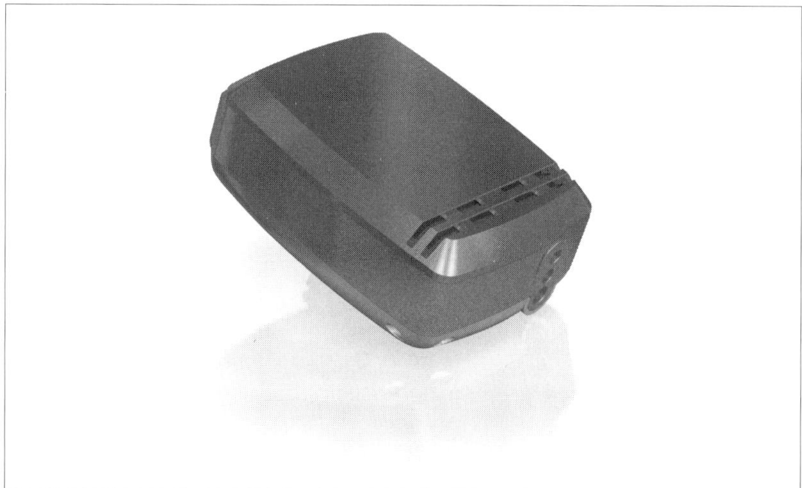

Figure 9.7. Bone-anchored hearing aid, provided by Cochlear Americas, Centennial, CO.

Cochlear Implant

A cochlear implant is a device that may be used for children who receive little or no benefit from hearing aids or for whom hearing aids do not allow sufficient access to spoken language. The cochlear implant does *not* restore normal hearing. In fact, the child "hears" in an entirely different manner. A microphone contained in the external processor picks up the speech signal. It then codes the signal and sends it to the transmitter coil. The coil is attached to the child's scalp with a magnet. The signal is transmitted across the scalp via a radio signal to the internal receiver, which is implanted in the mastoid bone behind the ear. This component receives this signal and sends it to the electrode array surgically implanted within the cochlea. Parts of the cochlear implant are seen in Figure 9.8.

OTHER ASSISTIVE LISTENING DEVICES

Unfortunately, hearing aids are generally not sufficient for a child with hearing loss to hear well in the poor listening conditions found in most classrooms. Anyone who has worn a hearing aid will tell you about the poor performance of many of these instruments in conditions with an abundance of background noise. This is because hearing aids generally amplify all sounds. They cannot differentiate between what the child wants to hear and what is "noise." To deal with the effects of background noise, reverberation or "echo," and the child's physical

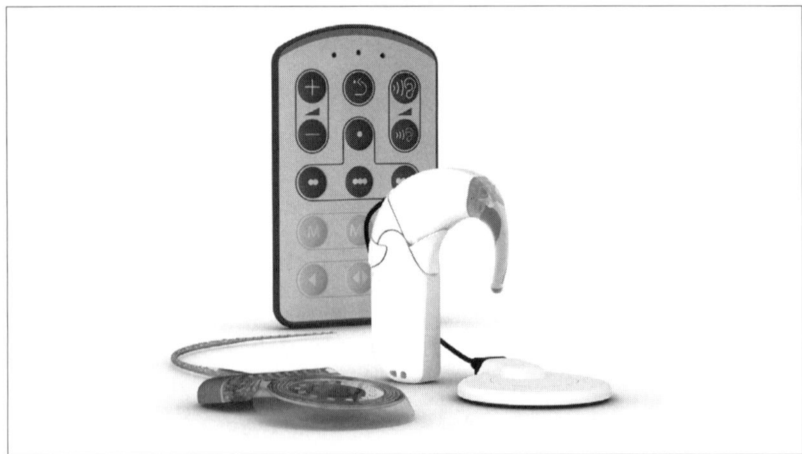

Figure 9.8. Behind-the-ear processor, including transmitter coil with internal receiver and electrode array as well as remote control, provided by MED EL Canada, Toronto, ON.

distance away from the person speaking—all of which are common in classrooms—a child may require more than personal hearing aids and/or preferential seating.

Background noise, reverberation, and distance all affect the signal-to-noise ratio (S/N). This is the relationship between the sound that the student wants to hear (signal) and all the other sounds present in the listening environment (noise). A person with difficulty hearing, whether wearing a hearing aid or not, needs a more positive S/N in order to understand speech than does a person without hearing loss. For those with normal hearing, speech is easily accessible as long as the speech signal is twice as loud as sounds in the background. For students who have difficulty hearing, speech needs to be almost ten times as loud as the background sounds to be perceived as intelligible (Flexer et al., 1989). This S/N ratio is often not possible in the classroom without the use of assistive listening devices.

A frequency modulated (FM) system is one type of assistive listening device commonly used in school settings. To envision how it works, think of a radio station. The teacher has a microphone worn close to his or her mouth. This serves to prevent the decrease in the speech signal as it travels from the teacher's mouth to the child's ear or hearing aid. The teacher's microphone may be attached to the FM transmitter via a wire or the microphone may be built into the transmitter as a single unit. The teacher's message is transformed into an electrical signal by the microphone. The transmitter, in turn, superimposes this signal onto a radio signal that is then transmitted into the child's FM receiver. Thus, using the radio analogy, the teacher would be similar to the announcer at a radio station speaking into the microphone. The student would be the radio listener tuned into the teacher's station. With this "direct connection," the effects of student distance from the teacher, background noise, and reverberation are all minimized. The student and teacher are not connected by wires and have free range of movement up to approximately 200 feet (Flexer et al., 1989). Figure 9.9 illustrates a teacher-worn FM transmitter and microphone.

PERSONAL FM EQUIPMENT

The FM signal can travel from the child's FM receiver to his or her ear in many different ways. Each has its advantages and disadvantages for the child within the classroom environment. There is not one solution that is best for all children, and many factors need to be considered before deciding on which one should be used for a given student.

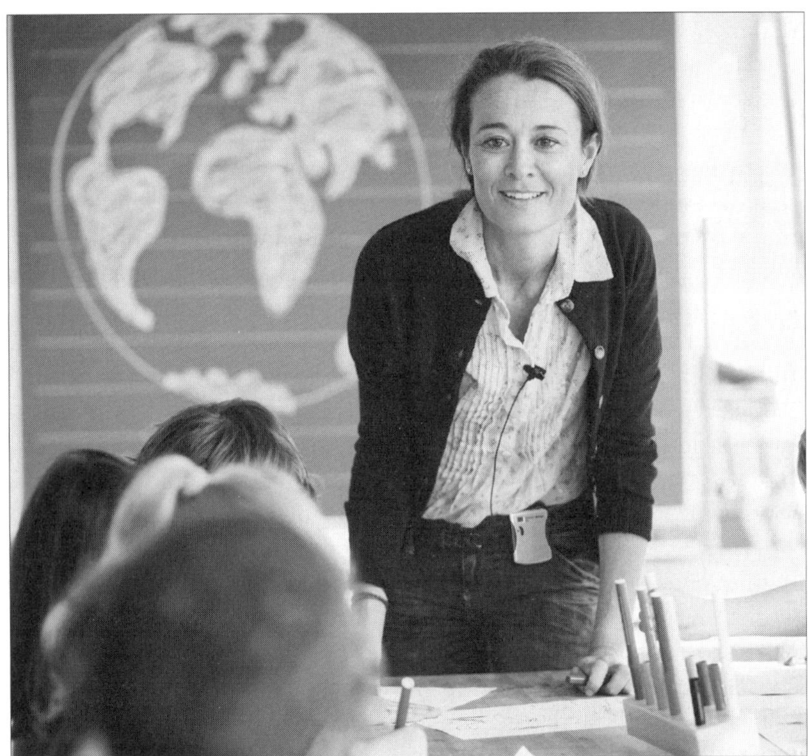

Figure 9.9. FM transmitter with microphone, provided by Oticon Canada, Mississauga, ON.

Direct audio input to the child's hearing aids applies mainly to traditional behind-the-ear hearing aids. A miniature FM receiver is built into an audio "shoe" or adaptor that fits over the bottom portion of the hearing aid and is powered by the battery of the child's hearing aid. The audio shoe can be removable or it can be more permanently integrated with the child's hearing aid. The sound reaches the child's ears through the child's own hearing aids and earmolds (see Figure 9.10).

A neckloop is a special strand of thick wire worn around the student's neck like a lanyard. The electrical signal from the FM receiver is delivered to the loop. The electrical current flowing through this loop creates a small magnetic field. The signal is picked up when the student's hearing aids are switched to the "T" (telecoil) position. The signal is converted back to sound and is delivered to the child through the hearing aids (see Figure 9.11).

A silhouette inductor arrangement or an inductive earhook operate similarly to the neckloop. The difference between the two lies in the device generating the magnetic field. With this arrangement,

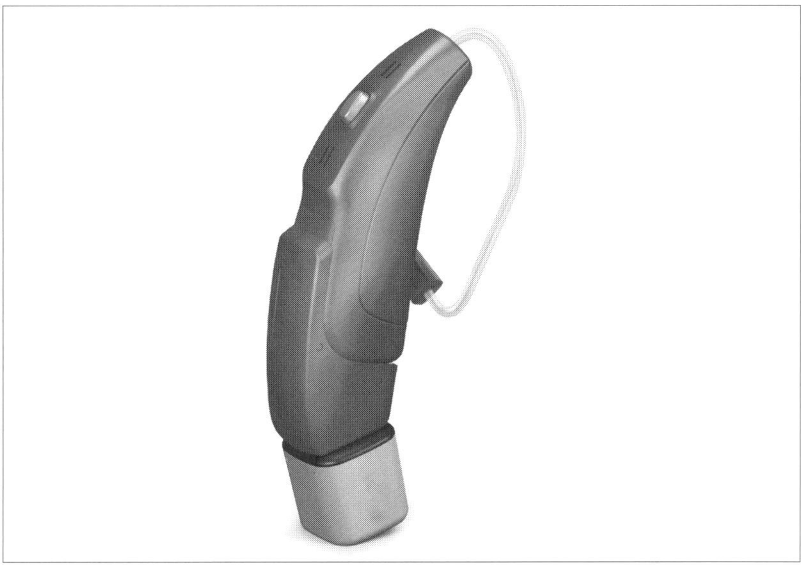

Figure 9.10. FM receiver attached to receiver in the canal (RIC) hearing aid, provided by Phonak, Mississauga, ON.

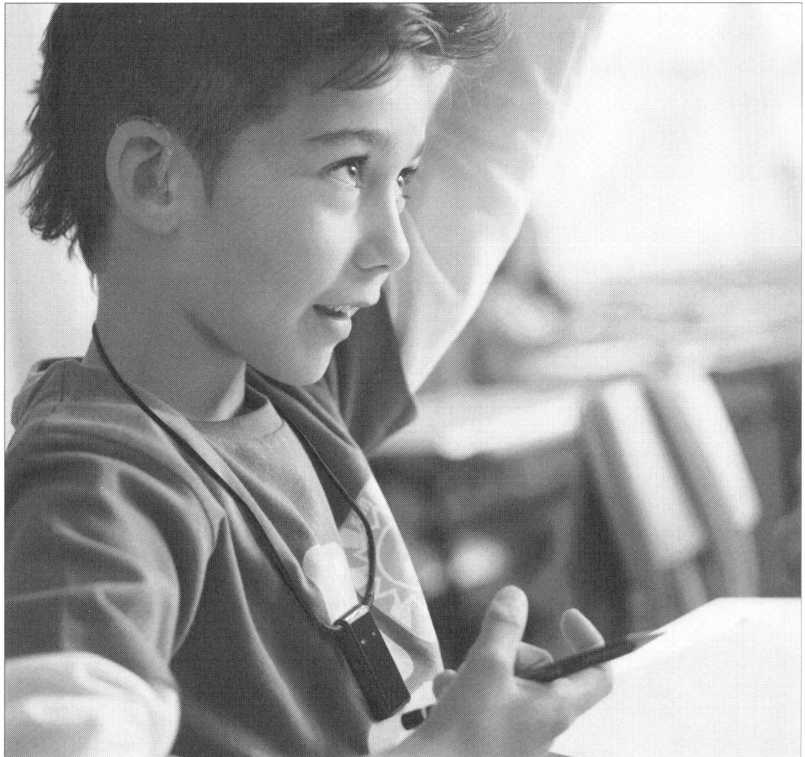

Figure 9.11. Neckloop FM receiver, provided by Oticon Canada, Mississauga, ON.

the magnetic field is created in a thin structure often resembling the shape of the behind-the-ear hearing aid itself. It is worn between the head and the hearing aids, and the student's hearing aids operate in the "T" position. The sound is again delivered to the child through the hearing aids.

An FM system can also deliver the signal to the child's ear using headphones of some sort if the child does not wear hearing aids. This arrangement looks similar to what many children are wearing for music listening or video gaming and, thus, may be more readily accepted by some children and by their peers. Unfortunately, many students find this arrangement uncomfortable when worn for extended periods of time.

The behind-the-ear FM system is another convenient alternative for children who do not wear hearing aids. For children with slight or mild hearing loss, fluctuating hearing loss, unilateral hearing loss, auditory neuropathy spectrum disorder, attention-deficit disorder, or central auditory processing disorders who do not wear hearing aids, a miniature behind-the-ear FM receiver exists (see Figure 9.12). This is worn in one or both ears just like other behind-the-ear devices.

It is important to remember that FM systems are not only for use when the teacher is talking. A pass-around microphone can be used by teaching assistants, classroom volunteers, and other students in the class. The FM system can also be connected to other sound sources, such as the television, computer, or MP3 player. Any device that the student needs to hear should be connected in one way or another to the FM system.

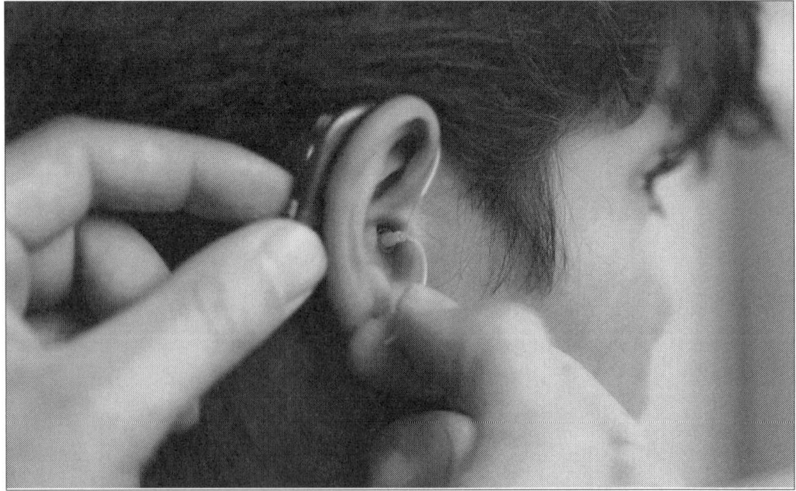

Figure 9.12. Behind-the-ear FM receiver, provided by Oticon Canada, Mississauga, ON.

SOUNDFIELD FM EQUIPMENT

A free-field or soundfield FM system works on the same premise as the personal FM system. The teacher speaks into a microphone that is worn close to the mouth. This is attached to an FM transmitter that sends the signal to a speaker or speakers strategically positioned in the classroom (see Figure 9.13). Soundfield FM systems facilitate the reception of the teacher's voice for all students. For example, children with unilateral hearing losses, fluctuating hearing losses, attentional difficulties, learning disabilities, articulation disorders, and developmental delays may all receive benefit from this device, as may children who are learning English as their second language. This may allow for more effective classroom instruction and management given the positive effects on student attention and engagement. Potential teacher benefits include decreased vocal strain (Rosenberg et al., 1999), decreased fatigue, and reduced stress.

TOTABLE FM SYSTEM

Basically, a totable FM system works in the same manner as a free-field or soundfield FM system. Rather than transmitting speech to strategically positioned speakers, however, the sound is transmitted to a small speaker, which is usually placed on the child's desk or table.

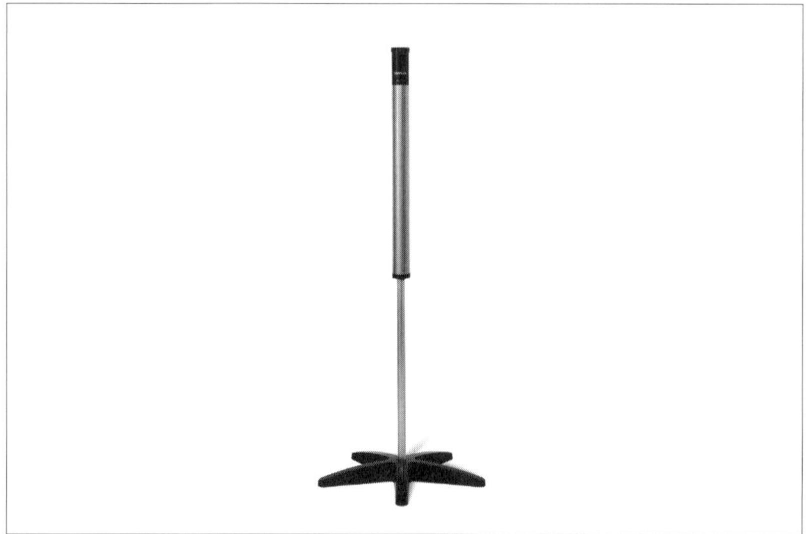

Figure 9.13. FM speaker with floor stand provided by Phonak Canada, Mississauga, ON.

In this way, the child can take the system to more than one location, which is not possible with a soundfield system (see Figure 9.14).

IN THE CLASSROOM

Daily Devices Check

Hearing aids and FM systems, like any pieces of electronic equipment, can malfunction. Given that much of a child's school day requires listening, these devices should be checked each morning before the child begins his or her day. At a relatively young age, most children can be responsible for at least some components of the daily check.

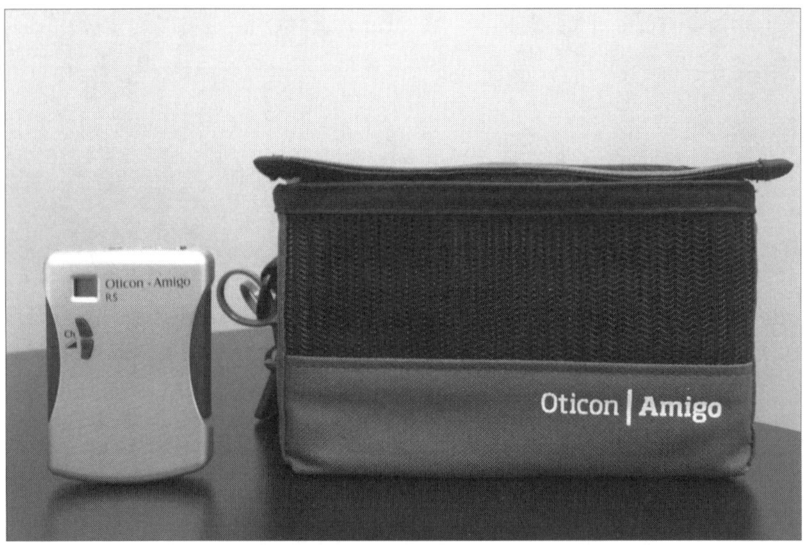

Figure 9.14. Totable FM receiver provided by Oticon Canada, Mississauga, ON.

Table 9.4
TEACHER TOOL KIT

Spare batteries
Battery tester
Listening tube or stethoscope
Hearing-aid dehumidifier
Hearing-aid air blower

Table 9.4 lists some things the teacher may find beneficial to have on hand, which would usually be provided by the parent. Table 9.5 lists the components of a daily hearing-aid check. This may be done by the teacher, educational assistant, a volunteer, or even a "hearing buddy."

FM systems must be monitored on a daily basis as well. Their benefit is minimized and they may actually hinder the child's performance if they are not working properly. Different types of FM systems require different test methods. Some ideas for ensuring that these systems are working properly are presented in Table 9.6.

MANAGEMENT STRATEGIES

Communication can be extremely challenging for culturally Deaf and hard-of-hearing students. Whether the student is using an interpreter, has an FM system with or without hearing aids, or uses hearing aids alone, listening for learning is difficult and tedious work. The student must concentrate intently and, because of this, may tire more easily than his or her hearing peers. It is important for the classroom teacher to be

Table 9.5

COMPONENTS OF A DAILY HEARING-AID CHECK

1. Test the hearing-aid battery with a battery tester. Replace the battery if dead or dying. (Parents should provide extras to keep at school.)
2. Visually check the device and earmold for cracks, dents, moisture, broken parts, or wax buildup.
3. Attach each hearing aid to the listening stethoscope. While speaking into the microphone repeat the sounds *oo, ah, ee, sh, s,* and *m*. This is called the Ling Six-Sound Test and will give an indication of the clarity of speech through the hearing aid. Consider the following: Does the hearing aid seem as loud as it usually is? Does the hearing aid sound as clear as it usually does?

   If the hearing aid has an active volume control, turn the volume up and down and listen for static, crackling, distortion, or intermittency. Return the volume to its original setting. If there are no numeric indicators, turn the hearing aid off and back on to get it back to the original volume setting. For some hearing aids, this may mean opening and closing the battery door.

   Send a note home to the parents if any step is eventful. It is even important for parents to know when a hearing-aid battery has been replaced, as some parents keep track of this.

Table 9.6
STRATEGIES FOR A DAILY FM SYSTEM CHECK

1. Different FM systems are powered differently. Check the power source daily and replace or recharge as necessary.
2. Check that both transmitter and receiver are on the same frequency, if this applies to your FM type. This is especially important if there is more than one FM system in a class or if the child travels from class to class with the FM system.
3. Ensure that the FM microphone is plugged into the correct port on the transmitter, if this applies to your FM type.
4. Connect the student's FM receiver to the hearing aids if they are not already permanently connected.
5. Set any FM controls either on the FM itself or on the hearing aid(s) (e.g., volume, on-off, T-switch) appropriately.
6. Engage the child in a listening activity that he or she can perform consistently. This should be something the child can do while wearing hearing aids in a quiet environment and sitting close to you. Carry out the same activity from a distance while wearing the transmitter and with the child wearing the FM to determine whether the signal is transmitting. The child can repeat words or sounds, or raise his or her hand when he or she hears a sound.

   If the child is not able to do this reliably, the microphone and the transmitter can be left close to a radio or with another student (or teacher or assistant), and the teacher can attach the child's hearing aids (which are already attached to the FM system) to a listening stethoscope to ensure that the FM system is transmitting properly.
7. For soundfield (and totable) systems, each speaker should be checked to ensure that it is functioning. This can be done by standing close to the speaker and listening to what is being transmitted.

aware of this and to make every attempt to arrange the lesson schedule such that it allows the student time to rest and rejuvenate so that he or she may continue for the entire day. Periods in which the student is not required to focus his or her attention on listening are imperative.

There are numerous strategies available to teachers that will help their culturally Deaf and hard-of-hearing students. Many of these will be beneficial not only to the aforementioned student but to all the other students in the classroom as well. Teachers themselves are also likely to enjoy the benefits following their implementation. With time and experience, many will become second nature. Most will benefit all students and the teacher as well. Several suggestions are discussed in the following section.

THE CLASSROOM ENVIRONMENT

When deciding on a child's classroom placement, traditional enclosed classrooms are preferred over those that are open concept. A classroom that is free from unnecessary noises and reverberation offers an environment that is conducive to both teaching and learning. It is beneficial for all students in the class and limits vocal strain for the teacher as well.

Minimize Reverberation

The noise or "echo," called reverberation, found in classrooms with an abundance of hard, flat surfaces needs to be minimized. The fewer hard surfaces in the classroom, the better. This includes the floor. A carpeted floor is one solution. If this is not feasible, throw rugs or area rugs will be helpful. In the event that carpet or rugs are not options at all, felt sliding pads or tennis balls placed on the legs of tables and chairs also reduce noise. Acoustic tile on the ceiling and absorbent material on the walls will reduce reverberation and absorb room noise too. Absorbent material can include the children's artwork displayed on the walls or a corkboard or bulletin board covering the walls. Long strips of felt can be hung on the walls. Students can even attach their artwork to these. To further reduce reverberant noise, teachers could teach with the curtains pulled shut to reduce the reflection of sound from the glass of the windows.

Maximize Lighting

Proper lighting in the classroom is imperative. Again, this is something that will be of benefit to all students. A shadow on the teacher's face makes speechreading extremely difficult. Light that shines from above and in front of the teacher's face is best to avoid shadows. Closing the curtains, as discussed earlier, also potentially reduces glare, which can negatively affect speechreading.

Minimize Extraneous Noise

There is enough noise in an average classroom without adding unnecessary sound sources. Ensure that equipment that is not in use is turned off. Computers, projectors, televisions, radios, and fans need to be off when not in use. Even though the hum of a single piece of equipment may seem harmless, the cumulative effect of several can be astounding. Buzzing or flickering lights will affect a student's ability to speechread and contribute unwanted extra noise to the classroom.

Open windows also increase noise in the classroom. Traffic noise from the street is extremely distracting to all students and an unwelcome noise source. If windows are the only sources of ventilation and must be left open, minimize external noise by ensuring that there is outdoor landscaping outside the windows such as hedges, trees, and earth mounds or solid fences as much as possible.

Classroom doors should be closed when teaching. Hallway noise or noise from the gymnasium, auditorium, cafeteria, or main office will again distract all students and create unwanted extra noise in the classroom.

Seating

Older children who are culturally Deaf or hard of hearing may have discovered the seating arrangement that works best for them. If this is the case, the teacher should allow the student to choose his or her own seat. In general, optimal seating is closest to where the teacher is speaking or the interpreter is translating. If the child has a better ear, this ear should be closest to and facing the teacher. It is important that the student is able to view the speaker's or interpreter's face. The view should be unobstructed, so that the child is not constantly fidgeting to get a better view. Culturally Deaf and hard-of-hearing students should be permitted to turn around in their seat to view classmates during group discussions. Furthermore, it is often a good idea to allow older students the freedom to change seats if the change allows them better access to the sound source.

If the classroom is arranged for learning centers or group discussions, the culturally Deaf or hard-of-hearing individual will function better if seated at a round table rather than one that is rectangular. At a round table the student has good visual access to all others seated at the table. This is not the case at a rectangular table. Circular or semicircular seating arrangements, in general, offer students who are culturally Deaf or hard of hearing the best advantage for seeing all class participants.

The student should be seated away from high-traffic areas, such as hallways, the entrance to the classroom, the route to the pencil sharpener, or any other such areas. He or she should not be seated near noise sources in the classroom such as fans, radiators, and aquariums, if at all possible. If there is a soundfield FM system in the classroom, a seat in close proximity to a speaker is ideal.

Teaching Strategies

The culturally Deaf or hard-of-hearing student needs access to the complete auditory and visual signal. Because of this, it is even more important with these students that the teacher face the class while speaking. Speaking while writing on the board is not recommended, nor is giving instructions while the lights are off during a video or computer presentation.

Keep instructions brief and uncomplicated. This will facilitate optimal comprehension for all students. Difficult concepts, in contrast, may benefit from being explained or demonstrated in multiple ways, including by leveraging visual and kinesthetic instructional strategies. This allows students several attempts at understanding what is presented.

Another difficult situation for the student is attempting to speechread a moving target. The teacher should try to avoid walking around the room while speaking. Speechreading an individual who is standing still is difficult enough. It is also important for teachers to keep their hands away from their face while speaking as this can obstruct the student's view. Chewing gum, drinking, or eating while teaching will also negatively affect student comprehension.

When talking to a culturally Deaf or hard-of-hearing student, it is not necessary to speak very slowly or to use exaggerated lip movements or an overly loud voice. In fact, all of those make speechreading and comprehension more difficult. It is best to use the same articulation patterns and vocal intensity that one would with anyone else. Speak clearly and at a reasonable and natural pace. The student's peers should be made aware of this as well.

A common complaint of teachers is that their culturally Deaf or hard-of-hearing student does not pay attention. In an attempt to prevent this, it is suggested that the teacher obtain the student's attention before beginning a lesson or giving instructions. It is not necessary to always call the individual's name to get his or her attention. Nonverbal cues such as gently touching or tapping the student or turning the lights quickly on and off could be used. This would help ensure that the culturally Deaf or hard-of-hearing student is not always the one singled out and could help other students to focus as well.

In classroom discussions, the teacher should encourage class members to wait until the culturally Deaf or hard-of-hearing student has made eye contact before beginning to speak. The teacher can facilitate this by identifying the student by name that is about to respond or to ask a question, as well as by pointing out this individual. It would also be beneficial for the teacher to restate or rephrase the comments and questions of other students as soon as the particular student has finished speaking. This will provide clarity in the event that all or part of the message was missed. A talking stick can be a useful teaching strategy. Use of a talking stick is based on the premise that the only individual who will be talking is the one with the stick. The FM microphone can be a convenient and student-appealing alternative. This teaches all of the students to only have one person speaking at a time and allows the culturally Deaf or hard-of-hearing student a visual cue to determine who is the current speaker.

Comprehension checks are also important for culturally Deaf or hard-of-hearing students as they allow the teacher to recognize when the student has been unable to follow the lesson. These can be overt, such as asking the student to restate a key point, or subtler, such as the teacher making eye contact with the student and the student nodding. Having the student paraphrase information is preferred to asking the student a question requiring a yes or no answer, but more subtle comprehension checks are often important for older students who do not want to stand out from the rest of the class. The teacher and the student can discuss these in advance. If the student is having difficulty understanding something, rather than simply repeating what was just said, it may sometimes be helpful for the teacher to restate the information in a different way.

The use of visual aids and visual information to complement lessons and announcements can greatly enhance comprehension for all students. Material that is presented auditorily is short-lived and requires immediate processing. Visually presented material by its very nature lasts longer and can be referred to even after the lesson is over. Key words and summaries can be written on flip charts, the blackboard, whiteboard, or Smart Board. Names of people and places, dates, page numbers, and new vocabulary will be especially difficult for culturally Deaf and hard-of-hearing individuals. Diagrams, illustrations, photographs, and charts should be used as much as possible as visual reinforcement of concepts presented auditorily and will again benefit all students in the classroom. Handouts will accomplish the same thing. PowerPoint presentations allow for a visual representation of the auditory message that is accessible to all students and can be made available by handouts or online. Ensure that closed-captioning is used for all videos presented in class.

Pre-teaching or pre-tutoring is often desirable with culturally Deaf and hard-of-hearing students. The day before a planned lesson, new words and concepts can be given to the student to investigate as part of the homework. As well, the child can practice these words at home with family members or in the mirror to become familiar with the lip movements required for each word. The student will be able to follow the lesson more easily because of his or her familiarity with the material. Comprehension and learning will be enhanced.

Post-teaching or post-tutoring can serve as a review of important lessons, consolidating the learning. In this way, the teacher can clarify misunderstandings and misinformation before it is too late. This can be facilitated by the teacher, an educational assistant, a resource teacher, a student "buddy," or a parent.

A "buddy system" can help the culturally Deaf or hard-of-hearing student immensely. The buddy can have a large or a small role, depending on his or her partner's needs and the buddy's abilities. The buddy may simply provide the student with brief explanations and provide clarifications. Alternately, he or she may have a bigger role, whereby the buddy writes out homework and assignments or is a notetaker for the culturally Deaf or hard-of-hearing student. Notetakers are especially important for older students, given the greater complexity of material. It is extremely difficult, if not impossible, to take good notes while attempting to speechread. As mentioned above, the buddy may help tutor the student as well. If the buddy is to act as a tutor, he or she should have a good knowledge of the subject area. Different tutors and, therefore, buddies may be required for different subject areas.

A student-specific lesson in self-advocacy may also be beneficial. The student with hearing loss needs to know that it is appropriate to ask for clarification when a spoken message is unclear. The student also needs to be confident that it will be patiently received. Lessons in self-advocacy will go a long way in empowering and motivating a student with hearing difficulty.

The student's peers are often very curious about their classmate who is "different." Teachers can use this opportunity to teach the children in the class about hearing and hearing loss. A lesson about sound and acoustics could also be beneficial. This can be a fun lesson in which demonstrations of the effects of many children talking at once are made evident. The use of a sound-level meter to measure actual sound levels is often a fun addition. Understanding peers will go a long way in creating a cooperative learning environment for all of the children in the class.

COMMON MISCONCEPTIONS ABOUT HEARING LOSS

A Hearing Aid Restores Normal Hearing

A hearing aid merely amplifies sound. Granted, it does so on a frequency-specific basis and is set to match the individual child's hearing loss, but speech is basically made *louder* and not necessarily *clearer*. Even though hearing aids are fit to compensate for a child's particular hearing loss, they do not give the child "normal hearing." Because hearing aids amplify sound and because even the most advanced hearing aids cannot precisely differentiate between speech and unwanted background noise (which is often also speech), hearing aids do not give children perfect access to the sounds that they need to hear. FM systems, directional microphones, and noise programs on hearing aids improve matters but do not restore normal hearing either.

People With Hearing Loss Are Good Lipreaders

Lipreading, more accurately referred to as speechreading, involves the interpretation of a spoken message through the observation of the speaker's lip and jaw movements, facial expressions, body language, and gestures. It is often assumed that because an individual is culturally Deaf or hard of hearing, that the individual will be a good speechreader. In fact, it is no easier for culturally Deaf or hard-of-hearing individuals to speechread than it is for hearing individuals. There will be hard-of-hearing and normal-hearing individuals who are good speechreaders and there will be hard-of-hearing and normal-hearing individuals who are poor speechreaders.

Speechreading is not an easy task. There are many sounds that look exactly the same on the lips (e.g., *b*, *p*, and *m*; *f* and *v*), and there are many sounds that are not visible on the lips (e.g., *k*, *g*, *h*). Because of this, very few people can rely on speechreading alone to understand a spoken message.

Audibility Is the Same as Intelligibility

This is often a difficult concept to understand. Many people assume that if a child can hear a spoken message, he or she can understand it. This is not always the case. Even though a child may be able to hear a teacher's voice, he or she may not be able to understand what is being said. To demonstrate this point, turn a radio on to a point where it is just audible. At this point, one is able to detect the fact that there is sound being produced, but the message is not intelligible. As one turns the radio louder, the message becomes easier and easier to understand. It is evident, then, that one cannot assume that simply because a child can *hear* the teacher, the child is able to *understand* what is being said. For this reason yes or no questions posed to the student like "Can you hear me?" are ineffective.

CONCLUSION

The educational needs of culturally Deaf and hard-of-hearing students are best served by a team of parents and professionals, all of whom have the individual child's best interests in mind. The classroom teacher is the professional most directly responsible for the child with a hearing loss in the school environment. A teacher with a basic understanding of hearing and the consequences of hearing loss will greatly facilitate the culturally Deaf or hard-of-hearing student's educational experience. Teachers should feel at ease with these students and realize that they, as teachers, perhaps more than any other single professional, have a great opportunity to contribute to the overall academic success and social and emotional growth of their culturally Deaf or hard-of-hearing students.

ADDITIONAL RESOURCES

Bess, F. H., Dodd-Murphy, J., & Parker, R. A. (1998). Children with minimal sensorineural hearing loss: Prevalence, educational performance, and functional status. *Ear & Hearing, 19*(5), 339–354.

Cole, E., & Flexer, C. (2011). *Children with hearing loss: Developing listening and talking, birth to six* (2nd ed.). San Diego, CA: Plural.

Crandell, C. C., Smaldino, J. J., & Flexer, C. (2005). *Sound-field amplification: Applications to speech perception and classroom acoustics* (2nd ed.). New York, NY: Thomson Delmar Learning.

Ertmer, D. J. (2005). *The source for children with cochlear implants.* East Moline, IL: LinguiSystems.

Rance, G. (2005). Auditory neuropathy/dys-synchrony and its perceptual consequences. *Trends in Amplification, 9*(1), 1–43.

REFERENCES

Flexer, C., Wray, D., & Ireland, J. (1989). Preferential seating is not enough: Issues in classroom management of hearing-impaired students. *Language, Speech, and Hearing Services in Schools, 20*, 11–21.

Rosenberg, G., Blake-Rahter, P., Heavner, J., Allen, L., Redmond, B., Philips, J., & Stigers, K. (1999). Improving classroom acoustics (ICA): A three-year FM sound field classroom amplification study. *Journal of Educational Audiology, 7,* 8–28.

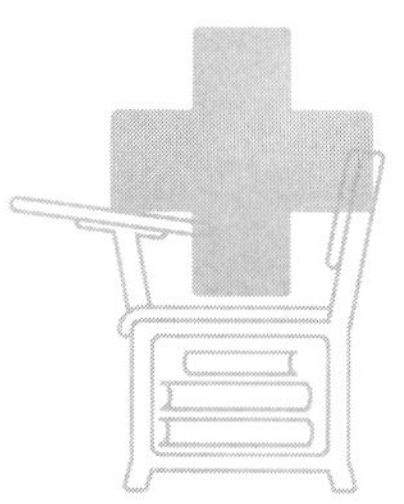

Chapter 10
Communication Disorders Associated With Medical Problems

Mary Anne Witzel

Speech and language disorders occur in 10%–15% of school-age children, and many of these problems are associated with an underlying medical illness or condition. Awareness and understanding of the communication disorders associated with medical problems by teachers, special educators, psychologists, speech–language pathologists, and other professionals in the educational system will enhance the curriculum planning and delivery as well as therapy intervention and classroom adaptation for these children. In some cases, previously unidentified medical conditions may be detected first by the communication disorders that they cause.

The purpose of this chapter is to provide teachers and other education professionals with a working knowledge of the types of communication disorders associated with various medical conditions and the role that teachers can play in the identification and management of these problems in the classroom. The medical conditions described were selected to cover the range of communication disorders that the classroom teacher may encounter. The Additional Resources list can be useful to individuals who wish to learn more about communication disorders associated with medical problems.

COMPONENTS OF SPEECH AND LANGUAGE

Articulation

Articulation is defined as a motor skill involving the use of the articulators, including the lips, tongue, teeth, vocal cords, and hard and soft palate, to form the consonant and vowel sounds of speech by shaping the air exhaled from the lungs as it flows through the vocal tract (see Figure 10.1). The articulation of speech sounds may be classified according to either the place in the vocal tract and the specific articulators used to form the sounds or the manner of formation, which is the degree of constriction of the airstream and the direction of the airflow, either oral or nasal (see Table 10.1). For example, /p/ and /b/ are classified as bilabial sounds for place of articulation because they are produced at the lips. They also are classified as stop sounds for manner of formation because the lip closure stops or occludes the airflow through the vocal tract for an instant to allow explosive air pressure to build up. When the lips are opened, the air is expelled with increased pressure, making the sound audible.

The place of production for /s/ and /z/ is lingual alveolar because the tongue (lingua) approximates the alveolar area of the hard palate. The manner of formation of these sounds is classified as fricative because the tongue approximates the alveolar area, narrowing the airstream and causing the turbulence and frication that makes these sounds audible and recognizable. Affricate sounds involve both an occlusion of the airstream and a narrow release of air; the glide and lateral sounds are produced with a relaxed narrowing of the vocal tract and less turbulent noise than the fricative sounds; and the nasal sounds are produced with an occlusion in the oral cavity and the airflow directed through the nose by an open soft palate. Almost all consonant sounds

Table 10.1

PLACE AND MANNER OF FORMATION OF CONSONANT SOUNDS IN THE VOCAL TRACT

		Manner of formation					
Sound	**Place**	**Stop**	**Fricative**	**Affricate**	**Glide**	**Lateral**	**Nasal**
/p, b, w, m/	Bilabial	/p, b/			/w/		/m/
/f, v/	Labiodental		/f, v/				
/th/	Lingual dental		/th/				
/t, d, l, n, s, z/	Lingual alveolar	/t, d/	/s, z/			/l/	/n/
/sh, zh, ch, j, y, r/	Lingual palatal		/sh, zh/	/ch, j/	/y, r/		
/k, g, ng/	Lingual velar	/k, g/					/ng/
/h/	Glottal		/h/				

are paired for both place and manner of formation (e.g., /p, b/, /t, d/, /s, z/). Voicing, or vibration from the vocal folds, distinguishes one sound from the other in a pair. For the paired sounds /s/ and /z/, place and manner of formation are identical; however, /s/ does not have vibration from the vocal folds since the larynx is open, whereas /z/ does (see Figure 10.2).

Voice

Phonation is the production of sound by the vibration of the vocal folds of the larynx as they are approximated or adducted (see Figure 10.2B). These sounds are known as voiced sounds. The characteristics of phonation of voice include quality, pitch, and loudness. Vowels are produced with phonation and changes in vocal tract shape by the tongue, lips, and soft palate. Some consonants (e.g., /p/, /t/, /s/) are produced

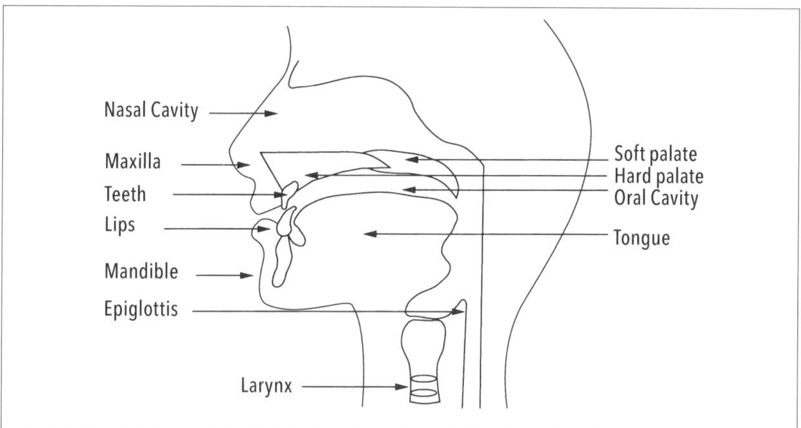

Figure 10.1. The human vocal tract.

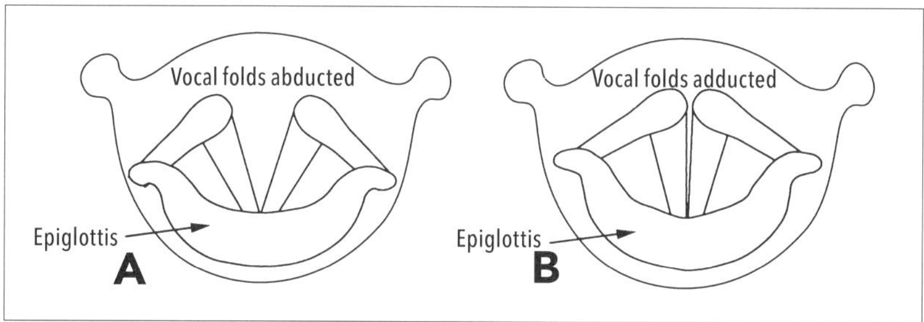

Figure 10.2. (A) Schematic drawing of vocal folds in open, or abducted, position for the voiceless consonant sound /s/. (B) Schematic drawing of the vocal folds in closed, or adducted, position for the voiced consonant sound /z/.

without phonation or voicing, since the vocal folds of the larynx are open, or abducted, and do not generate vibration during these sounds (see Figure 10.2A). These sounds, known as voiceless sounds, become audible because they have noise caused by hisses, clicks, and small explosions of air. The noise associated with these consonants is produced when the articulators (tongue and lips) narrow, or occlude, the airstream as it flows through the vocal tract. Other consonants (e.g., /b/, /d/, and /z/) are produced with both phonation and noise. They are referred to as the voiced consonants.

Resonance is defined as the amplification of sound waves generated by vibration of the vocal folds (phonation) and constrictions of the airstream in the vocal tract (noise), which increases the perception of specific vocal tones. Resonance varies according to vocal tract size and shape. The resonance required for the nasal sounds /m/, /n/, and /ng/ is achieved by using the entire vocal tract, including the nasal and oral cavities (see Figure 10.3A); the normal resonance required for the oral sounds—that is, vowels and all other consonants—is achieved by preventing airflow from entering the nasal cavity by closing the soft palate and surrounding musculature (see Figure 10.3B).

Fluency

Fluency is the flow of speech. Fluent speech is effortless, uninterrupted, and smooth. Fluent speech is free of abnormal pauses, hesitations, prolongations, and repetitions. In fluent speech, the rate or speed of speech does not detract from its intelligibility.

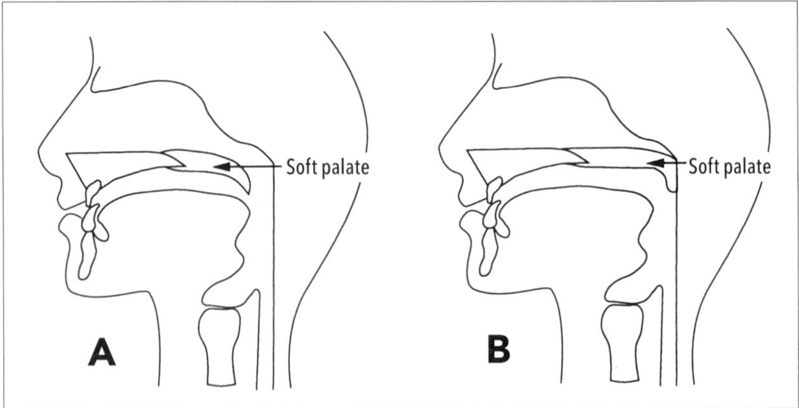

Figure 10.3. (A) Schematic drawing of the vocal tract with the soft palate open and tongue tip in position for the sound /n/. (B) Schematic drawing of the vocal tract with the soft palate closed and tongue tip in position for the fricative sound /s/.

Language

Language is defined as a communication system involving the use of words or meaningful units combined by a system of rules. It can be divided into two major components: receptive and expressive. Receptive language is the comprehension and understanding of spoken, written, or sign language, whereas expressive language is the verbal, written, or signed expression of an individual's thoughts, ideas, needs, and responses using the symbols and rules of a language. Expressive language consists of three major components: form, content, and use (Bloom & Lahey, 1978). *Form* includes phonology (rules that govern the sequencing and distribution of phonemes, sound units, and sound combinations of a language), syntax (rules that determine the form or structure of a sentence), and morphology (modification of word meanings by use of, for example, number, verb tense, possession, extension). *Content* includes semantics, or that aspect of language concerned with the meaning of words, whereas *use* involves pragmatics, or the social appropriateness and use of language within a communication situation.

SPEECH PRODUCTION AND DEVELOPMENT

Speech production is an integrated, complex process involving neurophysiology and respiration to make airflow from the lungs audible and recognizable by phonation, noise, resonance, and movements of the articulators. Speech development begins with the motor control abilities that emerge in the first year of life. During the first six months, the infant coos and babbles, which is followed by unintelligible speech utterances known as jargon. Simple, recognizable words occur around the child's first birthday. Vowel development is usually complete by the time the child is age 3 years, whereas consonant development often continues to age 5. The consistent correct pronunciation of consonants in blends (e.g., st as in *stop*) and clusters (e.g., *spr* as in *sprinkle*) may not be achieved in the normal speaking child until age 7 or 8. There is great variability in the normal development of speech in children, and the age of mastery of speech sounds may vary by as much as 3 years (Owens, 1994).

Neurophysiology

Speech production uses the nerves, muscles, cartilage, and bones of the head, neck, and trunk. Speech begins with nerve impulses that are fired from the brain to other areas of the nervous system, causing contraction of certain muscles. The nervous system consists of the central nervous system (CNS), which includes the brain and spinal cord, and the peripheral nervous system (PNS), which includes the cranial nerves and spinal nerves. The CNS and PNS are composed of a network of specialized cells known as neurons. Neurons may be motor or sensory. Motor neurons conduct impulses away from the CNS, usually to muscles in the periphery, and sensory neurons conduct impulses from the periphery toward the CNS. For example, when a person decides to close his or her lips, motor neurons carry the signal or impulse to the lip and jaw muscles, causing them to contract. When the lips contract, this stimulates the sensory receptors near the surface of the skin, and information that the lips have closed is carried along the sensory neurons to the brain (Borden, Harris, & Raphael, 1994).

Respiration

Respiration involves the spinal and thoracic peripheral nerves; the diaphragm, intercostal, and abdominal muscles; and sensory feedback to the CNS to allow the flow of air into and out of the lungs. Inspiration and expiration of air are necessary not only for breathing but also for speech. In general, the volume of air inspired and exhaled for speech sounds is greater than that needed for quiet breathing. Irregularities and abnormalities in respiratory patterns for breathing are often seen in those patients with speech problems. Inspiration occurs when the air pressure in the lungs is negative compared to atmospheric pressure and air is inhaled into the lungs through the respiratory–vocal tract to equalize the air pressure. Expiration occurs when the muscles of respiration contract, increasing the air pressure within the lungs compared to atmospheric pressure. Air is then exhaled through the tract to again equalize the air pressure with atmospheric pressure. The modulation or shaping of airflow exhaled from the lungs through the vocal tract produces the sounds of speech.

Phonation

For voiced sounds, nerve impulses from the brain bring the arytenoid cartilages of the larynx together, causing the vocal folds to approximate and putting them in position to vibrate (see Figure 10.2B). As air is exhaled from the lungs and passes between the folds, the increased air pressure causes the vocal folds to vibrate and produce sound. This vibration of the vocal folds is attributed to the pressure of the airstream rather than to nerve impulses. The vocal folds are positioned closer together for vowels than for voiced consonants.

Noise

For voiceless sounds, the nerve impulses from the brain keep the vocal folds open (see Figure 10.2A). Air then passes freely from the lungs into the oral cavity, where the articulators create noise by briefly stopping or narrowing the airstream to create turbulence.

Resonance

All objects have a capacity to resonate. The vocal tract (see Figure 10.1) functions as the resonating chamber for speech. It changes in shape and size depending on the position of the articulators and whether the soft palate musculature is open or closed (see Figure 10.3). When the soft palate musculature is open, the resonating chamber of the vocal tract is enlarged, because it includes the nasal cavity. This contributes to the differences in resonance that are perceived between the oral sounds and the nasal sounds (/m/, /n/, /ng/) of speech (see Figure 10.3). When specific vibrations from the vocal folds are similar in frequency to those of the individual vocal tract, these vibrations are enhanced. Those vibrations that are not similar are attenuated. This filtering of the vibrations from the vocal folds through the vocal tract results in the individual's vocal resonance, which helps to distinguish one individual's voice from another's.

Articulation

Articulation of vowels and consonants of speech results from the constriction of the vocal tract by the lips, tongue, jaws, and soft palate to either narrow or briefly stop the airstream. Movement of the articulators, particularly the opening and closing of the soft palate musculature, also directs the airstream through the nose for nasal sounds or through the mouth for oral sounds. Each sound of a language has a specific location in the vocal tract where it is produced, a specific degree of constriction of the vocal tract, and a specific direction of the airflow (see Figure 10.3 and Table 10.1).

LANGUAGE COMPETENCE

The brain and cortical function, in combination with adequate hearing, speech production, and appropriate social environment, is necessary for the development and use of language. Language is dependent on the individual's ability to learn and integrate the symbols and rule systems. Language development begins in the first months of life and is dramatic and rapid during the preschool years, with particular emphasis on semantics and pragmatics. By the time the child enters school, he or she exhibits the basic aspects of adult language, including a knowledge of the individual sound units and sound-symbol sequences, discrimination between sounds, extensive vocabulary development, and a solid knowledge of rules for combining units of meaning to convey specific ideas. The child is able to understand functional language and express thoughts, ideas, and desires. Growth of the five components of language continues in the school-age years, albeit at a slower rate, and even into adulthood. In the school-age years, refinements in the use of language are developed, particularly in the areas of semantics, syntax, and morphology. Metalinguistic abilities that allow the child to think about and reflect on language occur, and there is an emphasis on written language and reading. School-age children become increasingly able to deal with abstract concepts, attend to and follow complex directions, appreciate jokes, recognize the ambiguities of language, understand metaphors and similes, and narrate stories and thoughts (Landman, 1989).

TYPES OF COMMUNICATION DISORDERS

Speech

Articulation disorders consist of errors in the formation of individual sounds of speech. Errors may be classified as substitutions, omissions, or distortions. These errors are usually related to difficulties in the anatomy or physiology of the motor production system or in the neuromotor control system. For example, speech sound errors may be due to physical abnormalities of the vocal tract, as found in children with cleft palate or neuromotor impairments associated with cerebral palsy. An articulation disorder also may be known as a phonetic disorder.

Voice disorders include abnormalities in phonation (e.g., pitch, loudness, quality) and abnormalities in resonance. Abnormalities in pitch include excessively high or low pitch or unusual pitch fluctuations, abnormalities in loudness include excessively high or low volume of voice, and abnormalities in vocal quality include hoarseness (due to irregularities in the contact surface of the vocal folds) and breathiness (incomplete adduction of the vocal folds during phonation). Abnormalities in resonance include hypernasality (excessive resonance for oral sounds due to use of both the oral and nasal cavities as resonating chambers), which may occur in individuals with cleft palate, and hyponasality (decreased resonance of the nasal sounds due to partial or total blockage of the nasal cavity as a resonating chamber for the nasal sounds). This type of resonance also is heard when a head cold or allergies block a speaker's nasal passages. Voice disorders may be due to abnormalities in anatomy or function of the larynx, nasal cavity, or soft palate musculature during speech.

Stuttering and other disorders of fluency include abnormal pauses, hesitations, prolongations, interjections, repetitions, blockages, or excessive rates of speech that interrupt the flow of speech. Stuttering may be accompanied by secondary characteristics, such as excessive muscular tension in the vocal tract, eye blinking, and other abnormal body movements during speech. There are many theories about the causation of stuttering, including effects of genetics, neuroses, development, learning, and conditioning (Shames & Ramig, 1994).

Language

A *phonological disorder* is defined as abnormal organization of the individual's phonological system or a significant deficit in speech production or perception. Phonological disorders involve the cognitive and linguistic components of the speech sound system. Phonological disorders include (a) widespread patterns of errors (e.g., omissions of final consonants in words, production of one group of sounds for another), (b) severe limitations in the range of sounds produced (e.g., the child produces /t/ in place of a wide variety of consonants), (c) limitations in syllable structure of words produced (e.g., a child produces only the stressed syllables of words), and (d) interactions of sounds and syllable structures (e.g., a child ends all words with /s/) or production of words in which one sound influences the other sounds in the word (e.g., in words with more than one consonant, the two consonants are produced so that they are identical or nearly identical with no direct physical cause) (Schwartz, 1994).

Semantic disorders include poor vocabulary development, inappropriate use of word meanings, and an inability to comprehend word meanings. *Syntax difficulties* include abnormalities in average length of phrases and sentences and difficulty in interpreting word order and grammar. *Morphological difficulties* include abnormal use of prefixes and suffixes, abnormal structure of words, and abnormalities in use of tenses, plurals, and possessive forms. Finally, *pragmatics problems* involve the inability to comprehend or use language appropriately in context and inappropriate or inadequate use of language in conversation.

THE EFFECT OF ANATOMICAL ABNORMALITIES ON COMMUNICATION

Brain

Abnormalities in the structural, metabolic, or electrophysiological aspects of the brain or CNS may impair receptive and expressive language and speech production, as well as learning, reading, attention, and behavior. Congenital anomalies of the brain documented in various medical conditions include microcephaly (abnormally small brain), macrocephaly (abnormally large brain), holoprosencephaly (impaired midline cleavage of the forebrain), agenesis or absence of the corpus callosum, Arnold Chiari malformation, hydrocephaly, tumors, and encephaloceles. Seizures and increased intracranial pressure also may occur. Acquired conditions, such as traumatic head injury, tumors, infections, and seizures, also influence communication abilities, often resulting in regression of developed language abilities. Congenital and acquired conditions of the nervous system, such as myasthenia gravis and hypotonia, often affect the coordinated production of speech (Schaefer, Mathy-Lakko, & Bodensteiner, 1992).

Ear

Abnormalities in the anatomy and function of the components of the ear, including the inner ear, middle ear, eustachian tube, tympanic membrane, and outer ear, may cause varying types and degrees of hearing loss (see Chapter 9). Hearing loss can impede development and production of speech, development and competence of language, and behavior and learning.

Nose

Resonance of voice may be affected by abnormalities in the size and shape of the nose, because the nasal cavity is an important resonating cavity for speech. Deviation of the septum, enlarged nasal turbinates, or other blockages in the nose will increase nasal resistance in the nose. If this is significant, hyponasal resonance and an audible turbulent sound will occur during production of the nasal sounds.

Lips

Articulation of sounds such as /p/, /b/, /w/, and /m/, which require lip closure or rounding, or sounds such as /l/ and /v/, which require the lower lip to contact the upper teeth, may be affected if the lips are unable to close or contact the teeth as a result of abnormal position of the maxilla or mandible, abnormal nerve innervation, or a repaired cleft lip with severe scarring.

Jaws

If the size and position of the upper jaw (maxilla) or lower jaw (mandible) are in disproportion to each other, the articulation of bilabial, labiodental, lingual alveolar, and lingual palatal sounds may be affected. Speech may sound unusual if the lips and tongue assume abnormal positions for sound production.

Teeth

Occlusion

Abnormalities in the occlusion of the teeth are often implicated in articulation problems. When the upper incisor teeth are abnormally protrusive, the child may have difficulty achieving lip closure for the bilabial sounds. When the lower teeth are abnormally protrusive, the labiodental sounds /f/ and /v/ may be produced in reverse, with the lower incisors against the upper lip. When there is a space between the upper and lower incisor teeth during occlusion of the molar teeth (open bite), the lingual dental, lingual alveolar, and lingual palatal sounds may be distorted as the tongue protrudes through this space (see Figure 10.4).

Interdental Spacing and Missing Teeth

Missing, rotated, or abnormally spaced incisor teeth, resulting in large spaces in the dental arch, often cause abnormal tongue position for the lingual alveolar sounds /s/ and /z/. This may result in a lisp-type distortion of these sounds.

Tongue

In some craniofacial syndromes, the tongue may be abnormally large (macroglossia) or abnormally small (microglossia) or have abnormal function as a result of cranial nerve anomalies. In some cases these abnormalities are true growth anomalies, whereas in others they are relative anomalies due to the size of the oral cavity. For example, in Down syndrome the tongue often appears excessively large and protrusive. Some of these children have a relative macroglossia due to the small size of the oral cavity (see Figure 10.5). These abnormalities of

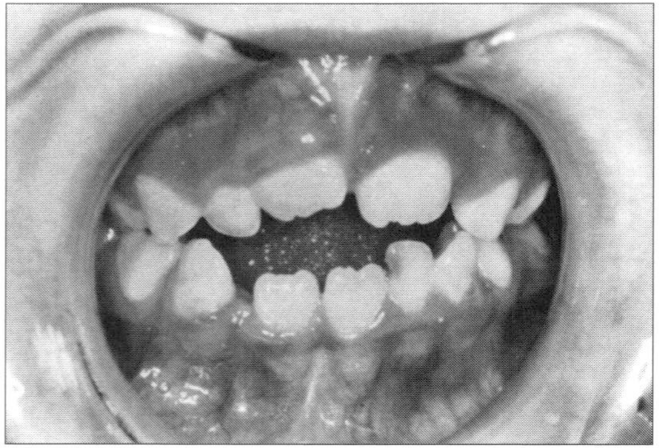

Figure 10.4. An open-bite malocclusion. From "Communicative Impairment Associated With Clefting," by M. A. Witzel, 1994, in *Cleft Palate Speech Management: A Multidisciplinary Approach* (p. 154), edited by R. J. Shprintzen and J. Bardach, St. Louis, MO: Mosby. Copyright 1994 by Mosby. Reprinted with permission.

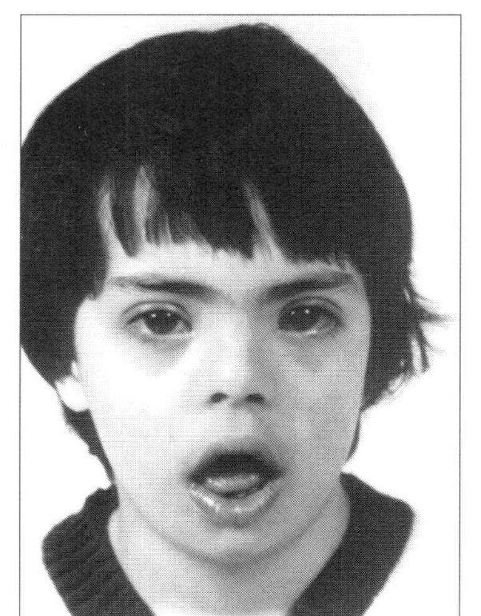

Figure 10.5. Child with Down syndrome and protrusive tongue. From "Speech Problems in Patients With Dentofacial or Craniofacial Deformities," by M. A. Witzel and L. Vallino, 1992, in *Modern Practice of Orthognathic and Reconstructive Surgery* (Vol. 2, p. 1700), edited by W. H. Bell, Philadelphia, PA: W. B. Saunders. Copyright 1992 by W. B. Saunders. Reprinted with permission.

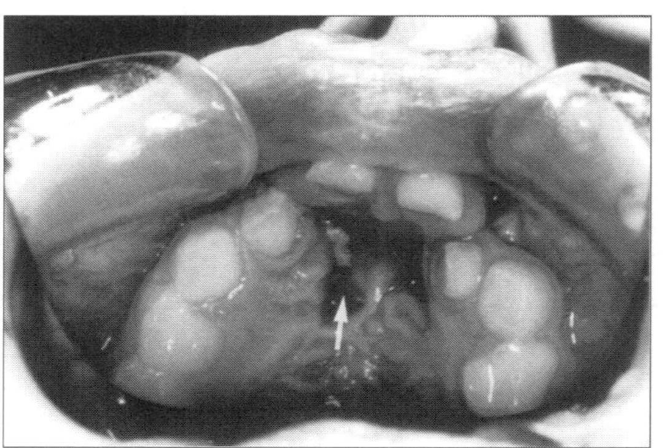

Figure 10.6. A fistula (*see arrow*) remaining in the hard palate of a child with repaired bilateral cleft lip and palate.

the tongue often affect articulation of the lingual dental, lingual alveolar, lingual palatal, and lingual velar sounds.

Hard Palate

Sometimes the hard palate has a fistula (hole or opening) due to an unrepaired cleft palate, incomplete surgical closure of the palate, maxillary collapse, or other abnormality. In such cases, the placement of the tongue for palatal sounds, as well as airflow through the oral cavity, is affected (see Figure 10.6).

Soft Palate and Velopharynx

An inability to close the soft palate and surrounding musculature that allows airflow into the nasal cavity during oral speech sounds results in hypernasal resonance of speech. This condition is known as velopharyngeal inadequacy, or VPI (see Figure 10.7). In addition to hypernasal resonance, the articulation of the oral sounds may be abnormal and sound weak, or there may be unusual substitutions or omission of sounds. This may occur in a child with a repaired cleft palate, submucous cleft palate (bifid uvula and muscle deficiency in the soft palate; see Figure 10.8), or, in rare cases, after adenoidectomy when there is an anatomical disproportion in the size of the structures. VPI also

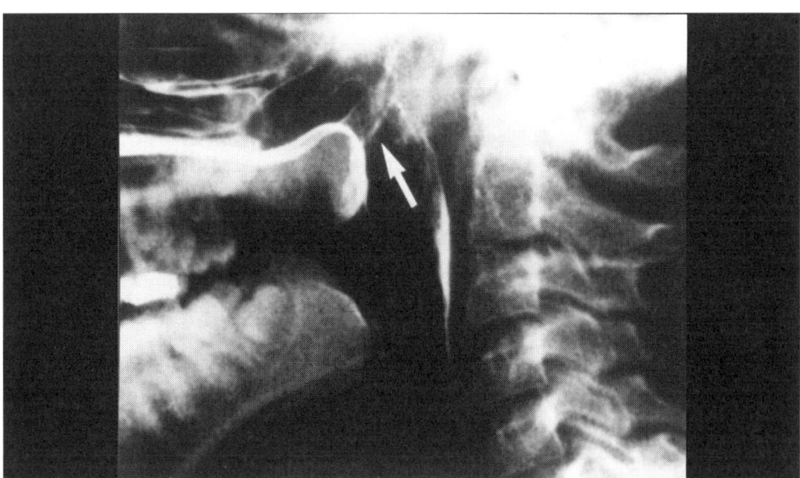

Figure 10.7. Child with velopharyngeal insufficiency. The soft palate fails to contact the pharynx during speech (see arrow). From "Speech Problems in Patients With Dentofacial or Craniofacial Deformities," by M. A. Witzel and L. Vallino, 1992, in *Modern Practice of Orthognathic and Reconstructive Surgery* (Vol. 2, p. 1704), edited by W. H. Bell, Philadelphia, PA: W. B. Saunders. Copyright 1992 by W. B. Saunders. Reprinted with permission.

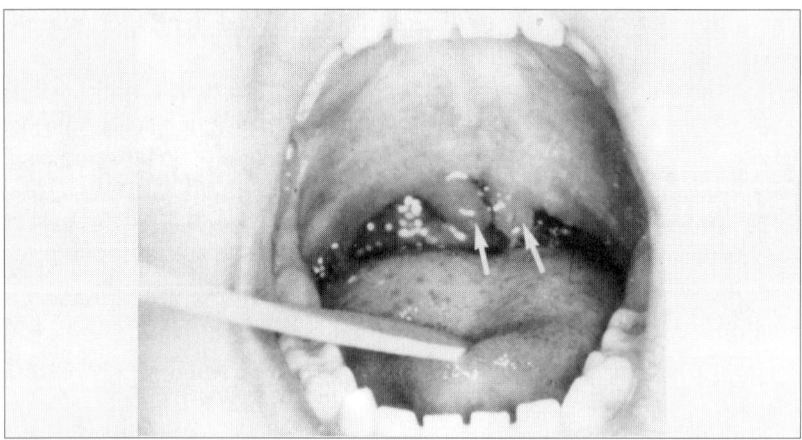

Figure 10.8. Submucous cleft palate. Note the bifid uvula (*see arrows*).

may be due to primary disorders of the central nervous system, which may alter the timing of velopharyngeal closure during speech.

Tonsils and Adenoids

Abnormally large tonsils often result in excessive tongue protrusion during speech, distorting the anterior tongue sounds. Abnormally large adenoids can impede the flow of air through the nose during speech, resulting in hyponasal resonance.

Larynx

Abnormalities in the anatomy and function of the larynx result in problems with the pitch, loudness, and quality of phonation of voice. A common voice problem in school-age children is hoarseness due to use of the vocal folds with excessive energy. This results in edema or swelling of the folds or, in more severe cases, vocal nodules or calluses on the vocal folds.

MEDICAL CONDITIONS AT RISK FOR COMMUNICATION DISORDERS

Medical conditions are either congenital (present at birth) or acquired after birth. The causes, or etiology, of medical conditions are various. Congenital conditions usually are classified as chromosomal, single-gene, polygenic–multifactorial, teratogenic, mechanically induced, or of unknown causation (Jones, 1988; Jung, 1989):

➜ **Chromosomal**

Human somatic cells normally contain 46 chromosomes (23 pairs). Chromosomal conditions occur due to abnormalities in the number or structure of one or more of these chromosomes. They are not usually inherited (see Chapter 2).

➜ **Single Gene**

A single-gene disease or condition is transmitted from one or both parents according to Mendelian laws of inheritance. These conditions are classified as autosomal dominant (individual has a single dose of an abnormal gene received from one parent, where one chromosome of a pair is affected) or autosomal recessive (individual has received the abnormal gene from each parent–thus a double dose).

➜ **Polygenic-Multifactorial**

A polygenic-multifactorial disease or condition is one whose likely cause is a combination of the environment and the effects of more than one gene.

➜ **Teratogenic**

Various teratogenic factors, such as exposure to drugs, infection, or environmental agents such as radiation during pregnancy, may cause abnormal development of an embryo or fetus.

➜ **Mechanically Induced**

An external factor such as an amniotic band impinges on the developing embryo or fetus, causing an abnormal shape or disruption to the developing body parts.

➜ **Unknown Causation**

Some conditions have no apparent cause. These cannot be categorized in any of the previous types of congenital conditions.

CONGENITAL MEDICAL CONDITIONS

All medical conditions have an associated *phenotypic spectrum*, or a series of abnormal observable features. Some individuals with a particular medical condition have all the features of the condition, whereas others have only a portion of the features. Some features occur more frequently than others, and the severity of phenotypic features is often variable from patient to patient. This is known as *variable expression*. The *natural history* of the condition refers to the progress of the condition as the individual develops and ages. *Prognosis* indicates the expected outcome or effect of the condition on the individual and the expected response to treatment.

The following is a partial list of congenital medical conditions due to abnormal chromosomes, single or multiple genes, or teratogenic causes. This list includes a brief description of the general phenotypic spectrum and a more detailed description of the spectrum of communication difficulties that these children may have or are at risk of having. Also included is information on the natural history of the condition and prognosis for improvement of communication skills with intervention. Prognosis is described as excellent (reasonable expectation of normal or near-normal speech and language), fair (reasonable expectation of functional communication skills), guarded (little improvement to be expected as a result of limiting factors of condition), or poor (no improvement expected because of limiting factors of the condition).

Chromosomal Disorders

Down Syndrome

Etiology: Chromosome disorder

Phenotypic Spectrum

General: Typical facies (see Figure 10.5), protruding tongue, cardiac malformations, gastrointestinal malformations, developmental delay, small ears, hearing loss, cleft palate

Communication

Articulation–substitutions, omissions, distortions, delayed onset

Voice phonation–breathy, husky, low pitch, increased loudness

Voice resonance–hypernasal

Fluency–stuttering, rapid rate of speech

Phonology–delayed onset

Semantics–delayed

Syntax–delayed

Morphology–delayed

Pragmatics–delayed, difficulty communicating abstract concepts

Natural History: Delayed motor, speech, and language development; cognitive deficits; frequent upper respiratory infections; increased risk for early Alzheimer's disease and psychological disorders. Protrusive tongue may influence eating and speech.

Prognosis for Communication Skills: Prognosis is excellent to guarded for communication skills. Infant stimulation programs are beneficial in helping the child reach his or her developmental potential. Speech and language therapy in the preschool and school-age years is beneficial in improving speech intelligibility, articulation, voice, fluency, and all aspects of language. Tongue reduction surgery may improve appearance and eating, but it has not been found to improve overall speech intelligibility (Klaiman, Witzel, Margar-Bacal, & Munro, 1988; Margar-Bacal, Witzel, & Munro, 1987).

Fragile X

Etiology: Chromosome disorder, X-linked

Phenotypic Spectrum

General: Typical facies (see Figure 10.9), including prominent lower jaw and large ears; cognitive impairment; testicular enlargement; speech and language disorders; emotional instability; autistic-like behaviors such as severe hand biting. Occurs primarily in males (Jung, 1989).

Communication

- **Articulation**–substitutions, omissions, distortions, delayed onset
- **Voice phonation**–difficulty monitoring loudness
- **Voice resonance**–normal
- **Fluency**–perseverations, cluttering
- **Phonology**–delayed onset
- **Semantics**–delayed

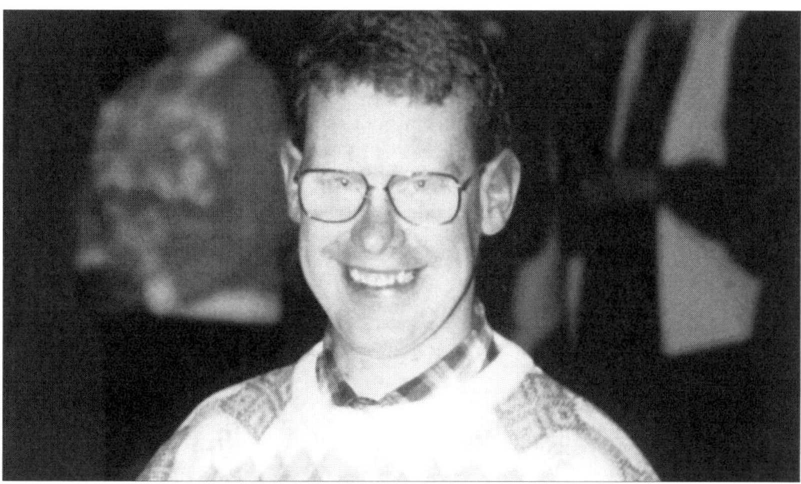

Figure 10.9. Adolescent with fragile X syndrome. (Photo courtesy of Dr. D. Chitayat.)

Syntax–delayed

Morphology–delayed

Pragmatics–delayed; difficulty communicating abstract concepts; use of jargon, echolalia, and/or self-talk

Natural History: Life span is normal. Cognitive abilities affect development of speech, language, behavior, and social interaction. Some individuals have normal intelligence; however, most have significant cognitive impairment. The symptoms of the condition are usually less severe in carrier females than in affected males. Speech problems are variable; most have a generalized language disability (Howard-Peebles, Stoddard, & Mims, 1979; Jung, 1989).

Prognosis for Communication Skills: Prognosis for speech and language abilities is primarily dependent on cognitive abilities and ranges from excellent to poor. Speech and language therapy is recommended to improve intelligibility of speech and functional use of language.

Single-Gene Disorders

Crouzon Syndrome

Etiology: Autosomal dominant, variable expression

Phenotypic Spectrum

General: Craniosynostosis, shallow orbits with exophthalmos (prominent eyes), hypertelorism, hearing loss, maxillary hypoplasia (underdevelopment) with significant malocclusion (see Figure 10.10), and attention problems. Some children require tracheostomy in the preschool years due to respiratory difficulties. Cleft palate or submucous cleft palate may occur, but this is not a frequent finding.

Communication

Articulation–substitutions, omissions, distortions, delayed onset

Voice phonation–normal

Voice resonance–hyponasal or hypernasal

Fluency–normal

Phonology–normal to delayed onset

Semantics–normal to delayed

Syntax–normal to delayed

Morphology–normal to delayed

Pragmatics–normal to delayed

Natural History: Although some children with Crouzon syndrome have delayed cognitive skills, many have normal development and cognitive function, particularly if craniosynostosis and hearing are surgically treated in infancy or in the preschool years. Poor development of the maxilla results in a significant malocclusion and forward positioning of the tongue, contributing to articulation difficulties. The nasal airway is reduced due to the abnormal anatomy of the nasal and pharyngeal cavity. This results in a hyponasal resonance quality. Hypernasal resonance will occur in those with velopharyngeal incompetency. Language abilities are variable and should be monitored. Speech and language therapy in the preschool and school-age years is recommended to optimize the child's potential (Witzel, 1983; Witzel & Vallino, 1992).

Prognosis for Communication Skills: The severity of expression of the syndrome will affect speech, language, and cognitive function. The prognosis for communication ranges from excellent to fair. Surgical and orthodontic treatment will improve the oral cavity for articulation.

Treacher Collins Syndrome

Etiology: Autosomal dominant, variable expression

Phenotypic Spectrum

General: Malar hypoplasia with down-slanting palpebral fissures; defect of the lower eyelid; mandibular hypoplasia and malocclusion; malformations of the

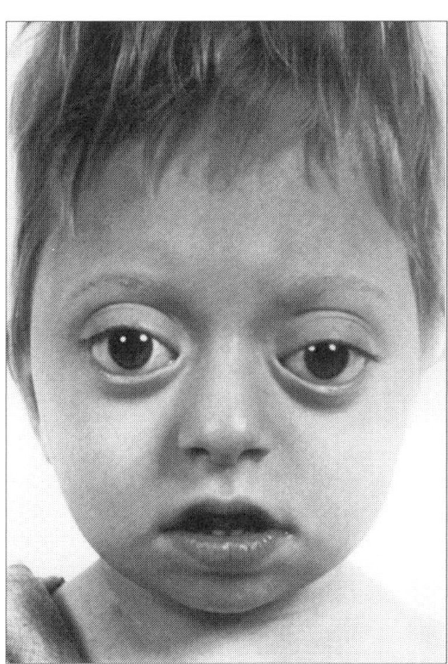

Figure 10.10. Child with Crouzon syndrome.

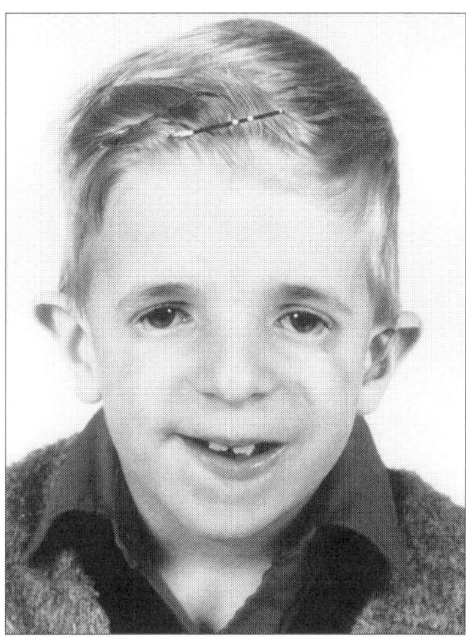

Figure 10.11. Child with Treacher Collins syndrome.

external ear, auditory canal, and middle- and inner-ear structures; hearing loss; cleft palate (see Figure 10.11).

Communication

- **Articulation**–substitutions, omissions, distortions, delayed onset
- **Voice phonation**–normal
- **Voice resonance**–hypernasal, muffled
- **Fluency**–normal
- **Phonology**–normal to delayed onset
- **Semantics**–normal to delayed
- **Syntax**–normal to delayed
- **Morphology**–normal to delayed
- **Pragmatics**–normal to delayed

Natural History: Life span is normal. Tracheostomy may be required in very severe cases in the preschool years due to small airway. Intelligence and cognitive function are usually normal, especially when hearing problems are managed early. Developmental delays may occur as a result of hearing loss and speech problems. Hearing problems are managed with surgery or hearing aids; speech and language problems are managed with therapy or surgery. Surgical closure of cleft palate, craniofacial surgery, and orthodontics improve appearance and oral function (Witzel & Vallino, 1992).

Prognosis for Communication Skills: Prognosis ranges from excellent to fair and is related to the severity of the condition and the timing of management of the facial, occlusal, and hearing problems. Early amplification is stressed. Surgery and orthodontic treatment improve appearance and function, articulation, and resonance. Cleft-palate repair may also improve resonance, although muffled resonance may persist. When speech and language problems occur, they can be successfully managed with therapy in the preschool and early school-age years. Surgery and orthodontic treatment to improve the occlusion and facial form will also benefit speech production.

Velocardiofacial Syndrome

Etiology: Autosomal dominant, variable expression

Phenotypic Spectrum

General: Most cases have a deletion on chromosome 22q11.2, learning disabilities, cleft palate and velopharyngeal insufficiency, cardiac malformations, asymmetric smile, behavior and attention-deficit difficulties, and fluctuating hearing loss due to middle-ear disease. More than 30 other phenotypic features have been described (Goldberg, Motzkin, Marion, Scambler, & Shprintzen, 1993). The syndrome is also known as Shprintzen (1997) syndrome or 22q11 deletion syndrome (see Figure 10.12).

Communication

Articulation–substitutions, omissions, distortions, delayed onset

Voice phonation–high pitch in preschool and early school years

Voice resonance–hypernasal

Fluency–normal

Phonology–delayed onset

Semantics–delayed

Syntax–delayed

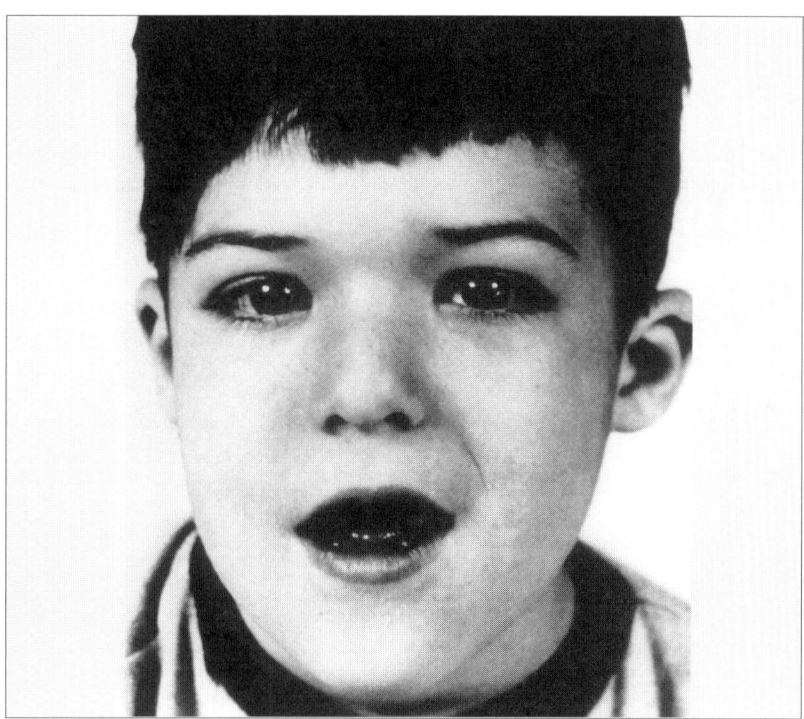

Figure 10.12. Six-year-old boy with velocardiofacial syndrome. From "Communicative Impairment Associated With Clefting," by M. A. Witzel, 1994, in *Cleft Palate Speech Management: A Multidisciplinary Approach* (p. 151), edited by R. J. Shprintzen and J. Bardach, St. Louis, MO: Mosby. Copyright 1994 by Mosby. Reprinted with permission.

Morphology–delayed

Pragmatics–delayed, difficulty communicating abstract concepts

Natural History: Life span is usually normal unless the cardiac condition or mental illness is severe. Attention and behavioral difficulties may present management problems for parents and educational professionals, particularly for children in the preschool and school-age years. Some young adults develop schizophrenia or other forms of mental illness.

Prognosis for Communication Skills: Prognosis is excellent to fair for speech and language. Speech problems respond well to therapy and surgical or prosthetic management. Language and attention difficulties are improved with therapy, particularly when a structured approach to therapy is emphasized.

Polygenic–Multifactorial Syndromes

Cleft Lip and Palate, Cleft Palate, Submucous Cleft Palate

Etiology: Multifactorial, variable expression

Phenotypic Spectrum

General: May occur as an isolated defect or as a phenotypic feature of a syndrome; cleft lip may be unilateral or bilateral; cleft palate and submucous cleft

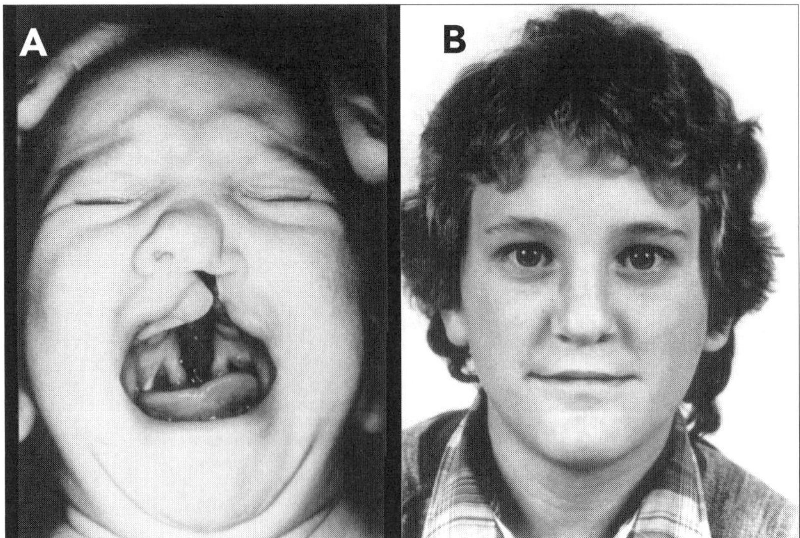

Figure 10.13. (A) Baby with unilateral cleft lip and palate prior to lip and palate repair. (B) The same child at 11 years of age. (Photos courtesy of Dr. W. K. Lindsay.)

palate may occur with cleft lip or as an isolated defect; feeding problems at birth; fluctuating hearing loss due to middle-ear disease; maxillary hypoplasia, malocclusion, velopharyngeal insufficiency, and reading and learning disabilities in some cases (see Figures 10.8 and 10.13).

Communication

Articulation–at risk for substitutions, omissions, distortions, delayed onset

Voice phonation–possible hoarseness

Voice resonance–hypernasal

Fluency–normal

Phonology–delayed onset

Semantics–normal, at risk

Syntax–normal, at risk

Morphology–normal, at risk

Pragmatics–normal, at risk

Natural History: Life span is normal, and intellect follows the distribution of the population in general. Surgical repair of the lip and palate in the first year of life improves feeding problems and assists speech and language development. Early management of middle-ear disease is necessary for speech and language competence. Secondary surgical treatment of velopharyngeal function in the school-age years is required in 10%–25% of cases. Definitive treatment of facial growth problems and malocclusion usually does not occur until teenage years. Secondary surgical treatment for the appearance of the lip and nose is usually undertaken in the school-age years. Early therapy intervention for speech and language problems is recommended; this also may be required in the primary grades (McWilliams & Witzel, 1994).

Prognosis for Communication Skills: Prognosis is excellent. Speech problems usually are resolved with surgical, orthodontic, and therapy interventions. Some cases require prosthodontic interventions. Language problems respond to therapy.

Teratogenic Syndromes

Fetal Alcohol Syndrome

Etiology: Maternal alcohol consumption during pregnancy

Phenotypic Spectrum

General: Growth deficiency, typical facies, microcephaly, cardiac defects, cleft palate, cognitive deficiency, learning and attention disabilities related to the

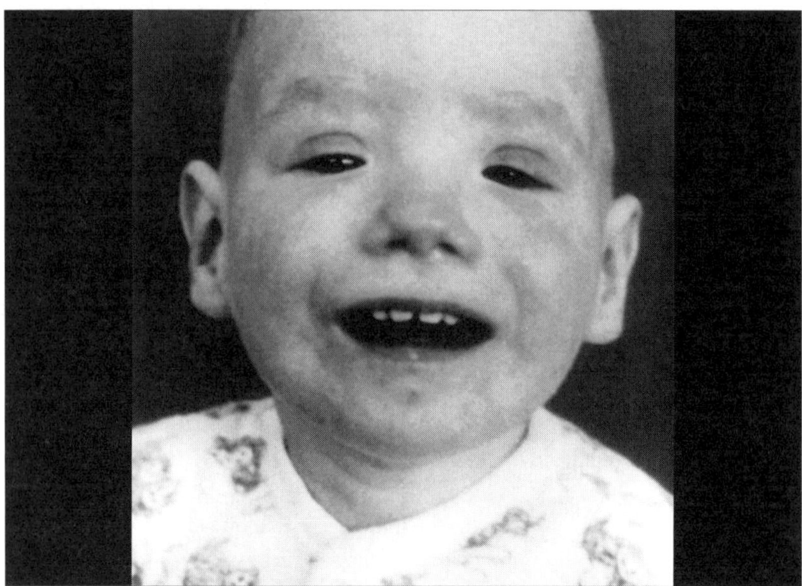

Figure 10.14. Child with fetal alcohol syndrome.

severity of the cognitive deficit (see Figure 10.14). In those cases with cleft palate or velopharyngeal insufficiency, surgical treatment may improve resonance and articulation.

Communication

Articulation–substitutions, omissions, distortions, delayed onset

Voice phonation–abnormal, may have hoarseness

Voice resonance–hypernasal

Fluency–stuttering

Phonology–delayed onset

Semantics–delayed

Syntax–delayed

Morphology–delayed

Pragmatics–abnormal

Natural History: Growth is deficient. Hyperactivity, behavior difficulties, and learning problems are common and related to cognitive function. Most children have speech and language problems, and individualized intervention in the preschool and school-age years is beneficial. For individuals who have velopharyngeal incompetency, surgical treatment is recommended to improve resonance and articulation.

Prognosis for Communication Skills: Prognosis is excellent to fair. Speech, language, and learning abilities and outcomes of therapy are influenced by the severity of the cognitive deficit and the psychosocial environment (Jung, 1989).

Other Conditions

Cerebral Palsy

Etiology: Brain insult due to hemorrhage and oxygen deprivation before, during, or after birth. The cause in most cases is unknown.

Phenotypic Spectrum

General: Neuromotor dysfunction, including flaccidity, hypertonia, hypotonia, hyperkinesia, hypokinesia, ataxia, respiratory system dysfunction, cognitive delay or deficiency; feeding and speech problems attributed to neuromotor abnormalities and cognitive deficiencies; language problems attributed to difficulties in speech production and cognitive deficits. There also is a high incidence of associated seizures (see Chapter 14).

Communication

Articulation–dysarthria (slurred speech), substitutions, omissions, distortions, delayed onset

Voice phonation–breathy; strained; inconsistent pitch, loudness, and syllable duration

Voice resonance–hypernasal

Fluency–normal

Phonology–delayed onset

Semantics–delayed

Syntax–delayed

Morphology–delayed

Pragmatics–delayed

Natural History: Hypotonia present in some newborns often develops into spasticity or dyskinesia. Speech and language development are often delayed because of a combination of cognitive deficits, neuromotor disorder, and difficulty in coordinating the respiratory and speech musculature. Early intervention to develop functional communication strategies is beneficial.

Prognosis for Communication Skills: Prognosis is excellent to guarded. The severity of the communication problem is related to the severity of the neuromuscular and cognitive problems. Some children have little difficulty in verbal communication, whereas others achieve functional oral communication with therapy. Some are unable to achieve intelligible oral speech; they communicate with the assistance of alternative or augmentative devices, such as picture symbols, electronic scanning systems, and digitized or synthesized speech. The very severe cases have limited communication abilities (Hardy, 1994).

Autism

Etiology: Chromosome abnormalities are present in at least 30% of cases. Further research will likely show an increase in subtle gene abnormalities.

Phenotypic Spectrum

General: Significant social deficits, inability to relate to other persons, failure to develop appropriate verbal and nonverbal communication skills, under- or overreaction to sensory stimuli, deficient play skills, repetitive or ritualistic behaviors, poor eye contact. Expression of the impairments is variable (see Chapter 16).

Communication

Articulation–substitutions, omissions, distortions, delayed onset

Voice phonation–monotone, grunting sounds, may be mute

Voice resonance–normal

Fluency–stuttering, unusual rhythm

Phonology–delayed onset

Semantics–delayed, severe echolalia

Syntax–delayed, pronoun confusions

Morphology–delayed

Pragmatics–abnormal, unable to initiate or maintain conversation

Natural History: Deviant social development, delayed or unusual language, ritualistic and repetitive behaviors. Some or all of these behaviors can be detected before the age of 3 years. Early intervention is beneficial in improving communication and reducing destructive behaviors.

Prognosis for Communication Skills: Prognosis ranges from excellent to poor, depending on the severity of the condition.

Acquired Brain Injury

Etiology: Cerebral vascular accident, hematoma, encephalitis, trauma, infection

Phenotypic Spectrum

General: Motor abnormalities; cognitive difficulties; difficulty with attention, perception, and memory; impulsivity; difficulty with abstraction, problem solving, judgment, decision making; and inappropriate social behavior.

Communication

Articulation–dysarthria, substitutions, omissions, distortions

Voice phonation–abnormal pitch with fluctuations

Voice resonance–hypernasal

Fluency–normal

Phonology–may be affected

Semantics–may be affected

Syntax–may be affected

Morphology–may be affected

Pragmatics–may be affected

Natural History: Acquired brain injury may involve brain lesions, hemorrhage within the brain, or swelling of the brain. Damage may be localized or pervasive, and there may be loss of consciousness or coma. Recovery is variable and may continue over a period of months or years. Motor, sensory, and cognitive functions may be impaired. Improvement in function from the time of the initial trauma often occurs both spontaneously and with interventions.

Prognosis for Communication Skills: Prognosis ranges from excellent to poor, depending on location and extent of head injury, rehabilitation program, family support, previous abilities, and individual motivation. Speech and language therapy is an important part of the rehabilitation program.

ASSESSMENT AND MANAGEMENT OF MEDICALLY BASED COMMUNICATION DISORDERS

Interdisciplinary Care

When a congenital or acquired medical condition affects one or more body systems and several health-care and education professionals are involved in the habilitation or rehabilitation of the child, interdisciplinary team assessment and treatment is beneficial in planning and delivering the most effective and efficient care. Interdisciplinary team care implies coordinated interaction among the professionals and with the child and family to improve the function and development of the child. This type of coordinated care is common for assessment and management of many medical conditions. Interdisciplinary teams are usually hospital based but also may be based in children's treatment or rehabilitation centers. More recently, interdisciplinary teams have been used in educational settings as an alternative model for service delivery. Teams involving classroom teachers, special education teachers, speech–language pathologists, psychologists, and parents facilitate the identification of children's language and speech problems and as a team are more likely to create a program that is relevant to the child in the classroom setting.

One of the most common interdisciplinary teams for medical conditions is the cleft lip and palate team. Hospital-based interdisciplinary team care for individuals with cleft lip or palate was developed in the 1940s, and this type of care is now the standard throughout the developed world for both cleft lip and palate and other craniofacial anomalies (Witzel, 1993, 1994). These teams provide assessment, diagnosis, intervention, referral, and follow-up. Children with cleft lip and palate usually are evaluated yearly or every other year by an interdisciplinary team until their late teens or early 20s. Surgical, orthodontic, and speech interventions occur at various stages and often are determined by the child's growth and development. Surgical and some medical interventions are conducted by the appropriate members of the hospital-based team; however, orthodontic and speech–language pathology interventions usually are conducted in the child's community. Therapy intervention for school-age children with cleft lip and palate who exhibit speech and language difficulties is often best undertaken in the school setting, as this reduces the time away from school, improves the frequency of attendance, and reduces the child's feeling of being different. For these cases, an open line of communication must be maintained between the team speech–language pathologist and his or her counterpart in the education system to ensure agreement on and understanding of the goals of management and the intervention techniques. Although professionals in education are not usually primary members of these teams, they are important secondary members, and timely and pertinent communication between the health-care and education professionals is important for effective and efficient management of the child's communication problems.

Assessment

The assessment of speech and language problems related to a medical condition is conducted primarily by the speech–language pathologist on the interdisciplinary team. However, input from parents and professionals in audiology, medicine, dentistry, psychology, and education is often necessary to determine the complete nature of the problem, the most effective intervention, the timing of the intervention, and the prognosis. Any assessment of a speech or language disorder must involve a detailed case history, screening of hearing abilities, and an examination of the child's mouth to determine the presence of structural anomalies that might explain the speech patterns.

Assessment of the components of speech involves perceptual ratings of articulation, phonation, resonance, and fluency using rating scales and analysis of speech samples; signal processing techniques to analyze the acoustic signals of speech using electronic instrumentation; and vocal tract imaging using X-ray or fiber optics to examine the anatomy and function of the vocal tract during speech. Although perceptual testing of speech can readily be accomplished in the school setting, the use of signal processing techniques and vocal tract imaging is usually done in a hospital or medical setting, as the technique and interpretation often involve an interdisciplinary approach.

Assessment of the components of language involves analyses of the child's phonology, semantics, syntax, morphology, and pragmatics in comparison to the expected performance for his or her age. This is accomplished through the administration of standardized norm-referenced tests and analyses of spontaneous conversational language samples. Most school boards provide complete assessment of language abilities. To complete the assessment, determine the diagnosis, and recommend appropriate intervention, the school, with the parent's approval, may refer the child for one or more of the following: neuropsychological testing, neurology examination, brain imaging, and genetic testing.

MANAGEMENT OF SPEECH AND LANGUAGE PROBLEMS

The goals of management of speech and language problems include early identification and elimination of the communication problem (secondary prevention) or reduction of the severity of the disorder to enhance or establish functional communication abilities (tertiary prevention; Witzel, 1990). The goals are selected for each child on the basis of the medical condition, its severity of expression, and the limiting factors such as neuromotor status and cognitive deficits. Management of articulation, specific voice problems, and stuttering includes direct individual or group therapy, often with an ongoing home program. Reconstructive craniofacial or orthognathic surgery is used to correct or improve anatomical or functional problems in the vocal tract, such as abnormalities of the larynx, cleft palate, velopharyngeal insufficiency, and severe jaw growth problems with malocclusion. Orthodontic treatment with or without surgery improves speech problems caused by malocclusion. A prosthetic speech obturator may be used to improve hypernasality due to velopharyngeal insufficiency in selected cases when surgical intervention is not possible.

Language problems in school-age children often are related to learning abilities. Management of language problems recently has involved a more holistic approach that emphasizes the interaction of language, cognition, and social context (Wiig & Secord, 1994). This type of approach involves the following:

- Collaborative consultation in which the speech–language pathologist, special educator, classroom teacher, and school psychologist plan and implement intervention as teams
- Contextual–pragmatic intervention in which language and communication training are provided in the contexts in which they are to be used
- Curriculum-related intervention in which language and communication training is related directly to the content and demands of the curriculum (e.g., stories, texts, poems, social studies, verbal math)
- Strategy-based intervention in which training involves active problem solving and decision making and focuses on teaching and learning effective approaches and strategies for using effective language in different contexts and for different purposes
- Whole-language approaches in which reading, writing, listening and speaking are integrated in whole situations, and the focus is on meaning and not on language itself in authentic speech and literacy events (Wiig & Secord, 1994, p. 240)

THE TEACHER'S ROLE

Teachers have an important role in the management of children with communication problems, particularly in schools where interdisciplinary teamwork is used for service delivery. Children who have speech and language disorders often benefit from coordinated programming by speech–language pathologists, teachers, and psychologists. In some cases, the teacher may discover previously undetected communication problems and assist the child and parents in referral to a speech–language pathologist or appropriate hospital-based interdisciplinary team. In other cases, the educator may assist the speech–language pathologist in the carryover aspects of therapy that can be conducted in the classroom. The teacher is often the ideal person to assist the family and speech–language pathologist in monitoring the outcome of therapy interventions and determining the need for continued therapy by observing the child's communication abilities in the educational setting and against the social demands of his or her peers.

For children with significant communication problems or observable medical conditions, such as cleft lip and palate, craniofacial anomalies, or cerebral palsy, the teacher can help to ease the social impact and isolation for the child and reduce teasing by educating other children in the classroom and school about the condition. For example, the AboutFace program (see Additional Resources) is a package that teachers can use to explain facial differences to children. Ability OnLine (see Additional Resources) is a support network that consists of forums and chat rooms, as well as role models and mentors. It provides a public forum where children, teens, and young adults with and without disabilities can share ideas, opinions, and knowledge electronically using a computer bulletin board system. Everybody looks and sounds the same online, and this computer network helps children with disabilities, including motor disorders, facial deformities, and communication problems, to feel less isolated from other children by promoting communication.

CONCLUSION

A child's speech and language problems may be associated with an underlying medical condition, which will affect the diagnosis, treatment, and predicted outcome of the communication disorder. Teachers may play a significant role in the identification and referral of children who would benefit from detailed assessment of their communication skills, coordinated interdisciplinary programming, and development of strategies within the classroom to enhance and improve communication and behavior. Intervention outcome in both communication disorders and education is improved by an understanding of the underlying pathology, its limitations, and its prognosis. The interaction among the family, teacher, other professionals in education, and health-care professionals is often critical to the improvement of the child's communication difficulties and his or her emotional health.

ADDITIONAL RESOURCES

PRINT

Anderson, N. B., & Shames, G. H. (2010). *Human communication disorders: An introduction* (8th ed.). New York, NY: Pearson.

Hennekam, R. C. M., Krantz, I. D., & Allanson, J. E. (2010). *Gorlin's syndromes of the head and neck* (5th ed.). New York, NY: Oxford University Press.

Paasche, C. L., Gorrill, L., & Strom, B. (2003). *Children with special needs in early childhood settings: Identification, intervention, mainstreaming.* Boston, MA: Cengage.

ORGANIZATIONS

Ability OnLine

1120 Finch Avenue West
Toronto, ON M3J 3H7
Canada
Phone 416/650-6207
Fax 416/650-5073
http://www.abilityonline.org

AboutFace International (for individuals with a facial difference and their families)

1057 Steeles Avenue West
PO Box 702
North York, ON M2R 3X1
Canada
Phone 800/665-3223
Fax 416/597-8494
info@aboutface.ca

AboutFace USA

PO Box 158
South Beloit, IL 61080-00158
Phone 888/486-1209
http://www.aboutfaceusa.org

American Cleft Palate-Craniofacial Association and Cleft Palate Foundation

1504 East Franklin Street, Suite 102
Chapel Hill, NC, 27514-2820
Phone 919/933-9044
Fax 919/933-9604
www.cleft.org

American Speech-Language-Hearing Association

2200 Research Blvd.
Rockville, MD 20850-3289
Phone 301/296-5700
http://www.asha.org

Canadian Association of Speech–Language Pathologists and Audiologists

1 Nicholas Street, Suite 1000
Ottawa, ON K1N 7B7
Canada
Phone 613/567-9968
Fax 800/259-8519
http://www.caslpa.ca

Canadian Hearing Society

271 Spadina Rd.
Toronto, ON M5R 2V3
Canada
Phone 877/347-3427
Fax 416/928-2506
http://www.chs.ca

Council for Exceptional Children

2900 Crystal Drive, Suite 1000
Arlington, VA 22202-3557
Phone 888/232-7733
http://www.cec.sped.org

Velo-Cardio-Facial Syndrome Educational Foundation

PO Box 12591
Dallas, TX 75225
Phone 855/800-8237
http://www.ucfsef.org

REFERENCES

Bloom, L., & Lahey, M. (1978). *Language development and language disorders.* New York, NY: Wiley.

Borden, G. J., Harris, K. S., & Raphael, L. J. (1994). *Speech science primer.* Baltimore, MD: Williams & Wilkins.

Goldberg, R., Motzkin, B., Marion, R., Scambler, P. J., & Shprintzen, R. J. (1993). Velo-cardiofacial syndrome: A review of 120 patients. *American Journal of Medical Genetics, 45,* 313–319.

Hardy, J. C. (1994). Cerebral palsy. In G. H. Shames, E. H. Wiig, & W. A. Secord (Eds.), *Human communication disorders: An introduction.* New York, NY: Merrill.

Howard-Peebles, P., Stoddard, G., & Mims, M. (1979). Familial linked mental retardation, verbal disability and marker X chromosomes. *American Journal of Human Genetics, 31,* 214–222.

Jones, K. L. (1988). *Smith's recognizable patterns of human malformation.* Philadelphia, PA: Saunders.

Jung, J. H. (1989). *Genetic syndromes in communication disorders.* Boston, MA: College-Hill.

Klaiman, P. G., Witzel, M A., Margar-Bacal, F. M., & Munro, I. R. (1988). Changes in aesthetic appearance and intelligibility of speech after partial glossectomy in patients with Down syndrome. *Plastic and Reconstructive Surgery, 82,* 403–408.

Landman, G. B. (1989). Language development from six to twelve. *Pediatric Annals, 18,* 373–379.

Margar-Bacal, F. M., Witzel, M. A., & Munro, I. R. (1987). Speech intelligibility after partial glossectomy in children with Down syndrome. *Plastic and Reconstructive Surgery, 79,* 44–49.

McWilliams, B. J., & Witzel, M. A. (1994). Cleft palate. In G. H. Shames, E. H. Wiig, & W. A. Secord (Eds.), *Human communication disorders: An introduction.* New York, NY: Merrill.

Owens, B. R., Jr. (1994). Development of communication, language and speech. In G. H. Shames, E. H. Wiig, & W. A. Secord (Eds.), *Human communication disorders: An introduction* (pp. 36–81). New York, NY: Merrill.

Schaefer, G. B., Mathy-Lakko, P., & Bodensteiner, J. B. (1992). Neurogenetic aspects of communication disorders. *Clinics in Communication Disorders, 2,* 9–19.

Schwartz, R. G. (1994). Phonological disorders. In G. H. Shames, E. H. Wiig, & W. A. Secord (Eds.), *Human communication disorders: An introduction* (pp. 250–291). New York, NY: Merrill.

Shames, G. H., & Ramig, P. R. (1994). Stuttering and other disorders of fluency. In G. H. Shames, E. H. Wiig, & W. A. Secord (Eds.), *Human communication disorders: An introduction* (pp. 336–386). New York, NY: Merrill.

Shprintzen, R. J. (1997). *Genetics, syndromes, and communication disorders.* San Diego, CA: Singular.

Wiig, E. H., & Secord, W. A. (1994). Language disabilities in school-age children and youth. In G. H. Shames, E. H. Wiig, & W. A. Secord (Eds.), *Human communication disorders: An introduction* (pp. 212–248). New York, NY: Merrill.

Witzel, M. A. (1983). Speech problems in craniofacial anomalies. *Communication Disorders, 8,* 45–49.

Witzel, M. A. (1990). Craniofacial anomalies. *Seminars in Speech and Language, 11,* 146–156.

Witzel, M. A. (1993). Cleft lip and palate and craniofacial treatment. *Magazine of the American Speech-Language-Hearing Association, 35,* 27–42.

Witzel, M. A. (1994). Communicative impairment associated with clefting. In R. J. Shprintzen & J. Bardach (Eds.), *Cleft palate speech management: A multidisciplinary approach.* St. Louis, MO: Mosby.

Witzel, M. A., & Vallino, L. (1992). Speech problems in patients with dentofacial or craniofacial deformities. In W. H. Bell (Ed.), *Modern practice in orthognathic and reconstructive surgery* (Vol. 2, pp. 1687–1735). Philadelphia, PA: Saunders.

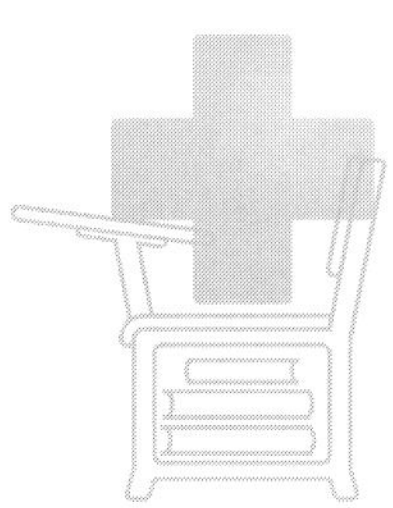

Chapter 11
Pediatric Obesity

Laurie Gaboury and Christine Orosz

The United States, along with the rest of the world, has witnessed a rapid increase in the prevalence of childhood obesity and subsequent early onset of physical and psychosocial health consequences for children and adolescents. Childhood overweight and obesity are complex, with genetic risks and metabolic mechanisms that are embedded in an "obesogenic" environment, with frequent opportunities for the consumption of food and sedentary behaviors (Barlow & Expert Committee, 2007; Golan & Crow, 2004). The cornerstone of current pediatric weight management interventions is a multidisciplinary team working with both the child and the family over an extended period of time (Barlow & Expert Committee, 2007; Lau et al., 2006). However, obesity prevention and treatment need to be conducted in a broader context and require support in the school and wider community (e.g., Lobstein & Jackson-Leach, 2006). Notably, in 2010, U.S. First Lady Michelle Obama initiated the Let's Move! campaign to promote a healthier nation. This chapter covers current understanding of the nature and risks associated with pediatric obesity, with a focus on illuminating the weight bias and stigmatization that children encounter in the school setting. It provides guidelines for the role of educators in ameliorating the significant emotional and social impact of obesity in children and adolescents, and the role of schools in promoting healthy lifestyle.

DEFINITION

Obesity and overweight are defined on the basis of age- and gender-specific body mass index (BMI) normative values. BMI is expressed as weight in kilograms divided by height in meters squared (kg/m2). On the basis of the 2000 CDC BMI-for-age-growth charts for the United States (Centers for Disease Control and Prevention, 2000), overweight for children is defined as a BMI at or above the 85th and less than the 95th percentile, and obesity is defined as a BMI greater than the 95th percentile for age and gender. Although these cutoff criteria are not diagnostic, elevated BMI for children denotes increased risk for future adverse health outcomes or development of disease (Ogden & Carroll, 2010).

PREVALENCE

Results from the 2007–2008 National Health and Nutrition Examination Survey (NHANES) indicated that approximately 17% (12.5 million) of American children and adolescents aged 2–19 years were obese (Ogden & Carroll, 2010). Since 1980, obesity prevalence among children and adolescents has nearly tripled. Among preschool children aged 2–5, obesity increased from 5.0% to 10.4%; among children aged 6–11, from 6.5% to 19.6%; among adolescents aged 12–19, from 5.0% to 18.1%. Significant racial and ethnic disparities also were noted. In 2007–2008 Hispanic adolescent boys (26.8%) were more likely to be obese than non-Hispanic white adolescent boys (16.7%). Among girls, non-Hispanic black adolescents (29.2%) were significantly more likely to be obese than non-Hispanic white adolescents (14.5%).

COMPLEX OBESITY FACTORS

There is a common belief that overweight individuals do not know the proper way to eat or lack self-discipline. However, body weight is affected by numerous factors, including genetic, metabolic, and hormonal influences that likely predispose some persons to obesity and may set the range of possible weights that an individual can achieve (Lustig, 2010). Davison and Birch (2001) suggested that three main ecological layers influence a child's weight status: individual characteristics and risk factors; parenting styles and family characteristics; and community, demographic, and societal characteristics. In addition to genetic and biological factors, influences at the individual and family levels include the meal environment, food availability, increased television and screen viewing, decreased leisure time for parents, cultural beliefs, parenting styles, sibling interactions, and emotional health. At the community level factors include urban designs that discourage walking; increased concerns over neighborhood safety; increased availability of fast food and high-fat, calorie-dense food; leisure and recreational facilities access; and seasonal influences, school lunch, and physical education programs. According to Yale University's Rudd Center for Food Policy and Obesity (http://www.yaleruddcenter.org/), American children typically watch about 15 food commercials daily, cueing cookies, chips, and high-calorie, high-fat snacks. Numerous studies report that exposure to advertising is associated with increased consumption of soft drinks and fast food among elementary school children. Societal factors also need to take into account peer interactions such as lack of social support for physical activity and healthy eating, and teasing (Wilfley, Vannucci, & White, 2010).

An obesogenic environment is a challenge for children and their families, and it likely contributes to a sense of personal failure related to weight control. Prevention of weight gain among normal-weight children requires similar policies as needed to support weight control among children with overweight and obesity. Measures proposed by the World Health Organization (2004) and other expert groups (e.g., Lobstein, Baur, & Uauy, 2004) target "downstream" policies in school, home, and neighborhood environments, as well as "upstream" policies for food supplies, commercial marketing, and promotion of healthier lifestyles. Addressing childhood obesity requires a multifaceted approach (Menon, 2007). The school setting provides opportunities to positively affect child health in both the short term and the long term, given the length of time spent in the education system. School psychologists are in a position to assess and design healthy lifestyle programs that are contextually and culturally relevant to their schools and to provide essential emotional health supports (McCarthy, Fallon, & Hagermoser Sanetti, 2012).

PHYSICAL HEALTH CONSEQUENCES

Childhood obesity causes a wide range of serious health complications and increases the risk of premature illness and death later in life (Ebbeling, Pawlak, & Ludwig, 2002). Children who are overweight or obese are at risk, for example, of impaired glucose tolerance, type 2 diabetes, high blood pressure, high cholesterol, cardiovascular disease, nonalcoholic fatty liver disease, sleep apnea, bone and joint problems, polycystic ovary syndrome, and other health issues. Children with obesity are more likely to become adults with obesity. Early onset of metabolic complications continues into adulthood and presents the risk of a shortened life expectancy.

COMORBIDITIES AND PSYCHOSOCIAL OUTCOMES

It is not in the scope of this chapter to review genetic conditions (e.g., Prader-Willi syndrome) and biological mechanisms (e.g., endocrine disorders) contributing to obesity. The majority of school-age children with obesity are not likely to be diagnosed with a specific genetic syndrome. Educators need to be aware of children with a traumatic brain injury (e.g., motor vehicle accident) or acquired brain injury (e.g., brain tumor requiring surgery or chemotherapy) who may have damage to their satiety center (i.e., hypothalamus). Some studies have reported an association between developmental coordination disorder (DCD), most pronounced in balance activities, and children with overweight and obesity (Wagner et al., 2011). A significant risk for these children also is avoidance of physical activities due to social stigmatization.

Children and adolescents who are overweight or obese often experience significant social and emotional outcomes, such as low self-esteem, anxiety, depression, social isolation, and weight stigmatization. In general, findings concerning psychological comorbidities of ADHD (attention-deficit/hyperactivity disorder), depression, and binge eating related to childhood obesity are mixed and equivocal (Lobstein et al., 2004; Ringham, Levine, & Marcus, 2009). In a large cohort study of adolescents in grades 7–12, Goodman and Whitaker (2002) found that elevated BMI was related to depression, and scores were highest in children with the greatest BMI. Although some research indicates that obesity, mood, and binge eating interact over time, the precise nature of these relationships is not clearly known. However, consistent findings indicate that a history of teasing or concerns about personal weight increase the association between obesity and depression, anxiety, low self-esteem, poor body image, and suicidality in children and adolescents (Eisenberg, Neumark-Sztainer, & Story, 2003; for a review, see Puhl & Latner, 2007). Obesity compromises peer relationships; overweight children often have fewer friends and more isolated and peripheral relationships than normal-weight children, who have more relationships with a central network of children (Strauss & Pollack, 2003). Compared with normal-weight peers, children and adolescents seeking treatment for weight have reported decreased quality of life in most domains of physical, mental, and social well-being (Forste & Moore, 2012).

BODY IMAGE

Body-image attitudes are influenced by societal and cultural factors. In the overall population, half of adolescent girls and one-fourth of adolescent boys are not satisfied with their bodies (Neumark-Sztainer, 2005). Although body dissatisfaction is commonly thought of as just part of growing up, it is linked to self-esteem issues and depression and is a risk factor for using unhealthy weight-control behaviors (Chaiton et al., 2009; Mond, van den Berg, Boutelle, Hannan, & Neumark-Sztainer, 2011). Body image is a common issue for children and adolescents who have been the victims of weight bias in their homes, schools, or communities. Self-evaluation of one's body image is affected by peer interactions and negative weight-related comments. Those who are frequently teased feel self-conscious or experience lower body image. Body-image issues are seen in adolescents regardless of race, gender, and socioeconomic status. However, differences exist regarding attitudes about eating and the pursuit of thinness between cultural groups (Ali, Rizzo, & Heiland, 2013; Kayano et al., 2008). For example, while both black and white adolescent females desired to be smaller in size and displayed body dissatisfaction, black adolescent girls chose a larger size as their ideal body size (Kelly, Bulik, & Mazzeo, 2011).

The media also has a significant impact on body image and self-esteem. Today's society idealizes a smaller body size, and children and adolescents are listening to these messages and are affected by them. Luff and Gray (2009) examined teen magazines aimed at girls published from 1956 to 2005 and found overall that these magazines were sending complex mixed messages to girls about the thin ideal. While the size of the cover model has increased and reflects a more realistic image of teen girls, more written information, such as information about dieting and exercise in the magazines, supports the thin ideal.

WEIGHT BIAS OR STIGMATIZATION

Much concern exists about stigmatization of children with overweight and obesity, most often in the form of teasing and bullying (Puhl, 2011), and its profound impact on the social development of youth (Gray, Kahhan, & Janicke, 2009). Studies indicate that peers, educators, parents and family members, strangers in public settings, and health-care professionals are sources of weight bias. Weight stigmatization begins as early as age 3 in childhood (Su & Di Santo, 2011) and is prevalent in the school setting by adolescence. The 2011 National Education Association (NEA) survey of educators identified the following percentage of teachers and support professionals reporting concerns for bullying based on a student's weight (23%), gender (20%), perceived sexual orientation (18%), race (18%), and disability (12%) (Bradshaw, Waasdorp, O'Brennan, & Gulemetova, 2011). Parents also reported significant concerns for weight-related teasing and identified a greater need to address psychosocial issues than healthy eating and physical activity (Haines, Neumark-Sztainer, & Thiel, 2007). Children with obesity are targeted regardless of their gender, race, socioeconomic status, social skills, or academic achievement (Lumeng et al., 2010), and the chances of being bullied increase with body weight (Rudd Center, 2013). Multiple forms of verbal, relational (e.g., social isolation), cyber, and physical teasing and bullying are documented, with verbal bullying occurring most frequently. In a study of 1,555 adolescents (Puhl, Luedicke, & Heuer, 2011), students reported witnessing overweight and/or obese peers being made fun of (92%), called names (91%), teased in a mean way (88%), teased during physical activities (85%), ignored or avoided (76%), excluded from activities (67%), verbally threatened (57%), and physically harassed (54%). Maladaptive coping strategies demonstrated by victims included avoidance (e.g., avoiding physical education class and physical activity), increased food consumption, and binge eating (Puhl & Luedicke, 2012). Weight-based victimization also contributed to poorer school performance and more absenteeism. Conversely, children with overweight and obesity also can be perpetrators of bullying behaviors (Janssen, Craig, Boyce, & Picket, 2004).

HEALTH IMPLICATIONS

Compared to overweight peers who are not teased, overweight children who *are* teased are more likely to experience higher levels of depression and to use unhealthy weight-control behaviors (Madowitz, Knatz, Maginot, Crow, & Boutelle, 2012). Weight-related teasing is inversely associated with health-related quality of life (Jensen & Steele, 2012). Children who were teased because of their weight had lower levels of psychological well-being, physical self-concept, and physical activity self-efficacy (Greenleaf, Petrie, & Martin, 2014). Notably lower scores on health-related measures of physical fitness indicated that teasing affected physical health as well as emotional health. In a large, nationally represented study (n = 7,825) of students aged 11–17 years, youth with overweight and obesity reported significant health-risk behaviors (Farhat, Iannotti, & Simons-Morton, 2010). Substance use (frequent smoking and drinking) was associated with overweight and obesity in girls; younger boys with obesity were more likely to be bullied; and older boys with obesity were more likely to carry weapons compared to boys of normal weight. These research studies indicate that overall health status of these children and adolescents is jeopardized.

NEGATIVE PEER EVALUATION

Numerous research studies have demonstrated that peers significantly influence perceptions of self-esteem for children with overweight and peers view obesity as one of the most stigmatizing and least acceptable conditions (DeJong, 1993; for reviews, see Haines & Neumark-Sztainer, 2009; Lobstein et al., 2004). Social marginalization is defined as youth excluding their peers as a result of perceptions of them as different or undesirable. In studies in which children rank ordered a series of drawings of children with various handicaps (crutches, wheelchair, missing a hand, facial disfigurement, obesity) on the basis of which child they "liked best," the drawing of an obese child was ranked lowest. Even when information explaining obesity was provided, it had minimal positive effect on children's attitudes and behavioral intentions toward a peer presented as obese (Bell & Morgan, 2000). Children and adolescents who experience weight stigma often suffer low self-esteem from damaging comments. Common negative stereotypes that are attributed to individuals with obesity include perceptions that they are lazy, lacking in self-discipline, less competent, and at fault for being overweight (Barnett, Sonnentag, Livengood, Struble, & Wadian, 2011). These stereotypes are communicated during teasing experiences (Puhl & Latner, 2007; Rudd Center for Food Policy and Obesity, 2013a, 2013b).

Educators need to challenge these stereotypes and to role-model behavior that it is not acceptable to treat others unfairly because of weight. To do so, educators need to question their own weight bias (i.e., ask, "What are my own attitudes and feelings about weight?"). Beliefs that obesity is under personal control and due to lack of willpower and discipline lead to lower expectations of students with overweight in physical, social, and academic abilities, and lead to stereotypes about students' character, intelligence, hygiene, and family life (Neumark-Sztainer, Story, & Harris, 1999). Such perceptions likely affect student scholastic performance, self-esteem, and emotional health.

PEER SUPPORT

Social support is a protective factor among children and adolescents with overweight and obesity. Perceived social support from school peers has shown to affect long-term, weight-related quality of life outcomes (Wu, Reiter-Purtill, & Zeller, 2014). Friendships may help support better psychosocial outcomes (Reiter-Purtill, Ridel, Jordan, & Zeller, 2010). For example, when children have a friend to play with on the playground or to hang out with, it can make a significant difference when others are being unkind. Friendship has shown a buffering effect on emotional well-being (Caccavale, Farhat, & Ianotti, 2012), such as protecting adolescent girls from developing body dissatisfaction. Social engagement was related to better body satisfaction compared to those who did not have that social engagement. Peer-support networks as part of a bullying intervention program have shown to mediate anxiety and depression in adolescents (Holt & Espelage, 2007). Improving a child's social network also had positive implications for physical activity (Salvy et al., 2009). Interventions using peers as role models and promoters of a healthy diet showed significant positive changes in dietary patterns (Field & Kitos, 2009).

Adolescents with overweight and obesity are more socially marginalized and isolated than their peers (Strauss & Pollack, 2003). Sometimes they withdraw from activities out of embarrassment or frustration due to their size (e.g., not fitting into a dance team uniform, being teased at a local pool by strangers, feeling out of breath when playing soccer). Consequently, rather than being out of the home socializing with peers, these adolescents often engage in solitary and sedentary activities, such as playing video games. Creating opportunities and encouraging students to be involved in social activities is likely to have a positive impact on their social relationships and emotional health.

MEDIA

The social acceptability of weight stigmatization as seen in media and social settings is compelling. Neumark-Sztainer (2005) described "weightism" as "the last of the socially acceptable 'isms,'" given the perception that weight is viewed as controllable and that individuals are responsible for their size. Individuals with overweight and obesity appear to be the "last acceptable targets of discrimination" (Puhl & Brownell, 2001, p. 788) and disparaging humor. They are frequently ridiculed and stereotyped in popular television shows and movies. One study demonstrated that the majority (72%) depicted in online news photographs were stigmatized (Heuer, McClure, & Puhl, 2011). Compared to non-overweight individuals, they were more likely to have their heads cut out of photos, to be portrayed with only their abdomens or lower bodies shown, to be partially clothed (e.g., bare stomachs showing), and to be eating or drinking. By isolating certain body parts and emphasizing excess weight, news photographs degrade these persons. Media also lacked positive portrayals of individuals with obesity wearing professional clothing or in professional capacities. Weight stereotypes are abundant in children's literature and media, including television programs, movies, and cartoons depicting children with obesity as lazy, having poor eating habits, being less intelligent, and having negative character traits. Such images may encourage children to devalue and stigmatize peers with above-average body weights (Latner, Rosewall, & Simmonds, 2007). Obesity stigma in the mass media contributes to the social acceptability of weight prejudice and its punitive consequences for those affected (Puhl & Heuer, 2009).

ACADEMICS

In studies of kindergarten children and elementary school-age children, respectively, the association between overweight and lower academic performance has been described as "a marker but not a causal factor" (Datar, Strum, & Magnabosco, 2004, p. 67), and differences were insignificant after adjusting for behavioral, socioeconomic, and maternal education variables (Judge & Jahns, 2007). Educators need to be responsive to a broad range of academic achievement and of learning challenges for all students. Students with overweight and obesity have additional risk factors for emotional challenges and school avoidance that likely impact learning opportunities. Educators' bias against weight also can affect their evaluations of students. MacCann and Roberts (2013) found that lower grades for students with overweight and obesity might reflect bias from teachers and peers rather than a lack of academic ability. The researchers found no difference between overweight or obese and normal-weight students on various tests of intelligence and achievement; however, there were discrepancies between the groups on school grades. Notably, some studies have shown that physical education teachers demonstrated a strong bias against persons with obesity and demonstrated lower expectations of students with obesity, leading to less participation in activities (Fontana, Furtado, Marston, Mazzardo, & Gallagher, 2013).

Overall diet quality is associated with academic achievement in children, as children with decreased diet quality are more likely to perform poorly on academic performance measures (Florence, Asbridge, & Veugelers, 2008). School nutrition programs have potential to increase student access to healthy food choices and improved diet quality, which can positively affect academic performance and health.

PHYSICAL ACTIVITY

Physical education in schools as typically provided has not been shown to reduce or prevent obesity (Casazza et al., 2013). Educators are faced with demands to include more learning goals in their curriculums and to reach expected achievement scores or learning outcomes. Time allocated to physical education may be reduced to accommodate academic goals, and allotted time percentage shows decline from middle school to high school programs (Johnston, Delva, & O'Malley, 2007). There is a mind–body connection that cannot be ignored. Physical activity improves learning by positively affecting functions like attention and motivation and affecting the body biology that is essential for learning (Ratey & Hagerman, 2008). Exercise can reduce stress-related diseases that affect health as well as help to manage anxiety, depression, and attention-deficit/hyperactivity disorder. Guidelines established by the National Association for Sport and Physical Education (NASPE, 2003) recommended that elementary schoolchildren should be active at least 60 minutes cumulative daily and include up to several hours of moderate to vigorous physical activity daily.

ROLE OF SCHOOLS AND GUIDELINES

Patino-Fernandez, Hernandez, Villa, and Delamater (2013) found that parents and educators were concerned about childhood obesity, although each identified the other as having the primary responsibility for addressing the issue, including causes of obesity, responsibility for the child's eating behavior, and barriers to healthy eating. They agreed on the necessity of working together to promote healthy environments for children both at school and at home. Educators can be important partners with families and health-care professionals in helping children with obesity by providing a healthy, supportive, and inclusive environment in the school. School psychologists play an important role in their knowledge about behavioral change and systems change (Menon, 2007). Administrators and elected school officials have influence in policies in mandating curricula and healthy lifestyle activities in the school. Actions taken in the school need to promote overall health and healthy lifestyle habits for all students, rather than giving the message of weight loss, especially for those who are dealing with weight issues. Schools should serve as healthy role models via what is taught in the curricula and via actions that provide a healthy environment for nutrition and physical activity. A salient goal for educators in supporting children is to maintain a psychologically healthy environment free of weight bias and weight-related teasing and bullying.

Role of the School in Promoting Health for All Students

Education and Promotion of Healthy Lifestyle

School programs have the potential to reach many children and to influence healthy lifestyle, including nutrition, physical activity, knowledge, and psychosocial factors. However, most school-based interventions have demonstrated only modest impact on weight management outcomes (for a review, see Gittelsohn & Park, 2010). A primary critique has been that school-centered programs need to be heavily reinforced by strong interventions in the community. There is evidence (e.g., Schwartz & Brownell, 2010) that children's diets are influenced by foods available in school cafeterias and vending machines, the schools' nutrition policies, and the availability of unhealthy snacks in school locales. As well, there is a vast branded marketing that occurs on school grounds. At the school level, strategies to limit high-fat and high-sugar foods and to increase physical education are recommended to influence children's healthy diet and physical activity patterns (Jago, Thompson, O'Donnell, Cullen, & Baranowski, 2009).

Schools can focus on educating all students about the benefits of living a healthy lifestyle with information that is age- or grade-level-appropriate. Emphasize healthy food choices, introduce a variety of physical activity options, and encourage other healthy behaviors such as adequate sleep, time management, and stress reduction skills. Nutrition information can be incorporated into the curriculum (Blom-Hoffman, 2004) and lessons supplemented with activities such as field trips to a local grocery store or farm.

Educators are advised to refrain from giving children with overweight and obesity specific health advice. Many children may have specific dietary needs that should be addressed by trained medical staff, such as dieticians. They may present with complex health issues and use medications, requiring the oversight of physicians. Attrition rates from multidisciplinary pediatric weight management medical programs are high (Skelton, Goff, Ip, & Beech, 2011), and families leave for a variety of reasons, including perceived lack of success. Given the complex nature of lifestyle change, educators are cautioned to stay within the scope of their training and practice.

Awareness of the Psychosocial Issues Associated With Obesity

Overweight and obesity have profound psychosocial consequences, including social isolation, weight stigmatization, association with mental health issues, and risk of unhealthy behaviors such as extreme dieting measures. Educators need to recognize signs of psychological distress, assess if children have a support system to deal with weight-based victimization, and proactively help obtain mental health supports or other resources (Puhl, Peterson, & Luedicke, 2012).

Media Literacy

Paradoxically, the media cues both excessive consumption of food and an obsession with thinness. Media literacy is needed to teach students to become critical viewers of all media forms, especially advertising. For students with overweight and obesity, developing critical thinking skills is needed so that students may evaluate stigmatization and refrain from internalizing negative comments. Education for all students is needed to promote development of empathy and compassion.

Communication With Parents

Obesity is a sensitive topic. Parents of children with overweight may not perceive their child to have an unhealthy weight. Educators could ask the parents if they have concerns about their child's health and if the parents have suggestions or requests for accommodations to support their child's learning, social interactions, and participation in school activities.

Talking About Obesity and Weight Bias

An expert committee (Barlow & Expert Committee, 2007) recommended talking about obesity by using a supportive, empathetic, and nonjudgmental attitude that does not place blame and by careful choice of words, using neutral terms such as "unhealthy weight" and "overweight." Educators need to address weight bias in the classroom, gymnasium, locker rooms, bathrooms, and school playgrounds. It is important to communicate to students that teasing is never acceptable, regardless of whether the teasing is directed at appearance, weight, race, accent, wealth, and so on.

Parents and Educators as Partners

Parents and educators need to collaborate to assist with building healthy environments and initiatives, such as through focus groups.

Inclusive Environment

Acknowledge Different Needs and Experiences

Children with overweight and obesity differ among themselves in terms of personal life experiences and perspectives. Some children are severely bullied, while others are quite popular with their peers in school and enjoy participating in extracurricular activities. Some dread gym class, while others are quite athletic and enjoy it. Some are ashamed of their bodies, while others feel confident and accepting of their larger size. Educators need to be aware of the potential special needs of all the children in their classroom and to be sensitive to the accommodations that a child with overweight or obesity may need.

Facilitate Social Interactions

Because children with obesity or overweight are at risk of social isolation and of being victimized, teachers are encouraged to help facilitate friendships and to help the children assume leadership roles when possible in their class or school.

Focus on Strengths and Talents

Many children with overweight or obesity may have lower self-esteem and body image when compared with average-sized peers. Educators are in a position to encourage these students to discover their strengths and interests (e.g., musical ability, participation in clubs).

Address Discrimination in General

Schools need to address weight bias in the context of addressing discrimination in general (e.g., weight, race, sexual orientation) rather than focusing specifically on obesity. Drawing attention to size can be humiliating. Students need strategies for building resiliency and for taking appropriate actions when confronted with teasing and bullying.

Create a Safe and Welcoming Environment Free of Weight Bias and Bullying

Weight-related interventions and prevention programs need to address psychosocial issues, especially weight bias and teasing (Haines et al., 2007). Weight stigmatization and negative peer evaluation begin at a young age and are sanctioned in society for humor and prejudice. Making students aware that "fat jokes" are not acceptable helps create an environment that is safe and welcoming for children and adolescents who are overweight or obese. When a child is victimized, actions need to be taken to remediate the situation, enlisting the help of administrators or outside resources if necessary.

Create a Safe and Supportive Environment for Physical Education

Educators are encouraged to design physical activity lessons in a way that children of all sizes can participate and enjoy the activity (Greenleaf et al., 2014). Educators may interpret below-average performance as laziness or lack of effort, when in fact the child is physically unable to meet certain physical standards, despite trying. A physical therapist could help adapt equipment or modify physical education curriculum. There are emotional challenges faced by children (e.g., embarrassment from not fitting into the largest-sized uniform; a field trip to a swimming pool creates stress for children who are embarrassed to wear a bathing suit). Often avoidance of physical activities becomes a coping strategy.

Provide a Safe and Appropriate Physical Environment

Does the child's large size prevent him or her from comfortably fitting in desks and chairs or using any other classroom spaces or equipment? Is the furniture sturdy enough to support the child's weight to prevent injury or collapsing furniture? An occupational therapist could ensure proper fit of furniture. The school environment also needs to be welcoming for family members who may be overweight or obese. Is there appropriate seating for interviews, school performances, or social and sports events?

Examine Own Beliefs

Educators need to examine their own beliefs about obesity and weight bias by asking the following:

- "Do I believe that individuals with obesity are lazy?"
- "Do I believe that individuals need only to eat less and exercise more to reach a healthy weight while ignoring the complex nature and causes of obesity?"
- "Do I laugh at 'fat jokes' or overlook this prejudicial humor in my classroom?"
- "Do I give less attention to or negatively evaluate students who are overweight or obese?"
- "Do I use respectful and sensitive language when discussing weight?"

School as Healthy Role Model

As a society, providing junk food to children has become "normalized" and often justified as "just one" snack (Freedhoff, 2013). People are offended when these practices of giving junk food as part of an activity are challenged. However, these "just one" snacks accumulate to have an impact on health. There are many temptations to eat unhealthy foods in schools or those brought home (e.g., candy sold for school fund-raisers; rewards with unhealthy food for a job well done; sweet snacks given during soccer games; school bus drivers giving candy for good behavior and special holidays; gym teachers giving candy for "working hard"). There is no doubt of the good intentions of adults in praising students or simply providing an enjoyable treat. Problems arise because treats accumulate over time and are perceived as "normal" consumption. Children also create strong positive memories associated with these unhealthy foods. Lifelong eating habits are developed at a young age, and the school is a major part of this learning environment. Thus, schools need to serve as healthy role models for students. Here are some examples:

- *Limit access to unhealthy foods and provide healthy food options.* Schools can ensure that healthy foods are provided in food sales, vending machines, and the cafeteria. Access to unhealthy food should be limited (e.g., sweets at an occasional party or celebration). A "sign up" sheet for school parties where a variety of healthy snacks (e.g., fruit, vegetables) are listed gives educators more control over the kinds of food brought into the classroom.
- *Healthy eating is for everyone.* Children who are overweight or obese should not be singled out as all students benefit from healthy lifestyle choices.
- *Healthy fund-raising.* Fund-raising should include ideas other than selling foods. Be creative!
- *Avoid using food for a reward.* Children learn to associate positive feelings with food rewards, which may lead to unhealthy coping strategies (e.g., eating a treat to feel better).
- *Promote daily physical activity.* Physical education, unstructured play at recess, and school and community sports are associated with greater levels of physical activity for children. Opportunities for organized sport and activities are particularly important for low-income children whose options may be limited elsewhere. Supervision and access to equipment and play areas in the school settings support the development of healthy physical activity behaviors.

Table 11.1
CHECKLIST TOOL FOR SCHOOLS

Does this school or classroom provide a psychologically healthy environment for all students?
☐ Is there a no-tolerance policy regarding bullying or teasing for weight and other differences?
☐ Does this school educate students about discrimination, weight bias, and respecting differences?
☐ Have staff members challenged any weight biases that they may hold?
☐ Is support provided for students to promote healthy friendships and involvement in social activities, which may serve as a buffer for poor psychosocial outcomes?
☐ Are referrals made to school psychologists or other professionals for students struggling with psychosocial or mental health aspects related to obesity?
☐ Are students' special talents and strengths celebrated and recognized in the school?
Does this school or classroom provide an inclusive environment?
☐ Does the physical environment fit the student (e.g., sturdy and comfortable desks and chairs)?
☐ Does the student need accommodations (e.g., academic, larger uniform size)?
☐ Are physical activities appropriate or modified for the student, to encourage participation?
☐ Do overweight visitors or family members feel welcome in the school?
Does this school or classroom serve as a healthy role model for students?
☐ Are there opportunities for daily physical activity at school?
☐ Are healthy food choices available in the school?
☐ Are unhealthy food choices at the school eliminated or limited?
☐ Are privileges or items other than food used as rewards?
☐ Does the school provide age-appropriate education about a healthy lifestyle?
☐ Do educators work collaboratively with parents and health-care professionals?

CONCLUSION

Childhood obesity is a complex health condition with serious implications for physical and mental health, and for social functioning. When implementing school-based programs to promote a healthy lifestyle, it is important to impose no further stigmatization on students. Key interventions need to educate about the complex nature of obesity, address weight bias, and focus on improved health for all students as outcomes. Table 11.1 includes a checklist that can be used to assist teachers in supporting children with obesity in the school setting. Educators have significant roles in these interventions and in creating partnerships with families and health-care professionals to promote health in their students.

ADDITIONAL RESOURCES

Hassink, S. G. (2006). *A parent's guide to childhood obesity: A road map to health.* Washington, DC: American Academy of Pediatrics.

U.S. Department of Health and Human Services Centers for Disease Control and Prevention

Yale Rudd Center for Food Policy and Obesity (www.yaleruddcenter.org)

REFERENCES

Ali, M. M., Rizzo, J. A., & Heiland, F. W. (2013). Big and beautiful? Evidence of racial differences in the perceived attractiveness of obese females. *Journal of Adolescence, 336*(3), 539–549.

Barlow, S. E. & the Expert Committee (2007). Expert committee recommendations regarding the prevention, assessment, and treatment of child and adolescent overweight and obesity: Summary report. *Pediatrics, 120*, S164–S192.

Barnett, M. A., Sonnentag, T. L., Livengood, J. L., Struble, A. L., & Wadian, T. W. (2011). Role of fault attributions and desire, effort, and outcome expectations in children's anticipated responses to hypothetical peers with various undesirable characteristics. *Journal of Genetic Psychology, 173*(3), 317–329.

Bell, S. K., & Morgan, S. B. (2000). Children's attitudes and behavioral intentions toward a peer presented as obese: Does a medical explanation for the obesity make a difference? *Journal of Pediatric Psychology, 25*(3), 137–145.

Blom-Hoffman, J. (2004). Obesity prevention in children: Strategies for parents and school personnel. National Association of School Psychologists (NASP). *Communique, 33*(3). Retrieved from http://www.nasponline.org/publications/cq/cq333obesity.aspx

Bradshaw, C. P., Waasdorp, T. E., O'Brennan, L. M., & Gulemetova, M. (2011). *Findings from the National Education Association's Nationwide Study of Bullying: Teachers' and education support professionals' perspectives.* Retrieved from http://www.nea.org/assets/docs/Nationwide_Bullying_Research_Findings.pdf

Caccavale, L. J., Farhat, T., & Iannotti, R. J. (2012). Social engagement in adolescence moderates the association between weight status and body image. *Body Image, 9*(2), 221–226.

Casazza, K., Fontaine, K. R., Astrup, A., Birch, L. L., Brown, A. W., Bohan Brown, M. M., . . . Allison, D. B. (2013). Myths, presumptions, and facts about obesity. *New England Journal of Medicine, 368,* 446–454. doi:10.1056/NEJMsa1208051

Centers for Disease Control and Prevention. (2000). *CDC BMI growth charts.* Retrieved from http://www.cdc.gov/growthcharts

Chaiton, M., Sabiston, C., O'Loughlin, J., McGrath, J. J., Maximova, K., & Lambert, M. (2009). A structural equation model relating adiposity, psychosocial indicators of body image and depressive symptoms among adolescents. *International Journal of Obesity, 33,* 588–596.

Datar, A., Strum, R., & Magnabosco, J. L. (2004). Childhood overweight and academic performance: National study of kindergartners and first-graders. *Obesity Research, 12*(1), 58–68.

Davison, K. K., & Birch, L. L. (2001). Childhood overweight: A contextual model and recommendations for future research. *Obesity Reviews, 2*(3), 159–171.

DeJong, W. (1993). Obesity as a characterological stigma: The issue of responsibility and judgments of task performance. *Psychological Reports, 73,* 963–970.

Ebbeling, C. B., Pawlak, D. B., & Ludwig, D. S. (2002). Childhood obesity: Public-health crisis, common sense cure. *Lancet, 360,* 473–482.

Eisenberg, M. E., Neumark-Sztainer, D., & Story, M. (2003). Associations of weight-based teasing and emotional wellbeing among adolescents. *JAMA Pediatrics, 157*(8), 733–738.

Farhat, T., Iannotti, R. J., & Simons-Morton, B. G. (2010). Overweight, obesity, youth, and health-risk behaviors. *American Journal of Preventive Medicine, 38*(3), 258–267. doi:10.1016/j.amepre.2009.10.038

Field, A., & Kitos, N. (2009). Social and interpersonal influences on obesity in youth: Family, peers, society. In L. J. Heinberg & J. K. Thompson (Eds.), *Obesity in youth: Causes, consequences, and cures* (pp. 59–76). Washington, DC: American Psychological Association.

Florence, M. D., Asbridge, M., & Veugelers, P. (2008). Diet quality and academic performance. *Journal of School Health, 78*(4), 209–215.

Fontana, F. E., Furtado, O., Marston, R, Mazzardo, O., & Gallagher, J. (2013). Anti-fat bias among physical education teachers and majors. *Physical Educator, 70,* 15–31.

Forste, R., & Moore, E. (2012). Adolescent obesity and life satisfaction: Perceptions of self, peers, family, and school. *Economics & Human Biology, 10*(4), 385–394. http://dx.doi.org/10.1016/jehb.2012.04.008

Freedhoff, Y. (2013). Why is everyone always giving my kids junk food? *U.S. News & World Report.* Retrieved from http://health.usnews.com/health-news/blogs/eat-run/2013/02/20/why-is-everyone-always-giving-my-kids-junk-food

Gittelsohn, J., & Park, S. (2010). School- and community-based interventions. In M. Freemark (Ed.), *Contemporary endocrinology: Pediatric obesity: Etiology, pathogenesis, and treatment* (pp. 315–335). New York, NY: Humana Press.

Golan, M., & Crow, S. (2004). Parents are key players in the prevention and treatment of weight-related problems. *Nutrition Reviews, 62*(1), 39–50.

Goodman, E., & Whitaker, R. C. (2002). A prospective study of the role of depression in the development and persistence of adolescent obesity. *Pediatrics, 110,* 497–504.

Gray, W. N., Kahhan, N. A., & Janicke, D. M. (2009). Peer victimization and pediatric obesity: A review of the literature. *Psychology in the Schools, 46*(8), 720–727. doi:10.1002/pits.20410

Greenleaf, C., Petrie, T. A., & Martin, S. B. (2014). Relationship of weight-based teasing and adolescents' psychological well-being and physical health. *Journal of School Health, 84*(1), 49–55.

Haines, J., & Neumark-Sztainer, D. (2009). Psychosocial consequences of obesity and weight bias: Implications for interventions. In L. J. Heinberg & J. K. Thompson (Eds.), *Obesity in youth: Causes, consequences, and cures* (pp. 183–201). Washington, DC: American Psychological Association.

Haines, J., Neumark-Sztainer, D., & Thiel, L. (2007). Addressing weight-related issues in an elementary school: What do students, parents, and school staff recommend? *Eating Disorders, 15,* 5–21. doi:10.1080/10640260601044428

Heuer, C. A., McClure, K. J., & Puhl, R. M. (2011). Obesity stigma in online news: A visual content analysis. *Journal of Health Communication, 16*(9), 976–987.

Holt, M. K., & Espelage, D. L. (2007). Perceived social support among bullies, victims, and bully-victims. *Journal of Youth and Adolescence, 36,* 984–994.

Jago, R., Thompson, D., O'Donnell, S., Cullen, K., & Baranowski, T. (2009). Prevention: Changing children's diet and physical activity patterns via schools, families, and the environment. In L. J. Heinberg & J. K. Thompson (Eds.), *Obesity in youth: Causes, consequences, and cures* (pp. 183–201). Washington, DC: American Psychological Association.

Janssen, I., Craig, W. M., Boyce, W. F., & Picket, W. (2004). Associations between overweight and obesity with bullying behaviors in school-aged children. *Pediatrics, 113*(5), 1187–1194.

Jensen, C. D., & Steele, R. G. (2012). Longitudinal associations between teasing and health-related quality of life among treatment-seeking overweight and obese youth. *Journal of Pediatric Psychology, 37*(4), 438–447.

Johnston, L. D., Delva, J., & O'Malley, P. M. (2007). Sports participation and physical education in American secondary schools. *American Journal of Preventive Medicine, 33,* S195–S207. doi:10.1016/j.amepre.2007.07.015

Judge, S., & Jahns, L. (2007). Association of overweight with academic performance and social and behavioral problems: An update from the early childhood longitudinal study. *Journal of School Health, 77*(10), 672–678.

Kayano, M., Yoshiuchi, K., Al-Adawi, S., Viernes, N., Dorvlo, N., Kumano, H., . . . Akabayashi, A. (2008). Eating attitudes and body dissatisfaction in adolescents: Cross-cultural study. *Psychiatry and Clinical Neurosciences, 62,* 17–25.

Kelly, N. R., Bulik, C. M., & Mazzeo, S. E. (2011). An exploration of body dissatisfaction and perceptions of black and white girls enrolled in an intervention for overweight children. *Body Image, 8*(4), 379–384.

Latner, J. D., Rosewall, J. K., & Simmonds, M. B. (2007). Childhood obesity stigma: Association with television, videogame, and magazine exposure. *Body Image, 4*, 147–155.

Lau, D. C. W., Douketis, J. D., Morrison, K. M., Hramiak, I. M., Sharma, A. M., & Ur, E. (2006). For members of the Obesity Canada Clinical Practice Guidelines Expert Panel: Canadian clinical practice guidelines on the management and prevention of obesity in adults and children. *Canadian Medical Association Journal, 176*, S1–S13.

Lobstein, T., Baur, L., & Uauy, R. (2004). Obesity in children and young people: A crisis in public health. [For the IASO International Obesity Task Force]. *Obesity Reviews, 5*(Suppl. 1), 4–85.

Lobstein, T., & Jackson-Leach, R. (2006). Estimated burden of paediatric obesity and co-morbidities in Europe. Part 2: Numbers of children with indicators of obesity-related disease. *International Journal of Pediatric Obesity, 1*, 33–41.

Luff, G. M., & Gray, J. J. (2009). Complex messages regarding a thin ideal appearing in teenage girls' magazines from 1956 to 2005. *Body Image, 6*, 133–136. doi:10.1016/j.bodyim.2009.01.004

Lumeng, J. C., Forrest, P., Appugliese, D. P., Kaciroti, N., Corwyn, R. F., & Bradley, R. H. (2010). Weight status as a predictor of being bullied in third through sixth grades. *Pediatrics, 125*(6), 1301–1307. doi:10.1542/peds.2009-0774

Lustig, R. (2010). The neuroendocrine control of energy balance. In M. Freemark (Ed.), *Contemporary endocrinology: Pediatric obesity: Etiology, pathogenesis, and treatment* (pp. 15–32). New York, NY: Humana Press.

MacCann, C., & Roberts, R. D. (2013). Just as smart but not as successful: Obese students obtain lower school grades but equivalent test scores to nonobese students. *International Journal of Obesity, 37*, 40–46.

Madowitz, J., Knatz, S., Maginot, T., Crow, S. J., & Boutelle, K. N. (2012). Teasing, depression and unhealthy weight control behaviour in obese children. *Pediatric Obesity, 7*, 446–452.

McCarthy, S. R., Fallon, L. M., & Hagermoser Sanetti, L. M. (2012). The link between obesity and academics: School psychologists' role in collaborative prevention. National Association of School Psychologists (NASP). *School Psychology Forum: Research in Practice, 6*(2), 29–38.

Menon, V. (2007). School-based interventions for childhood overweight. *National Association of School Psychologists Communiqué, 36*(2), 10–11.

Mond, J., van den Berg, P., Boutelle, K., Hannan, P., & Neumark-Sztainer, D. (2011). Obesity, body dissatisfaction, and emotional well-being in early and late adolescence: Findings from the Project EAT Study. *Journal of Adolescent Health, 48*(4), 373–378.

National Association for Sport and Physical Education. (2003). *Guidelines for appropriate physical activity for elementary school children: Update 2003*. Reston, VA: Author. Retrieved from http://www.aahperd.org/naspe/standards/nationalGuidelines/PAguidelines.cfm

Neumark-Sztainer, D. (2005). *"I'm, like, SO fat!": Helping your teen make healthy choices about eating and exercise in a weight-obsessed world.* New York, NY: Guilford Press.

Neumark-Sztainer, D., Story, M., & Harris, T. (1999). Beliefs and attitudes about obesity among teachers and school health care providers working with adolescents. *Journal of Nutrition Education, 31*(1), 3–9.

Ogden, C., & Carroll, M. (2010). *Prevalence of obesity among children and adolescents: United States, trends 1963–1965 through 2007–2008.* Retrieved from http://www.cdc.gov/nchs/data/hestat/obesity_child_07_08/obesity_child_07_08.htm

Patino-Fernandez, A. M., Hernandez, J., Villa, M., & Delamater, A. (2013). School-based health promotion intervention: Parent and school staff perspectives. *Journal of School Health, 83*(11), 763–770. doi:10.1111/josh.12092

Puhl, R. M. (2011). Weight stigmatization toward youth: A significant problem in need of societal solutions. *Childhood Obesity, 7*(5), 359–363.

Puhl, R. M., & Brownell, K. D. (2001). Obesity, bias and discrimination. *Obesity Research, 9,* 788–805.

Puhl, R. M., & Heuer, C. A. (2009). The stigma of obesity: A review and update. *Obesity, 17,* 941–964.

Puhl, R. M., & Latner, J. D. (2007). Stigma, obesity, and the health of the nation's children. *Psychological Bulletin, 133,* 557–580.

Puhl, R. M., & Luedicke, J. (2012). Weight-based victimization among adolescents in the school setting: Emotional reactions and coping behaviors. *Journal of Youth and Adolescence, 41*(1), 27–40.

Puhl, R. M., Luedicke, J., & Heuer, C. (2011). Weight-based victimization toward overweight adolescents: Observations and reactions of peers. *Journal of School Health, 81*(11), 696–703.

Puhl, R. M., Peterson, J. L., & Luedicke, J. (2012). Weight-based victimization: Bullying experiences of weight loss treatment–seeking youth. *Pediatrics 131*(1), e1–e9. doi:10.1542/peds.2012-1106

Ratey, J. R., & Hagerman, E. (2008). *Spark: The revolutionary new science of exercise and the brain.* New York, NY: Little, Brown.

Reiter-Purtill, J., Ridel, S., Jordan, R., & Zeller, M. H. (2010). The benefits of reciprocated friendships for treatment-seeking obese youth. *Journal of Pediatric Psychology, 35*(8), 905–914. doi:10.1093/jpepsy/jsp140

Ringham, R., Levine, M., & Marcus, M. (2009). Psychological comorbidity and childhood overweight. In L. J. Heinberg & J. K. Thompson (Eds.), *Obesity in youth: Causes, consequences, and cures* (pp. 115–134). Washington, DC: American Psychological Association.

Rudd Center for Food Policy and Obesity. (2013). *Weight bias: School climate and bullying.* Retrieved from http:/www.yaleruddcenter.org

Rudd Center for Food Policy and Obesity. (2013). *Weight bias is a major reason that students are bullied in schools: A fact sheet on school climate.* Retrieved from http://www.yaleruddcenter.org

Salvy, S.-J., Roemmich, J. N., Bowker, J. C., Romero, N. D., Stadler, P. J., & Epstein, L. H. (2009). Effect of peers and friends on youth physical activity and motivation to be physically active. *Journal of Pediatric Psychology, 34*(2), 217–225. doi:10.1093/jpepsy/jsn071

Schwartz, M., & Brownell, K. (2010). Local and national policy-based interventions: To improve children's nutrition. In M. Freemark (Ed.), *Contemporary endocrinology: Pediatric obesity: Etiology, pathogenesis, and treatment* (pp. 451–463). New York, NY: Humana Press.

Skelton, J. A., Goff, D. C., Ip, E., & Beech, B. M. (2011). Attrition in a multidisciplinary pediatric weight management clinic. *Childhood Obesity, 7*(3), 185–193. doi:10.1089/chi.2011.0010

Strauss, R. S., & Pollack, H. A. (2003). Social marginalization of overweight children. *JAMA Pediatrics, 157*(8), 746–752.

Su, W., & Di Santo, A. (2011). Preschool children's perceptions of overweight peers. *Journal of Early Childhood Research, 10*(1), 19–31. doi:10.1177/1476718X11407411

Wagner, M. O., Kastner, J., Petermann, F., Jekauc, D., Worth, A., & Bos, K. (2011). The impact of obesity on developmental coordination disorder in adolescence. *Research in Developmental Disabilities, 32*(5), 1970–1976.

Wilfley, D. E., Vannucci, A., & White, E. K. (2010). Family-based behavioral interventions. In M. Freemark (Ed.), *Contemporary endocrinology: Pediatric obesity: Etiology, pathogenesis, and treatment* (pp. 281–301). New York, NY: Humana Press.

World Health Organization. (2004). *Global strategy on diet, physical activity and health.* Geneva, Switzerland: Author.

Wu, Y. P., Reiter-Purtill, J., & Zeller, M. H. (2014). The role of social support for promoting quality of life among persistently obese adolescents: Importance of support in schools. *Journal of School Health, 84*(2), 99–105.

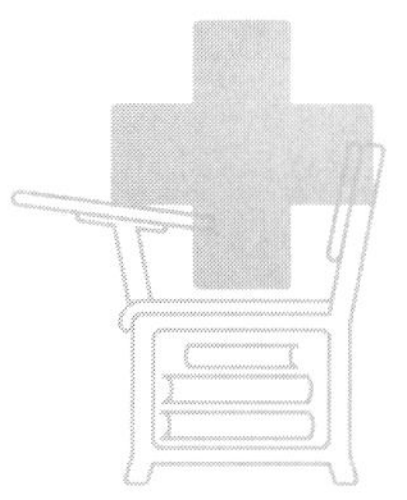

Chapter 12
Common Visual Problems in the Classroom

Caroline N. DeBenedictis and Alex V. Levin

Vision is one of the most important physical traits required for learning in traditional educational systems. Although today's "mainstreaming" projects allow children with low vision or blindness to be educated in the same setting as their peers, this chapter deals mostly with the common visual difficulties that most teachers encounter with sighted individuals who do not fit the definition for "legal blindness." In addition, the chapter covers symptoms and signs that teachers attribute to a visual disorder, or that prompt a referral for visual evaluation, that are nonocular in origin.

GLASSES AND CONTACT LENSES

"Normal" vision is arbitrarily designated as 20/20 (6/6 in the metric system). This means that a normal person can see letters of a certain size on a chart 20 feet away. The 20/20 eye focuses an image without assistance from glasses or contact lenses. The picture of the world we view enters the eye through the front crystalline domed surface of the eye (cornea) and passes through the pupil, and then the lens, which lies behind the pupil. The cornea and lens function similar to the lens on a camera, focusing an image onto film. In the case of an eye, the image is focused on the retina (the inner lining of the eye). In the normal 20/20 eye, this system works perfectly, with the cornea and lens focusing an image to fall precisely on the retina. However, just as some people are shorter or taller, many individuals have eyes that are microscopically longer or shorter but otherwise *perfectly healthy.* All corneas and lenses have approximately the same focusing power. If an eye is shorter or longer, the retina lies at a different distance behind the cornea and lens. In these cases, the cornea and lens do their jobs perfectly, but because the eye is a bit too short (farsighted) or long (nearsighted), the focused image falls behind or in front of the retina, thus creating a blurred image.

Glasses assist the cornea and lens to focus the image onto the retina when the eyeball is shorter or longer than the "normal" 20/20 eye. Because these eyes are otherwise perfectly healthy, once the image gets to its proper destination, the retina, it is in perfect focus and the patient sees 20/20. It is wrong to say that a person who is farsighted or nearsighted has "bad eyes," even if the glasses that person wears are very thick. These individuals have healthy eyes that simply need some assistance in focusing the light to achieve the 20/20 image. In fact, measuring a person's vision when he or she does not have glasses on is not a very important piece of information. It would be like taking a normal camera and trying to take a picture without a lens attached to the front. The camera is not broken and the film is good, yet the pictures will be very blurry. Instead of discarding the camera or sending it to a repair shop, you would screw on the appropriate lens, a situation analogous to wearing the appropriate pair of glasses and measuring the vision.

Refraction is when the eye focuses images. Nearsightedness, farsightedness, and astigmatism are called "refractive errors." Astigmatism is when the eye is of normal (average) length, but the front surface of the eye is not perfectly round. The front of the eye is shaped more like a football than a basketball. This microscopic alteration in the contour of the eye surface (cornea) causes distortion in vision, which can be corrected by wearing glasses. Once again, the eye is *perfectly healthy* and capable of seeing 20/20 with the assistance of glasses.

Contact lenses are the same as glasses, except they lie on the eye instead of in front of the eye. Today, people usually wear soft contact lenses or gas-permeable lenses (often referred to as "semisoft" or "semihard"). Some people are not able to wear contact lenses because of dryness in their eyes, allergies to cleaning solutions, or unusually high amounts of astigmatism. Most individuals can successfully wear contact lenses if they desire. Children can also wear contact lenses; no age is too young for contact lenses. For some eye conditions, contact lenses are prescribed in infancy. In these situations, parents learn to insert and remove the lenses daily. Other types of contact lenses can be worn for extended periods of time. The youngest age in which children may be able to insert and remove their contact lenses unassisted is approximately the age of 7 years. More commonly, children start around age 9. A general guideline is that children are able to manage their own contact lenses when they are old enough to manage their own person: cleaning their room, cleaning themselves, and caring for their own personal belongings. Although contact lenses do afford clearer vision, particularly for children who must wear very thick glasses, they are most often worn for cosmetic reasons or by individuals who do not like the inconvenience of glasses.

It is important for the schoolteacher to realize a few facts about contact lenses:

1. Any child who wears contact lenses and develops a red eye or eye pain should receive urgent care. In particular, the contact lens should be removed by the child, the school nurse, or the child's parent. Prompt evaluation by an ophthalmologist is suggested within 24 hours.

2. If a contact lens comes out accidentally in the classroom, the first thing to do is have everyone "freeze." Many contact lenses that could be found are lost or damaged during the search to find them. Contact lenses are sticky and adhere to surfaces on their way to the ground. Look carefully for the concave clear lens sticking to a piece of clothing or tabletop, or lying on the floor. They usually don't travel very far! Once found, soft contact lenses are easily recognizable by their extreme flexibility. Although all children should carry a spare contact lens case, in the absence of this, a contact lens can be placed in any container submersed in liquid. Although it is preferable to use contact lens solutions, in an emergency situation the lens can be placed in tap water. If the lens is gas permeable, only a drop or two of water is necessary to store the lens. Children should not reinsert the contact lens after it has fallen onto a dirty surface, or after it is in tap water, unless the lens is sterilized according to the protocol instructed by the child's eye caretaker. Most children can still function without one contact if the other eye sees well. If the child's vision is extremely poor without a contact lens in place, and the other eye does not see well, it is advisable for the child to have a spare pair of glasses at school, should a lost lens occur.

3. The wearing of contact lenses should not prevent a child from engaging in activities, including contact sports.

4. Contact lenses do not improve learning more than glasses.

5. Most children who wear contact lenses should have a backup pair of glasses either at home or at school.

Sometimes there is a concern regarding visual development (see section Amblyopia below). If this is the case, it is usually recommended the child wear glasses all the time to promote vision development. If this is not a concern, and the child is older (beyond the age of 7–9 years), most children need to wear their glasses only when they feel that doing so is helpful. Teachers usually write large enough on the blackboard that a child can perform normally in a classroom even if his or her vision is not 20/20. The hope is that a child wears glasses to optimize vision in order to learn more readily. Peer pressure is sometimes so strong that a child would rather sit in the front of a classroom to see the board more clearly than wear glasses and become subject to taunting by peers. This will not cause harm to the eyes. The child's parents or doctor can clarify when the child should wear glasses. It is important to keep in mind that young children run the risk of losing their glasses if they do not wear them all the time. Therefore, children often keep their glasses on full-time to avoid losing them.

There are many myths surrounding contact lenses and glasses. Children do not usually need reading glasses except in the rare instances of certain neurologic diseases (which would be obvious), after cataract removal, or in the case of accommodative insufficiency. In fact, children have an unusually strong focusing ability. They can read a newspaper attached to the end of their nose! Many children, especially those in the first few years of school, will place their heads very close to their reading material as a form of concentration. As long as they can see the blackboard normally, near vision is usually not an issue. Many children will even take their glasses off to read. This should not be discouraged as it is not harmful.

Wearing glasses does not make a person "addicted" to them. Keeping glasses on all the time will not make the eyes weaker or "dependent" on glasses. We often observe that people who wear glasses tend to wear them frequently. This is because they see better with the glasses and happen to like doing so, consciously or unconsciously. With the start of glasses treatment, they better appreciate how poorly they saw before and use the glasses more often. If they are in a situation where they do not need to see as clearly as the glasses allow them to (e.g., viewing something with large print), then going without glasses will do no harm.

If a teacher suspects that a child is having trouble with vision, appropriate referral is indicated. Signs that a child is having visual difficulty include squinting, always holding things very close, needing to sit in the front row, and having difficulties identifying letters or pictures from afar. Sometimes glasses are prescribed not to improve vision but to help straighten the eyes (see the section Strabismus below).

AMBLYOPIA

The term "lazy eye" is used by the lay public to refer either to an eye with amblyopia or to strabismus. Amblyopia refers to failure of the brain to develop vision normally. We are not born with good vision; we must develop good vision. For this to occur, we need two healthy eyes with relatively equal refractive errors, pointed in the same direction, to promote development. Anything that interferes with this process can cause amblyopia. This is not the same as having blurry vision as an adult and using glasses to clear the vision. Even with the correct glasses, an eye with amblyopia still sees blurry. Anything that causes the brain to prefer one eye over the other may result in amblyopia in the nonpreferred eye. One example is unequal refractive error between the eyes. If one eye is extremely nearsighted and the other eye is not, the brain favors the non-nearsighted eye and ignores development of vision in the very nearsighted eye. If glasses are not given at a young age in this situation, vision does not develop equally in the very nearsighted eye. In addition to unequal refractive errors, other abnormalities can lead to amblyopia. If a patient's eyes do not point in the same direction (e.g., crossed eyes), the brain may prefer to keep one eye straight for viewing while the other eye turns away. Vision development in the turned eye is ignored and full visual development does not occur.

Correction of amblyopia must begin as early as possible, before visual development comes to an end. By intervening at a time when the visual development is still proceeding, the brain is still "flexible" (or "plastic") in its ability to redevelop vision in an ignored eye. Treatment consists of correcting any underlying problem in the nonpreferred eye and then forcing the brain to use that eye by patching the good eye (see Figure 12.1). For the first example cited above, the child with unequal refractive error would be given glasses or contact lenses to correct the nearsightedness in the affected eye and might need to patch the good eye for a period of time each day. Sometimes the patching is done for just part of the day and at other times it is done all day. This decision is made by the ophthalmologist. As patching sometimes is a source of ridicule among peers, attempts might be made to do most of the patching when the child is not in school.

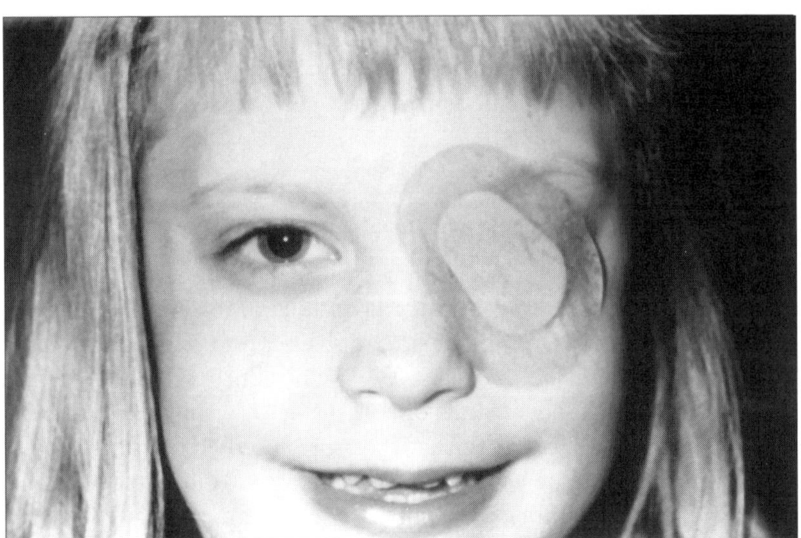

Figure 12.1 Patch commonly used in the treatment of amblyopia. The good left eye is patched to treat the amblyopia in the right eye.

Rarely, the brain can fail to develop vision adequately in both eyes (bilateral amblyopia). This might occur if both eyes have severe nearsightedness, farsightedness, or astigmatism that goes uncorrected for many years. Fortunately, this is usually picked up in school screening programs or by the simple observation that the child is having trouble with his or her vision. Once again, early intervention to correct such problems can lead to 20/20 vision in each eye.

Once a child reaches the age of 7–9 years, the failure of visual development may be irreversible. It is sometimes still possible to improve with treatment even into the teen years. The prognosis is best the younger the student is. If caught in older children, this may mean that even with glasses and patching, vision may not improve to 20/20. This fact emphasizes the need for early screening by pediatricians and family physicians to identify children who have poor vision at an early age, when intervention can best correct the deficiency. Unfortunately, most children who have poor vision in one eye are unaware they have a problem. A child's brain is "wired" in such a way that the brain automatically uses the better eye without any undo strain. Because children with one eye function normally (see the section The Monocular Child below), there is no way to detect a child with poor vision in one eye unless formal visual testing is performed. This is particularly true of children who are born with a problem in one eye, as they never know that it is abnormal for one eye to see less clearly than the other. The educator is wise to take seriously a child's complaint that he or she has all of a sudden noted that the vision in one eye is worse than the other. This can be confirmed by having the child first cover the bad eye and asking him or her to read the blackboard, and then covering the good eye to see if the child can perform the task equally. Should there be a discrepancy between the two eyes, prompt referral to an ophthalmologist is indicated.

Other treatments of amblyopia include the instillation of eye drops in the good eye to blur the vision, forcing the brain to use the nonpreferred eye. This will cause one pupil to be dilated as compared to the other. The pupil will also not constrict to bright light. Another alternative to patching is the placement of a suction-cup occluder on the back of the child's glasses, to act as a patch over the good eye.

STRABISMUS

"Strabismus" is a term that refers to any kind of misalignment of the eyeballs; the eyes are not pointing in the same direction. The eyes may be crossed (esotropia, or one or both eyes pointing toward the nose), turned out (exotropia, or "wall eyes," with one or both eyes pointing out toward the ears), or vertically misaligned (one eye pointing straight ahead and the other eye pointing up or down) (see Figures 12.2 and 12.3). Strabismus does not mean that a child sees poorly. In fact, many children with misaligned eyes will have one good eye that can see 20/20 while the other eye is misaligned, or the ability to alternate which eye is straight. This retains good vision in each eye as a result of equal visual stimulation during visual development. Although misaligned eyes have an abnormal appearance and can be the cause of peer ridicule, as long as the vision in at least one eye is normal, strabismus by itself does not interfere with school or athletic performance. There are many famous athletes and surgeons who have eyes that are misaligned. Straightening the eyes is usually undertaken to ensure normal visual development in both eyes and to reconstruct a child's facial appearance to normal.

There are three reasons children develop strabismus. It can be the result of an uncorrected refractive error. The eyes may cross as a result of farsightedness (Figure 12.2A) or turn out because of nearsightedness. Wearing glasses can straighten the eyes (Figure 12.2B). When these children remove their glasses, the eyes may return to misalignment (Figure 12.2A). This is of no concern. The analogy would be to people with diabetes who do not take their insulin. When they take their medication, their sugars are controlled. When they don't, their sugars are high. In strabismus, glasses are sometimes the

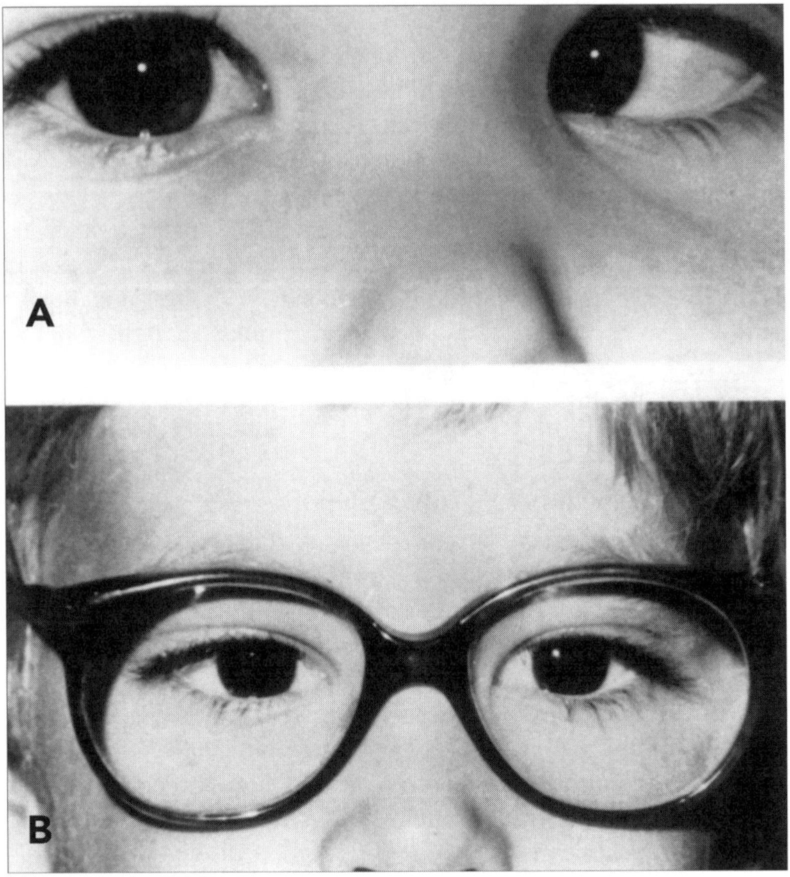

Figure 12.2 (A) Left esotropia (crossed left eye). (B) With farsighted glasses on, the crossed eye is now straightened.

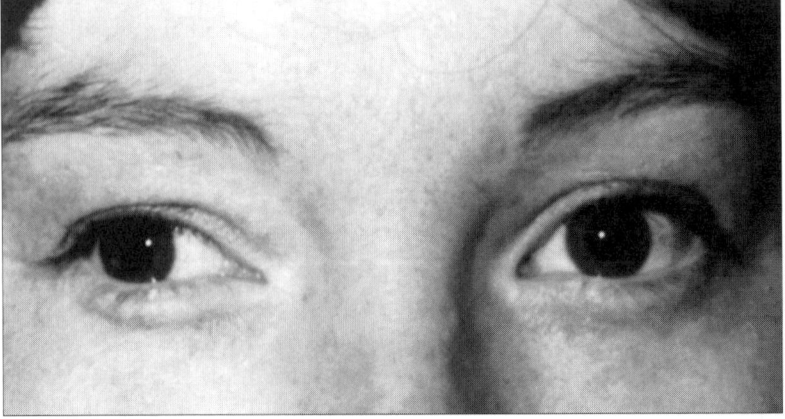

Figure 12.3 Right exotropia (turned-out right eye).

"medication" for the problem. When the glasses are off, the problem will manifest. Sometimes, these children will need the glasses to keep the eyes straight and promote vision development. Sometimes the child can see well without the glasses. These children must still wear the glasses all the time to keep the eyes straight and avoid amblyopia.

Although children do not outgrow strabismus, they can outgrow the need for glasses (or contact lenses). If they no longer need glasses to focus for them, the eyes can then be straight without the glasses.

Some children develop strabismus because the brain has difficulty with eye-muscle balance. We do not know why this occurs in most cases. These children usually do not need glasses to straighten their eyes, and surgery is often recommended and performed. This surgery is almost always an outpatient procedure in which the child is allowed to return to school in one or two days with virtually no restrictions. The eyes will be bloodred for many days, but many children are not sore and can perform most educational and athletic tasks normally. Sometimes a child may have double vision for one or two weeks after surgery, which often is not a cause for alarm. Approximately 15% of children will require two operations to straighten the eyes. Occasionally, three or more operations may be necessary. If a child wears glasses before strabismus surgery, then he or she will almost always need to wear glasses following surgery, as the operation only repositions the eyes and cannot change the refractive error (see above).

Strabismus can also be due to poor vision in one eye. The brain does not control the eye position in the poorly seeing eye after a period of time. If the poor vision is due to amblyopia, then patching the good eye and improving the vision in the weak eye might result in straightening the eye. However, strabismus may be the sign of poor vision due to other problems in the eye, such as a cataract. Therefore, all children with strabismus must be evaluated by an ophthalmologist to ensure that no serious abnormalities of the eyeball are present. The new development of strabismus in a child who has not previously shown any misalignment is of particular concern, and should result in a prompt referral to an eye physician.

Some myths surround strabismus. An eye cannot "get stuck" in a misaligned position. Most strabismus occurs in eyes that move normally. If one eye is preferred for vision, the other eye will appear to be "always turned." Correction of the underlying cause of the strabismus by glasses, surgery, or other means will return the turned eye to the normal position.

Children with a crossed eye are not less intelligent. Although they sometimes look like they are not focusing on their work, they are able to learn normally, provided that the vision in the nonturned eye is normal. Last, children rarely turn their eyes out of position "on purpose." Although this can occur, strabismus should not be ignored or attributed to child misbehavior.

THE MONOCULAR CHILD

Some children may have permanent loss of vision in one eye but normal vision in the other eye. These children are referred to as monocular. The poor vision can be the result of a number of abnormalities, including untreated amblyopia, cataract, and other conditions. Children with one eye function normally in school and athletics. A child with one normal eye does not require special seating or educational interventions. Many famous athletes, entertainers, scientists, and even surgeons have poor vision in one eye. This is particularly true when the poor vision in one eye develops at birth or in the very early years of visual development. Children have fantastic adaptive mechanisms. They develop unconscious strategies to give them virtually normal function, such as a wide range of peripheral vision, and monocular clues to obtain good functional depth perception. Many people falsely say that people with one eye have no depth perception. If you cover one eye and look across the room in which you are sitting, you could easily recognize which objects are in front of other objects. Although at first, as an adult, you may experience some trouble with fine depth-perception tasks (e.g., hammering a nail), you would quickly learn to adapt so that you could perform these tasks normally. Monocular children do this automatically and therefore have depth perception.

Some children have had an eye removed, most often as a result of trauma or tumor. Like all monocular children, if the remaining eye sees normally, these children will function normally. The difference is that they usually wear an artificial (prosthetic) eye. This is not a "glass eye." It is a porcelain shell that fits over the tissues left in the eye socket (Figure 12.4). If the shell is removed, there is no excavated hole where the previous eye existed. Rather, there is pink tissue covering the eye socket.

If the eye comes out during a classroom session, most children, even at a young age, can insert the eye themselves. If they are unable to do so, there is no harm in continuing the session with the eye wrapped in a tissue and placed in the child's pocket. The parent can then re-insert the prosthesis at home. If the child is concerned about appearance or is otherwise uncomfortable with the prosthetic eye out, the school nurse can place a patch for the remainder of the day's session. Patching should be done with the upper eyelid closed under the patch.

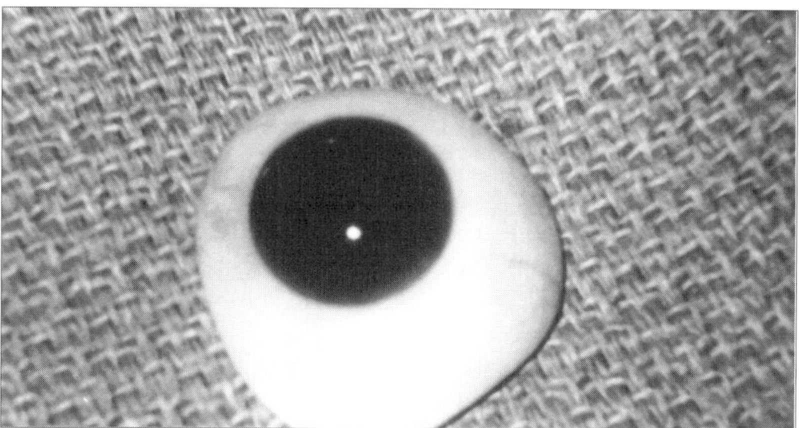

Figure 12.4. Prosthetic eye (artificial eye).

If the shell falls out repeatedly, the parent should return to the oculist who made the prosthesis to determine whether the fit is correct. Some children have been known to remove their eye prosthesis as a source of entertainment (positively or negatively) for their peers. If this becomes a problem, parents should be consulted.

The most important point in the management and care of the monocular child is protection of the good eye from accidental injury. All children who have one functional eye should wear glasses with lenses made out of shatter-proof polycarbonate plastic to prevent the good eye from becoming injured accidentally. Even if the child has no refractive error and sees 20/20 from the good eye without glasses, protective glasses should be worn. Likewise, all monocular children should wear appropriate protective eyewear for sports. This is particularly important for sports that involve balls or racquets. Monocular children do not need to be restricted from sports as long as they wear appropriate protective eyewear. A number of devices are available, usually through consultation with a local optician. Specific sport goggles are adequate for most sports, although visors (football), face masks (hockey, lacrosse), and chin guards (baseball batting helmets) are used in particular circumstances. A monocular child should not be viewed as "disabled."

LOW VISION

Legal blindness is defined in most jurisdictions as vision 20/200 or worse in the best eye, or a severe constriction of peripheral vision, with tunnel vision in the better eye (less than 20 degrees). Having vision of 20/200 means that the individual needs to stand at 20 feet to see what a normal person can see from 200 feet away. Remember that visual acuity refers to the best corrected vision: the vision with glasses on. If a person sees 20/200 with glasses off but 20/20 with glasses on, then there is no ocular problem.

There is a range of visual acuities between 20/20 and legal blindness (e.g., 20/40, 20/60, 20/80). To read normal-size print, most children need to have 20/50 or 20/60 vision. Remember, children have a very good ability to focus up close even when their distance vision is poor. To see a blackboard in school, vision of 20/60 or 20/80 might be sufficient, as most teachers write quite large, particularly in the elementary years. If the vision is worse, special visual aids may be necessary. These are beyond the scope of this chapter, and the educator facing a visually challenged child should consult his or her local ophthalmologist, optometrist, or school for the visually impaired for advice on managing the setting of the "mainstreamed" classroom. Children with significant visual impairment, even total blindness, can function remarkably well in a normal classroom setting with the help of visual aids such as Braille, small handheld telescopes, and large-print books. Other sources of information include the National Association for Parents of the Visually Impaired (http://www.napvi.org) and the Institute for Families of Blind Children (Mail Stop 111, 4650 Sunset Boulevard, Los Angeles, CA, 90027, USA). Teachers who work with visually impaired children should subscribe to the newsletters published by these agencies to learn more about methods of intervention, as well as the trials and tribulations of parenting a visually impaired child.

DYSLEXIA

Dyslexia is a collective term that refers to a number of learning problems, including problems with tracking, copying, letter reversal, word substitution, writing online, and other tasks of learning. It is important to remember there are many non-dyslexic causes of learning disability not related to dyslexia, including emotional immaturity, subnormal intellect, psychosocial problems, and attention-deficit disorder (see Chapters 5 and 17). In the absence of these problems, true dyslexia, a disorder found more commonly in boys than girls, can be a source of great difficulty in the classroom. Although the original understanding of dyslexia several decades ago referred to the eyes as the major cause, it is presently known that the eyes themselves are rarely an issue. Dyslexia, and all the learning disabilities that it encompasses, is a disorder of processing visual information. In other words, the eye allows perfect images into the brain, but the brain has difficulty making sense of the image and using it appropriately. We now understand that this processing also involves the speech and hearing centers of the brain. To illustrate this point, notice as you are reading these words, you hear the words spoken in your head. In fact, it is impossible to read "in silence." You cannot turn off this verbal and auditory part of visual processing. Studies show that it is the integration of these various brain functions that is abnormal in dyslexia. The eyes are normal in dyslexia, so interventions that attempt to train the eyes are not helpful. Unfortunately, a large and lucrative market has been created for the use of visual training in the correction of dyslexia and other learning problems. Such visual training is not offered at any medical children's hospital or medical eye hospital anywhere in North America. In nonphysician settings, this continues to be offered, often at great cost, which is not covered by insurance. Visual training may involve exercises in hand–eye coordination, balance boards, video games, eye exercises, the use of color overlays to treat "scotopic sensitivity syndrome," or prisms in glasses ("yoked prisms"). None of these treatments have withstood the trial of rigorous scientific testing. Unfortunately, unscientific anecdotal reports continue to emerge, claiming benefits to these unproven treatments and costing parents thousands of dollars as they search desperately for a solution for their child's learning problem. This conflict resulted in a statement issued jointly by the American Academy of Pediatrics, Section on Ophthalmology, Council on Children with Disabilities, American Academy of Ophthalmology, American Association for Pediatric Ophthalmology and Strabismus, and American Association of Certified Orthoptists (2009):

> Eye defects, subtle or severe, do not cause reversal of letters, words, or numbers. No scientific evidence supports claims that the academic abilities of dyslexic or learning-disabled children can be improved with treatment based on (a) visual training, including muscle exercises, ocular pursuit, tracking exercises, or 'training' glasses (with or without bifocals or prisms); (b) neurologic organizational training (laterality training, crawling, balance board, perceptual training); or (c) tinted or colored lenses. Some controversial methods of treatment result in a false sense of security that may delay or even prevent proper instruction or remediation. The expense of these methods is unwarranted, and they cannot be substituted for appropriate remedial educational measures. Claims of improved reading and learning after visual training, neurologic

> organization training or use of tinted or colored lenses are typically based on poorly controlled studies that rely on anecdotal information or testimony. (p. 1217)

All children who show learning difficulties should have a complete ophthalmic examination. Once this examination is found to be normal, further evaluation and treatment should rest within the educational system rather then in the hands of "visual trainers."

SYMPTOMS AND SIGNS OF POSSIBLE VISUAL DISORDERS

Educators often ask for guidelines to assess children with learning difficulties, to allow for early recognition of potential visual disorders. Some have been discussed above. Symptoms and signs listed below are often ascribed to the visual system—some correctly and others incorrectly.

Headaches

Headaches are only infrequently due to problems in the visual system. Most headaches are related to tension and stress or other disorders (see Chapter 13). It is more prudent to refer a child with headaches to the family physician or pediatrician before an ophthalmic examination, as the latter rarely results in the identification of a cause. Headaches that are prolonged, debilitating, associated with nausea or vomiting, and accompanied by visual symptoms such as aversion to bright lights (photophobia) or unusual visual phenomena, such as flashing lights or changes in the color or shapes of objects, might suggest a migraine with an ophthalmic component. Once again, although an eye examination might be part of the overall evaluation, it is suggested that this symptom first be evaluated by the pediatrician.

Eye Pain

If a child complains of a foreign-body sensation ("it feels like there is something in my eye"), this is rarely a visual disorder. It is a reflection of disruption of the ocular surface, such as a small scratch on the surface of the eye or a foreign particle resting somewhere on the eye or under the eyelids. Careful inspection by the school nurse or a medical caretaker may result in identification of the problem.

Dryness of the Eyes

Dryness is a symptom that affects adults much more than children. If a child has problems with dryness (or "stickiness"), the child should be referred for an eye examination.

Red Eye

Most red eyes are caused by local irritation and are noncontagious infections. However, some red eyes are due to viral conjunctivitis ("pink eye"), which can spread rapidly through a classroom. If a child develops a red eye, particularly a red eye that spreads from one eye to the other, it is prudent to have this child evaluated by his or her primary physician to see if further referral to an ophthalmologist is indicated. If viral conjunctivitis is suspected, a child may need to be out of the classroom for as long as 21 days to prevent infection of others. A history of multiple family members or classmates simultaneously affected is most consistent with a contagious conjunctivitis. Not every red eye represents a contagious problem, yet the potential for spread must be ruled out in each case when there is no clear cause for the redness, such as trauma or exposure to a noxious substance.

If there is a known exposure to a noxious substance (e.g., chemistry experiment), it is of great importance to irrigate the eyes *before medical consultation*. Any type of water can be used, including water from the nearest sink, to irrigate the eyes copiously. Even if this requires laying the child down and pouring water onto the eye's surface, it is essential to perform this treatment immediately to eliminate any ongoing contact with the offending agent as early as possible. School nurses should be well versed in this technique.

OTHER EYE DISORDERS

It is beyond the scope of this chapter to address the multitude of eye disorders that affect children. A few brief comments are made here regarding disorders that are seen commonly in the classroom.

Ptosis

A droopy eyelid may be present at birth or acquired later in childhood, particularly after trauma. If the droopy lid does not cross the center of vision (center of the pupil) and does not induce a large astigmatism, there may be no visual deficit. Once again, like all the ocular disorders discussed previously, if the other eye is entirely normal, then the child will function normally. Ptosis is usually repaired surgically.

Nystagmus

The term *nystagmus* refers to "shaky eyes." The eyes appear to jiggle in place. This is usually congenital and found in isolation or in combination with other ocular syndromes. Children with nystagmus do not see a shaky image. The brain is capable of taking microsecond samples of information to provide the child with a still image, similar to a computer. Nystagmus does cause visual blurring and can even lead to legal blindness. Many children with nystagmus hold their heads in an awkward position while looking straight ahead (e.g., a head turn or tilt). This position is found unconsciously to create the least amount of shaking. Children should be allowed to turn their face to seemingly awkward positions, as this will provide them with better visual acuity.

Cataract

A cataract is any opacity in the normally clear lens of the eye, which sits behind the pupil. Many cataracts are tiny and do not affect the vision. However, when a cataract becomes more significant, the vision is blurred. There is no harm in having a cataract in the eye, other than the effect on vision. However, in young children, cataracts are particularly dangerous, as they can lead to profound amblyopia. Surgery is necessary to remove the cataract. Cataract surgery requires removal of the entire lens. Postoperatively these children need something to replace the natural focusing mechanism of their eye (the lens). This can be accomplished with glasses, contact lenses, or insertion of an artificial lens. Provided that there is no significant amblyopia, once the cataract is removed and the patient is rehabilitated using one of these methods, visual function is restored to normal, although near-vision reading glasses may be necessary.

Albinism

Although we often think of albinism as a completely white individual with pink eyes, there are multiple kinds of albinism, many of which do not result in such a severe appearance. Albinism is a disorder in which the body cannot effectively make pigment. It may affect the skin, hair, and eyes, or the eyes alone. It causes nystagmus and reduced vision, and it is often associated with strabismus or a need for glasses. There is no treatment for albinism. These children may have difficulties with glare and bright lights. Therefore, seating that reduces glare on the blackboard may be helpful. Most children with albinism do well in a normal classroom setting, although they may need visual aids, particularly for distance vision.

Glaucoma

A microscopic increase in the fluid pressure that fills the inside of the eye can lead to damage to the optic nerve. The nerve sends the messages of vision between the eye and brain. Usually, people with glaucoma have no symptoms. Fortunately, it is a very rare disease in children. Many of these children will require eyedrops or oral medications, one dose of which may need to be taken during school.

Blepharitis

Blepharitis is microscopic crusting on the eyelashes. This can cause irritation of the eye surface, frequent blinking, and subjective blurry vision. This can be treated easily by an ophthalmologist.

INTERACTIVE WHITEBOARDS

There is no evidence that the use of devices with lighted backgrounds harm the eye. Many times children will complain of eye problems that are worse when viewing an interactive whiteboard in school. These complaints include vague subjective fatigue, blurriness, and difficulty concentrating. It is recommended that children be encouraged to look away from a lighted screen every 10–15 minutes to rest the eyes.

FUNCTIONAL VISION DISORDERS

Children may present with a variety of unusual symptoms with no true medical disease. These symptoms are not truly psychosomatic in the sense that they do not usually represent significant psychiatric disease. Many children, particularly between the ages of 5 and 12, will develop recurrent problems such as blinking, photophobia, intermittent visual loss, and eyelid pulling, which all represent a transient "habit." Although these children should be evaluated by an ophthalmologist to rule out the presence of true medical disease, most of these symptoms will resolve within three months after seeing the eye doctor. If symptoms persist, recur, or are replaced by other unusual symptoms (substitution), then further consultation with the child's pediatrician or family physician is indicated.

More information on all the above subjects and more is available on the websites for the American Association for Pediatric Ophthalmology and Strabismus (http://www.aapos.org) and the American Association of Ophthalmology (http://www.aao.org).

ADDITIONAL RESOURCES

American Academy of Ophthalmology (http://www.aao.org)

American Academy of Pediatrics, Section on Ophthalmology, Council on Children with Disabilities, American Academy of Ophthalmology, American Association for Pediatric Ophthalmology and Strabismus, and American Association of Certified Orthoptists. (2009). Learning disabilities, dyslexia, and vision. *Pediatrics, 124*, 837–844. doi:10.1542/peds.2009-1445

American Association for Pediatric Ophthalmology and Strabismus (http://aapos.org/)

Nelson, L. B. (Ed.). (2012). Wills Eye Institute: Pediatric ophthalmology. In C. R. Rapuano (Series Ed.), *Color atlas and synopsis of clinical ophthalmology*. Philadelphia, PA: Lippincott Williams & Wilkins.

Nelson, L. B., & Olitsky, S. E. (Eds.). *Harley's pediatric ophthalmology* (6th ed.). Philadelphia, PA: Wolters Kluwer/Lippincott Williams & Wilkins.

Riordan, P. R., & Cunningham, E. T. Jr. (2011). *Vaughan & Asbury's general ophthalmology* (18th ed.). San Francisco, CA: McGraw-Hill Medical.

Vrabec, T. R., Levin, A. V., & Nelson, L. B. (1989). Functional blinking in childhood. *Pediatrics, 83*(6), 967–970.

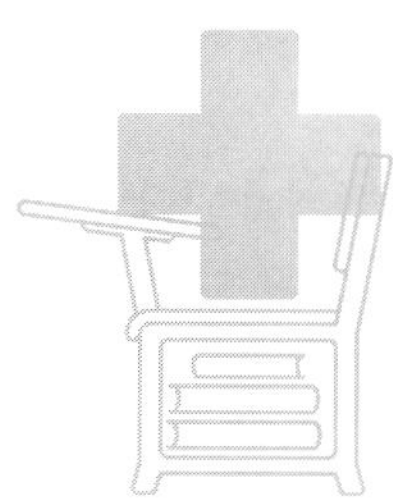

Chapter 13
Common Neurological Disorders in Children

Robert H. A. Haslam

The intent of this chapter is to outline three neurological disorders prevalent in children that teachers may encounter: headaches, epilepsy, and Tourette syndrome. The presenting symptoms are stressed to familiarize the educator with the clinical composition of these common conditions.

This brief account of common neurological conditions in children should serve to alert the teacher to the inherent complexities associated with disorders of the child's central nervous system. Cooperation on the part of the educator, physician, and parent in sharing knowledge and concerns about these sorts of problems will accomplish mutual understanding for the ultimate benefit of the child.

HEADACHE

Headache is a common condition in children and young adults. One study suggested that 48% of children experience headaches, albeit infrequently (Billie, 1962). Another found an incidence of approximately 15% in young adolescents (Hughes & Cooper, 1956). Oster (1972) suggested a prevalence of 20% in children of school age. A more recent Scottish study of all children from age 1 month to late adolescence showed a prevalence of 58% (Abu-Arafeh et al., 2010). The effect of headaches on children's academic performance, personality, memory, and interpersonal relationships, as well as school attendance, depends on their frequency, intensity, and etiology. Thus, if headaches are frequent and incapacitating, they may interfere with intellectual fulfillment and occasionally may represent a life-threatening symptom. For that reason, frequent headaches deserve careful medical scrutiny.

There are many reasons for headaches in the school-age child, but their cause is often difficult to delineate. Contrary to popular belief, refractive errors of vision, strabismus, sinusitis, and malocclusion of the teeth are not common causes. Any child who develops a high fever, for whatever reason, or has a systemic illness (e.g., pneumonia) may develop a headache that tends to parallel the severity of the illness. This headache always disappears with recovery from the primary sickness.

In this section, three major types of headache are discussed: migraine, tension (or muscle contraction) headaches, and headaches caused by increased intracranial pressure. For a comprehensive discussion of other possible sources of headache in children, the reader is referred to other texts (e.g., Barlow, 1984; Bonfert et al., 2013; Friedman & Harms, 1967; Gupta & Rothner, 2001; Shinnar & D'Souza, 1982; Stafstrom, Rostasy, & Minster, 2002).

Migraine

Migraine is defined as a recurrent headache accompanied by symptom-free intervals and at least three of the following symptoms or associated findings: abdominal pain, nausea or vomiting, throbbing headache, bilateral (unilateral more common in adults) location, associated aura (visual, sensory, motor), relief following sleep, and a positive family history (Prensky & Sommer, 1979). Migraines are relatively common in children. Because these headaches are rarely severe, medical advice is not always sought. The youngest child known to develop migraine was approximately 1 year old (Vahlquist, 1955). Migraine accounts for about 25% of all cases of headache in children. In an extensive, well-organized study in Uppsala, Sweden, Billie (1962) noted a 4% incidence of migraine in schoolchildren between the ages of 7 and 15. Prior to adolescence, the gender distribution is equivalent; however, later in life, girls are more frequently affected by migraine.

Precipitating Factors

In children, migraine headaches tend to have many characteristics that set them apart from migraine in adults. Migraine attacks are precipitated by a multitude of factors: tension; bright, flashing lights (photophobia) such as those from a movie or television screen; excessive physical exertion; mild head trauma; excessive noise (phonophobia), hunger, or alcohol consumption; and oral contraceptive use by the adolescent. One interesting finding is that some children develop migraine headaches following a stressful event, such as undergoing an examination, presenting a speech, participating in an athletic event, or performing in a school play. In contrast to tension headaches, migraine headaches frequently occur on weekend days. Migraine develops in children from all social strata and appears to be more common in compulsive, highly competitive children. Contrary to many reports, migraine can be found in the child with a disability as well as the very bright and intelligent student without a disability.

Prodome (Aura)

One possible reason for the difficulty in diagnosing migraine headaches in children is that they do not appear to have warning signs (*prodrome* or *aura*) as frequently as do adults. An alternative explanation may be that the child misinterprets these symptoms or gives little significance to them. *Prodromal* (precursory) symptoms are brief and most commonly visual, such as bright, flashing, and often colored lights in the form of stars, zigzag lines, or circles, as well as various crude visual shapes and distortion of body images. A graphic description of visual misinterpretation was depicted by Lewis Carroll, a migraine sufferer, in his *Alice's Adventures in Wonderland* (Carroll, 1865/1984, p. 58). As Alice explains to Caterpillar, "I can't remember things as I used—and I don't keep the same size for ten minutes together!" Other precursory symptoms may include numbness and tingling sensations in the extremities, dizziness, and aphasia.

Headache Symptoms

The prodromal symptoms are soon followed by the onset of the headache, which may begin in the posterior region of the skull but almost immediately tends to radiate to the forehead, often over an eye or the temple. The headache is described as pounding, pulselike, or throbbing. The headache is frequently not as severe in children as in adults and is usually of shorter duration. During this stage, the child may be extremely confused and belligerent and may prefer to lie down in a quiet, darkened room. Characteristic features that usually accompany the headache are nausea and vomiting, which often are more intense in children than the headache. Use of oral medication to alleviate the headache, therefore, is of little benefit to children with these symptoms. Vomiting may be associated with abdominal pain and fever; thus, other conditions such as appendicitis and infection may be incorrectly diagnosed.

The entire migraine attack usually lasts less than six hours and is almost always much shorter than what is commonly found in older patients. Afterward, the child awakens from a rather deep sleep in an alert state, asking to be fed and ready to resume normal activities as if nothing had transpired. If migraine attacks are frequent, significant absenteeism from school may result. This can produce anxiety in the child, particularly if school performance diminishes.

Common Migraine. The *common migraine* is the type that occurs most often in children and is not associated with an aura. A family history, particularly in the mother or her family, exists in approximately 90% of children with common migraine.

Classic Migraine. In classic migraine, an aura precedes the onset of the headache. The aura may consist of blurred vision, depressed vision within the visual field, flashes of light, brilliant white zigzag lines, or irregular distortion of objects. Sensory aura includes numbness of the lips, hands, and feet.

Variants. Some individuals experience cyclic vomiting or acute confusional states with migraine. Cyclic vomiting consists of periods of intense vomiting on a regular basis, beginning during infancy or the toddler stage. The vomiting may become protracted and lead to dehydration and electrolyte abnormalities, requiring hospitalization and intravenous fluids. Many children with cyclic vomiting have a positive family history of migraine and, as they grow older and become verbal, they describe a typical migraine headache in association with the vomiting. Thus, cyclic vomiting may be the initial manifestation of migraine headache in the preverbal child. Acute confusional states may occur during a migraine headache. The child may develop bizarre behavior characterized by confusion, memory disturbances, unresponsiveness, and lethargy, which may persist for several hours.

Complicated Migraine. There are three types of complicated migraine. Basilar migraine results when the blood vessels that supply the brain stem and cerebellum undergo vasoconstriction. Symptoms include vertigo, double vision, blurred vision, and unsteady gait. Some patients develop alterations in consciousness, such as a comatose state, associated with a seizure. Ophthalmoplegic migraine is a rare complication in children. It is characterized by a dilated pupil and drooping eyelid on the same side as the headache. Hemiplegic migraine is associated with temporary paralysis or weakness on one side of the body. Fortunately, these episodes are rare in children and do not tend to recur.

Treatment

Treatment for children with migraine headaches can be a challenge for the pediatrician. Before prescribing medication, the doctor must rule out other significant causes of headache. For example, because some symptoms of migraine are similar to epilepsy, an electroencephalogram (EEG) may be considered. Occasionally, the patient may require more specialized studies to rule out abnormalities in the blood vessels (arteriovenous malformation). Thus, a thorough history and physical examination are mandatory. Unfortunately, no laboratory tests ensure a diagnosis of migraine. Results from computerized tomography (CT) scans, magnetic resonance imaging (MRI), EEG, and blood tests are normal in the child with migraine, in contrast to a patient with epilepsy, arteriovenous malformations, or a brain tumor. Although a thorough psychological examination may demonstrate a compulsive, deliberate, and perhaps insecure student, these findings obviously are not conclusively diagnostic of migraine because they may also be found in many headache-free children. A child with typical migraine and a normal physical and neurological examination does not require further diagnostic testing.

The initial step in the management of migraine is to discuss with the parents and child the importance of lifestyle behaviors. A well-balanced and nutritious diet, good hydration, sufficient exercise, and adequate sleep are all known to decrease the frequency and intensity and in some cases prevent migraine attacks. In addition, alcohol, especially red wine, and birth-control pills in some adolescent girls may trigger a migraine. Some children experience a migraine headache following the ingestion of monosodium glutamate. This is often referred to as "Chinese restaurant syndrome."

Treatment of the Acute Attack. Most migraine headaches in children may be treated simply by the judicious use of ibuprofen, a nonsteroidal anti-inflammatory drug (NSAID), particularly if the headaches are relatively mild, infrequent, and of short duration. Overuse of the drug (i.e., more than three times a week) may cause "rebound headaches," which may be as debilitating as the migraine headache. Decreasing the frequent use of ibuprofen reverses the rebound headaches. For those children with more severe and debilitating headaches who do not respond to ibuprofen, treatment with a triptan agent (e.g., almotriptan) is usually extremely effective in aborting an attack. The drug may be given orally, subcutaneously, or nasally, a route of delivery that is favored by most children (Winner et al., 2000). The triptans are safe and associated with few side effects. As pernicious vomiting may be a major problem for these children during a headache, they may require treatment in a hospital with intravenous antiemetics.

Preventive or Prophylactic Therapy

Some children suffer from frequent and incapacitating migraine headaches and as a result are unable to attend school on a regular basis.

For these children a daily trial of prophylactic therapy is indicated. In most cases a trial of a drug is carried out for four to six months with careful observation and follow-up to detect unwanted side effects or lack of effectiveness. The drug flunarizine is the only prophylactic medication that has undergone scientific studies showing it to be very effective in the management of migraine headaches in older children and adolescents. Unfortunately, the drug may cause rare but serious side effects, including abnormal movements of the muscles. The drug amitriptyline, an antidepressant and analgesic, is also quite effective in the management of adolescent migraine. The side effects include dry mouth and drowsiness. A group of anticonvulsant drugs used primarily for the management of epilepsy is also quite effective in the treatment of migraine. These drugs include toprimate, valproic acid, and levetiracetam. As with most other drugs, children placed on these medications should be followed carefully for side effects. Fortunately, undesirable side effects are reversed with a decrease of the medication or its discontinuance. Additional drugs that have met with some success include propranolol and cyproheptadine. Finally, there is some evidence that riboflavin (vitamin B2) is a good alternative but probably less effective in the treatment of migraine than the above drugs. The physician should periodically reevaluate any child on continuous medication for possible harmful drug reaction, including drug dependence and abuse and, just as important, for the possibility that the child has discontinued the drug, unknown by the parents. Communication with the teacher regarding classroom behavior, medication, and unwanted side effects can be an important component of the management process.

Biofeedback

Pain management using relaxation techniques and behavior management is an effective treatment for some children and adolescents with migraine. Biofeedback and self-hypnosis programs can be mastered by most children older than 8 years of age and have shown positive results in many clinical trials (Olness, MacDonald, & Uden, 1987).

The teacher may assist the pupil during an acute migraine attack by providing a secluded, quiet, and darkened area in which to rest. In addition, reappraisal of the child's curriculum if headaches are frequent may demonstrate that undue pressures are being placed on the child. If absenteeism is frequent, steps should be initiated for medical reevaluation of the child.

Tension Headaches

Tension (muscle-contraction) headaches are a relatively common type of headache in children, as in adults. For most children, a tension headache is a rare occurrence and is so clearly related to a stressful but short-term situation that treatment is unnecessary. However, for some children these headaches may be frequent and prolonged.

Symptoms

Tension headaches appear most frequently during school hours, particularly during a test or similar anxiety-provoking circumstance. They rarely occur on weekends and usually have abated by the evening, but they may persist for weeks. Some children with tension headaches are found to have parents whose expectations for them—academically or athletically—are far too high. The most common cause of tension headaches in children appears to be unrealistic scholastic goals developed by the parents, teachers, or children themselves. If these headaches occur more often during a vacation period or other times when the child is in greater contact with the parents, parental marital discord or related phenomena may cause the child's anxiety. The student with severe tension headaches frequently has a parent who suffers from similar headaches.

Tension headaches are poorly described by children. They are usually located in the temples, over the forehead, or even in the base of the skull and neck muscles. The headache is usually a steady, dull, aching pain, and it is sometimes described as a pressure band constricting the skull. The student may complain of scalp tenderness, particularly during hair combing. These headaches probably are the result of prolonged, unconscious contraction of the muscles of the neck or temples that so often accompanies states of anxiety or tension. Unlike migraine, tension headaches are not associated with nausea or vomiting.

Diagnosis

The diagnosis of tension headache is made only after excluding other possible causes through use of a careful history and thorough physical and neurological examination. An EEG, CT scan, or MRI is not necessary in most cases because the history and physical examination usually suffice. The physician must then search for possible stressful situations. The teacher may be of great assistance during this phase of the evaluation. Most children have considerable insight into the origin of their emotional problems and, if given the opportunity to speak in confidence with a teacher or pediatrician, will share their concerns. Poor self-image, fear of school failure, and lack of confidence are oft-repeated apprehensions. Occasionally, a child who is depressed will complain of severe headaches (Ling, Oftedal, & Weinberg, 1970). Further questioning may uncover mood changes, lack of energy or excessive fatigue, poor appetite and weight loss, crying spells, and withdrawal from social activities. The term psychogenic headache is used to describe headaches caused by severe psychiatric disturbances; children who have this kind are in need of immediate psychiatric evaluation.

Treatment

The physician's and educator's major responsibility in treatment of tension headaches is to explain to the child that stressful events may culminate in a headache by unconsciously producing isometric contraction of the underlying forehead and temporal muscles. Steps should be taken to alter obvious anxiety-provoking situations. The teacher should be aware of his or her role in this regard. By careful interaction with the child, the teacher can help circumvent certain stressful situations to minimize tension-producing episodes. The child and family must be reassured that these headaches are not serious and that a healthy, normal life is to be expected. Acetaminophen, ibuprofen, or other mild analgesics may help in treating tension headaches, but tranquilizers and sedatives are rarely indicated (see earlier discussion of rebound headaches). The physician may choose to hospitalize the child with severe and recurrent tension headaches for observation, particularly if depression is suspected. Biofeedback techniques have proved useful for some children when the previously described measures have been unsuccessful (Baumann, 2002; Diamond, 1979).

Headaches Due to Increased Intracranial Pressure

Headache may be the earliest symptom of increased pressure within the skull. The causes of increased intracranial pressure in children include brain tumor, chronic lead poisoning, brain abscess, or an abnormal collection of blood clots (subdural hematoma) over the surface of the cortex. In addition, elevation of intracranial pressure may result from hydrocephalus, infection of the central nervous system (meningitis), vitamin A poisoning, water intoxication (the result of water retention and sodium depletion), or, in rare instances, a complication of drug therapy (e.g., tetracycline, an antibiotic, and isotretinoin used in treating acne and oral contraceptive agents in female adolescents). The characteristics of the pressure headache vary somewhat, depending on the individual's age and the underlying pathological condition. Sooner or later, other symptoms or neurological signs appear, implying a progressive, destructive process.

The increased pressure headache is the result of abnormal tension or stretching of the cerebral blood vessels and dura, the thick membranous covering of the brain. This kind of headache tends to occur in the early morning hours or shortly after rising. Most children have difficulty describing its location, but it tends to be a diffuse, generalized, often throbbing pain that may be more prominent over the forehead or the occipital region of the skull. Its onset is usually insidious, and in the beginning of the disease process, there may be days or even weeks when the child has no pain. The headache is often made worse by any activity that normally raises the intracranial pressure, such as coughing, sneezing, exercise, or straining during a bowel movement. Certain positions tend to influence the headache: Lying down may enhance the pain, and sitting up or standing may relieve it. Later, the headache becomes more frequent and intense. With increasing intracranial pressure, the child becomes lethargic, uncooperative, and finally comatose.

Vomiting may also occur. The child may awaken with a headache and vomit shortly thereafter. He or she usually will not complain of nausea, may eat a normal breakfast immediately following the episode of vomiting, and may remain symptom-free for the duration of the day. Unfortunately, some children who complain of morning vomiting and who appear normal in every other respect are accused of malingering or are thought to display a school phobia. These children require careful medical attention.

Diagnosis and Treatment

The treatment of intracranial pressure headaches depends on the cause. Every child suspected of increased intracranial pressure must have a thorough examination, including a history, blood pressure determination, and neurological evaluation that includes inspection of the retina (by using an ophthalmoscope and looking through the pupil to examine the retina) to determine whether the optic nerve is swollen.

More specific neuroradiological procedures may clearly outline a specific lesion (see Figures 13.1 and 13.2). The decision as to whether to proceed with further investigation, such as an MRI or arterial contrast studies (cerebral angiography), is dependent on the outcome of these noninvasive studies in conjunction with the patient's neurological findings. If an organic disease process is found, the appropriate medical or surgical therapeutic techniques can be used.

Symptoms Suggestive of an Organic Cause

Some headaches are worrisome and require prompt medical attention. A sudden, excruciating onset of head pain or an abrupt change in its characteristics suggests an underlying organic disorder, particularly if there is no past history of headache. Any headache that occurs in association with or shortly after head trauma may be extremely serious,

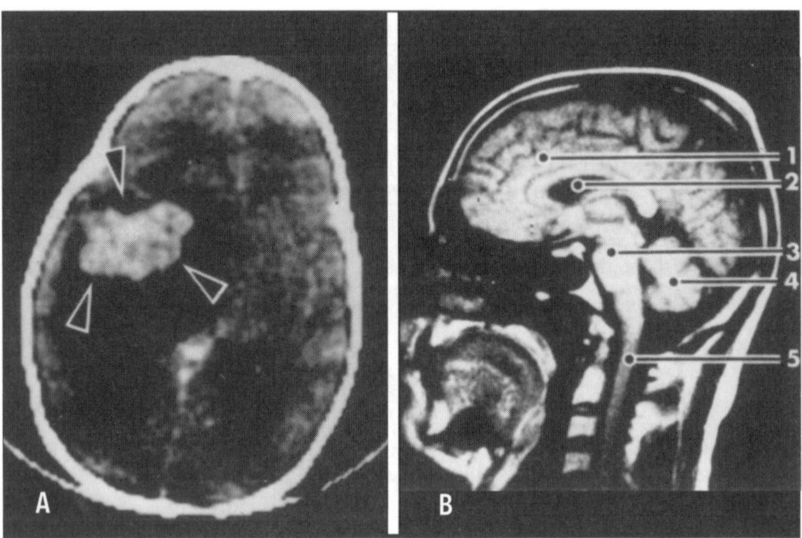

Figure 13.1. (A) A computerized tomogram (CT scan) on a child with headaches suggestive of increased intracranial pressure. The arrows outline a lobulated tumor that is protruding into the enlarged left lateral ventricle. The tumor, which proved a benign choroid plexus papilloma, was successfully removed. The CT scan is an extremely useful and noninvasive method of examining the brain structures. (B) Magnetic resonance imaging (MRI) produces lifelike images and, unlike the CT scan, does not expose the patient to radiation. This sagittal view of a normal patient's head clearly identifies the various components of the brain: 1 = cerebral cortex, 2 = lateral ventricle, 3 = pons, 4 = cerebellum, 5 = spinal cord.

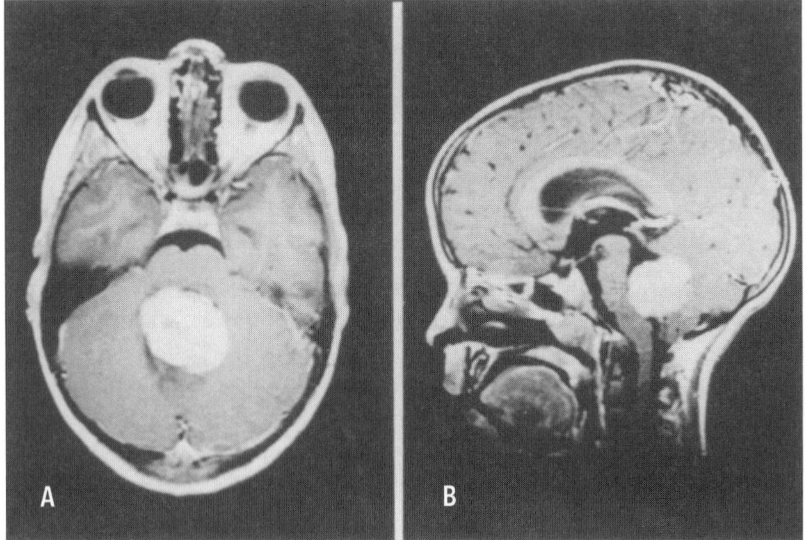

Figure 13.2. (A) Axial and (B) midsagittal magnetic resonance image (MRI) of a 6-year-old boy with a brain tumor (medulloblastoma) situated in the fourth ventricle. The midsagittal view shows that the tumor is pushing the brain stem forward.

no matter how trivial the injury may appear. All headaches suggestive of increased intracranial pressure justify immediate evaluation. They tend to become more frequent and intense and often are associated with other neurological symptoms in a relatively brief period. The prognosis of headaches due to increased intracranial pressure depends on the underlying abnormality. Early diagnosis and treatment are extremely important, as many of these conditions are life-threatening illnesses that can be cured by prompt medical or surgical management.

Children with recurrent headaches accompanied by other symptoms or signs are more likely to have organic pathology as a cause. A headache that awakens a child during sleep is always of concern. School failure, a change in behavior, or a falloff in linear growth (height) suggest underlying pathology. A seizure in association with a headache, the presence of neurological signs developing during a headache, or visual blurring at the peak of the headache all warrant further investigation by the physician.

Summary

The investigation and management of headaches in children can be taxing for physicians. A thorough understanding of a child is of considerable importance, particularly if migraine or tension headaches are to be treated successfully. Information from school officials concerning the child's change in personality, decline in school performance, or unusual behavior can be crucial in assisting the physician. The teacher can often initiate a referral to the pediatrician in cooperation with the parents if worrisome symptoms are noted.

Generally speaking, a pattern of recurrent headaches over a prolonged period, with normal behavior and intellectual functioning between episodes, suggests a benign process, such as migraine or tension headaches. The characteristics of the headache—including the inciting factors, location, duration, and associated symptomatology—usually differentiate the two. Many children in this category do not require medical attention because of the sporadic nature and insignificant consequences of their headaches. The educator must be aware of provoking events for the child with more troublesome headaches. Improvement can be expected if the appropriate causative factors can be established and reconciled. Such simple maneuvers as excusing a pupil subject to migraines from observing a movie or participating in functions productive of loud noises (e.g., the school band) may serve to prevent some headaches. Migraine headaches tend to be less severe in adolescence if their onset is prior to 10 years of age (Congdon & Forsythe, 1979). Tension or psychogenic headaches respond favorably to the relief of anxiety-provoking situations and the factors that promote them. Some patients must be taught how to live with their headaches.

EPILEPSY

Epilepsy is a common disorder in school-age children. Most teachers have experienced a student with epilepsy in the classroom; some are fearful of the condition and develop a negative relationship with the child, whereas others become overprotective and solicitous. Even in these modern times, epilepsy is considered by many well-educated but misinformed individuals to represent a host of incredible conditions and aberrations, including mental illness, cognitive impairment, evil spirits, and perverted thoughts. As a result, the patient with epilepsy may be shunned, shamed, and abused by friends, fellow students, teachers, and even parents.

A *seizure* can be defined as a recurrent involuntary disturbance of brain function that may be manifested as an impairment or loss of consciousness, abnormal motor activity, behavioral abnormality, sensory disturbance, or autonomic dysfunction. It is a symptom of an underlying disorder of the central nervous system. The term *epilepsy* is used to describe a wide variety of disorders due to many different causes and is defined as recurrent seizures unrelated to fever or to an acute cerebral insult. The clinical picture of epilepsy is partially dependent on the age of the child, the cause of the convulsion, and the area within the brain that is malfunctioning.

Epilepsy occurs in approximately 0.5% of the population, thus affecting about 1 million Americans. The initial presentation commonly occurs during the latter half of the first decade or at the time of adolescence. The causes of convulsions are numerous and include genetic and perinatal factors, complication of a head injury, infections of the central nervous system, congenital malformations, metabolic and degenerative diseases, tumors of the brain, and vascular diseases, as well as poisoning by exogenous substances (Livingston, 1972).

Classification

It is important for the physician to classify the patient's seizure disorder as precisely as possible as the anticonvulsant medication chosen depends on the seizure type. Some conditions may be confused with epilepsy, including breath-holding spells, temper tantrums, rage attacks, sleepwalking, night terrors, fainting, non-epileptic seizures (pseudoseizures), and hysteria. These paroxysmal events can only be differentiated from epilepsy by a thorough history, examination, and EEG. The classification of epilepsy as published in 2010 (Berg et al., 2010) presents a redefinition of generalized and focal seizures that simplifies these two major seizure types (Table 13.1).

Generalized Seizures

Tonic–clonic (grand mal) convulsions are the most common and, to the uninitiated, most frightening form of epilepsy. On occasion, the patient can anticipate a seizure minutes or hours prior to its occurrence. A severe headache, tired feeling, or clouding of the sensorium may be warning symptoms (aura). The convulsion is usually initiated by sudden loss of consciousness. The child may fall, the eyes roll upward, respirations momentarily cease, and the face becomes slightly dusky. At this point, rhythmic synchronous movements of

Table 13.1

CLASSIFICATION OF SEIZURES

Generalized seizures
Tonic-clonic (in any combination)
Absence
Typical
Atypical
Absence with special features
Myoclonic
Myoclonic atonic
Myoclonic tonic
Clonic
Tonic
Atonic
Focal seizures
Unknown
Epileptic spasms

Note. Adapted from A. T. Berg, S. F. Berkovic, M. J. Brodie, et al. (2010), ***Epilepsia 51***(4), 676–685.

the extremities and face may develop. These usually persist for a few minutes, but in rare cases for hours. During this phase of the convulsion, the person's arms and legs are rigid. Usually within minutes, the child becomes relaxed, moans, and may begin to move spontaneously. In most instances, the child is drowsy following a generalized seizure and prefers to sleep, although the child may be aroused.

If a child has persistent or repetitive seizures without regaining consciousness in the interval, for greater than 30 minutes, a medical emergency exists. The child must be immediately transported by ambulance to a hospital for treatment of this complication of epilepsy, known as *status epilepticus*. The most important cause of *status epilepticus* is failure of the person to take anticonvulsant medication on a regular basis, including unsupervised withdrawal from the drug.

Absence Seizures

Typical

Absence (petit mal) seizures commonly have an onset between the ages of 5 and 10 years and are more prevalent in girls. The seizure manifests as a brief episode of staring, usually less than 30 seconds, and is never associated with an aura. The child momentarily appears to be disinterested and out of contact with reality. There may be lapses of speech and fluttering of the eyelids, but the child does not fall. Automatisms (e.g., lip smacking) may also occur with absence seizures, confusing the diagnosis with focal seizures. Absence seizures may occur so frequently that they interfere with a child's concentration and school performance (Freemon, Douglas, & Penry, 1973). Frequent seizures undoubtedly interfere with memory.

The investigation of children with absence epilepsy is often initiated by the teacher. The physician may enhance or demonstrate an episode of this type of epilepsy by asking the child to take deep breaths (hyperventilation) for a period of several minutes. This technique is particularly useful in the EEG laboratory (see Figure 13.3). Unfortunately, absence epilepsy is not always diagnosed, and some children with this disorder are disciplined for their lack of academic interest and enthusiasm. This condition must be differentiated from daydreaming, which may occur during a boring classroom assignment, when tired, or with a longing anticipation for the events of the upcoming weekend.

Atypical

Children with atypical absence epilepsy share many of the symptoms observed with typical absence epilepsy. Children with atypical

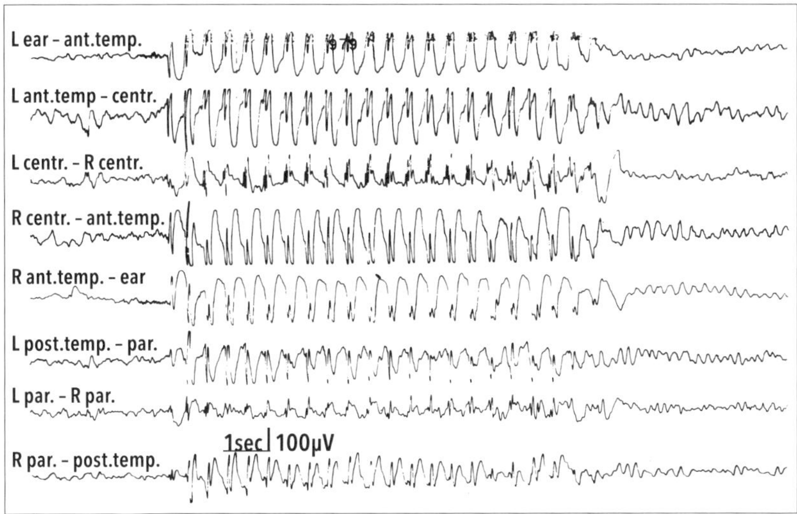

Figure 13.3. An electroencephalogram showing the typical three-per-second discharges of absence epilepsy. Note the sudden return to normalcy at the termination of the recording.

absence may not become unresponsive during the seizure, but they may have facial twitching and the EEG does not show the pattern seen in typical absence.

Myoclonic Epilepsies

Myoclonic seizures consist of repetitive, brief, symmetric muscular contractions with loss of body tone, which may cause the child to fall, resulting in trauma to the face and mouth. The subtypes of myoclonic epilepsy that most commonly develop during infancy and school-age years are discussed here.

Typical Early Childhood Myoclonic Epilepsy

Children with typical myoclonic epilepsy exhibit no symptoms prior to the onset of seizures, which occurs between 2 and 4 years of age. About 50% of children with this type of epilepsy also have occasional generalized tonic–clonic seizures. At least one third of children with this disorder have a positive family history of epilepsy, which suggests a genetic cause for the disorder. The long-term prognosis is relatively favorable, with at least half of the children becoming seizure-free several years later. Cognitive impairment develops in a few patients, but learning and language disabilities, as well as behavioral problems, occur in a significant number of these children and require management in a multidisciplinary setting.

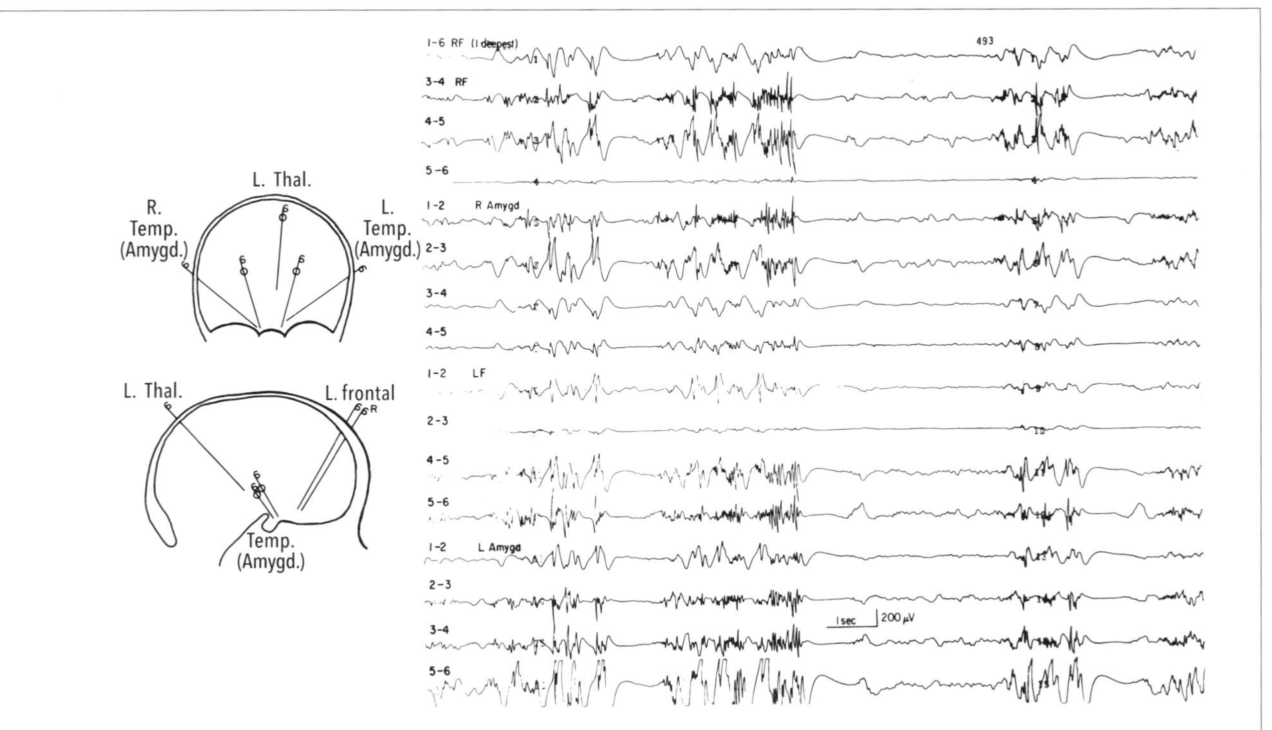

Figure 13.4. Intermittent bursts of spikes followed by slowing is a common finding in the electroencephalogram in patients with myoclonic seizures.

Complex Myoclonic Epilepsy

Complex myoclonic epilepsy begins with tonic–clonic seizures during the first year of life, followed by the development of myoclonic seizures (see Figure 13.5). Many children with this disorder have developmental delays prior to the onset of seizures. Complex myoclonic seizures are not associated with a positive family history of epilepsy. Unfortunately, these children have a poor prognosis. In spite of anticonvulsant therapy, the seizures persist and are associated with cognitive impairment and behavioral disabilities in 75% of cases.

Juvenile Myoclonic Epilepsy

Juvenile myoclonic epilepsy typically begins in early adolescence and is characterized by frequent myoclonic jerks, especially on awakening, which makes hair combing and brushing teeth difficult, as the comb or toothbrush is flung from the patient's hand during a seizure. Most of these patients also have generalized tonic–clonic seizures. This form of epilepsy is well controlled with the anticonvulsant valproic acid, and the long-term prognosis is excellent.

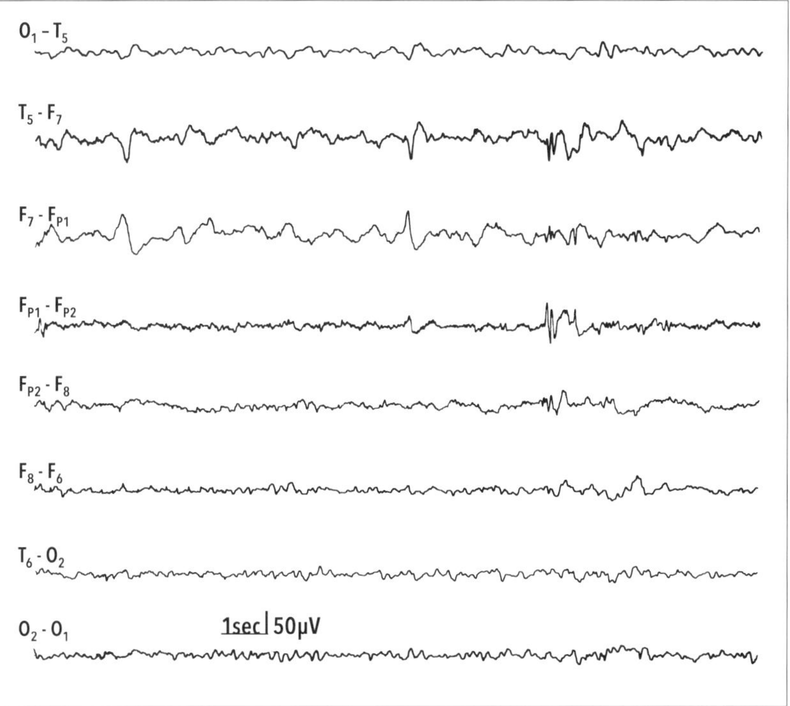

Figure 13.5. An abnormal electroencephalogram supporting the clinical diagnosis of complex partial epilepsy in a 10-year-old boy. Note the spikes or seizure discharges in T_5–F_7 and F_{P1}–F_{P2}.

Progressive Myoclonic Epilepsy

Progressive myoclonic epilepsy comprises a heterogeneous group of rare genetic disorders that uniformly have a grave prognosis. Tonic–clonic seizures develop in a previously normal child between 10 and 18 years of age. Within a short period of time, myoclonic seizures become evident. Deterioration of cognitive function and academic performance is apparent within one year of the onset of seizures. Neurological abnormalities, including ataxia and poor coordination, are associated with the seizure disorder. The myoclonic seizures are not controlled by anticonvulsants, but the tonic–clonic seizures are prevented by a combination of valproic acid and a benzodiazepine (i.e., clonazepam). This type of myoclonic epilepsy is slowly progressive and often leads to death within 5–10 years of the onset of seizures.

Focal Seizures

Previously, focal seizures were classified as partial, psychomotor, or temporal lobe epilepsy. Focal seizures (previously classified as simple partial seizures) are characterized by clonic (repetitive jerky movements) or tonic (tightening of the body) movements that involve the face, neck, or extremities. *Versive seizures*, which consist of the head and eyes turning to one side, are particularly common in this type of epilepsy. Some children complain of an aura, including chest discomfort or a headache, before the onset of the seizure. The entire seizure may persist for 10–20 seconds, and consciousness is maintained throughout the seizure.

Focal seizures may take a different form (previously called complex seizures). This type of focal seizure may or may not be preceded by an aura, and is always followed by a period of altered consciousness. The aura may be characterized by vague abdominal discomfort or fear, which may be present in approximately one-third of these children. During the period of impaired consciousness, the child may have a blank, "spacey" expression and be unresponsive to verbal commands. During the seizure, approximately 50%–75% of these children will have *automatisms*, which follow loss of consciousness and consist of lip smacking, chewing, and persistent swallowing movements. Automatisms in older children are characterized by semipurposeful, uncoordinated movements, such as pulling at clothing, buttoning and unbuttoning a garment, repetitive rubbing of objects, or running and clinging to a parent, friend, or object in an uncontrolled and frightened manner. The child may have a focal tonic–clonic or generalized grand mal seizure with spread of the epileptiform discharge (the burst of seizure activity in the brain). With these seizures, the head and eyes may turn to one side, the eyes may blink, and tonic–clonic movements may begin on one side of the body and then become generalized. Focal seizures are associated with EEG abnormalities in the majority of children, especially temporal-lobe sharp waves or spikes (see Figure 13.5). CT scanning and especially MRI studies may show a lesion in a temporal lobe in children with focal seizures, including scar tissue (the result of a head injury, previous prolonged seizure, birth injury, or meningitis), an arteriovenous malformation, or a slow-growing brain tumor.

Students with focal seizures are at a greater risk for learning disorders than are children without seizures. They may display a shortened attention span or inability to concentrate. A few children tend to display temper tantrums or acting-out behavior, which will require psychiatric consultation. Fortunately, with appropriate medication and counseling, the behavior outbursts and convulsions can usually be controlled.

Epilepsy Syndromes

A more recent approach to classifying epilepsy is by syndrome delineation. Many epilepsy syndromes result from a gene mutation, explaining the strong family history of seizures in some patients. Epilepsy syndromes are characterized by a typical age of onset, a specific seizure type, responsiveness to anticonvulsant drugs, and prognosis. The syndromic taxonomy of epilepsy provides a significant advantage compared to previous classifications by providing the physician with guidelines for selecting the most appropriate anticonvulsant, choosing those patients who are most likely to benefit from epilepsy surgery, and counseling patients and families with a reliable prognosis. Examples of epilepsy syndromes include infantile epileptic spasms (West syndrome), the Lennox-Gastaut (complex myoclonic epilepsy) syndrome, the Landau-Kleffner syndrome (acquired aphasia), and juvenile myoclonic epilepsy (Janz syndrome). Benign partial epilepsy with centrotemporal spikes (Rolandic epilepsy) is one of the most common epilepsy syndromes in school-age children. The peak onset is between 9 and 10 years of age, with a range from 2 to 14 years. The child's cognitive development and neurological examination are normal. There is often a positive family history of epilepsy. Seizures tend to occur during sleep or upon awakening and typically cause numbness of the tongue and cheek, unilateral tonic contractions of the face and extremities, guttural noises, and excessive salivation. The seizures are usually brief and infrequent and are associated with an excellent prognosis, as most children outgrow them by adolescence. The EEG shows a characteristic spike discharge pattern in the region of the temporal lobe.

Management

The successful management of a child with epilepsy is dependent on many factors. The patient who has a clear understanding of the disorder is in a better position to cope with frustrations as they occur. The child, physician, parent, and educator must appreciate the many facets of epilepsy to ensure that the child has a normal, happy, and fulfilling existence. The Epilepsy Foundation website (http://www.epilepsy.com) is an excellent resource for parents.

Emergency First Aid

The only type of epilepsy that warrants emergency assistance is the tonic–clonic variety. The others are often unrecognized and are rarely associated with complications. If a patient is actively convulsing, he or she should be moved from potentially dangerous areas, such as the Bunsen burner in the chemistry laboratory or the kitchen stove in the home economics class. The child should be placed in a horizontal position, preferably lying on his or her side, and tight or confining garments should be loosened. The patient must have a *free airway:* The mouth and nose should be uncovered and any substances in the oral cavity (including candy, chewing gum, or food) removed, if possible. Blunt objects such as a spoon, stick, or finger should not be forced into a patient's oral cavity during a seizure, as a tooth may be dislodged and aspirated into the lungs. If the convulsive movements are vigorous, the patient can be gently restrained. The majority of tonic–clonic convulsions may be managed in this fashion, and complete recovery is anticipated. If the seizure is prolonged (greater than 10 minutes), an ambulance should be summoned and the child given further care by a physician.

Medical Investigation

The physician initiates a course of management by seeking a cause for the seizure through taking a careful history and performing a physical examination. A complete description of the convulsion by a parent or teacher is an essential component of the investigation, as in most instances the seizure activity has ceased by the time the child reaches the hospital or doctor's office. Many parents will have captured a seizure on their cell phone, which may be important in confirming the diagnosis.

After the examination, the pediatrician may perform a variety of blood tests, including a fasting serum glucose and calcium test, and perhaps amino-acid and lead-level analyses. In addition, an MRI may be ordered, and the cerebrospinal fluid examined to determine whether the child has meningitis. These tests are carried out to seek a specific cause for the seizure, enabling the physician to provide a direct approach to its treatment. The interpretation and value of an EEG are misunderstood by many individuals. The physician orders this examination only to confirm the clinical impression. However, the EEG can be quite useful as a diagnostic tool when done in the proper context (see Figure 13.6 for a normal EEG reading).

Anticonvulsant Therapy

In recent decades, significant advances have been made for the treatment of epilepsy with the discovery of effective anticonvulsant drugs. Examples of useful anticonvulsants include valproic acid for the management of absence epilepsy, carbamazepine or levetiracetam for focal and generalized epilepsies, and gabapentin for refractory focal seizures. The majority of children with focal, absence, and tonic–clonic seizures can be expected to become seizure-free through the use of specific anticonvulsant drugs.

The principles of anticonvulsant therapy include the selection of an appropriate drug and the use of one drug (monotherapy), if at all

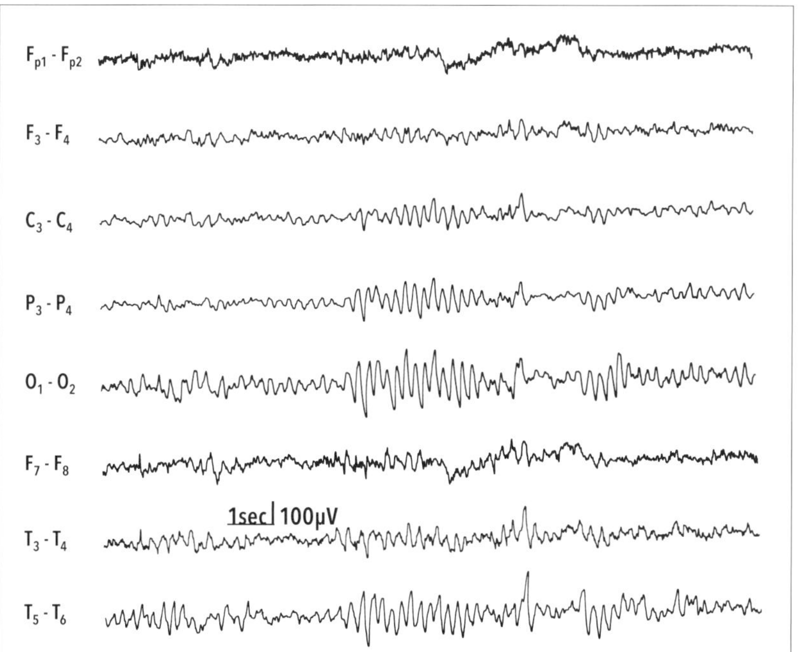

Figure 13.6. A normal electroencephalogram.

possible, to minimize untoward side effects and prevent drug interaction. It is the physician's responsibility to forewarn the parents and child of potential side effects and to explain the need for routine blood tests to monitor the drug's safety. Table 13.2 summarizes the more commonly used anticonvulsants, the seizure type(s) for which they are most effective, and the unwanted side effects that may be particularly evident in the classroom. A major advance in the management of epilepsy has been the ability to accurately measure the blood level of the anticonvulsant. If a child continues to have frequent seizures and the blood level for the specific drug is too low, adjustment of the anticonvulsant may control the convulsions.

Failure to direct therapy to the "whole child" eventually results in lack of cooperation, erratic intake of medication or noncompliance, and gradual reappearance of the seizures. The physician must be in contact with the patient at regular intervals to readjust the anticonvulsant medication, attempt to answer questions, alleviate fears, and assume responsibility for discontinuing the drug when medically feasible.

Ketogenic Diet

The ketogenic diet is usually reserved for the treatment of intractable seizures, especially complex myoclonic seizures, when anticonvulsants have failed. The diet restricts the amount of carbohydrate and protein; most calories are derived from fats. Because the preparation of the diet requires meticulous weighing of foodstuffs and is time consuming, some families find it difficult to implement. The mechanism of action is unknown but the anticonvulsant effect is thought to be related to elevated blood levels of beta-hydroxybutyric acid and acetoacetate, a byproduct of the fatty diet, resulting in ketosis. The diet is successful in controlling seizures in a significant number of these children and allows for a decrease in the anticonvulsant drugs, which often results in improvement in cognitive function and behavior.

Surgery

Surgery should be considered for those children with intractable seizures who are unresponsive to anticonvulsant therapy and who have EEG evidence of a focal onset of seizures. EEG recording with video monitoring for prolonged periods may be necessary to confirm the focal onset of seizures. Children are usually hospitalized for the procedure, and anticonvulsant use is lowered or discontinued in order to record several seizures. Special EEG recordings prior to surgery are complemented by neuropsychological studies and neuroimaging tests, including MRI, single-photon emission computed tomography

Table 13.2
ANTICONVULSANTS: USE AND SIDE EFFECTS

Generic drug (brand)	Seizure type	Side effects and toxicity
Carbamazepine (Tegretol)	Generalized tonic–clonic, focal	Dizziness, drowsiness, double vision, liver dysfunction, anemia, low white-blood cell count
Clobazam	Adjunctive therapy	Drooling, muscle fatigue, weight gain
Clonazepam (Rivotril, Klonopin)	Absence, myoclonic, focal	Drowsiness, irritability, behavioral abnormalities, depression, salivation
Ethosuximide (Zarontin)	Absence	Low white-blood count, liver dysfunction
Gabapentin (Neurontin)	Focal with secondary generalization	Somnolence, dizziness, ataxia, headache, tremor, vomiting, nystagmus, fatigue, weight gain
Lamotrigine (Lamictal)	Focal, absence, myclonic, tonic–clonic	Rash, dizziness, ataxia, headache, nausea, vomiting, somnolence
Levetiracetam (Keppra)	Tonic–clonic, absence, Lennox Gastaut syndrome	Irritability, anxiety, psychosis
Oxcarbazepine (Trileptal)	Focal and generalized seizures	Liver dysfunction
Phenobarbital	Generalized tonic–clonic	Hyperactivity, irritability, short attention span, temper tantrums, altered sleep pattern
Phenytoin (Dilantin)	Generalized tonic–clonic, focal	Gum swelling, increased body hair, unsteady gait, skin rash
Primidone (Mysoline)	Generalized tonic–clonic, focal	Personality changes, aggressive behavior similar to phenobarbital
Topiramate (Topamax)	Generalized, focal	Fatigue, cognitive depression
Valproic acid (Depakene)	Absence, generalized tonic–clonic, myoclonic	Occasional drowsiness, hair loss, weight gain, tremor, liver or pancreas dysfunction (rare)
Vigabatrin	Focal, infantile spasms	Peripheral visual loss, mental slowing, paresthesia, hyperthermia, liver and pancreas dysfunction (rare)

(SPECT), or positron emission tomography (PET), to determine if a lesion that coincides with the focal EEG abnormality can be identified. The results of epilepsy surgery are excellent for children with a well-defined focus of epileptogenic activity associated with a structural lesion identified by MRI scanning in the same region of the EEG abnormality (Engel, 1987).

Long-Term Management

Physicians know that certain events tend to precipitate or enhance seizures. For example, the child with seizures who is experiencing undue emotional stress or who is ill and not sleeping well is at a greater risk for worsening of the convulsive disorder. Some physicians believe that puberty is a particularly vulnerable period in the life of a child with epilepsy.

A concerted effort must be made to allow the child with epilepsy to lead as normal a life as possible. The reasons for long-term anticonvulsant medication should be stressed, and it should be explained that anticonvulsants are not addictive. Most children may be reassured that they will eventually "outgrow" their epilepsy and lead perfectly normal lives. Several studies suggest that a seizure-free period of two years in a neurologically normal child is associated with a good prognosis, so that the physician may elect to taper and eventually discontinue the anticonvulsant at that time (Emerson et al., 1981; Shinnar et al., 1994; Sirven, Sperling, & Wingerchuk, 2001; Thurston, Thurston, Hixon, & Keller, 1982). Children who have seizures that are well controlled should be allowed to engage in activities of all types, with the exception of unsupervised swimming or bathing and participation in contact sports such as football.

The Teacher's Role

Many parents do not inform school officials of their children's seizure disorders because of the concern that these children may be ostracized. Some schools resist the responsibility of dispensing the child's midday anticonvulsant medication. Thus, the pupil with epilepsy may face the embarrassment of his or her parent personally delivering the medication.

School administrators and educators must take a more positive attitude. Teachers must be aware of the fundamental principles of epilepsy and its management. The educator is in a position to help normalize the life of an epileptic child. The astute educator may use this opportunity to teach the facts of epilepsy to the entire class so that the social stigma of seizures will be lessened and epileptic children allowed to truly function as normal individuals.

Finally, the educator may play an active role in the management of a child with convulsions. The educator's observations of seizure activity in a child with epilepsy will enhance the physician's capability to prescribe accurately the proper quantity of an anticonvulsant drug for the child. Severe seizures may be adequately controlled in the hospital, but with a change in activity at home or at school the seizures may reappear. An educator's observations could be of considerable assistance in such a situation. Is the child excessively drowsy, which suggests too much medication? Has the pupil become hyperactive, combative, or recalcitrant, perhaps indicating an adverse reaction to the drug? Is the child alert, cooperative, and apparently seizure-free? Finally, these children require careful monitoring because learning disabilities are more common in children with epilepsy than in the general population. Most children with epilepsy will have their seizures well controlled by medication, will have normal intelligence, and can be expected to lead normal lives. Cooperation among patient, parent, physician, and educator provides a ready avenue for this goal.

TOURETTE SYNDROME

Tourette syndrome (TS), a common disorder with a prevalence of approximately 1 in 2,000 children, is inherited as an autosomal dominant trait (Pauls & Leckman, 1986). It occurs more commonly in boys than girls, by a ratio of 3:1. It is characterized by motor and vocal tics. The diagnosis of TS is made when a combination of these tics has been present for longer than one year, with an onset prior to 21 years of age and no medical causes such as drugs or central nervous system disease. *Motor tics* are brief, jerky, involuntary movements that typically are preceded by a sensation of increasing tension. Fatigue and anxiety exacerbate the motor tics; concentrating on a task usually decreases them. Motor tics tend to be localized to the head and shoulders and include head nodding, eyelid blinking, and shoulder shrugging. *Vocal tics* consist of throat clearing; sniffling and barking; and, rarely, coprolalia (the repetitive use of obscene words), echolalia (repetition of words addressed to the child), and palilalia (repetition of one's own words). Vocal tics tend to develop several months following the onset of motor tics, and the sniffling and throat clearing often are mistakenly ascribed to an allergy. The vocalizations are uncontrollable and may jeopardize the child's social interactions with classmates. The motor tics tend to wax and wane over time; for example, as eyelid blinking or sniffling disappear, a new tic such as head nodding or barking soon follows. The tics become most prominent and vexing during adolescence and on occasion are so severe that they can lead to self-mutilation. Fortunately, these tics become less intense and bothersome in the adult years, and some patients experience prolonged periods of remission.

Obsessive–compulsive behaviors, including uncontrollable licking, touching, repetitive thoughts, and motor actions, occur in approximately 60% of individuals with TS. In addition, attention-deficit/hyperactivity disorder (ADHD) is present in at least 50% of children with TS. In many cases, ADHD precedes the onset of motor and vocal tics by several years. Learning disabilities, particularly problems with mathematics, and behavioral problems including depression and anxiety are evident in approximately 25% of children with TS. Most children with severe ADHD and TS benefit significantly from stimulant medication. Several reports have implicated stimulant medication (e.g., methylphenidate) as the cause of TS; others have suggested that stimulants may unmask a latent tic disorder. The decision to begin or continue the medication will be determined by the severity of the ADHD and tic disorder (Sverd, Gadow, & Paolicelli, 1988). Recent reports indicate that stimulant drugs rarely enhance the frequency or severity of tics (Gillberg et al., 1997). However, if stimulant drugs are prescribed for a child with TS, it is mandatory that the child be closely followed for worsening of his or her tics and behavior. The cause of TS is unknown, but a genetic etiology is most likely. The symptoms of the condition and the response to specific medications suggest an abnormality in one or more neurotransmitter pathways, particularly the dopamine system (Felling & Singer, 2011).

Motor tics in children are not always due to TS. Transient tics, consisting of eyelid blinking or facial movements, are the most common movement disorder in children. They are most prevalent in boys, and there is often a positive family history. Unlike TS, these tics permanently disappear within one year of onset. Tics may also be observed in children following encephalitis, birth injury, or head trauma, and in rare genetic disorders such as Wilson and Hallevorden-Spatz diseases.

Most children with TS do not require treatment with medication because the symptoms are mild and do not interfere with scholastic or social activities. The physician should explain to the child and family that the tics are involuntary and not due to a psychiatric or emotional condition, and that punishment of the child or drawing attention to the tics will serve only to heighten the symptoms. Clonidine is effective in managing the tics, ADHD, and compulsive behavior, and it generally has few side effects. The anticonvulsant levetiracetam has also been studied but is less effective than clonidine (Hedderick,

Morris, & Singer, 2009). The neuroleptic group of drugs, especially haloperidol (a dopamine-blocking agent) and pimozide, are effective in the management of tics in approximately 50% of children with TS. However, their side effects may be severe and include cognitive impairment, lethargy, fatigue, and depression, which often preclude their use. All children with TS on medication require close medical supervision, especially for untoward side effects (Kurlan, 1989; Shapiro, Shapiro, Young, & Feinberg, 1988).

A teacher is likely to encounter a child with TS sometime during his or her career. A significant number of children display ADHD as the initial manifestation of TS. Ultimately, the characteristic symptoms of TS become evident, including motor and vocal tics. Some children with TS will also have severe learning problems requiring specific remediation. Not surprisingly, behavioral problems are prominent, probably due in part to the reaction of other children and adults to the TS symptoms. Fortunately, in most cases, TS does not significantly interfere with a child's academic achievement or social development; however, if the tics are severe or the ADHD incapacitating, medical management must be considered. As TS may be a chronic lifelong disorder, which may be associated with learning, behavioral, and social problems, the educator can play an important role in its multidisciplinary management by serving as an advocate for the child.

REFERENCES

Abu-Arafeh, I., Razak S., Sivaraman B., & Graham, C. (2010). Prevalence of headache and migraine in children and adolescents: A systemic review of population-based studies. *Developmental Medicine and Child Neurology, 52*(12), 1088–1097.

Barlow, C. F. (1984). *Headaches and migraine in childhood.* Philadelphia, PA: Lippincott.

Baumann, R. J. (2002). Behavioral treatment of migraine in children and adolescents. *Pediatric Drugs, 4*(9), 555–561.

Berg, A. T., Berkovic, S. F., Brodie, M. J., Buchhalter, J., Cross, J. H., van Emde, W., . . . Scheffer, I. E. (2010). Revised terminology and concepts for organization of seizures and epilepsies: Report of the ILAE Consensus in Classification and Terminology 2005–2009. *Epilepsia, 51*(4), 676–685.

Billie, B. (1962). Migraine in school children. *Acta Paediatrica Scandinavia, 51* (Suppl. 136), 1–151.

Bonfert, M., Straube, A., Schroeder, A. S., Reilich, P., Ebinger, F., & Heinen, F. (2013). Primary headache in children and adolescents: Update on pharmacotherapy of migraine and tension-type headache. *Neuropediatrics, 44*(1), 3–19.

Carroll, L. (1984). *Alice's adventures in Wonderland.* London, UK: Gollancz. (Original work published 1865)

Commission on Classification and Terminology of the International League Against Epilepsy. (1989). Proposal for revised classification of epilepsies and epileptic syndromes. *Epilepsia, 30*, 389–399.

Congdon, P. J., & Forsythe, W. I. (1979). Migraine in childhood: A study of 300 children. *Developmental Medicine and Child Neurology, 21*, 209–216.

Diamond, S. (1979). Biofeedback and headache. *Headache, 19*, 180–184.

Emerson, R., D'Souza, B. J., Vining, E. P., Holden, K. R., Mellits, E. D., & Freeman, J. M. (1981). Stopping medication in children with epilepsy: Predictors of outcome. *New England Journal of Medicine, 304*, 1125–1129.

Engel, J. E., Jr. (1987). *Surgical treatment of the epilepsies.* New York, NY: Raven.

Felling, R. J., & Singer H. S. (2011). Neurobiology of Tourette syndrome: Current status and need for further investigation. *Journal of Neuroscience, 31*(35), 12387–12395.

Freemon, F. R., Douglas, E. F. O., & Penry, J. K. (1973). Environmental interaction and memory during petit mal (absence) seizures. *Pediatrics, 51*, 911–918.

Friedman, A. P., & Harms, E. (1967). *Headaches in children.* Springfield, IL: Thomas.

Gillberg, C., Melander, H., von Knorring, A. L., Janols, L. O., Thernlund, G., Hagglof, B., . . . Kopp, S. (1997). Long term central stimulant treatment of children with attention-deficit hyperactivity disorder symptoms: A randomized double-blind placebo-controlled trial. *Archives of General Psychiatry, 54*, 857–864.

Gupta, A., & Rothner, A. D. (2001). Treatment of childhood headaches. *Current Neurological & Neuroscience Reprints, 1*(2), 144–154.

Hedderick, E. F., Morris, C. M., & Singer, H. S. (2009). Double-blind, crossover study of clonidine and levetiracetam in Tourette syndrome. *Pediatric Neurology, 40*(6), 420–425.

Hughes, E. L., & Cooper, C. E. (1956). Some observations on headache and eye pain in a group of schoolchildren. *British Medical Journal, 1*, 1138–1141.

Kurlan, R. (1989). Tourette's syndrome: Current concepts. *Neurology, 39*, 1625–1630.

Ling, W., Oftedal, G., & Weinberg, W. (1970). Depressive illness in childhood presenting as severe headache. *American Journal of Diseases of Children, 120*, 122–124.

Livingston, S. (1972). *Comprehensive management of epilepsy in infancy, childhood and adolescence.* Springfield, IL: Thomas.

Olness, H., MacDonald, J. T., & Uden, D. L. (1987). Comparison of self-hypnosis and propranolol in the treatment of juvenile classic migraine. *Pediatrics, 79*, 593–597.

Oster, J. (1972). Recurrent abdominal pain, headache, and limb pains in children and adolescents. *Pediatrics, 50*, 429–436.

Pauls, D. L., & Leckman, J. F. (1986). The inheritance of Gilles de la Tourette syndrome and associated behaviors: Evidence for autosomal dominant transmission. *New England Journal of Medicine, 315*, 993–997.

Prensky, A. L., & Sommer, D. (1979). Diagnosis and treatment of migraine in children. *Neurology, 29*, 506–510.

Shapiro, A. K., Shapiro, E. S., Young, Y. G., & Feinberg, T. E. (1988). *Gilles de la Tourette syndrome* (2nd ed.). New York, NY: Raven.

Shinnar, S., Berg, A. T., Moshe, S. L., Kang, H., O'Dell, C., Alemany, M., . . . Hauser, W. A. (1994). Discontinuing antiepileptic drugs in children: A prospective study. *Annals of Neurology, 35*(5), 509–510.

Shinnar, S., & D'Souza, B. J. (1982). The diagnosis and management of headaches in childhood. *Pediatric Clinics of North America, 29,* 79–94.

Sirven, J. I., Sperling, M., & Wingerchuk, D. M. (2001). Early versus late antiepileptic drug withdrawal for people with epilepsy in remission. *Cochrane Database Systems Review, 3,* CD001902.

Stafstrom, C. E., Rostasy, K., & Minster, A. (2002). The usefulness of children's drawings in the diagnosis of headache. *Pediatrics, 109*(3), 460–472.

Sverd, J., Gadow, K. D., & Paolicelli, L. M. (1988). Methylphenidate treatment of attention-deficit hyperactivity disorder in boys with Tourette's syndrome. *Journal of the American Academy of Child and Adolescent Psychiatry, 28*(4), 574–579.

Thurston, J. H., Thurston, D. L., Hixon, B. B., & Keller, A. J. (1982). Prognosis in childhood epilepsy: Additional follow-up of 148 children 15 to 23 years after withdrawal of anticonvulsant therapy. *New England Journal of Medicine, 306,* 831–836.

Vahlquist, B. (1955). Migraine in children. *International Archives of Allergy and Immunology, 7,* 348–355.

Winner, P., Rothner, A. D., Saper, J., Nett, R., Asgharnejad, M., Laurenza, A., . . . Peykamian, M. (2000). A randomized, double-blind, placebo-controlled study of sumatriptan nasal spray in the treatment of acute migraine in adolescents. *Pediatrics, 106,* 989–997.

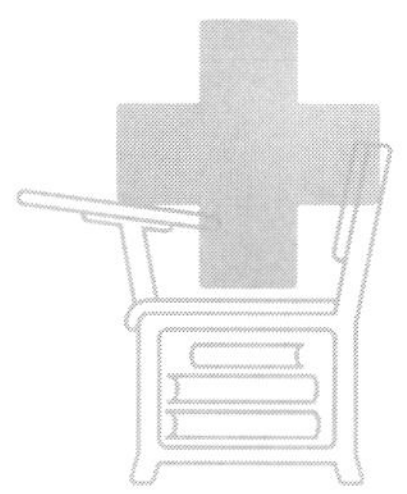

Chapter 14
Cerebral Palsy and Associated Dysfunction

Peter A. Blasco and Patricia M. Blasco

Parents of children with problems related to development typically describe nonspecific symptoms, such as "He doesn't talk," "He's not sitting (or walking) on time," or "She's too stiff [or floppy]." Sometimes the developmental problems of infants and toddlers are noticed first by early childhood personnel rather than by parents. Evaluation of a child with developmental problems may lead to a diagnosis of one or more neurodevelopmental disabilities (see Table 14.1 for prevalence statistics of various neurodevelopmental disorders). One of these disorders, cerebral palsy—a neurological condition that affects movement, balance, and posture—is the primary topic of this chapter, although other motor disabilities are also discussed.

Table 14.1
NEURODEVELOPMENTAL DISABILITIES AND PREVALENCE IN CHILDREN

Disability	Prevalence
Learning disabilities and/or attention-deficit syndromes	0.5%–0.7%
Intellectual disability	0.3%
Cerebral palsy	0.2%–0.5%
Deafness	0.1%
Blindness	0.05%
Autism and/or autism-spectrum disorders	0.08%–01.5%

Note. Prevalence is the proportion of a population that has a specific condition (e.g., cerebral palsy) in a given period.

AN APPROACH TO MOTOR IMPAIRMENT

When developmental specialists (e.g., developmental pediatricians, pediatric therapists, special educators) are asked to evaluate children with possible disabilities, the first approach should be to separate the developmental issues (concerns raised by caretakers and findings uncovered on evaluation) into three domains: motor dysfunction, cognitive deficits, and behavioral problems. Although closely interrelated, the three categories are independent. For example, children with severe motor disabilities may be intellectually normal or even gifted. Conversely, the majority of individuals with intellectual disability go through typical motor developmental milestones. Individuals with cerebral palsy, despite their physical (motor) limitations and associated medical problems, can be active participants in the classroom, the community, and the workplace. Integration into societal life, as fully as possible, is the ultimate goal, and the classroom is the source of much of this effort in the first two decades of the child's life.

CEREBRAL PALSY: HISTORICAL PERSPECTIVE

An English orthopedic surgeon, Sir William John Little, initially described the entity of cerebral palsy in 1843 (Little, 1853). He not only presented the first comprehensive clinical description of this motor disorder but also suggested modalities of therapy, such as manipulations, gymnastics, and braces. He emphasized birth trauma and premature delivery as etiologic factors. Subsequently, birth palsies of cerebral origin were referred to as "Little's disease." Sigmund Freud, one of the celebrated founders of psychiatry and psychoanalysis, started his career as a prominent neurologist and neuropathologist and was a pioneer in the field of cerebral palsy. In the 1890s, he published his clinical experience of children with Little's disease, described the neuropathology, and devised a classification system that was used during the early part of the 20th century and remains the foundation for what is used today. He suggested that there were prenatal causes of cerebral palsy that would be inappropriately attributed to difficulties occurring during delivery:

> Difficult birth and premature birth are not always accidental happenings, but may frequently be the result of a deeper cause or its expressions without being the actual etiological factor. Thus, it may well be possible that the same pathogenic factors that rendered in-

> trauterine development abnormal also extended their influence to parturition; abnormal birth is then the final result of an abnormal pregnancy. (Freud, 1897/1968, p. 208)

The term *cerebral palsy* was first coined by Sir William Osler in the late 19th century, but it was not commonly used until the 1930s, when Winthrop Phelps, an orthopedic surgeon, popularized it (Panteliadis, Panteliadis, & Vassilyadi, 2013). Over the course of three decades, Phelps oversaw the development of the field of cerebral palsy, demonstrating that these children could be successfully habilitated. He personally trained the lion's share of professionals from many disciplines who specialized in this chronic disorder.

In the late 1950s, Eric Denhoff, a developmental pediatrician, emphasized that cerebral palsy should be viewed as the motor manifestation of an extended spectrum of brain dysfunction. Thus, cerebral palsy was often coupled with cognitive deficits, convulsions, visual or hearing loss, speech difficulty, and behavioral and emotional disturbances (Denhoff & Robinault, 1960). He also made note of the "minimal" end of the spectrum, where the motor and cognitive disabilities are subtle and are frequently accompanied by a particular behavioral disorder, the hallmark of which is inattention. The child with a diagnosis of cerebral palsy needs ongoing surveillance for language development, cognitive abilities, visual motor ability, nutrition and growth, and seizure disorders. These associated deficits need to be delineated in order to provide the child with an educational plan most suitable for his or her needs.

Multidisciplinary and interdisciplinary approaches have been adopted in an effort to help identify all the specific problems and orchestrate all the needed services involved with the child and family. The goal of the team, including parents, is an educational placement that optimizes learning at a child's cognitive level, utilizing the child's strengths as well as his or her needs.

DEFINITION

Cerebral palsy is defined as a disorder of movement and posture—in other words, a motor disability—resulting from a permanent, nonprogressive insult involving the immature brain (Bax, 1964). Cerebral dysfunction can exist on the basis of a central nervous system (CNS) that has not developed properly from the start, which is referred to as a developmental malformation or CNS anomaly or, alternatively, can be the consequence of an injury to a previously normally developing nervous system. The insult of cerebral palsy is always static; that is, the lesion itself will not get worse. What often does change over time are the manifestations of the motor disorder and the emergence or recognition of associated deficits as the child grows and the nervous system matures. In instances where the brain insult does get progressively worse over time, we speak in terms of degenerative CNS disease.

PREVALENCE

The epidemiology of cerebral palsy has been confused because of different assumptions about the population being defined. For example, some studies exclude *all* cases that occur after birth, limiting the population to only prenatal and perinatal etiologies. Without a formal cerebral palsy registry in the United States, it is difficult to precisely define its prevalence. In developed countries, rates of cerebral palsy in children are generally quoted in the range of 0.1% to 0.3% of the pediatric population (Cans, 2000). We favor a rate of 0.5%—that is, about 1 in 200 children have cerebral palsy. This number takes into account milder cases and a broader age of onset.

There is some disagreement about whether the overall incidence of cerebral palsy is rising or staying stable. A possible rise has been attributed to the increased survival of children born with extremely low birth weights of less than 1,000 g (Allen, 2008). Twin gestations also present a much higher risk of cerebral palsy, and multifetal pregnancies have increased significantly in the past three decades (Rand, Eddleman, & Stone, 2005). Regardless of whether cerebral palsy incidence is rising or is remaining unchanged, the absolute number of cases is increasing because the overall survival of all high-risk infants has increased over time, thus resulting in larger numbers of healthy former preemies and multiple births, but also increased numbers of children with cerebral palsy (Allen, Cristofalo, & Kim, 2011).

Risk factors for cerebral palsy identified in a number of studies have included maternal age greater than 35 and younger than 20, children born to mothers who have had more than five pregnancies, multiple fetus gestations, intrauterine demise of one fetus in a twin pregnancy, birth weight less than 1,500 g (particularly birth weight less than 1,000 g), and African American racial background (Allen, 2008; McIntyre et al., 2013).

DIAGNOSIS

On average, cerebral palsy is diagnosed at 12 months of age (Lock, Shapiro, Ross, & Capute, 1986). The diagnosis is based on clinical examination findings. No laboratory or radiographic examination can make or even confirm the clinical diagnosis of cerebral palsy. The following are the criteria used for the clinical diagnosis of cerebral palsy:

- delayed motor milestones
- abnormal neurological examination
- aberrant primitive reflexes and postural reactions
- positive history for risk or evidence of insult
- no clinical progression based on history or repeat examination
- age of insult

To make a meaningful statement about a child's motor competence, the examiner should organize data gathered from the history, physical examination, and neurodevelopmental examination according to the following schema (Blasco, 1992):

1. Motor developmental milestones
2. The classic neurological examination
3. Markers of cerebral neuromotor maturation (the primitive reflexes and postural reactions)

Motor milestones are extracted from the developmental history, as well as from observations during the neurodevelopmental examination. A basic reference table of sequential gross and fine motor milestones is needed. Milestone assessment is best summarized as a single motor age (or narrow age range) for the child, allowing one to think of the child in terms of his or her level of motor function. The ratio of motor age to chronological age produces the motor quotient (MQ), giving a simple expression of deviation from the norm (Blasco, 1992). An MQ below 70 is considered abnormal.

Motor milestones do not take into account the quality of a child's movements. The motor portion of the *neurological examination*, including observations of station and gait (gross motor) and reach and grasp (fine motor), takes qualitative features into account. Neurological assessments of tone, strength, deep tendon reflexes, and coordination are difficult in the infant because of their subjective nature, compounded by the limited ability for cooperation. Muscle *tone* (passive resistance) and *strength* (active resistance) are a challenge to distinguish in the contrary subject. The best clues often come from observation rather than handling of the infant. Spontaneous or prompted motor activities (e.g., weight bearing in sitting or standing) require adequate strength. Weakness may be best appreciated from observing the quality of stationary posture and transition movements. It is important to understand that although the child's muscle *tone* (passive) may be extremely high, actual *strength* (voluntary) may be quite poor. Clinical experience is essential to gain accurate and useful information. After the child is 2 to 3 years of age, the neurological examination becomes easier and more meaningful, as cooperation improves.

Station refers to the posture (body alignment) assumed in sitting or standing and should be viewed from anterior, lateral, and posterior perspectives. *Gait* refers to walking and is examined in progress. Initially, the toddler walks on a wide base, slightly crouched, with the arms abducted and elevated a bit. Forward progression is more staccato than smooth. Movements gradually become more fluid, the base narrows, and arm swing evolves, leading to an adult pattern of walking by 3 years of age.

The motor *neuromaturational* markers include the *primitive reflexes,* which develop during gestation and generally disappear 3 to 6 months after birth, and the *postural reactions,* which are not present at birth but sequentially develop between 3 and 10 months of age. The Moro, tonic labyrinthine, asymmetric tonic neck, and positive support reflexes are the most clinically useful primitive reflexes. The appearance of postural reactions in sequence beginning after 1 to 2 months of age can provide great insight into the motor potential of young infants. Postural reactions are sought in each of the three major areas of righting, protection, and equilibrium, and they are easy to elicit in the normal infant. (See Blasco, 1992, for more detailed information on individual reflexes.)

Once a motor abnormality has been identified, further assessment as to its exact nature and etiology is essential. This almost always warrants referral to an appropriate subspecialty interdisciplinary team. Categories of motor disability fall into four general areas: static central nervous system disorders, progressive diseases, spinal cord and peripheral nerve injuries, and structural defects.

Motor dysfunction produced by a *static* (i.e., nonprogressive) *brain insult* is the etiology of cerebral palsy. The cerebral insult can happen during early fetal brain development, resulting in a central nervous system anomaly. The anomaly could be the result of improper genetic information (e.g., as in Down syndrome) or a very early biochemical or mechanical insult that permanently alters anatomical development of the brain. Alternatively, a brain developing in a normal fashion can be damaged before, during, or after birth by a variety of insults. Examples are infection (e.g., meningitis, encephalitis), trauma, ischemia (e.g., from dehydration or stroke), poisons (e.g., lead intoxication), metabolic diseases (e.g., phenylketonuria), and so forth. Brain injury resulting in neuron and axon destruction is mostly permanent—little true neuronal repair or regrowth takes place. However, the prevention of ongoing injury (Fleiss & Gressens, 2012) together with the continued development of intact areas during childhood allows some functional improvements to accrue up to a certain point. Maturation of motor areas in the brain has largely reached completion by 7 or 8 years of age. When a motor impairment is due to a brain anomaly or to a nonprogressive insult that took place before midadolescence (others would say before 7 to 8 years of age), the disorder is referred to as cerebral palsy. Specific types of cerebral palsy (e.g., spastic, athetoid) are diagnosed clinically and imply which motor control system in the brain has been primarily damaged. Establishing the type of cerebral palsy has great value in treatment planning and in prognosis. These diagnostic distinctions and the treatment plans based on them are best carried out by a coordinated team of physicians and therapists experienced in the care of children with motor impairments.

Progressive diseases of the brain, the nerves, or the muscles produce motor impairment that worsens with time. Although the number of diseases in this category is very large, each individual disease is extremely rare. Therefore, the fraction of all children whose motor impairments are caused by progressive diseases is quite small.

Spinal cord and peripheral nerve injuries and anomalies are all static conditions except the rare instance of a growing spine tumor. These conditions differ from cerebral palsy in that future functional loss is much easier to predict and they have different types of associated problems. In this category, the largest single group consists of children with spina bifida, specifically meningomyelocele.

Structural defects refer to situations in which some anatomical structure (e.g., a limb) is missing or deformed or in which some support tissue for the nerves and muscles is inadequate (e.g., connective tissue defects, biochemically abnormal bone). Structural defects are usually the most straightforward to understand of all motor-impairing conditions. On the mildest end of the spectrum are a wide variety of fairly common orthopedic deformities that may or may not affect motor development (e.g., club feet, developmental hip dysplasia), whereas other conditions (e.g., osteogenesis imperfecta, many varieties of childhood arthritis) are progressive in nature and may be extremely complex to manage.

Establishing the specific type of progressive disease, the level of spinal cord dysfunction, or the specific structural diagnosis is fundamental to developing a sound treatment program. In addition, the precise diagnosis will carry major implications for genetic counseling.

CLASSIFICATION

Different approaches have been employed as the basis for categorizing types of cerebral palsy, and the resulting classifications can be confusing. A simplified approach based first on the clinical neuromotor manifestations (spastic, extrapyramidal, or mixed) and then on the distribution of extremity impairment (topographical involvement) is favored by most:

Spastic (pyramidal)	Extrapyramidal	Mixed
Quadriplegia (tetraplegia)	Rigid	
Diplegia	Choreoathetoid	
Hemiplegia	Dystonic (dyskinetic)	
Triplegia	Ataxic	
Monoplegia	Tremor	
Paraplegia	Hypotonic	

Spastic (pyramidal) *cerebral palsy*, the most common type, is characterized by an increase in muscle tone that has a "clasp-knife" (spastic) quality, pathologically increased deep tendon reflexes, and a consistent pattern of agonist–antagonist muscle imbalance. For example, in the spastic lower extremity, it is difficult for the child to relax the leg muscles that allow him or her to straighten at the hip and knee and to dorsiflex at the ankle. Therefore, the child always tends to keep the leg postured or to move it in a pattern of flexion: flexed at the hip, flexed at the knee, and plantar flexed and turned in at the ankle. The term *pyramidal cerebral palsy* is derived from the location of the cerebral insult, which is in the pyramidal system involving the motor cortex in the gray matter of the brain and/or the pyramidal tract fibers leading from the cortex to the spinal cord. These cells usually innervate voluntary muscles (see Figure 14.1). Among spastic types of cerebral palsy, subclassification is based on topographical distribution, that is, which limbs are involved. Spastic quadriplegia involves all four extremities, typically the lower extremities more so than the uppers. In diplegia, all four extremities are again involved, but the lower extremities are dramatically more affected than the uppers. The term *paraplegia* should be reserved for those instances in which the legs are spastic and the arms are normal. Paraplegic cerebral palsy is very rare. *Spastic paraplegia* is primarily associated with spinal cord

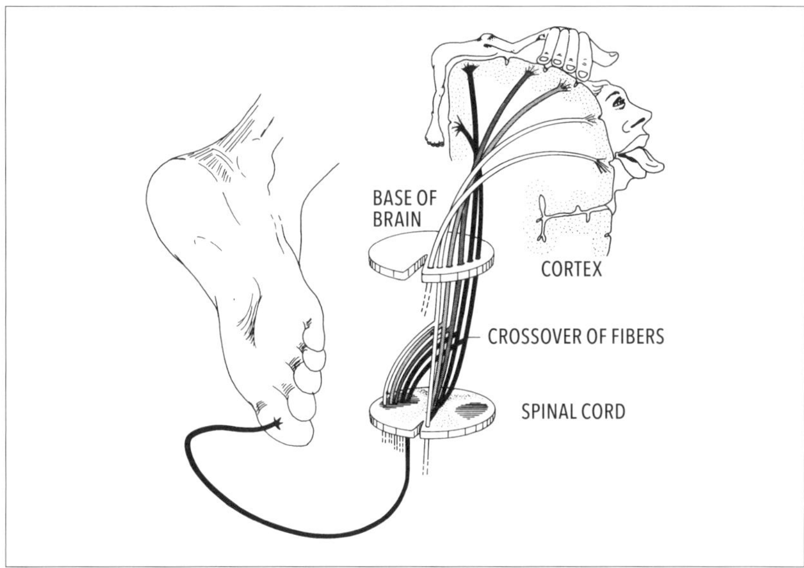

Figure 14.1 The pyramidal tracts: a schematic illustration of the motor cortex. Note the disproportionate representation of the lower face, tongue, lips, and hand on the motor area of the brain. Injury to the cerebral cortex in the region of the leg (*darkest line or tract*) will result in spasticity in the opposite extremity.

injury. Hemiplegia is confined to one half of the body, and the arm is usually more affected than the leg. When all four extremities are spastic, with the upper extremities clearly more involved than the lowers, the designation *double hemiplegia* is often used. Spastic *diplegia* and *quadriplegia* may be symmetrical in terms of severity of involvement but as often as not are somewhat asymmetric.

The second main type of cerebral palsy is classified as *extrapyramidal* (or nonspastic). In extrapyramidal cerebral palsy, the involvement is essentially always quadriplegic, so subclassification is determined on the basis of the dominant tone pattern or movement disorder features. *Choreoathetoid, dystonic,* ataxic, and *hypotonic* types of cerebral palsy are more commonly seen than *tremor* or *rigid* CP, which are quite rare. Sometimes the term *dyskinetic* is used in reference to the choreoathetoid and dystonic subtypes. Extrapyramidal types of cerebral palsy have their origin in the deep gray matter of the brain (the basal ganglia) or in the cerebellum (see Figure 14.2). Extrapyramidal types of cerebral palsy typically affect the upper extremities more than the lower extremities, and the character of increased extremity tone is of a "lead-pipe" (persistently rigid) rather than clasp-knife (i.e., spastic) quality. This lead-pipe or putty-like feel will tend to diminish

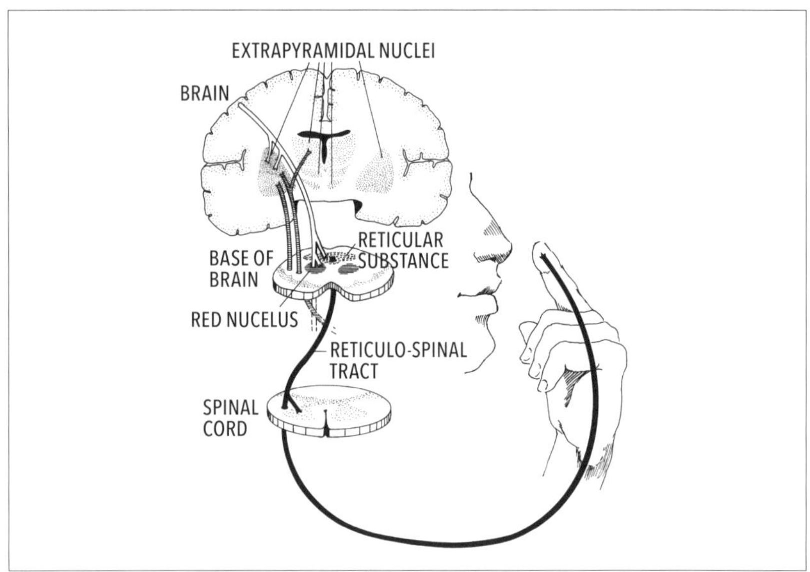

Figure 14.2 The extrapyramidal tracts: destruction of the various components of the extrapyramidal nuclei may result in a movement disorder (chorea, athetosis, rigidity, dystonia). The abnormal movements may become pronounced when the child performs certain tasks, such as pointing, writing with a pencil, and so on.

with repetitive active or passive movements. Oral-motor dysfunction is often a prominent feature in children with extrapyramidal cerebral palsy, with resultant difficulties in speaking and eating. In children with extrapyramidal cerebral palsy, extra movements and muscle tone become more evident when they become excited or nervous or attempt to perform tasks that require intense effort.

The final major category of cerebral palsy is *mixed*, a combination of both spastic and extrapyramidal patterns of involvement. About 60% of cerebral palsy is spastic, the majority of which is hemiplegic; about 15% is extrapyramidal; and 25% is mixed (Cans, 2000). Mixed cerebral palsy is underrecognized and often misclassified as spastic quadriplegic because the underlying choreoathetosis is unappreciated.

Understanding the classification of cerebral palsy, both the neuromotor manifestations and the topographic distribution, is useful clinically. The type of cerebral palsy often gives insight into the associated perceptual, sensory, and cognitive deficits. For example, children with hemiplegia have a higher incidence of seizures than those with quadriplegia or diplegia. Intelligence tends to be best preserved (generally normal) in spastic diplegia and is a little lower in hemiplegia (most often in the borderline to mild intellectual disability range). Children with spastic quadriplegia virtually always have intellectual disability

GMFCS E & R between 6th and 12th birthday: Descriptors and illustrations

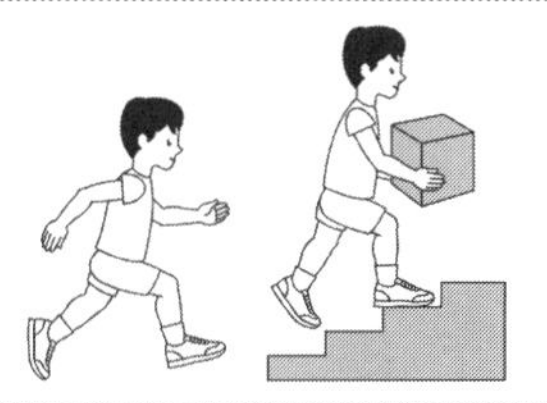

GMFCS Level I

Children walk at home, school, outdoors and in the community. They can climb stairs without the use of a railing. Children perform gross motor skills such as running and jumping, but speed, balance and coordination are limited

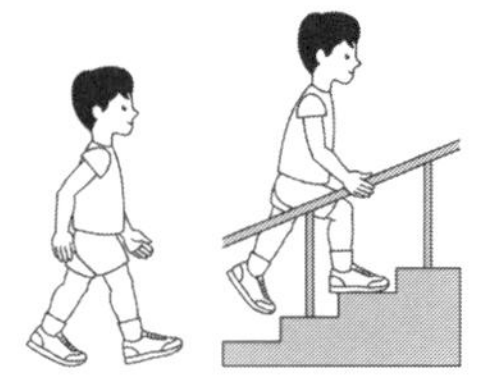

GMFCS Level II

Children walk in most settings and climb stairs holding onto a railing. They may experience difficulty walking long distances and balancing on uneven terrain, inclines, in crowded areas or confined spaces. Children may walk with physical assistance, a hand-held mobility device or used wheeled mobility over long distances. Children have only minimal ability to perform gross motor skills such as running and jumping.

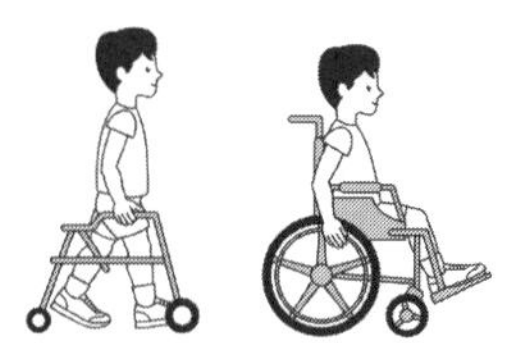

GMFCS Level III

Children walk using a hand-held mobility device in most indoor settings. They may climb stairs holding onto a railing with supervision or assistance. Children use wheeled mobility when traveling long distances and may self-propel for shorter distances.

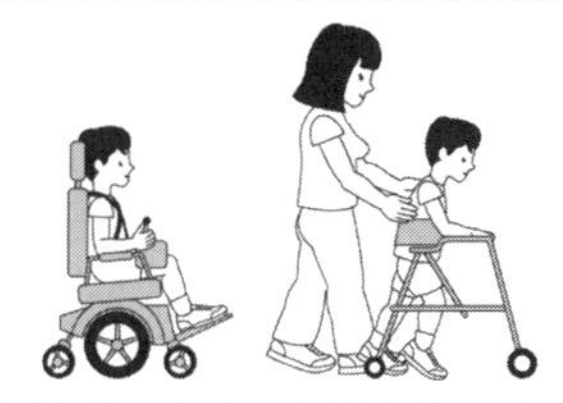

GMFCS Level IV

Children use methods of mobility that require physical assistance or powered mobility in most settings. They may walk for short distances at home with physical assistance or use powered mobility or a body support walker when positioned. At school, outdoors and in the community children are transported in a manual wheelchair or use powered mobility.

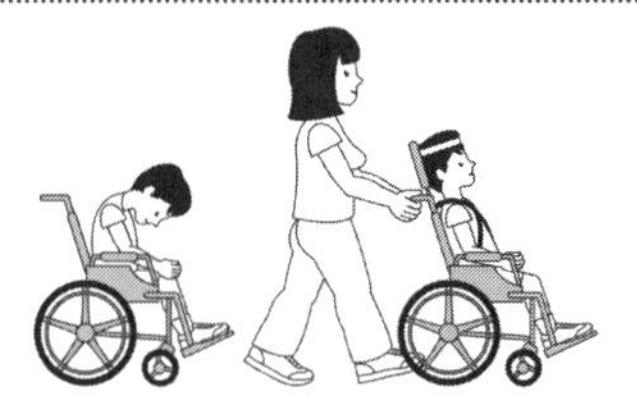

GMFCS Level V

Children are transported in a manual wheelchair in all settings. Children are limited in their ability to maintain antigravity head and trunk postures and control leg and arm movements.

GMFCS descriptors: Palisano et al. (1997) Dev Med Child Neurol 39:214-23
CanChild: www.canchild.ca

Illustrations copyright © Kerr Graham, Bill Reid and Adrienne Harvey, The Royal Children's Hospital, Melbourne

Note. To accurately classify gross motor function, see the full descriptions of the GMFCS in "Content Validity of the Expanded and Revised Gross Motor Function Classification System," by R. J. Palisano, P. Rosenbaum, D. Bartlett, and M. H. Livingston, 2008, *Developmental Medicine and Child Neurology, 50*, pp. 744–750. GMFCS descriptors from "Development and Validation of a Gross Motor Function Classification System for Children with Cerebral Palsy," by R. J. Palisano, P. Rosenbaum, S. Walter, D. Russell, E. Wood, and B. Galuppi, 1997, *Developmental Medicine and Child Neurology, 39*, pp. 214–223. Copyright 1997 by Robert Palisano, Peter Rosenbaum, Stephen Walter, Dianne Russell, Ellen Wood, and Barbara Galuppi. Adapted with permission. Illustrations © Kerr Graham, Bill Reid, and Adrienne Harvey, The Royal Children's Hospital, Melbourne. Reprinted with permission.

Figure 14.3 Pictorial representation of the gross motor function classification system (GMFCS).

to some degree. About 50% of children with hemiplegia have associated sensory impairment on the involved side. This is manifested by the child's inability to recognize an object by touch or feel (*astereognosis*), by diminished awareness of light touch or pain on the affected side, and by neglect of the involved side. This cortical sensory impairment may contribute as much or more to the child's failure to use the limb than does the motor impairment itself (Tizard, Paine, & Crothers, 1954). Additionally, approximately 25% of children with spastic hemiplegia have a loss of vision in a portion of the visual field toward the side of motor weakness (*homonymous hemianopsia*). For children with the choreoathetoid form of cerebral palsy, the motor involvement

Table 14.2
CAUSES OF CEREBRAL PALSY

I. Prenatal (congenital) A. Genetic (e.g., chromosome disorders such as trisomy 18; deletion syndromes; neurocutaneous syndromes such as tuberous sclerosis) B. Infectious (e.g., toxoplasmosis, rubella, cytomegalovirus, herpes, syphilis) C. Toxic/metabolic (e.g., maternal phenylketonuria, maternal iodine deficiency, fetal alcohol syndrome) D. Other (e.g., unexplained CNS malformations, prenatal cerebrovascular accidents
II. Acquired A. Perinatal (e.g., hypoxic-ischemic insult, prematurity, intraventricular hemorrhage) B. Postnatal (e.g., head trauma; hypoxia, as in near drowning) 1. Infectious: primary CNS infection such as meningitis, encephalitis, secondary effects on CNS 2. Toxic/metabolic: lead poisoning, inborn errors of metabolism, like phenylketonuria 3. Neoplastic (cancer) 4. Other diseases: cerebrovascular accidents, nutritional deficiency, collagen vascular disease

may be very severe in the face of normal or greater-than-normal intelligence (see Nolan, 1987).

As with any disorder, cerebral palsy occurs on a spectrum of severity from very mild to very severe. The most severely involved children may never achieve ambulation or develop intelligible speech. The most mildly involved walk late and, although awkward as children, experience little to no true motor limitation other than in competitive activities. The Gross Motor Function Classification System (GMFCS; see Figure 14.3) has been widely accepted as the best objective classification for cerebral palsy severity (Palisano et al., 1997). Children at the mildest end of the spectrum may or may not be identified as having cerebral palsy as infants and most often carry either no diagnosis or one of a variety of descriptive designations at school age (e.g., minor neuromotor dysfunction, developmental dyspraxia, developmental coordination disorder). Findings in the infant that fulfill the criteria for diagnosing cerebral palsy, albeit mild, often evolve into a more subtle picture in the older child. In that circumstance, the term *minimal* cerebral palsy is sometimes still used, but the preferred diagnostic term is *developmental coordination disorder* (Zwicker, Missiuna, Harris, & Boyd, 2012).

ETIOLOGY

Any brain injury to the areas governing motor control can cause cerebral palsy. No single etiology of cerebral palsy stands out above the others (see various causes listed in Table 14.2). Certain types of insult tend to result in specific types of motor dysfunction. For example, in the past, choreoathetoid cerebral palsy was most frequently ascribed to bilirubin encephalopathy (kernicterus), but with obstetric advances in the prevention of Rh factor disease, good neonatal surveillance, and improved management of hyperbilirubinemia in the past 50 years, choreoathetoid cerebral palsy is now rarely the result of hyperbilirubinemia. More frequently, it is linked to sudden and severe anoxic events in full-term infants. Spastic diplegia results from periventricular leukomalacia as a consequence of hypoxia and altered blood supply to especially vulnerable portions of the brain in premature infants.

Causes of cerebral palsy are conveniently divided into three categories based on time frame: prenatal, perinatal, and postnatal etiologies. Prenatal causes include CNS anomalies, which are structural abnormalities that occur during development of the brain. Prenatal injuries to the brain may result from intrauterine infection, such as from cytomegalovirus, toxoplasmosis, rubella, and so on. Additionally, exposure to toxins or drugs can have teratogenic effects on the fetus. Recent concerns relate to the use of cocaine during pregnancy or the existence of a familial predisposition to forming blood clots, either of which may cause strokes in utero, resulting in cerebral palsy. Birth asphyxia is a contributor to cerebral palsy, but improved obstetric care has reduced the risk of perinatal asphyxia. An infant may experience distress during or following a difficult delivery because of a central nervous system injury or a developmental brain defect that occurred antenatally but was undetected before birth. Thus, the prenatal defect and not the difficult delivery may be the actual cause of the cerebral palsy (as surmised by Freud many years ago). Sophisticated brain-imaging studies in many cases can pinpoint the nature and the timing of central nervous system lesions and thereby help in the identification of children who had brain pathology existing before delivery. Antenatal screening for specific chemical markers in amniotic fluid and chromosome studies from fetal cells can also help to identify etiologies such as structural anomalies, ischemic injuries, metabolic abnormalities, or specific genetic syndromes prior to birth. These tests are appropriate in pregnancies that are at risk for specific abnormalities because of a positive family history. Metabolic diseases can result in postnatal brain damage that will remain static once the disease is recognized and controlled. The types of cerebral palsy these insults produce are often unusual. They may yield atypical patterns of involvement with unusual progression, or additional insults may accrue due to episodes when the metabolic disease gets temporarily out of control.

In progressive neurological diseases, the motor disability may be described in the same terms used for cerebral palsy (e.g., quadriplegia, rigidity), but these disorders should not be lumped together with cerebral palsy because, by the nature of their etiologies, the motor disability will worsen with time. Brain tumors may create a picture of new or progressive motor deterioration as long as the tumor expands. If the tumor is successfully treated, the child may completely return to normal or may be left with a residual motor impairment that is static (i.e., cerebral palsy).

The cause of cerebral palsy cannot be precisely identified in about 10% of cases. The inability to identify a cause is disconcerting for physicians and frustrating for parents. Knowing the cause may not provide any information useful for treatment but still can be satisfying or relieving for parents who inevitably ask, "Why?" In addition, a particular pattern of disability coupled with radiographic findings may clearly support some causative insult, for example hypoxia, but the exact timing (prenatally, during birth, or shortly afterward) may still be unclear.

Table 14.3
CEREBRAL PALSY: ASSOCIATED DISORDERS

Orthopedic deformities
- Muscle and/or tendon contracture
- Bone deformities and/or misalignments
- Joint dislocation and/or degeneration
- Scoliosis
- Osteoporosis and fracture

Cognitive deficits
- Intellectual disability
- Learning disability

Poor growth and/or undernutrition

Sensory deficits
- Visual impairment
- Oculomotor disturbance
- Hearing loss
- Recurrent otitis

Oral-motor performance impairments
- Speech deficits (dysarthria)
- Feeding dysfunction (dysphagia)
- Drooling
- Aspiration

Gastroesophageal reflux

Bowel and bladder problems

Seizures

Cervical neuropathy

Behavioral and/or emotional disturbances
- Organic (e.g., attention-deficit/hyperactivity disorder)
- Acquired (e.g., low self-esteem, depression)

ASSOCIATED CONDITIONS

It is imperative that the child with cerebral palsy be recognized as being at very high risk for having associated deficits in neurological, cognitive, and perceptual abilities. The motor deficits are generally identified before delays in language or perceptual abilities are evident. Table 14.3 outlines the broad categories of the more common associated disorders, some of which are discussed in more detail below.

Orthopedic Deformities

Physical problems associated with cerebral palsy are deformities of the bones and contractures of the tendons and muscles, all of which result from the influence of excessively high or abnormally low muscle tone. Progressive contractures and at times joint dislocations (particularly the hips) are a major problem in spastic forms of cerebral palsy. Scoliosis is also fairly common and warrants careful attention to handling and positioning techniques in an effort to prevent development or progression of spine deformity. Children with cerebral palsy complain frequently of musculoskeletal discomfort and joint pain (Penner, Xie, Binepal, Switzer, & Fehlings, 2013).

Cognitive Deficits

The insult to the brain that causes cerebral palsy may also result in learning difficulties. Approximately 50% of children with cerebral palsy have varying degrees of intellectual disability. Special educators continue to play a primary role in their management, because these children should participate in educational programs appropriate to their level of cognitive functioning. Children with intellectual disability, despite the extent of their motor disability, should have as their goals the enhancement of self-help, social, and oral communication skills for living and, if possible, working in the environment that is least restrictive and most suitable to their capabilities. As these children approach their teenage years, they require vocational training through the school system and supported or sheltered work environments where they are allowed to practice their vocation while maintaining socialization as well as earning income to enhance self-esteem and assist in their financial support. They will often require planning for long-term supervision or guardianship.

Of the 50% of children with cerebral palsy who do not have intellectual disability, a significant but unknown portion have academic challenges due to borderline intelligence scores of 70–85 and/or uneven psychometric profiles indicative of specific learning disabilities, communication disorders, or both. Underlying perceptual and language disorders are common in this subgroup of children, and special teaching methods need to be part of their educational plan. Assistance from speech–language pathologists and occupational therapists should be employed to help with remediation planning and treatment. Because of the motor difficulties caused by cerebral palsy, experienced child psychologists must be available to differentiate abilities that are lacking because of physical limitations from those that are not present because of cognitive limitation. Physical limitations or other associated deficits that hinder cognitive testing may result in an underestimation of the child's intellectual potential. Experienced teachers know better than other professionals the need to allow extra time for the child with cerebral palsy to more fully comprehend and respond to the presented material, and they especially appreciate the great challenge of providing such accommodations in the busy classroom.

Sensory Deficits

Sensory loss is characteristic of almost every child with a myelomeningocele or a spinal cord injury but is uncommon among children with cerebral palsy. The exception is children with hemiplegia, among whom about 50% have cortical sensory impairments, not the complete loss of sensation seen in spinal cord dysfunction. Children with extrapyramidal cerebral palsy are suspected of having substantial oral and perioral sensory impairment, which promotes their tendency to drool. Some children with cerebral palsy seem to have oral sensory irritation (e.g., dysesthesia, tactile defensiveness) that further complicates feeding difficulties.

Strabismus (deviation of the eye) occurs in approximately 30%–35% of individuals with cerebral palsy, and there is a high incidence of refractory errors, which are twice as common in individuals having the spastic type than in those having the extrapyramidal type. Children with athetoid cerebral palsy are more prone to be farsighted, whereas children with spastic cerebral palsy can be either near- or farsighted. Visual field defects occur in approximately 25% of children with hemiplegia. In some children who use their eyes poorly, it is a great challenge to figure out whether visual acuity is the problem or whether visual *attention* is the issue. Again, classroom observations are invaluable.

Children with certain syndromes associated with cerebral palsy, who are born preterm, or who have prenatally or perinatally acquired infections are at high risk for hearing loss. In addition, many children with cerebral palsy, especially those related to genetic syndromes, have great difficulty with recurrent otitis and fluctuating conductive hearing losses. Audiological screening should be a routine practice for such children.

Oral-Motor Dysfunction

A continuum of problems related to involvement of the oral-motor and swallowing musculature exists in children with cerebral palsy (see Table 14.3). Mild articulation disorders are common; more severe dysarthria and dysphagia are usually associated with extrapyramidal or mixed types of cerebral palsy. There is often a history of poor suckle, difficulty with chewing and swallowing, or gastroesophageal reflux during infancy and the preschool years, the severity of which may preclude adequate nutrition or safe oral feeding. Oral sensory abnormalities, commonly manifested as oral aversion, can greatly aggravate feeding difficulties. Drooling is linked to poor swallowing and can be a major social problem, as well as distracting and even destructive in terms of classroom equipment and educational materials. Early referral to speech–language pathologists is important to establish a program of speech and language intervention, which can be carried out at home as well as in school.

Oral hygiene and dental care are challenges in children with cerebral palsy. Defective tooth enamel, malocclusion, dental caries, and especially periodontal disease are fairly common. Children with developmental disabilities are prone to facial and dental trauma as a result of accidental falls, seizures, or self-injurious and self-stimulatory behaviors such as biting and teeth grinding. Acid reflux from the stomach causes dental erosions. Good professional dental care for children with severe disabilities is often extremely difficult for families to access.

Seizures

Whereas seizure disorders occur in about 0.2% of all children, they develop in approximately 25% of individuals with cerebral palsy. The frequency of seizures is much greater in individuals with the spastic subtype than in those with the extrapyramidal subtype and is particularly more common in children with hemiplegia. Seizure medications, while invaluable for the suppression of active seizures, may have side effects that interfere with learning. The astute teacher's observations of both seizures and any behavioral changes that might be related to drug side effects are invaluable in the balancing act of finding the best medication dose for each child. When a child has a known seizure disorder, it is critical for the classroom teacher to be aware of the type, frequency, and duration of that child's spells so as to manage seizure events properly if needed, and to recognize when events deviate from their usual pattern.

Emotional and Behavioral Problems

Various behavioral problems are demonstrated by children with cerebral palsy. One subset consists of organically driven hyperactivity, emotional lability, attention deficits, perseveration, low frustration tolerance, impulsivity, and distractibility. These organic behavioral patterns may be observed in children with (or without) cerebral palsy who have normal global intelligence. The behavioral problems may have as significant an impact on the child's family or school environment as do the child's physical limitations. Aggressive environmental modifications, behavioral programming, and medication management may be of great benefit in ameliorating these issues.

Another set of behaviors are grounded more in learned responses to situations or people (e.g., refusals and opposition, temper tantrums, helplessness, etc.). Behavioral psychologists can provide considerable assistance by helping caretakers and others devise consistent management plans to modify or eliminate these undesirable behaviors and thus facilitate school performance and peace in the home. Because educators develop over time a working knowledge of the children's primary diagnoses and associated deficits, they can actively participate in the counseling rendered to these families and children.

During adolescence, some individuals with cerebral palsy occasionally lose capabilities in self-help as well as communicative, ambulatory, or social skills. Parents, teachers, and physicians should be concerned as to whether this apparent deterioration is of physical or psychogenic origin. During adolescence there may be a progression of orthopedic deformity or a spurt in bone growth that, when accompanied by insufficient muscular development, may result in the loss of physical skills such as walking. Occasionally, children gain excessive weight, a critical factor in compromising physical performance. The child's mental attitude may change, resulting in pseudo-deterioration after he or she has exerted considerable energy and mental effort for years to learn and perform certain skills, and at adolescence begins to seriously question whether the effort was worth it. The exact role of hormones is as yet unknown, but they undoubtedly affect emotional responses at this time. During adolescence, a child with cerebral palsy may experience a greater sense of social isolation as peers begin to date and attend dances, parties, and other events from which the child feels excluded. Perhaps for the first time the child realizes the social effects of having a disability, which can lead to depression, manifested in social and communicative withdrawal, as well as a loss of interest in physical activities. The child with average or superior intelligence who has involuntary movements of all extremities is probably the most prone to developing psychological disturbances during adolescence, with depression being fairly common, although this aspect of cerebral palsy morbidity has been poorly studied.

Mental health counseling should include anticipatory guidance to provide awareness and possibly prevention of emotional problems that may surface during adolescence. Furthermore, some of these youngsters become aware, during childhood, of their physical incapacities and limitations and have developed a poor self-image that may have been compounded by parental overprotection and unwillingness to allow them to participate in many of the social and recreational activities of other children their age. Most children with cerebral palsy need continuous emotional encouragement and sometimes environmental modifications to promote peer interactions in school settings and through extracurricular activities. The hope is for these interactive experiences to generalize socially. The parents and siblings of these children play central roles in rendering emotional support to the family member with a disability, which can lead to a whole spectrum of emotional difficulties for the siblings (Lobato, 1990). It may be possible to eliminate or at least diminish the psychological stress that may confront an adolescent with cerebral palsy by early (i.e., beginning in preschool), periodic mental health counseling for the child and family.

MANAGEMENT

The treatment of cerebral palsy begins with its identification and initial assessment. Because cerebral palsy is not easily identified in the neonate or young infant, it is important for all clinicians to do careful developmental surveillance on children at high risk for cerebral palsy. Early neonatal difficulties such as seizures, hypotonia, history of difficult delivery, and preterm birth should raise suspicion and increase the intensity of surveillance. Many centers have been established to closely monitor children at risk, such as neurodevelopmental follow-up clinics for the evaluation of infants discharged from neonatal intensive care. Infants with very low birth weights are automatically eligible for Supplemental Security Income (SSI) benefits and for early intervention evaluation and treatment services in all states.

Treatment interventions can be organized into five broad categories: counseling, hands-on therapy, equipment, medications, and surgery (see Table 14.4). Parents first of all look for guidance and support from their child's physicians, therapists, and teachers, mainly in the form of collaborative (sometimes creative) problem solving rather than

Table 14.4
INTERVENTIONS FOR CHILDREN WITH CEREBRAL PALSY

Counseling

Hands-on therapy

- Physical therapy
- Occupational therapy
- Speech
- Recreational therapy and/or adapted physical education
- Special education

Equipment

- Orthotics
- Adaptive devices
- Electronics

Drugs

- Oral
- Intramuscular
- Intrathecal

Surgery

- Orthopedics
- Neurosurgery

Ophthalmology

- Otolaryngology

ultimate decision conferring. Counseling refers to this type of advice, not only for parents but also for the children themselves and sometimes for siblings. Physicians should have a well-thought-out approach to "breaking the bad news" counseling. Kaminer and Cohen (1988) have offered guidelines for difficult counseling sessions, translating the information and knowledge base into language and concepts that are understandable to parents and that take into account educational, cultural, and ethnic characteristics of the family. The foundation for good communication skills is sensitivity, patience, and—especially—good listening skills.

Parents frequently ask for literature to clarify a new diagnosis. Such educational material is a desirable and useful adjunct to direct verbal counseling. Because much written literature, as well as information available on the Internet, is inaccurate, misleading, or otherwise unacceptable (Blasco, Baumgartner, & Mathes, 1983), professionals need to be familiar with the literature generally available and to be prepared to recommend the best resources to families. Among our favorites are *Exceptional Parent* magazine and *Children With Cerebral Palsy: A Parent's Guide* by Geralis (1998).

Physicians and other health-care professionals can greatly assist parents to effectively and efficiently meet their children's needs and to address the needs of the *entire* family. A popular term (and important concept) is *empowerment,* that is, providing parents the encouragement and, where needed, skills to become more effective case managers and advocates. Parents are unable to do this unless they have extensive information regarding the medical, developmental, and psychoeducational interventions their children should be receiving. They are being taught to ask more questions, seek literature, attend professional conferences, and join parent support groups so they can learn as much as possible about disabilities and their management.

The management team for children with cerebral palsy includes a variety of professionals. Physical therapists concentrate on the child's posture and locomotor skills, with particular emphasis on ambulation. They direct and monitor exercise programs to promote strength and endurance and to prevent contractures. They work in conjunction with the orthopedist to determine which orthotic supports are best suited to help the child ambulate. Orthotics may be needed for stability, prevention of deformity, or reduction of extraneous movements. Orthotics, canes, walkers, and wheelchairs are often used for mobility assistance.

Occupational therapists focus on posture and upper extremity control as a prelude to enhancement of self-help skills and activities of daily living. They focus on such self-help abilities as eating, dressing, and toileting. Children with cerebral palsy of the extrapyramidal type commonly have difficulties with oral-motor control and the swallowing mechanism. Occupational therapists, in conjunction with speech and physical therapists, develop seating and positioning systems to reduce tongue thrust and enhance the ability to swallow, to accommodate adaptive equipment that provides the child with greater independence in activities of daily living and in accessing electronic interfaces, and to facilitate mobility.

Speech–language pathologists and assistive technology personnel are important to the child's management team, especially as attention to communication abilities is added to concerns about motor ability. Communication depends not only on oral-motor skills but also on use of the upper extremities. The most efficient and preferred means of communication is verbal; however, children with significant oral-motor dysfunction may be frustrated by unsuccessful efforts to improve their articulation and speech intelligibility. These children may benefit greatly from augmentative means of communication, such as communication boards and electronic devices.

Recreational therapists and adaptive physical educators often get left out in therapy considerations, yet they have a tremendous amount to offer the child with cerebral palsy. Recreational activities, such as hydrotherapy, swimming, and therapeutic horseback riding, not only offer therapy but also boost self-esteem.

The physician managing the child with cerebral palsy may consider the use of medications to reduce muscle tone or involuntary movements. A long list of drugs has been anecdotally reported to be beneficial. For example, diazepam (Valium), trihexyphenidyl (Artane), and baclofen (Lioresal) are helpful in reducing some of the spasticity of pyramidal cerebral palsy or the dystonia of extrapyramidal cerebral palsy. In truth, the majority of children do not benefit substantially from medication. No good data are available, but probably 10% or less of all children with cerebral palsy genuinely benefit from long-term use of oral medications. In the short term, postoperative use of muscle relaxant medications can be extremely helpful following orthopedic surgery. The side effects of medications should not be underestimated because sedation, lethargy, and depression may result, therefore compromising a child's mental capabilities. The local injection of botulinum toxin into specific muscle groups decreases spasticity but also weakens muscles. An implantable pump device has been developed to infuse baclofen into the spinal cord (intrathecal baclofen) and greatly diminish spasticity with very low medication doses.

Surgical interventions employed by orthopedists consist most commonly of tendon release or lengthening and bone reconstruction procedures. The intent is to improve function and prevent deformity. On occasion, cosmesis is a factor, but rarely is it the primary indication for orthopedic surgery. Neurosurgeons have also developed techniques, such as selective posterior rhizotomy of the spinal nerve roots, to eliminate spasticity and thereby enhance ambulation in the child with spastic diplegia. In rare instances, stereotactic brain surgery targeting the basal ganglia has been used to inhibit severe movement disorders. The neurosurgeon is also involved if the child requires a shunt for the treatment of hydrocephalus. Because of the high prevalence of eye problems and hearing deficits, surgeons in ophthalmology and otolaryngology are often involved in the care of children with cerebral palsy at irregular intervals, mostly early in the child's life.

Thus, the management of the child with cerebral palsy requires the skills and coordinated collaboration of physical and occupational therapists, the recreational therapist or adaptive physical educator, speech–language pathologists, nurses, psychologists, social workers, the orthopedist, the neurosurgeon and other subspecialty surgeons, dentists, the orthotist, sometimes the nutritionist, general pediatricians or family physicians, and neurodevelopmental pediatricians or similar medical subspecialists. The coordination of these professionals, as well as educational and community social and mental health services, is always an enormous challenge.

PROGNOSIS AND OUTCOME

Most individuals with cerebral palsy are able to live in the community independently or in a somewhat protected environment and to work on their own or in supported situations. A smaller subgroup needs total care throughout life. In Sweden, among adults with cerebral palsy but not intellectual disability, 75% either lived on their own or with a partner, 54% felt they were not limited in their ability to get around in the community, and 24% reported working full-time (Andersson & Mattsson, 2001). With aging, some adults have a hard time with progressive foot deformities and joint pain from osteoarthritis. These changes conspire to cause a deterioration in walking, leading to falls and additional injuries (Opheim, Jahnsen, Olsson, & Stanghelle, 2009).

The life span of individuals with cerebral palsy is somewhat diminished, but the great majority live well into adulthood. The degree of life shortening is related directly to the severity of motor involvement plus the number and severity of associated deficits. The most profoundly affected individuals have greatly reduced life expectancies and often are predicted to die before or by adolescence. This is an extremely small group, and prediction is unreliable for individual cases because it is based on chance of survival in a population of similar individuals.

THE TEACHER'S ROLE: SUPPORTING CHILDREN WITH CP IN THE CLASSROOM

In years past, many children and adults with cerebral palsy lived out their lives secluded at home or in large institutions. This sense of exclusion was depicted in the biographical movie *My Left Foot* (1989), the life story of the intellectually gifted Christy Brown who, despite severe cerebral palsy, learned to paint and write using his only controllable limb, his left foot (see Brown, 1970).

Today, society embraces inclusion into all aspects of community living in large part as a result of changes in public laws, including the Americans With Disabilities Act (ADA, 1990, http://www.ada.gov). The ADA is an equal-opportunity law for persons with disabilities. In addition, IDEA, the Individuals With Disabilities Education Act, has its roots in the original law—Public Law No. 94-142, the Education for All Handicapped Children Act—passed in 1975. IDEA requires a free, appropriate education in the least restrictive environment. In other words, children should be educated with their peers to the greatest extent possible. States must follow the guidelines of IDEA under Part B of the law (children ages 3 to 21) and Part C (infants and toddlers ages birth to 2) (http://idea.ed.gov).

Inclusion of all children in early learning and education is the goal of both the Division for Early Childhood (DEC) of the Council for Exceptional Children and the National Association for the Education of Young Children (NAEYC). In a joint position statement, these agencies endorse inclusion in the following way:

> Early childhood inclusion embodies the values, policies, and practices that support the right of every infant and young child and his or her family, regardless of ability, to participate in a broad range of activities and contexts as full members of families, communities, and society. The desired results of inclusive experiences for children with and without disabilities and their families include a sense of belonging and membership, positive social relationships and friendships, and development and learning to reach their full potential. (DEC/NAEYC, 2009, p. 2)

This statement defines three important concepts to ensure that all children receive the best possible outcomes for learning and education:

1. *Access* is interpreted as providing a variety of activities as well as settings (learning environments, home, community) for every child by not only removing physical barriers but also promoting strategies to ensure that children with disabilities have the opportunity to learn with their peers. An example of removing physical barriers would be installing a ramp at a child-care preschool for wheelchair access. An example of access to learning opportunities would be adaptive equipment and assistive technology, which are great equalizers for children with cerebral palsy. Children can use communication devices to socially interact with their peers and engage in learning experiences within the classroom.

2. *Participation* means using a range of instructional approaches to facilitate active engagement in all learning activities and thereby promote a sense of belonging for the child. An example of participation follows:

   Joey has cerebral palsy and uses a wheelchair and a stander in his preschool classroom. Today the children are preparing milkshakes, using this fun activity to teach multiple concepts such as measuring ingredients, discussing nutritional value, and encouraging social turn-taking. The blender is hooked up to an assistive device that will allow Joey to operate it using his joystick. The children all participate in naming and measuring the ingredients. Once all the ingredients are in the blender, the children ask Joey to press the "on" button, activating the blender. Everyone cheers!

3. *Supports* refers to systematic implementation of inclusion strategies such as professional development and opportunities for collaboration among families and professionals to assure high quality inclusion. All professionals and administrators need to "buy in" to inclusion and have a shared understanding of what it means. Without access, participation, and supports, children will not be fully included and their educational goals will not be met.

THE ROLE OF FAMILY IN SUPPORTING LEARNING OUTCOMES

Special educators, therapists, and other professionals are transient in the child's life while families provide ongoing influence (Basu, 2007). Early intervention recognizes the important role of the family through the Individual Family Service Plan (IFSP), which is tailored to meet the unique interests, priorities, resources, and concerns of the family. It is used to develop, implement, and evaluate appropriate early intervention in natural settings, including the home. Through the IFSP process, family members, early childhood personnel, service coordinators, and early interventionists, including related therapy services (physical and occupational and speech), work together as a team. The teamwork develops goals and objectives that are functional, meaningful, and age-appropriate for the child in the least restrictive environment. Goals and objectives are based on the student's present level of performance. The IFSP is guided by the language in Part C of IDEA. By focusing on the child's interests and strengths and the family's priorities, the team identifies outcomes to impact the child's learning and development. The IFSP is reviewed annually; however, ongoing assessment ensures that children's needs will be met during the year by adjusting activities as goals are either met or need to be reevaluated.

All children identified through state-required assessment procedures have an IFSP or, if they are over 3 years of age, an Individualized Education Program (IEP). Family members are included in all decision-making aspects of the IEP/IFSP development process. They have the right to due-process proceedings if they disagree with the rest of the team on placement or educational decisions. Parent advocacy groups such as Parent Advocacy Coalition for Education Rights (PACER; http://www.pacer.org) are available to help parents locate resources and services. Family members often find additional information on the Internet or through social media that can be incorporated into plans when appropriate. Family-to-family support through social media helps family members feel validated in their own experiences with their child as well as establishing a sense of companionship with other families.

The provision of services from birth provides a safety net for children diagnosed early with cerebral palsy. Many of these children and families are referred for services as they leave the hospital. With early intervention, children with cerebral palsy receive the supports they need to develop to their fullest potential. These supports are best delivered using a coordinated, interagency team-based approach. Teams are most effective when they work in partnership with parents to ensure the very best services for the child with cerebral palsy (Turnbull, Turnbull, & Wehmeyer, 2010). Children with cerebral palsy have a wide range of intellectual abilities, and the team must consider cognitive and other associated impairments that may affect the child's learning when determining services and placement. Early recognition of learning strengths and needs by the team will enhance learning outcomes. The IEP should include objectives for teaching academic, adaptive, and social skills, in addition to recommendations for the use of adaptive equipment and assistive technology in the classroom.

The special educator, in collaboration with occupational, physical, and speech–language therapists and with the family, should address both the strengths and needs of the child to determine functional goals as well as techniques that will increase classroom participation and mobility. Special educators and classroom aides should know how to remove and apply orthoses, position children in various mobility or positioning devices, and help operate augmentative communication systems. Special educators also assist with activities during daily routines that are essential for the child to be successful in the home and in the community. They are the logical advocates with school authorities to provide modifications within the classroom and the school to accommodate the child with special needs. For the child who is taking medication, the special educator plays a vital role in informing parents and physicians whether or not there are positive or negative effects of the medication observed in the classroom setting.

Special educators and therapists work closely with general education teachers, classroom staff, and parents so children develop the necessary skills to be effective learners across all environments in the school and in the community. Collaborative consultation means that educational and therapy specialists coach other school personnel on carrying out goals and objectives developed by the IEP team (Dinnebeil & McInerney, 2011; Knackendoffel & Thurston, 2009).

Inclusion of children with cerebral palsy can be facilitated with the use of assistive technology. When physical limitations prohibit participation, adaptive devices become a powerful equalizer, providing the means for a child to accomplish classroom assignments and to communicate with peers. Careful assessment of the learner (including, for example, positioning, physical ability, visual ability), the environments, and the tasks expected of the child within each environment will provide a firm basis for selecting assistive technology devices to use. Technology changes rapidly, and it is the responsibility of the team to monitor and evaluate the technology used by the child (Mihaylov, Jarvis, Colver, & Beresford, 2004; Østensjø, Carlberg, & Vøllestad, 2005). It is very important to consider family factors when making education and technology plans for children with disabilities (Raina et al., 2005). Caregivers carry out therapeutic and education strategies at home and in the community. Taking into account how the family copes with these responsibilities cannot be understated.

Special educators are encouraged to join organizations that help determine and advocate for recommended practices in the field of special education. The Council for Exceptional Children (CEC) is the largest international professional organization in support of children with disabilities and their families. CEC provides not only guidelines on professional practices but also advocacy and ethical standards for professionals working with children. DEC is a division of CEC that provides recommended practices and leadership in early intervention and early childhood special education.

ADDITIONAL RESOURCES

Exceptional Parent magazine

http://www.eparent.com

United Cerebral Palsy (UCP)

A parent support organization committed to progress for persons with disabilities to ensure the inclusion of persons with disabilities in every facet of society. UCP's mission is to advance the independence, productivity, and full citizenship of people with cerebral palsy and other disabilities, through the principles of independence, inclusion, and self-determination.

United States site (with links to state sites)

http://ucp.org

Canada (each province has its own site): see, e.g., CP Association of Manitoba

http://www.cerebralpalsy.mb.ca

American Academy for Cerebral Palsy and Developmental Medicine (AACPDM)

A multidisciplinary professional society devoted to the study of cerebral palsy and other childhood onset disabilities. The site includes libraries, news, research, conferences, and membership opportunities.
http://www.aacpdm.org

Early Childhood Technical Assistance Center (ECTA Center)

A national technical assistance consortium working to support states, jurisdictions, and others to improve services and outcomes for young children with disabilities and their families.
http://ectacenter.org

AbleData

A national database covering information on assistive technology and rehabilitation equipment. The database contains detailed information on more than 27,000 assistive technology products, noncommercial prototypes, customized and one-of-a-kind products, do-it-yourself designs, assistive technology fact sheets, and consumer guides.
http://www.abledata.com

Assistive Technology and Augmentative Communication

Provides handouts describing the general philosophical basis for using augmentative communication and assistive technology with young children, directions for adapting existing products, books, selected vendors, and Internet resources.
http://www.lburkhart.com

CP Mini-Module

A training module developed for early childhood educators working in inclusive settings with young children who have cerebral palsy. The module provides definitions and information to enable professionals to work successfully with young children with CP. (Blasco, 2012, *Mini-module on cerebral palsy*. Oregon Early Childhood Inclusion Collaborative. Monmouth, OR: Western Oregon University, Teaching Research Institute.)
http://www.centeroninclusion.org/CP_Module

REFERENCES

Allen, M. C. (2008). Neurodevelopmental outcomes of preterm infants. *Current Opinions in Neurology, 21*, 123–128.

Allen, M. C., Cristofalo, E. A., & Kim, C. (2011). Outcomes of preterm infants: Morbidity replaces mortality. *Clinical Perinatology, 38*, 441–454.

Americans With Disabilities Act of 1990, 42 U.S.C. § 12101 et seq.

Andersson, C., & Mattsson, E. (2001). Adults with cerebral palsy: A survey describing problems, needs, and resources, with special emphasis on locomotion. *Developmental Medicine and Child Neurology, 43*, 76–82.

Basu, S. (2007). *Assessing collaboration between therapists and caregivers during early intervention service delivery.* Ann Arbor, MI: ProQuest.

Bax, M. C. O. (1964). Terminology and classification of cerebral palsy. *Developmental Medicine and Child Neurology, 6*, 295–297.

Blasco, P. A. (1992). Normal and abnormal motor development. *Pediatric Rounds, 1*(2), 1–6.

Blasco, P. A., Baumgartner, M. C., & Mathes, B. C. (1983). Literature for parents of children with cerebral palsy. *Developmental Medicine and Child Neurology, 25*, 642–647.

Brown, C. (1970). *Down all the days.* New York, NY: Stein and Day.

Cans, C. (2000). Surveillance of cerebral palsy in Europe: A collaboration of cerebral palsy registers. *Developmental Medicine and Child Neurology, 42*, 816–824.

DEC/NAEYC. (2009). *Early childhood inclusion: A joint position statement of the Division for Early Childhood (DEC) and the National Association for the Education of Young Children (NAEYC).* Chapel Hill, NC: University of North Carolina, FPG Child Development Institute.

Denhoff, E., & Robinault, I. P. (1960). *Cerebral palsy and related disorders.* New York, NY: McGraw-Hill.

Dinnebeil, L., & McInerney, B. (2011). *A guide to itinerant early childhood special education services.* Baltimore, MD: Brookes.

Education for All Handicapped Children Act of 1975, 20 U.S.C. § 1400 et seq.

Fleiss, B., & Gressens, P. (2012). Tertiary mechanisms of brain damage: A new hope for treatment of cerebral palsy? *Lancet Neurology, 11*, 556–566.

Freud, S. (1968). *Infantile cerebral paralysis* (Trans. L. A. Russin). Coral Gables, FL: University of Miami Press. (Originally published 1897)

Geralis, E. (Ed.) (1998). *Children with cerebral palsy: A parent's guide* (2nd ed.). Rockville, MD: Woodbine House.

Individuals With Disabilities Education Act of 1990, 20 U.S.C. § 1400 et seq.

Kaminer, R. K., & Cohen, H. J. (1988). How do you say, "Your child is retarded"? *Contemporary Pediatrics, 5*, 36–49.

Knackendoffel, A., & Thurston, L. P. (2009). *Collaboration, consultation, and teamwork for students with special needs.* Upper Saddle River, NJ: Pearson/Merrill.

Little, W. J. (1853). *On the nature and treatment of the deformities of the human frame: Being a course of lectures delivered at the Royal Orthopedic Hospital in 1843 with numerous notes and additions.* London, UK: Longman, Brown, Greene, and Longmans.

Lobato, D. J. (1990). *Brothers, sisters, and special needs: Information and activities for helping young siblings of children with chronic illnesses and developmental disorders.* Baltimore, MD: Brookes.

Lock, T. H. M., Shapiro, B. K., Ross, A., & Capute, A. J. (1986). Age of presentation of developmental disabilities. *Journal of Developmental and Behavioral Pediatrics, 7*, 340–345.

McIntyre, S., Taitz, D., Keogh J., Goldsmith, S., Badawi, N., & Blair, E. (2013). A systematic review of risk factors for cerebral palsy in children born at term in developed countries. *Developmental Medicine and Child Neurology, 55*, 499–508.

Mihaylov, S. I., Jarvis, S. N., Colver, A. F., & Beresford, B. (2004). Identification and description of environmental factors that influence participation of children with cerebral palsy. *Developmental Medicine and Child Neurology, 46*, 299–304.

Nolan, C. (1987). *Under the eye of the clock.* New York, NY: St. Martin's Press.

Opheim, A., Jahnsen, R., Olsson, E., & Stanghelle, J. K. (2009). Walking function, pain, and fatigue in adults with cerebral palsy: A 7-year follow-up study. *Developmental Medicine and Child Neurology, 51*, 381–388.

Østensjø, S., Carlberg, E. B., & Vøllestad, N. K. (2005). The use and impact of assistive devices and other environmental modifications on everyday activities and care in young children with cerebral palsy. *Disability Rehabilitation, 27*, 849–861.

Palisano, R., Rosenbaum, P., Walters, S., Russell, D., Wood, E., & Galuppi, B. (1997). Development and reliability of a system to classify gross motor function in children with cerebral palsy. *Developmental Medicine and Child Neurology, 39*, 214–223.

Panteliadis, C., Panteliadis, P., & Vassilyadi, F. (2013). Hallmarks in the history of cerebral palsy: From antiquity to mid-20th century. *Brain and Development, 35*, 285–292.

Penner, M., Xie, W. Y., Binepal, N., Switzer, L., & Fehlings, D. (2013). Characteristics of pain in children and youth with cerebral palsy. *Pediatrics, 132*, e407–e413.

Raina, P., O'Donnell, M., Rosenbaum, P., Brehaut, J., Walter, S. D., Russell, D., & Wood, E. (2005). The health and well-being of caregivers of children with cerebral palsy. *Pediatrics, 115*(6), e626–e636.

Rand, L., Eddleman, K. A., & Stone, J. (2005). Long-term outcomes in multiple gestations. *Clinical Perinatology, 32*, 495–513.

Tizard, J. P., Paine, R. S., & Crothers, B. (1954). Disturbances of sensation in children with hemiplegia. *JAMA, 155*, 628–632.

Turnbull, A., Turnbull, R., & Wehmeyer, M. L. (2010). *Exceptional lives: Special education in today's schools* (6th ed.). Upper Saddle River, NJ: Merrill.

Zwicker, J. G., Missiuna, C., Harris, S. R., & Boyd, L. A. (2012). Developmental coordination disorder: View and update. *European Journal of Paediatric Neurology, 16*, 573–581.

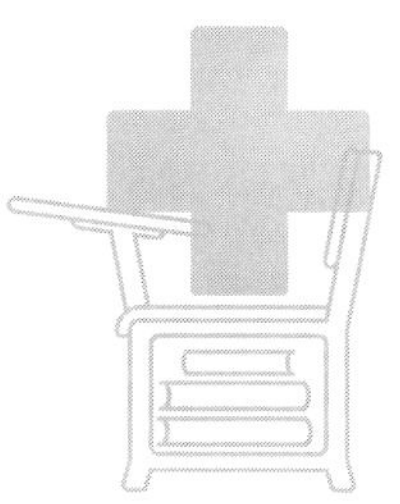

Chapter 15
Teacher Awareness of Drug and Substance Abuse

Constance Mackenzie, Jesse Godwin,
and Margaret Thompson

Substance abuse is a major problem, with the prevalence of illicit drug use increasing globally. A number of different government and social service agencies conduct regular surveys of drug use in selected populations. The National Survey on Drug Use and Health (Substance Abuse and Mental Health Services Administration, 2013) reported that, in 2012, 9.2% of the population admitted to illicit drug use in the previous 30 days, representing approximately 23.9 million Americans. This has increased from the 2002 rate of 8.3% of the population. Similarly, the *World Drug Report 2013* (UN Office on Drugs and Crime, 2013) estimated illicit drug use at 5.2% of the worldwide population. For further resources on the scope of the drug problem in youth, see Table 15.1.

A pattern of illicit drug use is usually established during youth, in parallel with tobacco use and alcohol drinking, and tends to be carried on into adulthood. In children and adolescents, the use of illicit substances is often associated with educational underachievement, school dropout, serious medical consequences, and various criminal or self-inflicting activities. Also, increased mortality and morbidity (risk of a disease) continue to pose major problems, not only for users themselves in later life but also for the society to which they belong. Because substance abuse behavior often begins in the preteen or teen years, understanding of and education about this problem in the school setting is particularly crucial.

For educators, the first step in the prevention of and intervention in this hazardous behavior is to acknowledge its existence and

Table 15.1

STATISTICS ON SUBSTANCE ABUSE

National Institute on Drugs of Abuse (http://www.nida.nih.gov/Infofax/HSYouthtrends.html) "DrugFacts: High School and Youth Trends": Contains articles on U.S.-specific drug trends
Canadian Centre on Substance Abuse (http://www.ccsa.ca/Eng/Pages/default.aspx) Links to Canadian reports on the costs of drug abuse, and drug abuse patterns, on a regional and Canada-wide basis
Centre for Addiction and Mental Health Ontario Student Drug Use and Health Survey 2013 (http://www.camh.ca/en/research/news_and_publications/ontario-student-drug-use-and-health-survey/Documents/2013%20OSDUHS%20Docs/2013OSDUHS_Detailed_DrugUseReport.pdf) "Drug Use Among Ontario Students": Contains Ontario-specific statistics on drug use trends

to address the problem in an honest and knowledgeable fashion. Although there are many different approaches, which are sometimes mutually exclusive (e.g., for and against legalizing marijuana use), nobody can argue against the importance of knowing facts. This chapter is designed to provide educators with basic information on this complicated issue. Historical aspects of substance abuse, recent statistics, and medical issues are discussed. An attempt was made to avoid the use of technical terms, but those that are included are fully explained. Drug and chemical names, as well as commonly used street names, are given in the text. Table 15.2 provides websites listing street drug names. We searched all web addresses listed and found them to be reliable and current sites. Street terms may also be regional; not finding a term on one site may reflect that it is not used in a particular region of the world. Several sites may need to be searched.

DEFINITIONS

The term *substance abuse* is defined as the self-administration of any substance in a way that oversteps the social norms of a culture. This definition implies that there are medical, social, and cultural con-

Table 15.2
GLOSSARIES OF STREET DRUG NAMES

Center for Substance Abuse Research (http://www.cesar.umd.edu/cesar/drug_info.asp) "Drug Information": Searchable site for common street names of drugs of abuse
Erowid drug slang pages (http://www.erowid.org/psychoactives/slang/slang.shtml) "Drug Slang & Terminology Vault": Alphabetically organized dictionary of terms for street drugs
No Slang (http://www.noslang.com/drugs/dictionary.php) "Drug Slang Dictionary": Searchable dictionary of drug slang

texts to the substance abuse problem. For instance, once a substance is legalized or well accepted, modest use of it may no longer be seen as abuse by society. In contrast, use of currently legal substances may be regarded as abuse in the future. Some children who start substance abuse or use of potentially addictive legal substances develop physical and/or psychological dependence on the substance.

Although addiction and drug dependence are often used interchangeably, there are distinctions between these terms. *Addiction* implies psychological dependence on the substance, characterized by poor control over drug use, compulsive drug use, cravings for the drug, and continued use of the drug despite physical, mental, and social harm (American Psychiatric Association, APA, 2013). *Dependence* refers to the normal body response or adaptation to a drug. It is characterized by the features of tolerance and withdrawal. *Tolerance* is defined as either a need for markedly increased amounts of the substance to achieve intoxication or desired effect, or markedly diminished effect with continued use of the same amount of the substance. When tolerance to the effects of a substance develops, the user needs more and more of the substance to acquire the effects previously experienced. By using more, substance abusers are at a higher risk for the toxic, often fatal effects of the substance. *Withdrawal* manifests as a characteristic withdrawal syndrome for the substance (substance dependent), or the same (or a closely related) substance is taken to relieve or avoid withdrawal symptoms (APA, 2013). Sudden discontinuation of drugs after frequent exposure for a sufficiently long period often causes a withdrawal syndrome or abstinence symptoms, which are disturbing and sometimes life threatening, especially in the cases of alcohol and sedatives or hypnotics.

The medical community uses clearly defined criteria to make the diagnosis of substance-related disorders, including use disorders, intoxication, and withdrawal for 10 separate classes of drugs: tobacco, alcohol, caffeine, cannabis, hallucinogens, inhalants, opioids, sedatives, hypnotics and anxiolytics, and stimulants, and other (or unknown) substances (APA, 2013). Although the specific criteria vary slightly between substance classes, the general criteria are similar. The diagnosis of a substance-related disorder requires at least two of the following criteria over a 12-month period (APA, 2013):

1. The substance is taken in larger amounts or over a longer period than was intended.
2. There is a persistent desire or unsuccessful efforts to cut down on or control the substance use.
3. A great deal of time is spent in activities necessary to obtain the substance (e.g., visiting multiple doctors or driving long distances), use the substance (e.g., chain-smoking), or recover from its effects.
4. Craving, or a strong desire or urge to use the substance.
5. Recurrent use of the substance resulting in a failure to fulfill major obligations at school, home, or work.
6. Continued use of the substance despite having persistent or recurrent social or interpersonal problems caused or exacerbated by the effects of its use.
7. Important social, occupational, or recreational activities are given up or reduced because of use of the substance.
8. Recurrent use of the substance in situations in which it is physically hazardous.
9. Use of the substance is continued despite knowledge of having a persistent or recurrent physical or psychological problem that is likely to have been caused or exacerbated by the substance (e.g., current cocaine use despite recognition of cocaine-induced depression, or continued drinking despite recognition that an ulcer was made worse by alcohol consumption).
10. Tolerance, as defined earlier.
11. Withdrawal, as defined earlier.

EVOLVEMENT OF SUBSTANCE ABUSE IN AN INDIVIDUAL

Adolescents and young adults commonly experiment with mood-altering substances, including nicotine, alcohol, and drugs. However, the American Academy of Pediatrics emphasizes that experimentation should not be trivialized, facilitated, or condoned by adults including parents, teachers, and health-care providers. Drug and alcohol use are a leading cause of morbidity and mortality in the United States, and even first-time use can potentially result in injury or death (American Academy of Pediatrics, 2011). Experimentation is the most common initial motive for using illicit substances or drugs for nonmedicinal purposes. This is especially true in adolescents, who often lack the ability to exercise mature judgment and whose peer circle tends to have its own internal standards. Experts in substance abuse recognize that very few abusers correctly predicted that their substance-abusing behavior would result from experimentation. Experimenters believe that they will be in full control of using illicit drugs and that they will be able to stop using them anytime they want to. Unfortunately, some eventually become drug abusers, despite initial confidence in their behavioral immunity against addiction. Adolescence is a critical period of neurodevelopment, which makes this age group vulnerable to developing addictions (Chambers, Taylor, & Potenza, 2003).

In general, children and adolescents who progress to drug addiction experiment with such substances as alcohol and tobacco, which are legal for adults, before initiating use of illicit substances. Among illicit drugs, use of marijuana usually precedes that of cocaine and other substances. Although alcohol, tobacco, and marijuana are typically viewed as "gateway" substances, there is some variability in the order of drug initiation between countries and contexts that reflects local background prevalence of drug use (Degenhardt et al., 2010). In the United States in 2012, approximately 2.9 million persons aged 12 or older used an illicit drug for the first time in the previous 12 months. More than half of these first-time users were younger than 18 (55.1%). The majority reported that their first drug was marijuana (65.6%), 26% initiated with nonmedical use of psychotherapeutics (including 17.0% with pain relievers, 4.1% with tranquilizers, 3.6% with stimulants, and 1.3% with sedatives), 6.3% reported inhalants as their first illicit drug, and 2% used hallucinogens (including LSD, ecstasy, PCP). Cocaine and heroin account for only a small percentage of first-time drug users (0.1% each) (Substance Abuse and Mental Health Services Administration, 2013). In a similar 2013 survey of students in Ontario, Canada, the majority of new substance users (including tobacco, alcohol, and drugs) were in Grades 9, 10, or 11 (Boak, Hamilton, Adlaf, & Mann, 2013).

The age of onset for cigarette smoking and alcohol drinking is also a predictor for subsequent involvement with other abused substances (Kandel & Yamaguchi, 1993). In the study by Kandel and Yamaguchi, adolescents using cocaine reportedly began smoking tobacco, drinking alcohol, or both two years earlier than those who did not progress to using cocaine (mean age 11 years vs. 13 years). Similarly, cocaine-using adolescents on average began using marijuana two years earlier (13 years of age) than those who did not go on to use cocaine (15 years of age). Although this earlier initiation of the behavior may not be a *cause* of subsequent use of more toxic substances, this is certainly an important marker for identifying children at greater risk of advanced substance abuse. Other studies have shown that the risk of developing drug dependence appears to be related to the extent of prior use of *any* drug (not just tobacco, alcohol, and marijuana), early age of first drug use, and mental health problems. This suggests that all types of drug use should be targeted for prevention efforts instead of particular "gateway drugs" (Degenhardt et al., 2010).

RISK FACTORS

Much of the current knowledge about substance abuse has come from studies using animal models. Experimental animals *self-administer* substances of abuse in a similar way to that of humans who abuse drugs. In humans, prevention of initial experimentation and subsequent development of addiction may be the result of many counteracting factors, including social disapproval, family norms against their use, and knowledge about the grave consequences of substance abuse. However, certain family and peer environments may provide children with an atmosphere convenient for experimenting with substances of abuse. Friends, rather than strangers, almost always entice adolescents into substance abuse; hence, family and peer environments that fail to denounce substance abuse undoubtedly are strong risk factors for children.

A number of risk factors for substance use and mental health problems in youth have been identified, including having family members with mental health disorders, concurrent developmental disabilities and chronic medical conditions, uncertainty around sexual identity, and adolescents (particularly girls) in the juvenile justice system. Environmental factors such as stress and psychological trauma (including abuse, neglect, or violence) can contribute to the risk. Conversely, family stability, strong and supportive relationships, communities, and faith organizations can have a protective effect (Substance Abuse and Mental Health Services Administration, 2011).

It is widely accepted that a vulnerability to alcoholism is partly inherited (Cloninger, Dinwiddie, & Reich, 1989), although environmental factors also play an important role, and the mode of inheritance seems extremely complex (Holden, 1991). Genetic predisposition to other substances of abuse is less clear, but there seem to be susceptible personalities, such as those who display rebelliousness, risk taking, low self-esteem, aggressiveness, and other antisocial characteristics, who are predisposed to drug addiction. Overall rates of substance abuse seem to differ among different ethnic groups; however, when social and environmental conditions are controlled, there are no genetic differences in rates of abuse in different races (Lillie-Blanton, Anthony, & Schuster, 1993).

RECOGNITION OF SUBSTANCE USE

Educators are in a unique position to recognize physical and behavioral indicators of substance abuse in students. Substance abuse is associated with both mental and physical health problems, which makes early recognition and intervention important. Despite an estimated 6.1 million youths aged 12–17 needing treatment for an illicit drug use problem in 2001, only 1.1 million received treatment, which suggests that there is a huge gap between the number of youths who need and who actually receive treatment (Substance Abuse and Mental Health Services Administration, 2011).

A number of screening tools have been developed for healthcare professionals to help identify alcohol and substance use. The CRAFFT test (Figure 15.1.) is a validated, brief screening tool specifically developed to identify alcohol and drug problems among adolescent medical patients (younger than age 21). This test has been successfully used in school settings to assess problem drug and alcohol use in students. When administered anonymously, it can be a quick and inexpensive tool to assess the prevalence of problem drug and alcohol use within a school district (Falck, Nahhas, Li, & Carlson, 2012). CRAFFT is a mnemonic acronym of the first letters of key words in the screening questions. Questions should be asked exactly as written or can be self-administered in paper format. Each yes answer is scored as 1 point, with a score of 2 or more indicating the need for further assessment (Knight, Sherritt, Shrier, Harris, & Chang, 2002). Further guidelines on the use of the CRAFFT test are outlined in an American Academy of Pediatrics (2011) Policy Statement on substance use. The U.S. Substance Abuse and Mental Health Services Administration has a guideline available for appropriate and effective identification of substance use problems in children and adolescents, including information about requesting consent prior to screening, other screening tools, and interventions (Substance Abuse and Mental Health Services Administration, 2011).

Poor school performance, truancy, and dropping out-of-school activities such as music and sports can be signs of alcohol or drug use. Other signs include changes in appearance or mood, hostile or aggressive outbursts, anxiety, hyperactivity, depression, sleepiness, lack of

The CRAFFT v.2.0 Screening Interview

Begin: "I'm going to ask you a few questions that I ask all my patients. Please be honest. I will keep your answers confidential."

Part A

During the PAST 12 MONTHS, did you:	**No**	**Yes**
1. Smoke any cigarettes or use any other tobacco product, including smokeless tobacco?	☐	☐
2. Drink any alcohol (more than a few sips)? (Do not count a few sips of alcohol taken during family or religious events)	☐	☐
3. Smoke any marijuana or hashish?	☐	☐
4. Use anything else to get high? (This includes other illegal drugs, prescription or non-prescription medicines or things that people sniff or inhale)	☐	☐

For clinic use only: Did the patient answer "yes" to any questions in Part A?

No ☐ → **Ask CAR question only, then stop**

Yes ☐ → **Ask all 6 CRAFFT questions**

Part B	**No**	**Yes**
1. Have you ever ridden in a **CAR** driven by someone (including yourself) who was "high" or had been using alcohol or drugs?	☐	☐
2. Do you ever use alcohol or drugs to **RELAX**, feel better about yourself, or fit in?	☐	☐
3. Do you ever use alcohol or drugs while you are by yourself, or **ALONE**?	☐	☐
4. Do you ever **FORGET** things you did while using alcohol or drugs?	☐	☐
5. Do your **FAMILY** or **FRIENDS** ever tell you that you should cut down on your drinking or drug use?	☐	☐
6. Have you ever gotten into **TROUBLE** while you were using alcohol or drugs?	☐	☐

SCORING INSTRUCTIONS (FOR CLINIC STAFF USE ONLY)
Each "yes" response in **Part B** scores 1 point.
A total score of 2 or higher is a positive screen, indicating a need for additional assessment.

Figure 15.1. CRAFFT Screening Interview. From "Validity of the CRAFFT Substance Abuse Screening Test Among Adolescent Clinic Patients," by J. R. Knight, L. Sherritt, L. A. Shrier, S. K. Harris, and G. Chang, 2002, *Archives of Pediatrics & Adolescent Medicine, 156*(6), 607–614. Copyright John R. Knight, MD, Boston Children's Hospital, 2014. All rights reserved. Reproduced with permission. For more information, contact ceasar@childrens.harvard.edu

motivation, or forgetfulness. Table 15.3 lists physical findings and behaviors associated with the use and withdrawal of different classes of substances of abuse that may be observed in the classroom. The section below on abused substances provides more in-depth information about the most common abused substances.

PREVENTION AND TREATMENT

There are many drug abuse prevention programs, some of which are incorporated in school systems. Students must be taught the consequences of experimentation and abuse of these substances, although this approach alone is not sufficient. A model program that appears to be successful in school settings provides opportunities for students to become familiar with external and internal pressures leading to substance abuse and to learn how to disregard the pro-drug arguments and pressures. If supported by other approaches aimed at parents and the community, this kind of program can be even more effective.

Long-term medical complications and acute overdose require medical treatment, but behavioral and psychological interventions play more crucial roles in sustaining drug-free lifestyles. Medical attention to acute problems of substance abuse should always be followed by the above-mentioned approaches, of which drug rehabilitation programs are important components.

Table 15.4 lists multiple reliable web addresses for drug education programs and curricula.

ROUTES OF ADMINISTRATION

Drugs of abuse can be taken by multiple different routes. For any drug to have an effect, it must be absorbed, either through the gastrointestinal tract, lungs, mucous membranes, or skin, or directly injected under the skin (also known as skin popping), into muscle, or into blood vessels (mainlining). Drugs of abuse can be taken by mouth, smoked, inhaled by mouth (huffing, bagging, dusting), insufflated through the nose (sniffing, snorting), injected (intravenous or intramuscular), or applied to the skin or mucous membranes (mouth, genital area). Some medications intended for use by one route may be used by another route when being abused. For example, bupropion (Wellbutrin, Zyban) is normally an oral antidepressant and smoking cessation medication that is abused by snorting or injection. Fentanyl patches containing a high-potency opioid, normally applied to the skin for chronic

(text continues on p. 374)

Table 15.3

PHYSICAL FINDINGS AND BEHAVIORS ASSOCIATED WITH DRUGS OF ABUSE

Drug class	Examples	Physical appearance and findings	Behavior
Stimulants	Cocaine Amphetamines Methamphetamine Bath salts Ritalin Caffeine Buproprion MDMA	Dilated pupils Rapid heart rate or palpitations Sweaty skin Raw, dripping nostrils and cough from snorting Jaw clenching (MDMA) Weight loss Tremors Seizures	Elevated mood Restlessness Anxiety Irritability Erratic, aggressive behavior Hallucinations Paranoia Fatigue Insomnia
Sedatives–hypnotics	Alcohol Benzodiazepines Barbiturates Marijuana Synthetic cannabinoids Solvent use GHB	Dazed appearance Red eyes Slowed breathing Paint or oil stains on hands, face, clothing (solvent use) Sores around mouth and runny nose (solvent use)	Disinhibited behavior: talkativeness, spontaneous laughter Sleepiness Labile mood, irritable or excitable Slowed thinking and poor memory Confusion Slurred speech Uncoordinated or clumsy Psychosis Hallucinations
Narcotics or opioids	Percocet Oxycontin Heroin	Pinpoint pupils Low heart rate, blood pressure, slowed breathing Cool, moist skin	Sleepiness Depressed mental status Decreased motivation

Table 15.3 (*continued*)

Drug class	Examples	Physical appearance and findings	Behavior
Hallucinogens	LSD Mescaline Mushrooms PCP Ketamine	Dilated pupils Blurred vision Seizures (PCP)	Labile mood Vivid visual and auditory illusions Hallucinations Paranoia Disturbed memory Altered speech and personality
Anticholinergics	Gravol Benadryl Jimson weed	Dilated pupils Blurred vision Rapid heart rate Flushed, dry skin Nausea/vomiting Seizures	Confusion Agitation Hallucinations Psychosis
Withdrawal syndromes	Alcohol Sedatives–hypnotics Opioids Solvents	Rapid heart rate Tremors Seizure Vomiting Diarrhea Yawning Sweaty skin Gooseflesh	Irritability or anxiety Jitteriness Agitation Sleep disturbance Disorientation Hallucinations (e.g., sensation of crawling insects all over body) Constant scratching or picking at skin and hair

Table 15.4

DRUG EDUCATION MATERIALS AND RESOURCES

National Institute of Health (http://science.education.nih.gov) "NIH Curriculum Supplements for K-12 Science Teachers": Links to science education resources, for teachers, curriculum supplements, drug abuse and addiction
National Institute on Drug Abuse (http://www.drugabuse.gov) Provides current research on drug abuse
Mind Over Matter (http://www.drugabuse.gov/publications/mind-over-matter/complete-set) "Mind Over Matter: Complete Set": An eight-part series directed at children in grades 5–9 regarding the brain's response to common drugs of abuse, complete with teacher's guide with activities, word finds, and more
National Institute on Drug Abuse (http://www.drugabuse.gov/parents-educators) "Parents and Educators": Follow links to teacher information and slide-teaching packets for downloadable slides for classroom use.
Science Education Enhances Knowledge (SEEK) About Tobacco (http://www.rise.duke.edu/seek/) Module on tobacco products and nicotine addiction
Pharmacology Education Partnership (http://www.thepepproject.net/Load/) "PEP Project": Online modules for students and teachers
UN Office on Drugs and Crime (http://www.unodc.org/pdf/youthnet/handbook_school_english.pdf) "Schools-Based Education for Drug Prevention": Curriculum guide to teaching about drugs of abuse

pain control, may be applied to mucosal membranes or injected for increased absorption by abusers.

ABUSED SUBSTANCES

Recreational substances that are abused can usually be categorized in four groups. These include stimulants, sedatives–hypnotics, narcotics, and hallucinogens. Common drugs of abuse are discussed in each category. Special mention is also made of "club" or "rave" drugs, natural or "legal" drugs, the growing problem of over-the-counter and prescription medication use for nonmedicinal purposes, and adolescent steroid abuse in sports. For more information on specific substances, Table 15.5 gives reliable websites with information on common drugs of abuse that follow.

Stimulants

Tobacco

Cigarette smoking and use of smokeless tobacco are closely associated with adolescent alcohol and drug use. About 90% of adults and adolescents who abuse drugs or alcohol also smoke cigarettes (Myers & Brown, 1994). Every day in the United States, nearly 3,200 persons younger than 18 years of age smoke their first cigarette, and 2,100 persons in this age group become new daily cigarette smokers (Centers for Disease Control and Prevention, 2013). Findings of the Monitoring the Future survey (Johnston, O'Malley, Miech, Bachman, & Schulenberg, 2014) indicated that approximately 4.5% of children in Grade 8, 9% in Grade 10, and 16% in Grade 12 admitted to cigarette use in the previous 30 days. Daily tobacco use was 1.8%, 4.4%, and 8.5%, respectively, for the same grade cohorts. Despite a steady decline in tobacco use for all ages over the past 10 years, young adults aged 18–25 continue to have the highest rate of current tobacco use (38%) compared with youths (aged 12–17) and adults (older than 26) (8.6% and 27%, respectively) (Substance Abuse and Mental Health Services Administration, 2013). Many of these young smokers carry this habit into adulthood, probably because of a combination of nicotine dependence and a reinforcing environment, unless intervention is implemented. Indeed, 90% of adults who smoke started smoking before age 19 (Jacobs et al., 2001).

Youths aged 12–17 who smoked in the previous month are more likely to have also used an illicit drug (54.6% compared to 6.4% of nonsmoking youths). The same association exists between smoking and alcohol use (including binge and heavy alcohol use) (Substance Abuse and Mental Health Services Administration, 2013).

In experiments (Cox, Goldstein, & Nelson, 1984), animals have been shown to self-administer nicotine repeatedly, indicating the reinforcing actions of the substance (strengthening effects on its own use). In humans, one puff of smoke reaches the brain within 10 seconds of inhalation and stimulates the reward centers of the brain by increasing a brain substance known as dopamine. Nicotine may further facilitate

Table 15.5
GENERAL INFORMATION ON DRUGS OF ABUSE

National Institute on Drug Abuse (http://www.drugabuse.gov/drugs-abuse) A comprehensive resource with information for teachers, parents, and students. It includes descriptions of drugs of abuse, links to educational materials, and information about related medical conditions.
Center for Substance Abuse Research (http://www.cesar.umd.edu) This site contains specific information and photographs on selected drugs of abuse.
Erowid (http://www.erowid.org) Private but balanced website with some valuable information and pictures on numerous drugs of abuse. The information on this site is largely gathered from forum postings, so it must be interpreted with caution. Links to "Experiences" are subjective users' accounts of a particular substance.
Streetdrugs.org (http://www.streetdrugs.org/index.html) Private site with limited information on web about drugs of abuse. Does have reliable teacher's resource guide and CD-ROM of pictures for purchase.
Government of Canada: National Anti-Drug Strategy (http://www.nationalantidrugstrategy.gc.ca) An official Canadian website that offers resources for parents and teens, as well as basic descriptions of the most common drugs of abuse.
Partnership for Drug-Free Kids (http://www.drugfree.org/drug-guide) This website contains basic descriptions of more than 40 drugs of abuse.
Resources Specific to Ontario **Ontario Drug and Alcohol Helpline** (http://www.drugandalcoholhelpline.ca/) A website that offers confidential phone and Internet chat lines that provide information about drug and alcohol addiction services in Ontario.
Centre for Mental Health and Addiction (CAMH) (http://www.camh.ca/EN/HOSPITAL/HEALTH_INFORMATION/A_Z_MENTAL_HEALTH_AND_ADDICTION_INFORMATION/Pages/default.aspx) This website includes Ontario-centered information about drugs of abuse and mental illness as well as links to resources.
Toronto Drug Strategy Report/City of Toronto Drug and Alcohol Pages (http://www.toronto.ca/legdocs/mmis/2014/hl/bgzd/backgroundfile-73557.pdf)
Canadian Law Controlled Drug and Substances Act (http://laws-lois.justice.gc.ca/eng/acts/C-38.8/) Food and Drugs Act (http://laws-lois.justice.gc.ca/eng/acts/F-27/)

memory and attention, enhance composure, and reduce appetite, leading to decreased weight gain. Another strong reinforcing factor is the positive image of tobacco use endorsed by actors, celebrities, athletes, or other role models for children and adolescents.

The main active component in tobacco is nicotine. During cigarette smoking, nicotine stimulates the body by increasing noradrenaline and adrenaline levels. Mild increases in heart rate, blood pressure, and respiratory rate, comparable to those resulting from mild exercise, occur. Nausea, vomiting, and tremors (typically, fine shaking of hands and fingers) may be seen more frequently in some people, especially first-time or occasional smokers. This same increase in adrenaline levels can lead to the adverse effects of nicotine, including severe blood-vessel disruption, causing loss of limbs, gangrene, heart attacks, or blindness.

Tobacco smoke has ill effects distinct from those of nicotine. Various health hazards also result from other combustion substances, such as polycyclic aromatic hydrocarbons (some of which may cause cancer) and carbon monoxide. About 4,000 compounds are estimated to exist in tobacco smoke. Smoke contains substances capable of inducing cancer (i.e., carcinogens). This deadly effect becomes apparent only several decades after the initiation of the smoking habit. Another important clinical implication is that infants and children in a smoker's household, as well as smokers themselves, are at risk for respiratory illness, stunted growth, and learning difficulties due to secondhand smoke.

Cigarette smoking during pregnancy poses risks of growth retardation in the fetus. The fetus is exposed to nicotine, carbon monoxide, and other toxic chemicals when the mother smokes. In fact, the fetus is exposed to nicotine when someone other than the mother exposes the child to secondhand tobacco smoke (Fried & Watkinson, 2001). Tobacco use should be strongly discouraged in school settings, where the next generations of parents begin forming their social habits.

Cocaine

Cocaine (street names include coke, crack, C, candy, lady, and line) comes from the leaves of the *Erythroxylon coca* tree. Natives of the South American Andes have chewed coca leaves for more than 5,000 years to gain feelings of well-being. Medical use of cocaine as a local anesthetic and for various other indications began in the 19th century in Europe, although local anesthesia to the nose for surgical procedures is the sole remaining medical indication for cocaine hydrochloride. Sigmund Freud, the founder of modern psychoanalysis, was one of the first Europeans who studied the clinical uses of cocaine. Interested in brain effects of cocaine, Freud gave the drug to one of his colleagues in an attempt to wean the person from morphine (a potent narcotic). The weaning was successful, but the patient became one of the first-known cocaine addicts. Cocaine was an ingredient in Coca-Cola from 1888 until 1901, when it was removed from the formulation. Cocaine was banned for use in the United States in 1914. Since then, the medicinal use of cocaine is under strict governmental control in most countries.

In the illegal market, cocaine is supplied either as a hydrochloride powder, which is sniffed or injected intravenously after being dissolved into water, or as freebase cocaine ("crack"), which also can be smoked. Because cocaine hydrochloride decomposes under heat from a match or lighter, it cannot be smoked. The name crack stems from the cracking sound generated when clusters of freebase cocaine break upon heat. Crack is sold in small dosage units of "rocks," approximately $20 each. This relatively low price makes crack cocaine within the reach of adolescents.

Data from Monitoring the Future (Johnston et al., 2014) indicated that 2.6% of high school seniors, 1.9% of 10th graders, and 1% of 8th graders in the United States had used cocaine hydrochloride in the previous year. Between 0.6% and 1.1% of those from all grades surveyed had used crack in the previous year. This compares to a high in 1986 of approximately 13%.

Peak blood concentrations of cocaine are achieved 30–60 minutes after intranasal application (e.g., sniffing), which suggests that absorption is not completed immediately after sniffing. Inhalation of cocaine smoke produces more intense and instantaneous effects, and heavy users may repeat the smoking every 10–15 minutes. After intravenous or inhalation application, cocaine is rapidly eliminated from the bloodstream. Although there are substantial variations in cocaine-use behaviors, taking the drug in bouts or binges is common. Binge users may be totally dependent on the drug and out of control in their drug-seeking behavior, even if they do not use it on a daily basis.

Cocaine is also a stimulant. Similar to nicotine, it increases the amount of noradrenaline and adrenaline released. Acute effects of cocaine use include elated mood and increased self-confidence, increased heart rate and blood pressure, dilated pupils, and erratic or aggressive behavior. Headache, seizures, fever, chest pain, irregular heart rhythm, and even heart attack may occur in toxic cases. When the acute effects of cocaine have gone, the user often becomes severely fatigued and mentally depressed.

Symptoms commonly seen in chronic adolescent cocaine users are fatigue, insomnia (sleeplessness), loss of appetite, weight loss, and a chronic cough. Because users of cocaine, especially crack cocaine, are often polysubstance abusers, they may have other health problems attributable to multiple substance exposures.

Cocaine use is associated not only with higher homicide rates but also with increased rates of suicide, which is the second leading cause of death among U.S. adolescents. Among high school students, suicide ideation and attempts are more common in drug users, particularly crack cocaine users (Felts, Chenier, & Barnes, 1992). Moreover, in New York City, cocaine was detected in 64% of fatalities by "Russian roulette" and in 35% of those who committed suicide by handgun, which suggests a link between cocaine use and potentially fatal risk-taking behaviors (Marzuk, Tardiff, Smyth, Stajic, & Leon, 1992).

Amphetamines and "Look-Alikes"

Amphetamines are a group of drugs with chemical structures related to ephedrine and adrenaline. These include *amphetamine* (known as beans, bennies, uppers, and hearts), *dextroamphetamine* (known as Dexedrine), *methamphetamine* (known as speed, ice, crystal, and crystal meth), and *methylphenidate* (known as Ritalin). Modifications of the parent structure contribute to differing effects of these substances. In general, these drugs affect chemicals in the brain known as dopamine and serotonin to varying degrees. Except for mescaline, the amphetamines are not hallucinogenic as much as stimulants. They have medical uses in the treatment of narcolepsy (uncontrollable periodic attacks of sleepiness) and attention-deficit/hyperactivity disorder. They are abused orally or intravenously. Over-the-counter weight-reduction medications (or mail-order drugs) containing phenylpropanolamine and caffeine also are used in sufficiently high doses to gain stimulant effects similar to those of amphetamines. These "look-alike" drugs are easily available. Abuse problems with amphetamines include use for weight reduction (not medically indicated), stress, and binges for pleasure. Similar to cocaine, amphetamines are stimulants that produce mood elevation, a sense of well-being, energy, and decreased appetite. At the same time, some users experience anxiety, irritability, and sleeplessness. The agitated mood is usually followed by anxiety, fatigue, and sustained feelings of depression. In contrast to cocaine, with its short half-life of one hour, it takes 5–10 hours to eliminate half of the amphetamine in the bloodstream.

Overdosing results in confusion, assaultiveness, restlessness, hallucinations, excessive sweating, palpitations, and collapse. Suicidal or homicidal tendencies may appear. Convulsions and coma occur in fatal intoxication. Chronic toxicities include hallucinations, paranoid behaviors, and delusions, resembling schizophrenia. These psychotic reactions usually subside after cessation of the drugs but may not disappear in some individuals.

Two chemically modified amphetamines—MDMA (3,4-methylenedi-oxy-methamphetamine, or ecstasy) and MDEA (3,4-methylenedioxy-ethamphetamine, or Eve)—are sold on the illicit drug market. Designed and manufactured in unauthorized laboratories, they are called designer drugs. They produce elated feelings without inducing hallucinations or alterations of visual images. Ecstasy has the unique property of causing spasm of the jaw muscles; to prevent tooth damage, the user is often seen carrying a baby pacifier for use during intoxication. In the United States in the year 2013, more than 4% of adolescents in Grade 12, more than 3% in Grade 10, and more than 1% in Grade 8 admitted to having used ecstasy in the previous year (Johnston et al., 2014). In the setting of increased physical activity (e.g., dancing all night), dehydration (inadequate replacement of water loss), and warm external environments (inadequately ventilated settings), individuals may be more susceptible to the adverse effects of ecstasy. Some individuals also have a predisposition to the adverse effects of ecstasy. These factors may contribute to the increasing number of ecstasy deaths.

Particularly potent amphetamines have also been introduced in the recent past. One of these, PMA (para-methoxy-amphetamine), is also known as "death" on the streets. Not surprisingly, there is no quality control in the illicit drug world. It is possible that what is sold as one product may be contaminated with or substituted with another.

High-caffeine energy drinks (e.g., Red Bull, Monster, Rockstar, Amp) are readily available and contain high doses of caffeine, up to 242 mg per serving (equivalent to 2.5 8-ounce cups of coffee or 5 cans of cola) (*Consumer Reports*, 2012). In 2013, nearly 40% of Ontario high school students in Grades 7–12 reported drinking a high-caffeine energy drink at least once in the previous year, ranging from 26% in Grade 7 to 50% in Grade 12. Approximately 12% reported drinking an energy drink at least once in the week before the survey (Boak et al., 2013). The prevalence of daily caffeine use including cola drinks, energy drinks, coffee, and tea in adolescents is approximately 75%. Caffeine use in adolescents has been associated with disrupted sleep, daytime sleepiness, and poorer academic performance (James, Kristjánsson, & Sigfúsdóttir, 2011). In addition to this, energy drink consumption by young adults has been associated with higher alcohol use (both frequency and volume) and dependence, and tobacco and illicit drug use (Terry-McElrath, O'Malley, & Johnston, 2013). The caffeine in energy drinks can mask impairment associated with alcohol and other substance use, which makes them a popular method to extend the ability to "party" (Terry-McElrath et al., 2013). Caffeine withdrawal symptoms can appear six to eight hours after the last caffeine ingestion and include sleepiness, lethargy, lack of attention, and decreased cognitive performance (James et al., 2011).

Sedatives–Hypnotics

Alcohol

Alcoholic beverages have been part of human culture for more than 8,000 years and generally are considered socially compatible. Many current societies view drinking alcohol as an acceptable behavior in adulthood. In the United States, about 60% of all adults drink alcohol at least occasionally, and 10% are considered heavy drinkers. Although it is illegal in most countries for minors to consume alcoholic beverages, enormous numbers of adolescents do drink. In a 2013 U.S. survey, 39% of high school seniors, 26% of 10th graders, and 10% of 8th graders said they had used alcohol in the previous month (Johnston et al., 2014).

The main component of alcoholic beverages is ethyl alcohol (or ethanol), concentrations of which range from 4% to 5% in regular beer, 11% to 15% in wine, and 45% in liquor. As the concentrations of ethanol increase in one's blood, toxic effects occur proportional to concentration, although sensitivity can differ considerably among individuals. The most imminent health hazards to young drinkers are impaired judgment and motor skills, which often lead to various forms of accidents and suicide attempts. As blood alcohol levels rise into the toxic range, death can occur as a result of inability to protect one's airway and the vomiting of stomach contents into one's lungs.

Although ethanol is metabolized (or broken down by the body) relatively quickly, because the liver has a finite amount of enzyme available to detoxify it, only a fixed amount per unit of time can be eliminated; hence, the greater the amount ingested, the greater the time required for elimination. Consider that an average adult male is able to break down approximately 10 g of alcohol per hour, and that one bottle of 5% beer contains 13.4 g of ethyl alcohol per bottle. At the rate of one beer per hour, after three hours, 10 g of alcohol will remain in the body and require a further hour to be eliminated, even if consumption is stopped. Activity levels of the enzymes responsible for ethanol detoxification can differ significantly among people. In general, younger children have slower alcohol metabolism. This translates into prolonged intoxication or influence of alcohol from equivalent amounts.

Tolerance develops when one is exposed to ethyl alcohol repeatedly. The chronic drinker is not as impaired as a naive drinker with any particular blood alcohol concentration, to a limit. Greater amounts of alcohol are required to achieve the same intoxicating effect, setting the stage for dependence. One cannot become tolerant to the lethal concentrations of alcohol, however. Alcohol withdrawal syndrome, which occurs in ethanol-dependent persons one to three days after stopping drinking, can be life threatening, although a case has not been reported in adolescents.

Alcohol is a potent toxin for the unborn child. If the mother drinks significant amounts of alcohol (2 g/kg ethanol per day, corresponding to about six to eight drinks per day) during pregnancy, the fetus is often permanently damaged. *Fetal alcohol syndrome* is characterized by cognitive impairment, delayed growth and development, birth defects, and various behavioral problems such as hyperactivity and learning disabilities (see Chapter 10). In women who drink regularly but to a lesser extent, the fetus may be less severely affected, suffering mainly from behavioral problems, with no obvious physical characteristics of the syndrome. This condition is referred to as *fetal alcohol effects.* Although occasional mild drinking during pregnancy does not seem to pose these risks, safety levels concerning amount of consumption and the mode of drinking during pregnancy (e.g., whether to drink a large amount occasionally or a small quantity constantly) have not been defined clearly. Pregnant women who have a drinking problem need thorough medical consultation.

Marijuana

In Johnston et al.'s (2014) survey, 13% of 8th graders reported use of marijuana in the past year, and 1.1% admitted to daily use; 30% of 10th graders and 36.4% of 12th graders had used marijuana in the last year, with 6.5% of the latter reporting daily use. This compares to 13% of 10th graders in Europe (Hibell et al., 2012) and 24.5% of 10th graders in Ontario, Canada (Boak et al., 2013), who used marijuana during the previous year.

The term *marijuana* (street names include MJ, Mary Jane, weed, joint, ganja, grass, jay, and pot) refers to any part of the hemp plant (*Cannabis sativa*) or its extract prepared for illicit use. Cannabis, obtained from the flowering tops of the hemp plant, is one of the oldest and most widely used psychoactive substances. Recorded use of cannabis goes back thousands of years in China and India. The hemp plant produces more than 60 related compounds called cannabinoids, of which *l*-delta-9-tetrahydrocannabinol (Δ^9-THC) is the main active substance. Currently, Δ^9-THC is used medically as a drug to control nausea and vomiting that are unresponsive to other drugs. Because marijuana is commonly smoked rather than ingested, toxic combustion substances may be clinically important in the development of long-term toxicity, as is the case with tobacco.

The Δ^9-THC contents of marijuana vary substantially, ranging from 0.5% to more than 30%. Also, the smoking technique and the effects of *pyrolysis* (the chemical reaction caused by the high temperature of burning) influence the amount of Δ^9-THC that may reach important body organs. In addition, possibilities for contamination by herbicides, fungi, and, in some regions, mercury, also exist.

Marijuana usually causes an enhanced sense of well-being, a subjective feeling of relaxation, talkativeness, spontaneous laughter, and altered perception of time. Slowed thinking (often inaccurate and irrelevant) and sleepiness are also common, and emotional control becomes fragile. These conditions resemble mild ethanol intoxication. High doses of Δ^9-THC may result in acute toxic psychosis, characterized by hallucinations, delusions, and panic reactions, which often need to be handled as psychiatric emergencies. Effects of Δ^9-THC include increased heart rate, decreased standing blood pressure, and congestion of the blood vessels of the eyes, resulting in redness.

Heavy marijuana users develop many chronic health problems. It is difficult to distinguish chronic effects of cigarette smoking from those of marijuana smoking because both behaviors often go together. However, chronic bronchitis has been observed in heavy marijuana users, which may be partly due to a much higher tar content in marijuana smoke than in tobacco smoke.

Chronic heavy users of marijuana also may display altered mental conditions, such as apathy (extreme indifference), mental slowing, memory loss, impairment of judgment, loss of drive, and emotional flatness (i.e., amotivational syndrome). Although this condition may be due partly to other risky behaviors (e.g., other drug use, malnutrition) or be a result of preexisting behavioral problems, experiments in rats have shown that heavy chronic exposure to Δ^9-THC can cause structural changes in the brain (Landfield, Cadwallader, & Vinsant, 1988).

Organic Solvents

Organic solvents is a collective term denoting a volatile liquid that may dissolve water-insoluble organic compounds. Examples are toluene, xylenes, various forms of alcohol, acetone, ether, trichloroethylene, trichloromethane, and other petroleum-derived compounds or mixtures such as gasoline. These are part of many household products, including some types of glue, spray paints, lacquer thinners, and cleaning fluids. They are relatively inexpensive and easy to obtain. Sniffing of these substances has been a substance abuse problem for decades because they create a high that is similar to that produced by drinking alcohol. In North America, gasoline sniffing is more prevalent in communities of First Nations populations than in other ethnic groups. This does not necessarily indicate the existence of a genetic or biologic predisposing factor toward gasoline sniffing in this particular ethnic group; rather, the social and economic environment appears to be the crucial factor. In some of these communities, children as young as 6 years old have been found sniffing gasoline, with 70% of third-grade students having tried sniffing gas (Eggertson, 2014). Overall, about 11% of U.S. students in eighth grade reported an experience with inhalant abuse, decreasing to 7% in high school seniors (Johnston et al., 2014).

Almost immediately after inhalation, these volatile substances exert effects lasting for 5–10 minutes. Sudden death, probably due to acute heart failure, is not uncommon because lethal arrhythmias (severe forms of irregular heartbeat) can be induced by the organic solvents, especially when abusers are startled during use. Signs of solvent abuse include paint or oil stains on clothes or skin, sores and dry, cracked skin around the mouth, red eyes, runny nose, dazed appearance, and a chemical odor. Chronic detrimental effects include liver and kidney dysfunction, brain damage, memory loss, learning disabilities, and peripheral nerve toxicity. In the past, gasoline contained various amounts of lead, a toxic heavy metal, which may have contributed to brain and nerve damage. Children born to heavy organic solvent abusers show health problems similar to the fetal alcohol syndrome effects (see the previous section on alcohol).

Organic nitrites (isobutyl, butyl, or amyl nitrite), another group of volatile compounds, have been abused as aphrodisiacs (to enhance sexual experiences), primarily in the male homosexual community. These compounds are available in pornography or "head" shops and from mail-order stores. Amyl nitrite is used clinically to treat acute angina. The nitrites can cause lowered blood pressure, headaches, and fainting. They may also alter the hemoglobin (an oxygen-carrying protein) in red blood cells, resulting in decreased ability of the blood to carry oxygen.

Tranquilizers

This category of drugs, which is widely used in clinical medicine, includes antipsychotic drugs with little reinforcing or addictive propensity. Drugs discussed in this section include minor tranquilizers with habit-forming characteristics. The two main groups of addictive drugs in this category are *barbiturates* (phenobarbital, pentobarbital) and *benzodiazepines* (diazepam, or Valium, and lorazepam, or Ativan).

Most abusers take these drugs orally, with the exception of barbiturates, which can also be injected intravenously or intramuscularly. An estimated 3%–8% of high school students have had an experience with sedative or hypnotic abuse (Johnston et al., 2014). These groups of drugs are often taken with opioids and alcohol by polysubstance abusers to enhance the experience. Another form of sedative or hypnotic abuse is seen in individuals who initially were prescribed these drugs (e.g., for the treatment of anxiety) and who later developed dependence on them.

Sedation is a common effect of this group of drugs. Acute intoxication leads to mental confusion, slurred speech, *ataxia* (impaired balance and coordination of movement), slow respiration, coma, low body temperature, and death. The effects of chronically taken sedatives or hypnotics may not necessarily be evident. Regular use of these drugs as sleeping pills may cause sleeping difficulties and anxiety when the drugs are discontinued. Heavier use may lead to a chronic intoxicated state resembling ethanol intoxication. The withdrawal syndrome following dependence may result in seizures and *delirium* (i.e., visual hallucinations, disorientation, and mental confusion), which can be a medical emergency.

Gamma Hydroxybutyrate

Gamma hydroxybutyrate (GHB; street names include G, Grievous Bodily Harm, and liquid E) is one of three chemicals—the other two being gamma butyrolactone (GBL) and 1,4 butanediol (both of which are metabolized in the body to GBH)—that have been implicated as "date rape" drugs. GHB is a naturally occurring substance in the body that affects the release of dopamine in the brain. Intoxication with GHB results in effects similar to those of alcohol. At lower doses, relaxation occurs, as well as loss of inhibition, increased appreciation for music, and mood elevation. At increasing doses, coordination is impaired, consciousness is depressed, and breathing is slowed. Deaths due to intoxication with GHB are usually in the setting of large recreational doses (GHB is a liquid sold in varying concentrations) or in combination with some other sedative, such as alcohol.

GHB was first developed as an anesthetic. Side effects limited its use. It then became available as an over-the-counter sleeping aid and as a dietary supplement to enhance muscle bulk. Although illegal to possess or sell in most countries, recipes of the product are available over the Internet. With increased use, one does develop tolerance to its effects. Similarly, once tolerant, if use ceases abruptly, withdrawal syndromes have been described. This state can result in severe symptoms with hallucinations, paranoia, and abnormalities in blood pressure and heart rate requiring urgent medical intervention (Sivilotti, Burns, Aaron, & Greenberg, 2001).

Narcotics

There are several terms, including *narcotic, opioid,* and *opiate,* used to designate a group of chemicals with characteristic effects on brain function; the main effect is a decrease in one's perception of pain. The word *opium* stems from the Greek word for "juice" because historically the source of opium was the milky juice derived from the unripe seed capsules of the poppy plant (*Papaver somniferum*). In the early 19th century, one of the compounds isolated from opium was called morphine after Morpheus, the Greek god of dreams. Soon after the discovery of morphine, other biologically active compounds, such as codeine, were isolated from crude opium as well. The relatively obsolete term *opiate* designates such drugs obtained from opium (e.g., morphine and codeine) and those obtained by chemical modification of morphine (e.g., heroin). Both chemically modified opium extracts and synthetic compounds with morphine-like actions (e.g., methadone, meperidine) soon became available. It is now widely known that the human body also synthesizes proteins called endorphins that produce morphine-like activities by operating on the same brain-cell sites as do morphine and related drugs. The term *opioid* denotes all the naturally occurring compounds, including chemically modified ones, and the synthetic drugs that exert morphine-like effects. Opioid use often leads to a habit (i.e., addiction), but clinical use for pain control under appropriate medical supervision rarely does so.

Heroin, the most commonly abused opioid, is snorted or injected. Heroin abuse reached a peak in the 1960s and 1970s and then decreased. An accurate estimation of the rate of heroin abuse in adolescents is difficult to determine because heroin addicts are most likely to have dropped out of the school system and are therefore unavailable to answer school surveys. Intravenous heroin abuse also poses risks of various serious infections such as hepatitis viruses and HIV (human immunodeficiency virus), due to the lack of hygienic procedures and the sharing of needles; this risk is common in any injectable substances of abuse.

Opioids, which are sought due to their euphoric effects, depress brain function, resulting in drowsiness, reduced pain sensation, and decreased behavioral and motivational drive. These drugs often cause nausea and vomiting by activating the center in the brain that controls nauseous sensation. Various degrees of tolerance develop to these effects. Because the tolerance usually disappears upon withdrawal, restarting opioid use at the same dose often results in fatality.

Acute intoxication with opioids is usually characterized by small pupils; coma; slow and irregular breathing; cool, moist skin; slow heart rate; and potentially death. Overdosing is always a possibility for heroin addicts because the strength of the heroin formulation in the illegal market varies significantly. Opioid overdose is a medical emergency that should be managed by intensive supportive care and administration of opioid antagonists to counteract the effects.

Upon discontinuing chronic use of opioids, the user will develop a withdrawal (abstinence) syndrome characterized by anxiety, restlessness, insomnia (inability to sleep), muscle pain, gooseflesh, sneezing, tearing, yawning, nasal congestion, vomiting, diarrhea, and rapid heart rate. Because heroin is eliminated from the body relatively quickly, the withdrawal syndrome tends to be intense, although rarely life threatening. Because methadone has less sedative effects and longer elimination time from the body, it is substituted for heroin or morphine to circumvent an opioid withdrawal syndrome in the long-term medical management of opioid addicts.

Unauthorized production of chemically modified opioid drugs has increased the number of opioids introduced into the illicit drug market. There have been reports of deaths due to overdose of potent opioids such as α-methylfentanyl and 3-methylfentanyl, both of which are obtained by chemical modification of a potent anesthetic, fentanyl. Another tragic example is 4-phenyl-4-propionoxy-piperidine (MPPP), which is produced by chemical modification of a synthetic opiate, meperidine. A group of young drug addicts in California had some MPPP that was contaminated with a compound used as a catalyst in the chemical reaction that happened to be toxic to a specific part of the brain. This toxic chemical destroyed a group of brain cells called *substantia nigra*, resulting in a severe brain disorder known as Parkinson's disease (Langston, Ballard, Tetrud, & Irwin, 1983). These drugs, designed and produced in unauthorized laboratories (i.e., designer drugs), will probably continue posing a serious challenge to society.

Hallucinogens

Mescaline

The prototype hallucinogen is mescaline (street names include mesc and button), derived from the cactus plant peyote, which grows in the deserts of Mexico and the U.S. Southwest. Typically the plant is dried and smoked to produce physical, visual, and perceptual hallucinations. Its use probably dates back thousands of years to the natives of Mexico. Because it takes years for the plant to mature, it is relatively unavailable and very expensive to purchase. It is probable that anything sold on the streets as mescaline is actually LSD or PCP, discussed next.

LSD (Lysergic Acid Diethylamide)

LSD (street names include acid and blotter) is a chemical derived from the fungus or mold called ergot that grows on rye. It and similar naturally occurring compounds, such as those found in the seeds of the morning glory plant (LSA, or lysergic acid amide) and nutmeg, are hallucinogens or psychedelics. LSD is made as a liquid; blotting paper is soaked in the liquid and dried. A dose (50–150 mg) is sold as a 1-cm-square "blotter" for $3–$5. The blotter is placed on the tongue and sucked for release of the hallucinogen. In the survey by Johnston et al. (2014), 1.4% of 8th graders, 3.7% of 10th graders, and 3.9% of 12th graders admitted to having used LSD at some time in their life, considerably lower than in 2001, when previous LSD use was reported as 3.9%, 7.6%, and 11.1% in grade 8, 10, and 12 students, respectively.

LSD is the most potent of all hallucinogens. After minute doses of the drug, LSD alters perception of time and space, visual images, and sound. Visual information is often perceived as sound images, and sound provokes colorful visual images. Mood may fluctuate, although pleasurable feelings tend to dominate. Because most, if not all, users correctly recognize these effects as drug induced, the psychological boundary between reality and fantasy appears to be somehow maintained, despite the vivid illusions; strictly speaking, therefore, these are not hallucinations, because they are not confused with reality. These effects occur over three to four hours and are called a "trip." The illegal use of LSD is typically repeated in weeks or months to reexperience the trip. However, unpredictable episodes of panic ("bad trips") can occur with use of the drug. Moreover, in more than 15% of users, a disturbing phenomenon occurs that is called "flashbacks," which is an unexpected repetition of the drug experience in the absence of the drug, even several years after the last dose of LSD.

Phencyclidine (PCP)

Although no longer in use medically, PCP (street names include angel dust) originally was developed as an anesthetic for human and animal use in the 1950s. Phencyclidine began to be abused in the late 1960s. Statistics about PCP use are unreliable because it is sometimes contaminated with or mistaken for LSD, mescaline, or marijuana. In general, it is now rare to find PCP available on the streets.

PCP can be injected intravenously, snorted, ingested, or smoked. The effects, lasting 12 hours or more, include an elated feeling, emotional instability, staggering gait, slurred speech, muscle stiffness, confusion, and drowsiness. Higher doses may cause panic reactions, anesthetic effects, auditory hallucinations, coma, and seizures. Disturbed memory and speech and altered personality may be observed in chronic users.

Ketamine

A synthetic analogue of phencyclidine, ketamine (street names include K, special K, and vitamin K), was developed and is currently used in the medical profession as a dissociative anesthetic, especially in children. Emerging from a ketamine anesthetic has the common side effects of nausea, vomiting, and paranoid delusions. Despite this, however, ketamine has found its place as a drug of abuse. At low doses, it causes a sense of euphoria, increased sociability, and pleasant perceptual distortions. At higher doses, complete dissociation from one's surroundings and near-death experiences have been described.

Nonmedicinal Use of Medication

A growing problem is the use of over-the-counter and prescription medications taken for nonmedicinal purposes. Of Ontario students, 10% reported using over-the-counter cough and cold medications containing dextromethorphan to "get high" during the previous year (up from 7.2% in 2009) (Boak et al., 2013). In this same study, 12% of all students used a prescription opioid pain medication (e.g., Tylenol #3, Codeine, Percocet, Demerol, Percodan) in the previous year without a prescription. Use of these opioids increased with grade level and peaked at 16% in grade 12 students. Overall, the use of any nonmedicinal prescription drug was reported in 15.2% of these 9th–12th graders (Boak et al., 2013). In the survey by Johnston et al. (2014), 21.5% of high school seniors reported having used prescription drugs for nonmedicinal purposes at any time in their lifetime. These include over-the-counter cough medications (5%), the stimulants Ritalin (2.3%) and Adderall (7.4%), narcotics (11.1%) (e.g., Vicodan, Oxycontin), or tranquilizers (7.7%), including the "date rape" drug Rohypnol (a potent benzodiazepine, used by 0.9% of grade 12 students in the previous year). The majority (70%) reported obtaining the drug from someone at home (Boak et al., 2013).

Another over-the-counter medication abused by youth is diphenhydramine, the active ingredient in Gravol, Benadryl, and a number of over-the-counter sleep aids. This seemingly harmless antihistamine is marketed for its antinauseant or sedative properties, but it is sometimes abused by youth for recreational purposes to achieve a "cheap high." The resulting symptoms are typical for a drug with anticholinergic properties and include dilated pupils, rapid heart rate, dry mouth, unsteady gait, euphoria, hallucinations, and agitation.

"Legal" Highs

In an effort to avoid problems with the law, youth may experiment with substances that are considered "natural" or "legal" drugs. The plant-based substance *Salvia divinorum* is an herb with hallucinogenic properties. In 2013, 3.4% of U.S. 12th graders (Johnston et al., 2014) and 4.4% of Ontario 12th graders (Boak et al., 2013) reported having used Salvia in the past year. It is smoked or taken orally as a tea. Hallucinations can be vivid and extreme, resulting in traumatic physical injuries.

Jimson weed (*Datura stramonium*; devil's apple, fireweed, stinkweed, stinkwort) is a plant that grows naturally in many parts of North America. All parts of this plant have potent anticholinergic properties (similar to diphenhydramine) and are used recreationally. The seeds and leaves can be eaten, taken as a tea, or smoked. Symptoms include dilated pupils, blurred vision, rapid heart rate, dry mouth, hallucinations, seizures, and agitation that can occasionally be severe and dangerous to the users.

New synthetic substances such as mephedrone or "bath salts" can initially appear on the market as "legal" products. Often the packaging is labeled as "not for human consumption." However, once they are recognized as having abuse and harm potential by regulatory authorities, they inevitably become listed as controlled substances and become "illegal." Exposures to bath salts reported to the American Poison Control Centers peaked in 2011 at 6,137, with preliminary data suggesting a decline to less than 1,000 calls in 2013 (American Association of Poison Control Centers, 2013), possibly coinciding with their reclassification as illicit substances, although they are still available online. Extremely low use estimates from youth surveys in Ontario, Canada, suggest that these drugs have not become part of mainstream student culture (Boak et al., 2013). They can be injected, taken orally, or snorted. The effects are similar to amphetamines, including hallucinations and violent behavior, and have been reported to be as addictive as cocaine (Antoniou & Juurlink, 2012).

Synthetic cannabinoids known as "K2" or "Spice" are often marketed as incense, "natural" or plant-based products, despite being synthetic drugs. Although many synthetic cannabinoids are already considered illegal, new formulations continue to be made available and are readily purchased via the Internet. Packages contain shredded plant material that may look like potpourri with a synthetic additive that produces the psychoactive effect. It is usually smoked like marijuana, taken orally as an herbal infusion, or used rectally. In 2013, 2% of 7th–12th graders in Ontario, Canada, reported using these substances within the previous year, representing about 17,300 students (Boak et al., 2013). The synthetic cannabinoids bind to the cannabinoid receptors but are stronger than natural cannabis. Chronic abuse of "Spice" can result in an addiction syndrome and withdrawal symptoms similar to those observed in marijuana abuse. Effects of synthetic cannabinoids are similar to marijuana, but can be accompanied by more agitation, psychotic effects, violence, hallucinations, paranoia, and seizures (Antoniou & Juurlink, 2014).

Anabolic Steroids

Steroids denote compounds that have a specific chemical structure in common. Several of them are important hormones that are synthesized in the human body. *Anabolic steroids* designate those steroids with enhancing actions on protein synthesis and accumulation, possibly leading to an increase in functional muscle mass in some populations. This group of steroids is abused largely for the muscle-enhancing effects. However, a pure anabolic steroid without other effects, such as androgenic effects (see below), has not been, and probably never will be, discovered.

Some athletes, both women and men, use anabolic steroids because they expect them to increase physical competence. Since weight lifters and bodybuilders began using these drugs in the 1950s, the trend has become widespread, from professional to college and high school athletes. Anabolic steroids are not addictive in the same sense as are psychoactive drugs such as cocaine and heroin, but the expectation of becoming more physically fit is reinforcing. It has never been proved that anabolic steroids in medically used doses actually promote muscle growth over the levels achieved by normal levels of naturally occurring male sex hormones in the mature man. In women and sexually immature men, muscle growth is promoted by use of these steroids. The doses of anabolic steroids used for muscle-increasing purposes are 10–100 times higher than those used for medical indications.

In 2013, about 2% of 12th graders reported at least one use of an anabolic steroid (Johnston et al., 2014). In a study conducted in Georgia among 9th graders, 5.4% of boys and 1.5% of girls had tried anabolic steroids (DuRant, Rickert, Ashworth, Newman, & Slavens,

1993). Importantly, the more often they used anabolic steroids, the more likely they were to abuse cocaine, smokeless tobacco, marijuana, cigarettes, and/or alcohol. Sharing needles to inject anabolic steroids is a common phenomenon, posing risks of life-threatening infections such as HIV and hepatitis.

Testosterone, a naturally occurring male sex hormone (women also produce testosterone in smaller amounts), is a prototypical anabolic steroid used for muscle-increasing potential, although it has other natural androgenic (male) effects, such as the growth of body hair and coarsening of the voice. Many other synthetic anabolic steroids exist. These synthetic drugs were designed to be purely anabolic, although other androgenic effects are unavoidable. Many anabolic steroids used for "doping" purposes lack human safety data, as they are designated for animal use. Adverse effects of the anabolic steroids are mental changes; liver diseases, including hepatitis and tumors; damages to the testes; and menstrual changes.

CONCLUSION

Substance abuse problems in children and adolescents range from experimentation with gateway substances to full-blown addiction to potent drugs. The younger the experimenting child, the more serious the consequences. Whereas many experimenters do not go on to abuse more potent substances, some eventually become fully addicted despite initial confidence in their ability to control such behavior. These victims of substance abuse should be identified immediately, supported, and treated through appropriate medical and behavioral programs. Commitment of the family is essential. It is important for teachers to educate students to promote the prevention of drug use, to intervene in early-stage substance-abusing behavior, and to take immediate actions on emergent situations of advanced substance abuse. Continuous anti–drug abuse activities in school settings, combined with more broad-based community models, should help create an atmosphere that makes vulnerable minors more resistant to substance abuse.

REFERENCES

American Academy of Pediatrics. (2011). Substance use screening, brief intervention, and referral to treatment for pediatricians. *Pediatrics, 128,* e1330–e1340.

American Association of Poison Control Centers. (2013). *Bath salts data December 31,* 2013. Retrieved from https://aapcc.s3.amazonaws.com/files/library/Bath_Salts_Web_Data_through_12.2013_3.pdf

American Psychiatric Association. (2013). *Diagnostic and statistical manual of mental disorders* (5th ed.). Retrieved from http://www.dsm.psychiatryonline.org

Antoniou, T., & Juurlink, D. N. (2012). Five things to know about "bath salts." *Canadian Medical Association Journal, 184*(15), 1713.

Antoniou, T., & Juurlink, D. N. (2014). Synthetic cannabinoids. *Canadian Medical Association Journal, 186*(3), 210.

Boak, A., Hamilton, H. A., Adlaf, E. M., & Mann, R. E. (2013). Drug use among Ontario students, 1977–2013: *Detailed OSDUHS findings* (CAMH Research Document Series No. 36). Toronto, ON: Centre for Addiction and Mental Health.

Cloninger, C. R., Dinwiddie, S. H., & Reich, T. (1989). Epidemiology and genetics of alcoholism. *Annual Review of Psychiatry, 8*, 331–346.

Centers for Disease Control and Prevention. (2013). *Smoking and tobacco use: Fast facts.* Retrieved from http://www.cdc.gov/tobacco/data_statistics/fact_sheets/fast_facts/

Chambers, R. A., Taylor, J. R., & Potenza, M. N. (2003). Developmental neurocircuitry of motivation in adolescence: A critical period of addiction vulnerability. *American Journal of Psychiatry, 160*, 1041–1052.

Consumer Reports. (2012). *The buzz on energy-drink caffeine.* Retrieved from http://consumerreports.org/cro/magazine/2012/12/the-buzz-on-energy-drink-caffeine/index.htm

Cox, B. M., Goldstein, A., & Nelson, W. T. (1984). Nicotine self-administration in rats. *British Journal of Pharmacology, 83*, 49–55.

Degenhardt, L., Dierker, L., Chiu, W. T., Medina-Mora, M. E., Neumark, Y., Sampson, N., . . . Kessler, R. C. (2010). Evaluating the drug use "gateway" theory using cross-national data: Consistency and associations of the order of initiation of drug use among participants in the WHO World Mental Health Surveys. *Drug and Alcohol Dependence, 108*, 84–97.

DuRant, R. H., Rickert, V. I., Ashworth, C. S., Newman, C., & Slavens, G. (1993). Use of multiple drugs among adolescents who use anabolic steroids. *New England Journal of Medicine, 328*, 922–926.

Eggertson, L. (2014). Children as young as six sniffing gas in Pikangikum. *Canadian Medical Association Journal, 186*(3), 171–172.

Falck, R. S., Nahhas, R. W., Li, L., & Carlson, R. G. (2012), Surveying teens in school to assess the prevalence of problematic drug use. *Journal of School Health, 82*, 217–224.

Felts, W. M., Chenier, T., & Barnes, R. (1992). Drug use and suicide ideation and behavior among North Carolina public school students. *American Journal of Public Health, 82*, 870–872.

Fried, P. A., & Watkinson, B. (2001). Differential effects on facets of attention in adolescents prenatally exposed to cigarettes and marihuana. *Neurotoxicology and Teratology, 23*, 421–430.

Hibell, B., Guttormsson, U., Ahlström, S., Balakireva, O., Bjarnason, T., Kokkevi, A., & Kraus, L. (2012). *The 2011 ESPAD report: Substance use among students in 36 European countries.* Stockholm, Sweden: Swedish Council for Information on Alcohol and Other Drugs.

Holden, C. (1991). Probing the complex genetics of alcoholism. *Science, 251*, 163–164.

Jacobs, E. A., Joffe, A., Knight, J. R., Kulig, J., Rogers, P. D., Boyd, G. M., . . . Smith, K. (2001). Tobacco's toll: Implications for the pediatrician. *Pediatrics, 107*(4), 1025–1029.

James, J. E., Kristjánsson, A. L., & Sigfúsdóttir, I. D. (2011). Adolescent substance use, sleep, and academic achievement: Evidence of harm due to caffeine. *Journal of Adolescence, 34*(4), 665–673.

Johnston, L. D., O'Malley, P. M., Miech, R. A, Bachman, J. G., & Schulenberg, J. E. (2014). *Monitoring the Future national results on drug use: 1975–2013: Overview, key findings on adolescent drug use.* Ann Arbor, MI: Institute for Social Research, University of Michigan. Available at http://www.monitoringthefuture.org

Kandel, D., & Yamaguchi, K. (1993). From beer to crack: Developmental patterns of drug involvement. *American Journal of Public Health, 83*, 851–855.

Knight, J. R., Sherritt, L., Shrier L. A., Harris, S. K., & Chang, G. (2002). Validity of the CRAFFT substance abuse screening test among adolescent clinic patients. *Archives of Pediatrics & Adolescent Medicine, 156*(6), 607–614.

Landfield, P. W., Cadwallader, L. B., & Vinsant, S. (1988). Quantitative changes in hippocampal structure following long-term exposure to delta 9-tetrahydrocannabinol: Possible mediation by glucocorticoid systems. *Brain Research, 443*, 47–62.

Langston, J. W., Ballard, P., Tetrud, J. W., & Irwin, I. (1983). Chronic Parkinsonism in humans due to product of meperidine-analog synthesis. *Science, 219*, 979–980.

Lillie-Blanton, M., Anthony, J. C., & Schuster, C. (1993). Probing the meaning of racial/ethnic group comparisons in crack cocaine smoking. *Journal of the American Medical Association, 269*, 993–997.

Marzuk, P. M., Tardiff, K., Smyth, D., Stajic, M., & Leon, A. C. (1992). Cocaine use, risk taking, and fatal Russian roulette. *Journal of the American Medical Association, 267*, 2635–2637.

Myers, M. G., & Brown, S. A. (1994). Smoking and health in substance abusing adolescents: A two-year follow-up. *Pediatrics, 93*, 561–566.

Sivilotti, M. L. A., Burns, M. J., Aaron, C. K., & Greenberg, M. J. (2001). Pentobarbital for severe gamma-butyrolactone withdrawal. *Annals of Emergency Medicine, 38*(6), 660–665.

Substance Abuse and Mental Health Services Administration. (2011). *Identifying mental health and substance use problems of children and adolescents: A guide for child-serving organizations* (HHS Publication No. SMA 12-4670). Rockville, MD: Author. Retrieved from http://www.samhsa.gov/children/508compliant_Identifying_MH_and_SU_Problems_1-30-2012.pdf

Substance Abuse and Mental Health Services Administration. (2013). *Results from the 2012 National Survey on Drug Use and Health: Summary of National Findings.* Retrieved from http://www.samhsa.gov/data/NSDUH/2012SummNatFindDetTables/NationalFindings/NSDUHresults2012.htm

Terry-McElrath, Y. M., O'Malley, P. M., & Johnston, L. D. (2013). Energy drinks, soft drinks, and substance use among United States secondary school students. *Journal of Addiction Medicine, 8*(1), 6–13.

UN Office on Drugs and Crime. (2013). *World drug report 2013.* Retrieved from http://www.unodc.org/unodc/secured/wdr/wdr2013/World_Drug_Report_2013.pdf

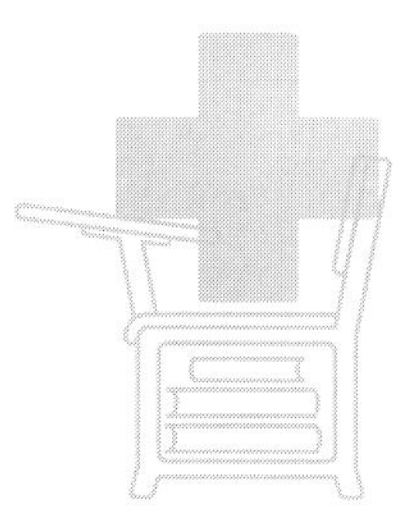

Chapter 16
Autism-Spectrum Disorders

Lonnie Zwaigenbaum and Susan Bobbitt

Autism-spectrum disorder (ASD) is a form of developmental disability characterized by difficulties with communicating and interacting with others, and a pattern of restricted and repetitive interests and behaviors that further interfere with social relationships and general adaptability. The field has recently transitioned to a new clinical definition of ASD, with the implementation of the 5th edition of the *Diagnostic and Statistical Manual of Mental Disorders* (DSM-5; American Psychiatric Association, 2013). Currently, ASD is a single diagnostic category that comprises a diverse group of individuals who share challenges in social communication and behavioral flexibility but differ in developmental course, symptom pattern, and severity, as well as language, cognitive, and learning abilities. Previously, the "autism spectrum" included specific subtypes including autistic disorder, the prototypic form, Asperger syndrome, which was characterized by less severe cognitive and language handicaps, and pervasive developmental disorder not otherwise specified (PDD-NOS), characterized by subthreshold symptoms and/or later onset (see DSM-IV; American Psychiatric Association, 2000). Assessments completed prior to the implementation of DSM-5 may refer to these diagnostic subtypes. Although there has been concern about shifts in criteria and the potential for children to be reclassified and lose services (Zwaigenbaum, 2012), the DSM-5 specifies that individuals with previously established DSM-IV diagnoses of autistic disorder, Asperger syndrome, or PDD-NOS are automatically considered to have ASD.

The clinical features of ASD, as defined in the DSM-5 (American Psychiatric Association, 2013), occur on a continuum. Social and communication challenges in individuals with ASD affect their ability to participate in back-and-forth interaction (e.g., two-way conversation, play activities) in a flexible manner that takes into account the perspective of their social partner. They have difficulties with nonverbal aspects of communication, for example, use of eye gaze and gestures, and the quality of how these different modalities are coordinated. They also experience difficulties in developing, maintaining, and understanding relationships appropriate to their developmental level. Some students with ASD appear to have reduced interest in peers, but they are often interested in having friends and being part of group activities. However, they are often unsure of how to make the initial approach, or they do so in ways that are inappropriate, given their reduced awareness of social expectations. Also, individuals with ASD are often preoccupied with interests that are unusual in their intensity or focus, which also interferes with their ability to interact appropriately with peers. Even when they have interests that are shared by other children their age, their tendency to perseverate on a topic or fixate on highly specific aspects (e.g., the exact horsepower of their favorite cars), may make it difficult for them to use that shared interest as an effective launching pad for interactions with peers. As well, their difficulties coping with minor changes in routine, transitions between activities, and with various aspects of the sensory environment (e.g., sounds, odors, tactile sensations) can lead to emotional dysregulation and meltdowns. These extreme reactions often further interfere with peer relationships and contribute to challenges with behavioral management in the classroom. Some students with autism also display unusual speech patterns (e.g., repeating phrases from favorite movies) and/or repetitive motor habits (e.g., hand flapping) and actions with objects (e.g., tapping or spinning classroom items). Such narrow, repetitive interests and behavioral rigidity compound difficulties with social communication to strain peer relationships, and reduce the child's ability to meet classroom expectations. In addition, students with ASD, even those with above-average intellectual abilities, frequently have specific learning disabilities and difficulties with attention and self-monitoring, which interfere with their academic performance. Thus, children with ASD often experience myriad social, emotional–behavioral, and academic challenges in the classroom.

ASD is among the most common developmental disorders, currently diagnosed in more than 1% of all school-age children in Canada and the United States (Centers for Disease Control, 2014; Lazoff, Zhong, Piperni, & Fombonne, 2010). ASD is three to four times more commonly diagnosed in boys than in girls. There has been a marked increase in the estimated rates of ASD over the past 30 years, which has been attributed, at least in part, to broader case definition, greater awareness among professional groups, and improved tracking systems (Fombonne, 2009). ASD tends to run in families, with a 10%–20% risk to children who have an older sibling with ASD (Ozonoff et al., 2011; Risch et al., 2014; Sandin et al., 2014). There is a strong genetic component, with substantial progress in recent years in both the sophistication of genetic testing methods in clinical labs and the identification of specific genes responsible for vulnerability to ASD in some families (Carter & Scherer, 2013). However, there is also growing evidence that vulnerability to ASD is not due entirely to genetics; that is, it could be due to environmental factors and/or interactions between genetic vulnerability and environmental exposures. For example, there are some families in which one identical twin is diagnosed with ASD and the other twin is not (Sandin et al., 2014), although the second twin may have other developmental challenges. The same is true of younger siblings of children with ASD: Even among those who do not develop ASD, there are high rates of milder developmental and/or social-emotional difficulties (Messinger et al., 2013). Regardless of whether the main influences are genetic or other factors, parents of students with ASD often need supports for their other children as well.

The clinical spectrum of ASD has changed over time. In the past, a substantial proportion of children with ASD had limited speech and significant intellectual disabilities and rarely completed high school or functioned independently as adults (Lotter, 1974). In contrast, currently the majority of individuals with ASD can communicate verbally, and function within or above the average range of intellectual functioning, although many have specific learning disabilities. An increasing number of adolescents complete high school and some move on to postsecondary education and the workforce, although they face many challenges in those environments. Rising rates as well as concerted efforts to raise awareness and advocate for the needs of the broad spectrum of affected individuals has brought ASD increasingly into the public spotlight. Indeed, ASD was once regarded as a rare condition and received minimal attention in health and educational and professional training programs. Currently, most teachers will encounter students with ASD in their classrooms or as part of the broader school community, and there is increasing need to incorporate ASD-related topics into training curricula. Working with students with ASD can be extremely rewarding, but the complexities of this multifaceted condition have implications for instructional approaches, management of the classroom environment, and supporting peer relationships.

In this chapter, we discuss the defining features of ASD and how these may be expressed in different age groups, common associated physical and mental health conditions and implications for management at school, general strategies to promote successful integration of children with ASD, and common learning challenges and strategies for promoting success. We also discuss strategies for fostering positive relationships between students with ASD and their peers, and for addressing negative interactions that can occur, including bullying.

AUTISM-SPECTRUM DISORDER: SYMPTOM EXPRESSION ACROSS THE AGE RANGE

Parents of children with ASD typically recall initial concerns in the first two years of life—frequently, late speech and/or lack of social engagement—and recent research involving at-risk infants suggests that the earliest behavioral signs may be detected by 12 months of age (for a review, see Zwaigenbaum et al., 2009). However, the average age at which ASD is diagnosed is around 4 years, and children with more subtle symptoms or less severe language and/or intellectual delays may not be diagnosed until much later (Daniels & Mandell, 2013). As such, there are many children with ASD who are not diagnosed until they have entered school. There is considerable diversity among children with ASD in terms of their behavioral symptoms, and each child's symptoms can also change considerably over time. As such, there is no single clinical profile that be considered "typical" for a child with ASD at any age; indeed, there is an oft-quoted saying in the ASD community: "If you've seen one child with autism, you've seen one child with autism." However, there are some features that may be more prominent than others in particular age groups, and variation in the types of behaviors that raise concerns regarding those children with ASD who have not yet been diagnosed. Although one should be sensitive to the full range of ASD-related symptoms, and keep in mind that there is no single symptom that confirms the diagnosis (or if absent, excludes the possibility), the following descriptions may help identify children with ASD and some of their greatest challenges at different ages.

Preschool (≤5 Years)

Although impairments in verbal communication are common in preschool children with ASD, there are specific features that distinguish

ASD from isolated language delay. Deficits in *nonverbal* communication are more specific to ASD. These deficits include reduced eye contact and use of gestures, such as pointing, and/or difficulty with coordinating eye gaze with other communication. For example, in contrast to typically developing toddlers and preschoolers, children with ASD may not point to show something of interest and then look back at another person to draw their attention to it (referred to as initiating joint attention; Mundy, Gwaltney, & Henderson, 2010). There may also be unusual patterns of *verbal* communication, such as use of scripts or lengthy phrases or sentences memorized from favorite videos (or from listening to parents or teachers), or abnormalities in the pitch or rhythm (prosody) of speech (McCann et al., 2007). Examples of the latter are speaking in monotone and ending every statement as if it were a question. Although there are many typically developing young children who have difficulty transitioning between activities and thrive on structure and predictability, children with ASD may be distinguished by what can be catastrophic reactions to what seem like minor changes in routine and/or any interference with repetitive play activities, such as lining up or arranging toys and other objects. Unusual reactions to aspects of the sensory environment, either fascination (e.g., watching objects spin) and/or aversion (extreme distress to specific sounds) are also common in preschool children with ASD, and they may be accompanied by repetitive motor behaviors, such as hand flapping.

Some preschool children with ASD have more subtle features, which can contribute to delays in diagnosis. Indeed, the DSM-5 (American Psychiatric Association, 2013) does not include a minimum age of onset, but rather, symptoms that are "present early in development but may not become fully manifest until social demands exceed ability to compensate" (p. 50). Some children with ASD have less overt impairments in basic aspects of social communication (e.g., eye gaze, efforts to direct others' attention to topics or objects of interest) but still tend to interact with others in a manner that is unusually one-sided. For example, such a child may dominate conversations by perseverating on topics of special interest, regardless of the context or listener, or greet others in a friendly albeit highly stereotyped manner, such as asking the same sequence of questions each time. Such a child, especially if they are highly verbal and enjoy sharing their interests with adults (who are more likely to accommodate to a child's idiosyncrasies than their peers might), may be viewed as charming and precocious rather than as having a disability. Keen interests and an ongoing personality might mask difficulties with reciprocal social interaction and behavioral flexibility until they are somewhat older, and unable to cope with increasing expectations to adapt to rules and routines outside of their control, and engage in cooperative activities with peers.

School Age (6–12 Years)

Older children with ASD may exhibit features similar to those described in the first paragraph above describing preschoolers. However, follow-up studies tend to report that the communication and social skills of children diagnosed in the preschool years gradually improve (Soke et al., 2011; Szatmari et al., 2003), even if levels of restricted interests and repetitive behavior remain relatively stable (Joseph, Thurm, Farmer, & Shumway, 2013; Soke et al., 2011). Children with severe symptoms tend to be diagnosed during the preschool years (APA, 2013), so children with ASD who are not detected until after entering elementary school may have less obvious features. This resonates with the notion that ASD may not be "fully manifest until social demands [exceed] (a child's ability) to compensate" (p. 50). In part because of increasing expectations for independent work and to follow classroom rules and routines, children with ASD who enter the school system without a diagnosis may be identified because of attention and/or emotional-behavioral problems rather than because of social difficulties. They may appear inattentive for a number of reasons. They may have difficulty shifting from narrow interests or be distracted by aspects of the sensory environment (e.g., background noise) that other children are able to ignore. They may also not fully understand their teachers' instructions. Children with ASD often have weaker comprehension than their expressive language level (Tager-Flusberg & Caronna, 2007; Volden et al., 2011) and struggle to interpret abstract or figurative language. The child may have emotional outbursts and/or refuse to comply with the teacher's instructions, giving the impression of oppositional–defiant behavior. Yet the child may actually be reacting to minor changes in routine that go unnoticed by classmates or be experiencing anxiety related to interrupted rituals or having to shift from obsessional interests. Social difficulties may be more apparent during less structured interactions with peers on the playground, yet they may also come to attention because of conflicts or inappropriate behavior (e.g., aggression) rather than because of the child's social difficulties (e.g., understanding the perspectives of others). The longer the child's ASD diagnosis remains undetected, the greater the risk that repeated negative experiences in the classroom and on the playground will lead to increasing anxiety and/or depressed or irritable mood, which may fuel a vicious cycle of worsening behavior and deteriorating relationships with peers and teachers. The same set of criteria used to diagnose ASD in preschool children applies to older children, but recognizing the social communication deficits and cognitive rigidity that underlie the more obvious disruptive behaviors can be challenging.

Adolescents (13 Years and Older)

Although most individuals with ASD are diagnosed during early childhood, there are some who are not diagnosed until adolescence or adulthood. As with school-age children, individuals with later diagnoses generally have more subtle symptoms and less language and/or intellectual impairment. Diagnostic assessment in this age group may be complicated by secondary mental health problems. In fact, even among adolescents who were diagnosed with ASD earlier in childhood, comorbid anxiety and depression are common, occurring in as many as 50% of those diagnosed (Mattila et al., 2010). Core social communication symptoms may be less obvious than at earlier ages but still cause significant impairment to day-to-day functioning. Many adolescents with ASD continue to have difficulty understanding abstract language, such as humor and sarcasm, and as a result they may misinterpret what others are saying. Although they may learn the basic conventions of back-and-forth conversation, they may continue to dwell on their own special interests and have difficulty with small talk and adapting their conversational style to various partners and contexts (de Villiers, Fine, Ginsberg, Vaccarella, & Szatmari, 2007). Many adolescents with ASD have ongoing difficulty recognizing nonverbal cues (e.g., facial expression, body language; Koning & Magill-Evans, 2001), which leads to further confusion about others' intentions. These factors all contribute to difficulty interacting with others and developing peer relationships. Some adolescents with ASD are able to make friends, albeit often with other individuals with ASD, and of poorer quality with respect to closeness (e.g., trust and emotional intimacy) compared to friendships reported by their typically developing peers (Locke, Ishijima, Kasari, & London, 2010). Sometimes these friendships center on participating in specific recreational activities of shared interest (e.g., online gaming; Kuo, Magill-Evans, & Zwaigenbaum, 2014) and do not involve social contacts beyond that activity. Recent data from the U.S. National Longitudinal Transition Study show that as adolescents with ASD approach adulthood, they frequently find themselves without regular social contacts. A discouraging 66.7% of young adults with ASD report less than monthly communication from a friend, and 48.1% report never being invited to social activities (Orsmond et al., 2013). These are much higher rates than what young adults with intellectual or learning disabilities reported. Recent interventions aimed at helping children and adolescents with ASD improve their social skills and become more proactive in initiating social contacts show promise (reviewed by Laugeson, 2013). These interventions (e.g., Program for the Education and Enrichment of Relational Skills, or PEERS; Laugeson, Frankel, Gantman, Dillon, & Mogil, 2012) can be delivered either at home by parents or at school by teachers (Laugeson, Ellingsen, Sanderson, Tucci, & Bates, 2014) and lead to sustained improvement in social skills and the frequency of get-togethers with peers. However, it remains to be seen whether such interventions will lead to lasting effects, helping adolescents with ASD establish friendships that carry on past high school. Supporting friendships and broader social engagement should be considered an important priority in educational planning for children and adolescents with ASD, as there are significant long-term implications (Orsmond et al., 2013). Adolescents should also be given opportunity for work-related experiences during high school, to gain relevant skills and experience to help open doors for future competitive employment.

ASSOCIATED HEALTH CONDITIONS

Although ASD is defined based on symptoms related to social communication and repetitive interests and behaviors, it is also recognized that functional impairments associated with the disorder reflect a broader range of associated (or comorbid) health conditions (Coury, 2010). These conditions can significantly affect students' classroom performance and emotional-behavioral state, and thus they are important to recognize and treat. Although details regarding medical management are beyond the scope of this chapter, there are excellent, evidence-based resources available online for both parents and professionals (e.g., at the Autism Speaks website, http://www.autismspeaks.org/family-services/tool-kits).

Epilepsy

Students with ASD are at higher risk of epilepsy than their typically developing peers. Epilepsy is a chronic brain disorder characterized by recurrent seizures: brief episodes of involuntary shaking and/or loss of consciousness. These episodes result from abnormal electrical discharge in the brain. Children most commonly have their first seizure during the preschool years or during adolescence (in contrast to typically developing students with epilepsy, in whom adolescent onset is uncommon). Recent data suggest that approximately one in four children with ASD is diagnosed with epilepsy by age 17, in contrast to less than 1% of the general population (Viscidi et al., 2013). Epilepsy is more common among children with ASD who have intellectual disabilities, but occurs across all cognitive levels.

As with other students with epilepsy, seizures in children with ASD can range from brief lapses in attention or muscle jerks to severe and prolonged convulsions. Characteristics of seizures depend on where in the brain the abnormal electrical discharge starts and where it spreads. Complex partial seizures, or focal seizures (often associated with prolonged staring or loss of awareness, sometimes with repetitive movements, such as of the mouth), are most common, but any seizure type can occur in children with ASD. Untreated seizures can lead to marked disruption in concentration and academic performance, and prolonged generalized seizures can compromise the child's breathing ability and lead to risk of injury as a result of jerky movements. Unexplained staring spells, episodes of reduced responsiveness (even to touch), and/or involuntary movements should prompt an urgent assessment by the child's physician for possible epilepsy. Epilepsy may be managed by the child's physician or by referral to a specialist (e.g., child neurologist), and the overall treatment plan should include guidance to school staff regarding seizure management. Even when seizures are well controlled, students with ASD and epilepsy may be at higher risk of irritable mood and/or hyperactivity (Viscidi et al., in press). Medications used to treat epilepsy may also affect mood and concentration. However, most children with ASD and epilepsy are able to return to their previous level of functioning once seizures are well controlled (see Chapter 13).

Sleep Disorders

Sleep problems are common among typically developing children and adolescents, but even more so among those with ASD. Elevated rates of sleep problems (as high as 50%–80%; Coury, 2010; Goldman, Richdale, Clemons, & Malow, 2012) may relate to both behavioral symptoms (e.g., responses to the sensory environment, difficulties with transition) as well as the underlying biology of ASD (e.g., abnormalities in the "clock genes" regulating the melatonin biosynthesis pathway; Bourgeron, 2007). Moreover, there are serious medical conditions that occur in children with ASD that can initially present with disrupted sleep, such as epilepsy (see above), obstructive sleep apnea, and restless-leg syndrome. However, the types of sleep problems experienced by children and adolescents with ASD are generally similar to those of typically developing similar-aged peers (Goldman et al., 2012). For example, difficulties settling and staying asleep are common among young preschool and school-age children with ASD, whereas teens with ASD often experience delayed sleep-phase disorders (i.e., get stuck in the pattern of staying up too late and having trouble getting up in the morning). Disrupted sleep can lead to reduced attention span, irritable mood, and worsening behaviors (e.g., hyperactivity, emotional outbursts, aggression) (Sikora, Johnson, Clemons, & Katz, 2012) and add to family stress, as parents' sleep is also likely to be disrupted if their children are awake at night. Thus, impaired sleep should be considered as a possible contributor when students with ASD exhibit worsening behavior or attention span, especially after a major change in routine (e.g., following a school holiday break). Families should follow up with their child's community physician for assessment and discussion of treatment options (Malow et al., 2014). Parent-mediated interventions to help restore healthy sleep habits, modeled on successful approaches used in typically developing children, can also be effective in children with ASD (Malow et al., 2014).

Gastrointestinal Issues

Children with ASD have more parent-reported gastrointestinal symptoms than children who are typically developing or who have other developmental delays (Chaidez, Hansen, & Hertz-Picciotto, 2014). Constipation is most common, but other symptoms are reported as well, including recurrent abdominal pain, bloating, gaseousness, and diarrhea. It is not yet clear whether these symptoms are secondary to unusual patterns of food intake, or stem from gastrointestinal dysfunction inherent to ASD. Many children with ASD have a limited repertoire of food preferences (Marshall, Hill, Ziviani, & Dodrill, 2014), and some families place their children on restrictive diets (e.g., the gluten-free, casein-free) in hopes of improvement in ASD-related symptoms despite limited evidence of efficacy (Dosman et al., 2013). However, a recent study suggested that gastrointestinal symptoms in children with ASD were unrelated to dietary habits (Gorrindo et al., 2012). Regardless, common gastrointestinal symptoms such as constipation in children with ASD respond to conventional treatments, and families should be advised to speak to their community health provider if they have concerns (Furuta et al., 2012). Untreated constipation and other uncontrolled symptoms can be associated with irritable mood and restlessness in students with ASD (Chaidez et al., 2014), as in other children.

Associated Emotional–Behavioral Conditions

Anxious tendencies (e.g., in relation to the sensory environment and/or changes in classroom routine), behavioral inflexibility, and difficulty modulating attentional focus are common correlates of ASD symptoms and are almost invariably part of the overall clinical profile of students with ASD (Georgiades et al., 2011). In addition, there are many students with ASD who meet full criteria for additional diagnoses such as attention deficit hyperactivity disorder, anxiety, and/or mood disorders, which creates additional challenges for learning, socializing, and behavioral adaptation. Indeed, rates of emotional–behavioral disorders across the diagnostic spectrum are higher among students with ASD than among typically developing students (Kim et al., 2000; Mattila et al., 2010). This is also the case among intellectually disabled students: Rates across a range of emotional–behavioral disorders are generally higher among intellectually normal youth with ASD than among those with intellectual disability alone (Bradley, Summers, Wood, & Bryson, 2004). Treatment strategies that are effective in students with these disorders who do not have ASD can be helpful for students who have both ASD and these other diagnoses. For example, both behavioral management strategies and medications used in other children with ASD can be effective for children with ASD plus ADHD (Mahajan et al., 2012). Children with ASD plus anxiety disorders can respond to therapeutic approaches that are effective for children with anxiety alone; specifically, to cognitive behavioral therapy, which helps children develop coping and perspective-taking skills to allow them to manage anxious thoughts and feelings (Sukhodolsky, Bloch, Panza, & Reichow, 2013). However, the presence of ASD symptoms (e.g., communication impairments) can make these therapies more difficult to implement, and in some communities there may be limited access to therapists who have experience in working with children and youth with ASD.

Learning Challenges

The intellectual abilities of individuals with ASD vary from the severely handicapped range to the highest levels of giftedness, and accordingly, learning and academic skills also vary across a broad continuum. There are also specific challenges related to core symptoms that can impair learning and lead to underachievement relative to overall intellectual capacity (reviewed in Jordan, 2005). For example, young students with ASD may not as intuitively orient when their teacher is talking and may not detect nonverbal aspects of their teacher's communication (e.g., facial expression and tone of voice, gestures). As a result, these students may not understand what is expected of them on a given task, and also not benefit from their teacher's efforts to cue the class to important topics and activities. Children with ASD may attend suboptimally because of difficulties shifting their attention from special interests, or because of distress and/or distractions related to aspects of the sensory environment (e.g., noise level, visual stimuli). There are also specific related neuropsychological deficits associated with ASD that can have a negative effect on academic achievement, particularly as children progress through the school system. For example, even highly intelligent children and youth with ASD often have specific deficits in the executive functions, which include self-monitoring, the ability to shift attention between one aspect of a task to another, working memory, and planning and organizational skills (O'Hearn, Asato, Ordaz, & Luna, 2008). These challenges become more apparent as students move through the school system and are faced with completing projects that require multiple stages of preparation, and tests or exams that require studying outside of class.

Although there has been relatively little research on specific learning disabilities in students with ASD, it does appear that students with ASD tend to have a more uneven learning profile than their peers and often have at least one area of academic achievement that is lagging behind. For example, Jones et al. (2009), in a study of 100 youths with ASD (14–16 years old), reported that 73% had at least one area of literacy or mathematical achievement that was discrepant from general intellectual ability by at least a full standard deviation. The most common profile was characterized by poor reading comprehension. This finding is consistent with previous research on language arts skills in students with ASD, which has consistently identified that a substantial proportion (though not all) experience weak comprehension, despite adequate reading skills (Ricketts, 2011). It is also important to note that weaknesses in reading comprehension are not limited to students with ASD with overt delays in expressive and receptive language skills (Norbury & Nation, 2011). Moreover, weak reading comprehension may correlate with severity of social communication symptoms in students with ASD (Jones et al., 2009; Ricketts, Jones, Happé, & Charman, 2013). Given that social deficits in ASD extend to understanding the mental states of others, it may be difficult for students with ASD to read between the lines and interpret the intentions and preferences of the characters in a story that are not explicitly stated (Ricketts, 2011). There are also some students with ASD who experience specific difficulties in math skills (Chiang & Lin, 2007; Jones et al., 2009). It should be noted that the presence of "splinter" or "savant" skills (islets of exceptional ability), such as the ability to make mental calculations, generally does not correlate with overall understanding of math concepts or problem-solving skills. However, some students with ASD genuinely have exceptional mathematical reasoning abilities (generally, without savant skills) (Chiang & Lin, 2007; Grigorenko, Klin, & Volkmas, 2003; Jones et al., 2009). Likewise, although weak comprehension skills are common, there are some students with ASD with genuine strengths in this area (Jones et al., 2009; Ricketts, 2011). Ultimately, there is no single learning profile that is consistently associated with ASD, and many factors influence a student's performance on academic tasks, including their ASD symptoms, comorbid emotional–behavioral symptoms, and aspects of the classroom environment (including available supports and accommodations). An individualized approach that takes account of these various factors is needed to optimize success.

STRATEGIES TO PROMOTE SUCCESSFUL INTEGRATION OF CHILDREN WITH ASD

Children with ASD can be, and have been, successfully included within mainstream classrooms. This is usually most successful when schools and classroom teachers have had opportunities to understand the presentation and manifestations of ASD, and to explore and try different classroom strategies and interventions. Students with ASD may need different strategies from those employed for other children in the classroom (Kasari, Rotheram-Fuller, Locke, & Gulsrud, 2012). A close working relationship with the parents of the child with ASD is important and essential to ensure consistency and mutual support both inside and outside of the classroom. In addition, input from therapists from various disciplines with special expertise in working with students with ASD can be extremely helpful in developing and implementing a comprehensive support plan. For example, speech–language pathologists are critical in fostering the student's development of functional communication skills and ensuring that the student can make him- or herself understood to peers and classroom staff, and vice versa. This may include implementation of augmentative and alternative communication strategies and supports (see below). Occupational therapists can help the child more fully participate in classroom activities and achieve social and academic success by addressing motor deficits, maladaptive behaviors, and the child's sensory processing and potential need for modification of the classroom environment (Arbesman, Bazyk, & Nochajski, 2013). Behavioral consultants can provide further support to analyze what factors trigger and perpetuate maladaptive behaviors, and develop a tailored management plan (Crosland & Dunlap, 2012). Current best practice focuses on positive behavioral supports, which emphasizes reinforcing preferred behaviors (e.g., with praise, or using a token system) and setting up the child for success by setting achievable short-term goals, which are modified as the child progresses (Crosland & Dunlap, 2012). Clinical psychologists may serve this role and/or provide in-depth psychoeducational assessments to help inform an individualized learning plan and supports aimed at promoting academic success. Resource teachers and other school-board consultants also address many of these areas, working in partnership with classroom teachers to promote the child's learning as well as social and emotional development. Although the planning process needs to be individualized, in this section, we summarize some general principles and strategies that are often helpful for students with ASD (also see Jordan, 2005).

Structure, Routine, and Visual Supports

Many children with ASD prefer a structured environment. It is important for the classroom teacher to establish a routine and strive to keep it consistent. Routines should be clearly defined and demonstrated. It is often helpful to break down the routine into smaller, more discrete steps, to make it less overwhelming and easier to understand. For example, a possible morning routine could look like this:

> Enter the classroom.
> Say "Good morning" to the teacher.
> Say "Good morning" to the friend standing next to you.
> Hang up your jacket.
> Place your backpack and your lunch kit where they belong.
> Sit down at your desk and wait for class to begin.

Each of these steps could be matched with a specific visual to help make the routine easier for the child to follow and remember. Multiple-step lists can also be used to help the student with ASD successfully complete a wide range of classroom tasks and activities, from the bathroom routine to specific helping roles (e.g., handing out a snack), story writing, and more complex tasks. Pairing these steps with specific visuals, particularly for younger or less verbal students, helps make each step clearer and easier to remember. Visual schedules that list the activities of the school day and calendars that identify on what days of the week certain activities occur can be very effective in helping orient and prepare the child to follow classroom routines. Children with ASD know what to expect and can put more attention toward learning when visuals are used. Other examples of classroom supports employing visual aids are summarized below (Schreibman & Stahmer, 2014).

Social Stories

A Social Story illustrates situations, skills, or concepts in terms of appropriate social cues, perspectives, and common responses in a specifically defined style and format. Social Stories were created by Carol Gray to help individuals with ASD break down tasks or social situations into smaller steps with descriptive words and pictures (Gray & Garand, 1993). In a recent systematic review of six clinical trials that evaluated the effectiveness of Social Stories, Karkhaneh et al. (2014) concluded that the use of Social Stories was associated with improvements in a variety of aspects of social interaction, including facial emotion learning and labeling and adopting specific social skills addressed in the stories (e.g., introducing oneself to another person, saying kind things to others, following rules in a turn-taking game). In the classroom, Social Stories can be used to describe a classroom routine. Teachers and teaching assistants can include potential modifications to the routine to better enable a child with ASD to recognize and anticipate that sometimes routines and transitions in the classroom may not go as smoothly as hoped (Thompson & Johnston, 2013).

Picture Exchange Communication System (PECS)

The PECS system (Bondy & Frost, 1998) is a form of augmentative and alternative communication that might be considered (in consultation with the school board's speech–language pathologist) to provide nonverbal students with ASD with the ability to communicate with others using pictures. The PECS system can be implemented and used in a variety of ways. The system can help a child with ASD communicate with those around him or her. It can also be used to provide visual schedules and communicate with the child in an organized, easy-to-understand manner. Beginning to use the PECS system generally starts with pictures of a favorite, desired object to capture the attention and cooperation of the child. For example, if cookies are among the child's preferred stacks, one might introduce the picture symbol:

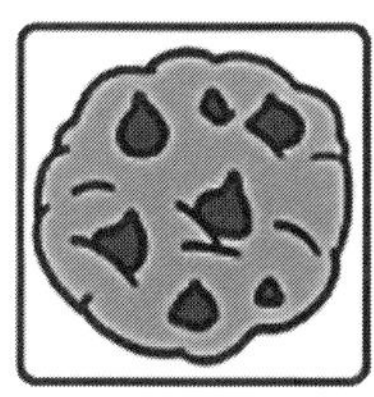

Cookie.

Over time, the system progresses to pictures with sentence strips:

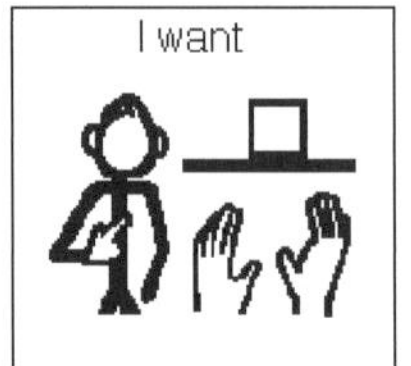

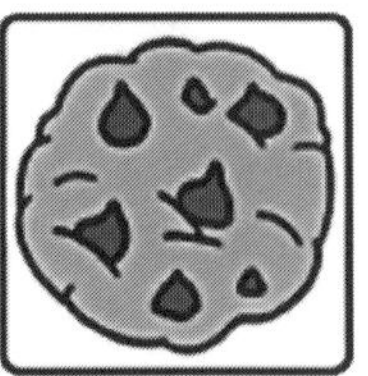

I want a cookie.

The child then builds a vocabulary that is relevant to him or her, and communicates desires, feelings, or observations by using the pictures consistently. It is important to note that although PECS is based on visual pictures, verbal reinforcement is a major component and verbal communication is encouraged as much as possible.

Supports for Transitions

All children must move from one activity to another and from one setting to another throughout their day. Whether at home or school, or during extracurricular activities, transitions occur constantly during the average day. Students with ASD may have greater difficulty with shifting their attention from one task or environment to another. The underlying reasons may vary among individuals and across contexts, but they often include a greater need for predictability, difficulties in understanding what will be coming next, or fear of the unknown, which can increase stress and anxiety and set the stage for a negative behavioral reaction.

Strategies to help students with ASD cope with transitions can be used before a transition occurs, during a transition, and/or after a transition. Visual timers can be helpful as an initial strategy for young children, especially for those who have strengths in visual processing. It should be explained that when the timer goes off, it is time to move to a new setting or move on and start a new activity. Then, the child is informed periodically approximately how much time is left to better prepare them for the buzzer going off. As well, using visual cue cards during a transition can decrease challenging behaviors and increase adherence to transitioning demands.

Other strategies, such as transition objects, can reduce the child's reluctance to move from one activity to another. It can be helpful for the student to carry the transition object, be it a photograph, card, and the like, with him or her to the next activity or location. This allows the student to continually reference information about where he or she is headed or what he or she will be doing as the transition is occurring. Once arriving at the destination or next activity, consider creating a designated space for the student to place the transition object. This indicates to the student that they have transitioned and can begin the next activity. For younger students or nonverbal students who do not understand that pictures can represent upcoming activities, or for whom engaging in verbal cuing is difficult, it may be helpful to show them an actual object relating to the upcoming activity to prepare them for the transition. For example, you could give them a soccer ball to carry to the scheduled gym class.

If the student is having difficulty with a particular transition, it can be useful to let him or her hold on to a "transitional object," such as a special object of their choice. This can help the student feel more in control by having something comforting and familiar in his or her presence. It is also helpful to remove visual distracters from a student's immediate environment. By doing so, you reduce the extraneous visual input and make it easier for the student to identify visual clues that are relevant to whatever he or she is engaging in.

Fostering Positive Peer Relationships

It is increasingly recognized that although students with ASD may struggle to understand the "unspoken rules" of social conduct and become part of their peer group, most children and youth with ASD desire social contact and would like to have friends. Indeed, many students with ASD describe feeling lonely, and the resulting stress from feeling that they don't "fit in" can lead to a vicious cycle of increasing anxiety, depression, and further social withdrawal (White & Roberson-Nay, 2009). Social skills groups for students with ASD are typically designed to help them learn behaviors that better prepare them to participate in friendships (Laugeson, 2013). However, there is some evidence that there is also considerable learning that occurs naturally in the context of a friendship, such as greater interpersonal awareness and prosocial behaviors that place the child with ASD on a trajectory toward enhanced social interaction skills (Bauminger et al., 2008). Thus, while structured, adult therapist-directed social skills groups can be extremely helpful, particularly for older children and adolescents (Laugeson et al., 2012), fostering friendships through get-togethers with peers and participation in recreational activities with other children who share similar interests is also critical, and should begin as early as possible. Teachers and other staff can play an extremely helpful role in promoting positive peer interactions at school (e.g., helping structure an enjoyable turn-taking activity with a classmate) and in helping parents make informed choices about potential play dates outside of school. Classmates as young as 6 years can also be engaged as buddies or mentors and even as assistants in social skills training programs for students with ASD (Kasari et al., 2013; Chung et al., 2007), which can help lead to greater social involvement among the students with ASD and opportunities for typically developing students to become more sensitive and helpful to peers with different developmental needs (Kasari et al., 2013).

It is also important for teachers and principals to be aware of both the prevalence and negative impacts of bullying as experienced by students with ASD (Sterzing, Shattuck, Narendorf, Wagner, & Cooper, 2012). As many as 65%–94% of children and youth with ASD report being bullied at school (van Roekel, Scholte, & Didden, 2010), which exceeds rates among other students in Canadian schools (Vaillancourt et al., 2010). Children with ASD may be even more vulnerable to bullying than other special needs populations, in part because of their core symptoms (including social impairments) and comorbid emotional–behavioral problems. With less opportunity to establish positive relationships with peers, students with ASD then may be misunderstood, overlooked, and more prone to bullying by peers. Children and youth with ASD may be at particular risk to bullying by persons who lack such understanding or compassion, and who may be inclined to assert power over a more vulnerable peer. Individuals with ASD often exhibit behaviors (e.g., repetitive motor mannerisms) that may be seen as unusual or inappropriate by their typically developing peers and adults, and thus they are viewed negatively. Extreme emotional and/or aggressive outbursts are also more common in children and youth with ASD than in their peers, presenting significant challenges in the classroom and on the playground, and leading to further isolation from peers. These behaviors may be exacerbated by difficulties that students with ASD face as they react to rejection and/or overt aggression by peers and various other challenges in everyday interactions and environments.

Responding to these behaviors with greater understanding, acceptance, and targeted intervention invites consideration of the multilayered challenges facing children and youth with ASD (Schroeder, Cappadocia, Bebko, Pepler, & Weiss, 2014). In general, interventions aimed at reducing bullying are most effective when implemented at the level of the entire school and focused on fostering a school climate in which peer victimization is unacceptable in any context, and when there is consistent playground supervision and specific classroom strategies for detecting and addressing bullying (Ttofi & Farington, 2011; also see Vaillancourt's chapter 18 in this book). Ultimately, bullying needs to be both acknowledged and addressed at multiple levels (i.e., peer-to-peer, classroom, school, and community) to promote positive and healthy social relationships for all children and youth.

REFERENCES

American Psychiatric Association. (2000). *Diagnostic and statistical manual of mental disorders* (4th ed.). Arlington, VA: Author.

American Psychiatric Association. (2013). *Diagnostic and statistical manual of mental disorders* (5th ed.). Arlington, VA: Author.

Arbesman, M., Bazyk, S., & Nochajski, S. M. (2013). Systematic review of occupational therapy and mental health promotion, prevention, and intervention for children and youth. *American Journal of Occupational Therapy, 67*(6), e120–e130.

Bauminger, N., Solomon, M., Aviezer, A., Heung, K., Gazit, L., Brown, J., & Rogers, S. J. (2008). Children with autism and their friends: A multidimensional study of friendship in high-functioning autism spectrum disorder. *Journal of Abnormal Child Psychology, 36*(2), 135–150.

Bondy, A. S., & Frost, L. A. (1998). The picture exchange communication system. *Seminars in Speech and Language, 19*(4), 373–388.

Bourgeron, T. (2007). The possible interplay of synaptic and clock genes in autism spectrum disorders. *Cold Spring Harbor Symposium Quantitative Biology, 72*, 645–654.

Bradley, E. A., Summers, J. A., Wood, H. L., & Bryson, S. E. (2004). Comparing rates of psychiatric and behavior disorders in adolescents and young adults with severe intellectual disability with and without autism. *Journal of Autism and Developmental Disorders, 34*(2), 151–161.

Carter, M. T., & Scherer, S. W. (2013). Autism spectrum disorder in the genetics clinic: A review. *Clinical Genetics, 83*(5), 399–407.

Chaidez, V., Hansen, R. L., & Hertz-Picciotto, I. (2014). Gastrointestinal problems in children with autism, developmental delays or typical development. *Journal of Autism and Developmental Disorders, 44*(5), 1117–1127.

Chiang, H. M., & Lin, Y. H. (2007). Mathematical ability of students with Asperger syndrome and high-functioning autism: A review of literature. *Autism, 11*(6), 547–556.

Chung, K. M., Reavis, S., Mosconi, M., Drewry, J., Matthews, T., & Tassé, M. J. (2007). Peer-mediated social skills training program for young children with high-functioning autism. *Research in Developmental Disabilities, 28*(4), 423–436.

Coury, D. (2010). Medical treatment of autism spectrum disorders. *Current Opinions in Neurology, 23*, 131–136.

Crosland, K., & Dunlap, G. (2012). Effective strategies for the inclusion of children with autism in general education classrooms. *Behavior Modification, 36*(3), 251–269.

Daniels, A. M., & Mandell, D. S. (2013). Explaining differences in age at autism spectrum disorder diagnosis: A critical review. *Autism, 18*(5), 583–597.

Developmental Disabilities Monitoring Network Surveillance Year 2010 Principal Investigators & Centers for Disease Control and Prevention. (2014). Prevalence of autism spectrum disorder among children aged 8 years: Autism and developmental disabilities monitoring network, 11 sites, United States, 2010. *MMWR Surveillance Summaries, 63*(2), 1–21.

de Villiers, J., Fine, J., Ginsberg, G., Vaccarella, L., & Szatmari, P. (2007). Brief report: A scale for rating conversational impairment in autism spectrum disorder. *Journal of Autism and Developmental Disorders, 37*, 1375–1380.

Dosman, C., Adams, D., Wudel, B., Vogels, L., Turner, J., & Vohra, S. (2013). Complementary, holistic, and integrative medicine: Autism spectrum disorder and gluten- and casein-free diet. *Pediatrics in Review, 34*(10), e36–e341.

Fombonne, E. (2009). Epidemiology of pervasive developmental disorders. *Pediatric Research, 65*(6), 591–598.

Furuta, G. T., Williams, K., Kooros, K., Kaul, A., Panzer, R., Coury, D. L., & Fuchs, G. (2012). Management of constipation in children and adolescents with autism spectrum disorders. *Pediatrics, 130*(Suppl. 2), S98–S105.

Ganz, J. B., Davis, J. L., Lund, E. M., Goodwyn, F. D., & Simpson, R. L. (2012). Meta-analysis of PECS with individuals with ASD: Investigation of targeted versus non-targeted outcomes, participant characteristics, and implementation phase. *Research in Developmental Disabilities, 33*(2), 406–418.

Georgiades, S., Szatmari, P., Duku, E., Zwaigenbaum, L., Bryson, S., Roberts, W., . . . Pathways in ASD Study Team. (2011). Phenotypic overlap between core diagnostic features and emotional/behavioral problems in preschool children with autism spectrum disorder. *Journal of Autism and Developmental Disorders, 41*(10), 1321–1329.

Goldman, S. E., Richdale, A. L., Clemons, T., & Malow, B. A. (2012). Parental sleep concerns in autism spectrum disorders: Variations from childhood to adolescence. *Journal of Autism and Developmental Disorders, 42*(4), 531–538.

Gorrindo, P., Williams, K. C., Lee, E. B., Walker, L. S., McGrew, S. G., & Levitt, P. (2012). Gastrointestinal dysfunction in autism: Parental report, clinical evaluation, and associated factors. *Autism Research, 5*, 101–108.

Gray, C. A., & Garand, J. (1993). Social stories: Improving responses of individuals with autism with accurate social information. *Focus on Autistic Behavior, 8*, 1–10.

Grigorenko, E. L., Klin, A., & Volkmar, F. (2003). Annotation: Hyperlexia: Disability or superability? *Journal of Child Psychology and Psychiatry, 44*, 1079–1091.

Jones, C. R., Happé, F., Golden, H., Marsden, A. J., Tregay, J., Simonoff, E., . . . Charman, T. (2009). Reading and arithmetic in adolescents with autism spectrum disorders: Peaks and dips in attainment. *Neuropsychology, 23*(6), 718–728.

Jordan, R. (2005). Managing autism and Asperger's syndrome in current educational provision. *Pediatric Rehabilitation, 8*(2), 104–112.

Joseph, L., Thurm, A., Farmer, C., & Shumway, S. (2013). Repetitive behavior and restricted interests in young children with autism: Comparisons with controls and stability over 2 years. *Autism Research, 6*(6), 584–595.

Karkhaneh, M., Clark, B., Ospina, M. B., Seida, J. C., Smith, V., & Hartling, L. (2010). Social Stories to improve social skills in children with autism spectrum disorder: A systematic review. *Autism, 14*(6), 641–662.

Kasari, C., Rotheram-Fuller, E., Locke, J., & Gulsrud, A. (2012). Making the connection: Randomized controlled trial of social skills at school for children with autism spectrum disorders. *Journal of Child Psychology and Psychiatry, 53*(4), 431–439.

Koning, C., & Magill-Evans, J. (2001) Social and language skills in adolescent boys with Asperger syndrome. *Autism, 5*, 23–36.

Kuo, M., Magill-Evans, J., & Zwaigenbaum, L. (2014). Parental mediation of television viewing and videogaming of adolescents with autism spectrum disorder and their siblings. *Autism*.

Laugeson, E. A. (2013). Review: Social skills groups may improve social competence in children and adolescents with autism spectrum disorder. *Evidence-Based Mental Health, 16*, 11.

Laugeson, E. A., Ellingsen, R., Sanderson, J., Tucci, L., & Bates, S. (2014). The ABC's of teaching social skills to adolescents with autism spectrum disorder in the classroom: The UCLA PEERS Program. *Journal of Autism and Developmental Disorders, 44*(9), 2244–2256.

Laugeson, E. A., Frankel, F., Gantman, A., Dillon, A. R., & Mogil, C. (2012). Evidence-based social skills training for adolescents with autism spectrum disorders: The UCLA PEERS program. *Journal of Autism and Developmental Disorders, 42*, 1025–1036.

Lazoff, T., Zhong, L., Piperni, T., & Fombonne, E. (2010). Prevalence of pervasive developmental disorders among children at the English Montreal School Board. *Canadian Journal of Psychiatry, 55*(11), 715–720.

Locke, J., Ishijima, E. H., Kasari, C., & London, N. (2010). Loneliness, friendship quality and the social networks of adolescents with high-functioning autism in an inclusive school setting. *Journal of Research in Special Educational Needs, 10*, 74–81.

Lotter, V. (1974). Factors related to outcome in autistic children. *Journal of Autism and Child Schizophrenia, 4*(3), 263–277.

Mahajan, R., Bernal, M. P., Panzer, R., Whitaker, A., Roberts, W., Handen, B., . . . Autism Speaks Autism Treatment Network Psychopharmacology Committee. (2012). Clinical practice pathways for evaluation and medication choice for attention-deficit/hyperactivity disorder symptoms in autism spectrum disorders. *Pediatrics, 130*(Suppl. 2), S125–S138.

Malow, B. A., Adkins, K. W., Reynolds, A., Weiss, S. K., Loh, A., Fawkes, D., . . . Hundley, R. (2014). Parent-based sleep education for children with autism spectrum disorders. *Journal of Autism and Developmental Disorders, 44*(1), 216–228.

Malow, B. A., Byars, K., Johnson, K., Weiss, S., Bernal, P., Goldman, S. E., . . . Glaze, D. G. (2012). A practice pathway for the identification, evaluation, and management of insomnia in children and adolescents with autism spectrum disorders. *Pediatrics, 130*(Suppl. 2), S106–S124.

Mandelberg, J., Frankel, F., Cunningham, T., Gorospe, C., & Laugeson, E. A. (2014). Long-term outcomes of parent-assisted social skills intervention for high-functioning children with autism spectrum disorders. *Autism, 18*, 255–263.

Marshall, J., Hill, R. J., Ziviani, J., & Dodrill, P. (2014). Features of feeding difficulty in children with autism spectrum disorder. *International Journal of Speech and Language Pathology, 16*(2), 151–158.

Mattila, M. L., Hurtig, T., Haapsamo, H., Jussila, K., Kuusikko-Gauffin, S., Kielinen, M., . . . Moilanen, I. (2010). Comorbid psychiatric disorders associated with Asperger syndrome/high-functioning autism: A community- and clinic-based study. *Journal of Autism and Developmental Disorders, 40*, 1080–1093.

McCann, J., Peppé, S., Gibbon, F. E., O'Hare, A., & Rutherford, M. (2007). Prosody and its relationship to language in school-aged children with high-functioning autism. *International Journal of Language and Communication Disorders, 42*(6), 682–702.

Messinger, D., Young, G. S., Ozonoff, S., Dobkins, K., Carter, A., Zwaigenbaum, L., . . . Sigman, M. (2013). Beyond autism: A baby siblings research consortium study of high-risk children at three years of age. *Journal of the American Academy of Child and Adolescent Psychiatry, 52*(3), 300–308.

Mundy, P., Gwaltney, M., & Henderson, H. (2010). Self-referenced processing, neurodevelopment and joint attention in autism. *Autism, 14*(5), 408–429.

Norbury, C., & Nation, K. (2011). Understanding variability in reading comprehension in adolescents with autism spectrum disorders: Interactions with language status and decoding skill. *Scientific Studies of Reading, 15*(3), 191–210.

O'Hearn, K., Asato, M., Ordaz, S., & Luna, B. (2008). Neurodevelopment and executive function in autism. *Developmental Psychopathology, 20*(4), 1103–1132.

Orsmond, G. I., Shattuck, P. T., Cooper, B. P., Sterzing, P. R., & Anderson, K. A. (2013). Social participation among young adults with an autism spectrum disorder. *Journal of Autism and Developmental Disorders, 43*(11), 2710–2719.

Ozonoff, S., Young, G. S., Carter, A., Messinger, D., Yirmiya, N., Zwaigenbaum, L., . . . Stone, W. L. (2011). Recurrence risk for autism spectrum disorders: A baby siblings research consortium study. *Pediatrics, 128*(3), e488–e495.

Ricketts, J. (2011). Research review: Reading comprehension in developmental disorders of language and communication. *Journal of Child Psychology and Psychiatry, 52*(11), 1111–1123.

Ricketts, J., Jones, C. R., Happé, F., & Charman, T. (2013). Reading comprehension in autism spectrum disorders: The role of oral language and social functioning. *Journal of Autism and Developmental Disorders, 43*(4), 807–816.

Risch, N., Hoffmann, T. J., Anderson, M., Croen, L. A., Grether, J. K., & Windham, G. C. (2014, June 27). Familial recurrence of autism spectrum disorder: Evaluating genetic and environmental contributions. *American Journal of Psychiatry*. [Advance web publication]. doi:10.1176/appi.ajp.2014.13101359.

Sandin, S., Lichtenstein, P., Kuja-Halkola, R., Larsson, H., Hultman, C. M., & Reichenberg, A. (2014). The familial risk of autism. *JAMA, 311*(17), 1770–1777.

Schreibman, L., & Stahmer, A. C. (2014). A randomized trial comparison of the effects of verbal and pictorial naturalistic communication strategies on spoken language for young children with autism. *Journal of Autism and Developmental Disorders, 44*(5), 1244–1251.

Schroeder, J. H., Cappadocia, M. C., Bebko, J. M., Pepler, D. J., & Weiss, J. A. (2014). Shedding light on a pervasive problem: A review of research on bullying experiences among children with autism spectrum disorders. *Journal of Autism and Developmental Disorders, 44*(7), 1520–1534.

Sikora, D. M., Johnson, K., Clemons, T., & Katz, T. (2012). The relationship between sleep problems and behavior in children of different ages with autism spectrum disorders. *Pediatrics, 130*(Suppl. 2), S83–S90.

Soke, G. N., Philofsky, A., Diguiseppi, C., Lezotte, D., Rogers, S., & Hepburn, S. (2011). Longitudinal changes in Scores on the Autism Diagnostic Interview—Revised (ADI-R) in pre-school children with autism: Implications for diagnostic classification and symptom stability. *Autism, 15*(5), 545–562.

Sterzing, P. R., Shattuck, P. T., Narendorf, S. C., Wagner, M., & Cooper, B. P. (2012). Bullying involvement and autism spectrum disorders: Prevalence and correlates of bullying. *Archives of Pediatric and Adolescent Medicine, 166*, 1058–1064.

Sukhodolsky, D. G., Bloch, M. H., Panza, K. E., & Reichow, B. (2013). Cognitive-behavioral therapy for anxiety in children with high-functioning autism: A meta-analysis. *Pediatrics, 132*(5), e1341–e1350.

Szatmari, P., Bryson, S. E., Boyle, M. H., Streiner, D. L., & Duku, E. (2003). Predictors of outcome among high functioning children with autism and Asperger syndrome. *Journal of Child Psychology and Psychiatry, 44*(4), 520–528.

Tager-Flusberg, H., & Caronna, E. (2007). Language disorders: Autism and other pervasive developmental disorders. *Pediatric Clinics of North America, 54*(3), 469–481.

Thompson, R. M., & Johnston, S. (2013). Use of social stories to improve self-regulation in children with autism spectrum disorders. *Physical and Occupational Therapy in Pediatrics, 33*(3), 271–284.

Ttofi, M., & Farrington, D. (2011). Effectiveness of school-based programs to reduce bullying: A systematic and meta-analytic review. *Journal of Experimental Criminology, 7*, 27–56.

Vaillancourt, T., Trinh, V. I., McDougall, P., Duku, E., Cunningham, L., & Cunningham, C. (2010). Optimizing population screening of bullying in school-aged children. *Journal of School Violence, 9*(3), 233–250.

van Roekel, E., Scholte, R. H., & Didden, R. (2010). Bullying among adolescents with autism spectrum disorders: Prevalence and perception. *Journal of Autism & Developmental Disorders, 40*(1), 63–73.

Viscidi, E. W., Johnson, A. L., Spence, S. J., Buka, S. L., Morrow, E. M., & Triche, E. W. (in press). The association between epilepsy and autism symptoms and maladaptive behaviors in children with autism spectrum disorder. *Autism.*

Viscidi, E. W., Triche, E. W., Pescosolido, M. F., McLean, R. L., Joseph, R. M., Spence, S. J., & Morrow, E. M. (2013). Clinical characteristics of children with autism spectrum disorder and co-occurring epilepsy. *PLoS One, 8*(7), e67797.

Volden, J., Smith, I. M., Szatmari, P., Bryson, S., Fombonne, E., Mirenda, P., . . . Thompson, A. (2011). Using the Preschool Language Scale, fourth edition to characterize language in preschoolers with autism spectrum disorders. *American Journal of Speech and Language Pathology, 20*(3), 200–208.

White, S. W., & Roberson-Nay, R. (2009). Anxiety, social deficits, and loneliness in youth with autism spectrum disorders. *Journal of Autism and Developmental Disorders, 39*(7), 1006–1013.

Zwaigenbaum, L. (2012). What's in a name: Changing the terminology of autism diagnosis. *Developmental Medicine and Child Neurology, 54*(10), 871–872.

Zwaigenbaum, L., Bryson, S., Lord, C., Rogers, S., Carter, A., Carver, L., . . . Yirmiya N. (2009). Clinical assessment and management of toddlers with suspected autism spectrum disorder: Insights from studies of high-risk infants. *Pediatrics, 123*(5), 1383–1391.

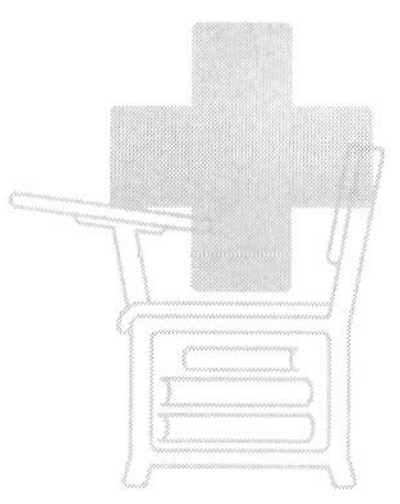

Chapter 17
The Science of Reading and Dyslexia

Sally E. Shaywitz and Bennett A. Shaywitz[1]

Dyslexia (or specific reading disability) is the most common and most carefully studied of the learning disabilities, affecting 80% of all individuals identified as learning disabled. Not only is dyslexia the best characterized of all learning disabilities; it is historically the oldest. In fact, the first description of dyslexia in children preceded the first mention of "learning disability" by more than 60 years—dyslexia was first described in 1896, whereas the term "learning disability" was not used until 1962! This chapter reviews recent advances in our knowledge of the epidemiology, etiology, cognitive influences, neurobiology, clinical manifestations, and management of dyslexia in children and adults.

Dyslexia first came to attention in the latter part of the 19th century, when physicians began to report on a puzzling group of children who seemed to have all the factors present to be good readers: They were bright and motivated, their parents were caring and concerned, they had received intensive reading instruction and tutoring, and yet they continued to struggle to learn to read (Morgan, 1896).

The definition of dyslexia as an *unexpected* difficulty in reading (Critchley, 1970; Lyon, 1995; Peterson & Pennington, 2012) has remained invariant over the century since its first description (Morgan, 1896), and this concept of an unexpected difficulty has also been the hallmark of learning disability from its origins in 1962 continuing to

[1]Portions of this chapter appeared in and are similar to other reviews by us (B. Shaywitz et al., 2000; S. E. Shaywitz & Shaywitz, in press-a, in press-b; S. Shaywitz, 1998; S. Shaywitz & Shaywitz, 1999).

the present day. Thus, in the earliest descriptions of learning disability authors noted a "discrepancy between the capacity for reading and actual achievement" (Kirk & Bateman, 1962, p. 73) and "a discrepancy between potential and actual success in learning" (Myklebust, 1968, p. 1). The most current definition of dyslexia is that proposed by the U.S. Congress (2013–2014) in Resolution 456: "Defined as an unexpected difficulty in reading in an individual who has the intelligence to be a much better reader, dyslexia reflects a difficulty in getting to the individual sounds of spoken language which typically impacts speaking (word retrieval), reading (accuracy and fluency), spelling, and often, learning a second language."

There is now empirical support for defining dyslexia (and by extension, other learning disabilities) as an unexpected difficulty in reading. Using data from the Connecticut Longitudinal Study, we demonstrated that in typical readers, reading and IQ development are dynamically linked over time (Ferrer, Shaywitz, Holahan, Marchione, & Shaywitz, 2010). Not only do reading and IQ track together over time; they also influence each other. In contrast, such mutual interrelationships are not perceptible in dyslexic readers, which suggests that reading and cognition develop more independently in these individuals (Figure 17.1).

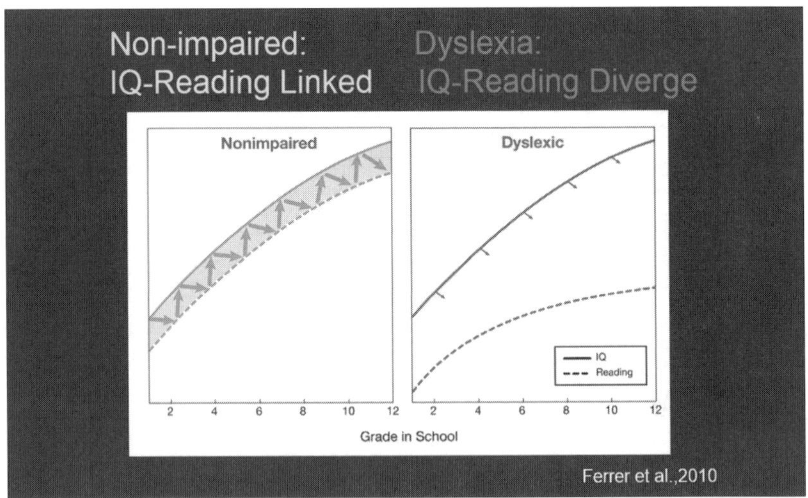

Figure 17.1. Uncoupling of reading and IQ over time: Empirical evidence for a definition of dyslexia. The left panel shows that in typical readers, reading and IQ development are dynamically linked over time. In contrast, the right panel, dyslexic readers, shows that reading and IQ development are dissociated and one can be highly intelligent and still struggle with reading. Data adapted from "Uncoupling of Reading and IQ Over Time," by E. Ferrer, B. Shaywitz, J. Holahan, K. Marchione, and S. Shaywitz, 2010, *Psychological Science, 21*(1), 93–101. Copyright 2010 by E. Ferrer, B. Shaywitz, J. Holahan, K. Marchione, and S. Shaywitz. Adapted with permission.

EPIDEMIOLOGY

Epidemiological data indicate that, like hypertension and obesity, dyslexia occurs in gradations and fits a dimensional model. In other words, within the population, reading ability and reading disability occur along a continuum, with reading disability representing the lower tail of a normal distribution of reading ability (Gilger, Borecki, Smith, DeFries, & Pennington, 1996; S. Shaywitz, Escobar, Shaywitz, Fletcher, & Makuch, 1992), with prevalence rates ranging from 5% to 17.5% (Interagency Committee on Learning Disabilities, 1987; S. Shaywitz, 1998). Data from the 2013 National Assessment of Educational Progress (U.S. Department of Education, 2013) indicate that overall, only about one in three students is proficient in fourth-grade or eighth-grade reading. And among some groups of students, the numbers are far worse. About one in five African American, Latino, and Native American students are proficient in fourth- and eighth-grade reading. Longitudinal studies, both prospective (Francis, Shaywitz, Stuebing, Shaywitz, & Fletcher, 1996; B. Shaywitz et al., 1995) and retrospective (Bruck, 1992; Felton, Naylor, & Wood, 1990; Scarborough, 1990), indicate that dyslexia is a persistent, chronic condition; it does not represent a transient developmental lag (Figure 17.2). Over time, poor readers and good readers tend to maintain their relative positions along the spectrum of reading ability—children who early on function at the 10th percentile for reading and those who function at the 90th percentile and all those in-between tend to maintain their positions. Dyslexia is found in readers of all languages including both alphabetic and logographic scripts.

ETIOLOGY

Dyslexia is both familial and heritable (Pennington & Gilger, 1996). Family history is one of the most important risk factors, with 23% to as much as 65% of children who have a parent with dyslexia reported to have the disorder (Scarborough, 1990). A rate among siblings of affected persons of approximately 40% and among parents ranging from 27% to 49% (Pennington & Gilger, 1996) provides opportunities for early identification of affected siblings and often for delayed but helpful identification of affected adults.

Given that dyslexia is familial and heritable, initial hopes that dyslexia would be explained by one or just a few genes have been disappointing. Thus, along with a great many common diseases, genome-

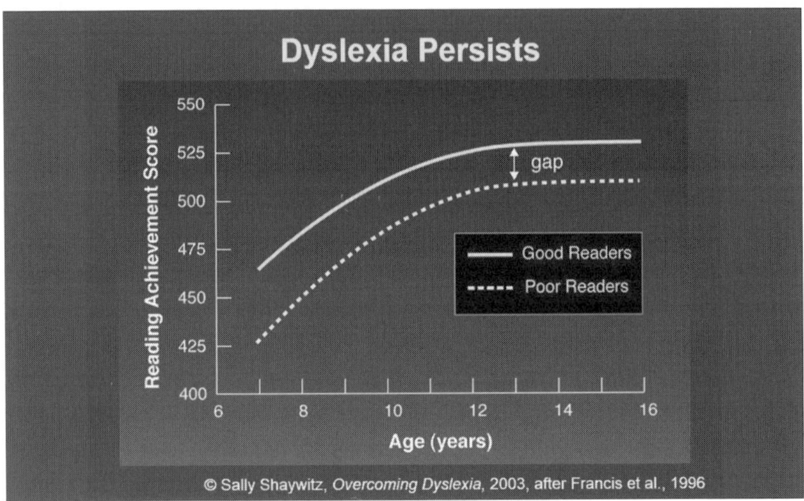

Figure 17.2. Trajectory of reading skills over time in nonimpaired and dyslexic readers. Ordinate is Rasch scores (W scores) from the Woodcock-Johnson reading test (Woodcock & Johnson, 1989), and abscissa is age in years. Both dyslexic and nonimpaired readers improve their reading scores as they get older, but the gap between the dyslexic and nonimpaired readers remains. Thus dyslexia is a deficit and not a developmental lag. Adapted with permission from data from "Developmental Lag Versus Deficit Models of Reading Disability: A Longitudinal, Individual Growth Curves Analysis," in D. Francis, S. Shaywitz, K. Stuebing, B. Shaywitz, and J. Fletcher, 1996, *Journal of Educational Psychology, 88*(1), 3–17, and reprinted from "Neural Systems for Compensation and Persistence: Young Adult Outcome of Childhood Reading Disability," in S. Shaywitz, B. Shaywitz, R. Fulbright, P. Skudlarski, W. Mencl, and R. Constable, 2003, *Biological Psychiatry, 54*(1), 25–33. Reprinted with permission.

wide association studies (GWAS) in dyslexia have so far identified genetic variants that account for only a very small percentage of the risk, less than 1% (Meaburn, 2008). Current evidence suggests "that common diseases involve thousands of genes and proteins interacting on complex pathways" (Duncan, 2009, p. D3) and that, similar to experience with other complex disorders (heart disease, diabetes), it is unlikely that a single gene or even a few genes will identify people with dyslexia. Rather, dyslexia is best explained by *multiple* genes, each contributing a small amount of the variance. Thus, current evidence suggests that the etiology of dyslexia is best conceptualized within a multifactorial model, with multiple genetic and environmental risk and protective factors leading to dyslexia.

COGNITIVE INFLUENCES

Among investigators in the field, there is now a strong consensus supporting the phonological theory. This theory recognizes that speech and language are acquired naturally, whereas reading must be taught. To read, the beginning reader must recognize that the letters and letter strings (the orthography) represent the sounds of spoken language. To read, a child has to develop the insight that spoken words can be pulled apart into the elemental particles of speech (phonemes) and that the letters in a written word represent these sounds (S. Shaywitz, 2003); such awareness is largely missing in dyslexic children and adults (Bruck, 1992; Fletcher et al., 1994; Liberman & Shankweiler, 1991; S. Shaywitz, 2003). Results from large and well-studied populations of students with dyslexia confirm that in young school-age children (Fletcher et al., 1994; Stanovich & Siegel, 1994) and in adolescents (S. Shaywitz et al., 1999), a deficit in phonology represents the most robust and specific correlate of dyslexia.

Difficulties with phonological processing are the most commonly reported problem in dyslexia (Morris et al., 1998). Phonological processing includes phonological awareness, a component of oral language ability that encompasses the abilities to attend to, discriminate, and manipulate individual speech sounds. This metacognitive understanding involves the realization that spoken language is composed of a series of discrete speech sounds (phonemes) that are arranged in a particular sequence (Clark & Uhry, 1995). Phonemic awareness refers to the ability to discern and identify the smallest individual speech sounds or phonemes, whereas phonological awareness is a broader term that includes phonemes, as well as all types of larger elements of speech that can be assessed by asking a child to rhyme words or count the number of syllables in a word. Both types of awareness involve the understanding that speech can be divided into sounds, and these sounds can then be sequenced into a series to form syllables and words.

Weaknesses in phonological processing play a critical role in dyslexia (S. Shaywitz, 2003; Willcutt, Pennington, Olson, Chhabildas, & Hulslander, 2005). Whereas spoken language is natural and instinctive, print or written language is artificial and must be learned (S. Shaywitz, 2003). Brain mechanisms are in place to process the sounds of language automatically but not the letters and words that make up print. Accordingly, these printed elements must link to something that is accepted by the neural machinery and has inherent meaning: the sounds of spoken language. To read, a child first must pull apart the written words into their individual sounds, link the letters to their appropriate sound (phonics), and then blend the sounds together. Thus, the awareness that spoken words come apart and the ability to notice and identify phonemes, these smallest elements of sound, allow the child to link letters to sound. To read, a child first must master what is referred to as "the alphabetic principle," that is, develop the awareness that the printed word has the same number and sequence of sounds as the spoken word. Phonemic awareness abilities have their primary impact on the development of phonics skills, or knowledge of the ways that letters represent the sounds in printed words (Torgesen & Mathes, 2000), as well as on encoding or spelling development (Bailet, 2001).

Reflecting the core phonological deficit, a range of downstream effects is observed in spoken and written language (S. E. Shaywitz & Shaywitz, 2008). Phonological processing is critical to both spoken and written language. While most attention has centered on print difficulties, the ability to notice, manipulate, and retrieve phonological elements has an important function in speaking. For example, uttering a spoken word requires a two-step mechanism involving first semantic and then phonological components (Levelt, Roelofs, & Meyer, 1999). In dyslexia, it is the second step involving phonology that is affected (Hanley & Vandenberg, 2010). First, one must generate the concept of what one wants to communicate; this in turn triggers activation of the semantic or meaning-based representation of the word in the speaker's lexicon. However, to speak the word, once the concept and associated semantic form are activated, the lexical representations must be transformed into their phonological codes. To accomplish this, in the second step, the speaker accesses and retrieves the phonological representations (phonological codes) that link to the semantic structures, a necessary step to generate the articulatory (motor) patterns that are ultimately put into action by the articulatory muscles, which result in the production of the spoken word. In dyslexia, activation of the concept and its semantic representation proceeds smoothly; however, it is the second step, the transformation of the semantic (meaning) into the phonological (sound) code that is disrupted. A feedback mechanism enables the speaker to monitor his or her own speech and exercise some output control to correct errors. However, if the individual is anxious, as often is the case in dyslexia, word retrieval is further negatively affected.

NEUROBIOLOGICAL STUDIES IN DYSLEXIA

Although brain imaging studies of dyslexia are relatively recent, neural systems influencing reading were first proposed over a century ago by Dejerine (1891) in studies of adults who suffered a stroke with subsequent acquired alexia, the sudden loss of the ability to read. Dejerine proposed at least two brain regions in the left hemisphere, one in the parieto-temporal region, the other more inferior in the occipito-temporal region. It has only been within the past two decades that neuroscientists using noninvasive brain imaging, particularly functional magnetic resonance imaging (fMRI), have been able to confirm the importance for dyslexia of the posterior brain regions proposed by Dejerine.

THE READING SYSTEMS IN DYSLEXIA

With the use of functional magnetic resonance imaging (fMRI), converging evidence from many laboratories around the world has demonstrated a neural signature for dyslexia, that is, an inefficient functioning of posterior reading systems during reading real words and pseudowords (see Figure 17.3). This evidence from fMRI has for the first time made visible what previously was a hidden disability. For example, in one of the first studies of fMRI in dyslexia, B. Shaywitz and colleagues (2002) used fMRI to study 144 children, approximately half of whom had dyslexia and half were typical readers. Our results indicated significantly greater activation in typical readers than in

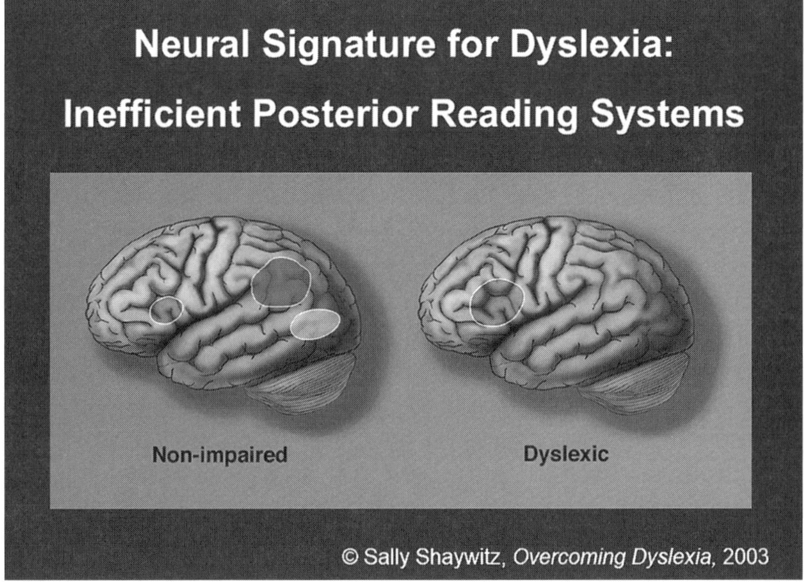

Figure 17.3. Neural signature for dyslexia. A neural signature for dyslexia is illustrated in this schematic view of left-hemisphere brain systems in (*left*) nonimpaired and (*right*) dyslexic readers. In dyslexic readers, the anterior system is slightly overactivated compared with systems of typical readers; in contrast, the two posterior systems are underactivated. This pattern of underactivation in left posterior reading systems is referred to as the neural signature for dyslexia. Adapted from *Overcoming Dyslexia: A New and Complete Science-Based Program for Reading Problems at Any Level*, by S. Shaywitz, 2003, New York, NY: Knopf. Copyright 2003 by S. Shaywitz. Adapted with permission.

dyslexic readers in posterior reading systems during a task tapping phonologic analysis.

These data from fMRI studies in children with dyslexia reported by our group have been replicated in reports from many investigators and show a failure of left-hemisphere posterior brain systems to function properly during reading, particularly the systems in the left hemisphere's occipito-temporal region (for reviews, see Peterson & Pennington, 2012; C. Price & Mechelli, 2005; Richlan, Kronbichler, & Wimmer, 2009, 2011; S. Shaywitz & B. Shaywitz, 2005). Similar findings have been reported in German (Kronbichler et al., 2006) and Italian (Brambati et al., 2006) readers with dyslexia. Studies in Chinese readers with dyslexia show some differences, although the systems are generally the same. For example, in both typical Chinese readers and Chinese readers with dyslexia, there is more involvement of the left middle frontal, superior parietal, and bilateral posterior visual regions and less involvement of the inferior frontal and superior parietal regions (Perfetti, 2011).

Although readers with dyslexia exhibit an inefficiency of functioning in the left occipito-temporal word-form area, they appear to develop ancillary systems in other brain regions (B. Shaywitz et al., 2002). While these ancillary systems allow the reader to read accurately, readers with dyslexia continue to read dysfluently. Inefficient functioning in this essential system for skilled reading has very important practical implications for individuals with dyslexia: It provides the neurobiological evidence for the biological necessity for the accommodation of additional time on high-stakes tests (see Figure 17.4).

Results from several lines of investigation indicate that the system responsible for the fluent, automatic integration of letters and sounds, in the anterior lateral occipito-temporal system, a system known as the visual word-form area (VWFA), is the neural circuit that develops with age in typical readers. Just how the VWFA functions is the subject of intense investigation. Price and Devlin (2011), in what they term the integrative account, suggest that the VWFA acts to integrate phonologic, orthographic, and semantic information.

Connectivity analyses of fMRI data represent the most recent evolution in characterizing brain networks in dyslexia. Measures of functional connectivity are designed to detect differences in brain regions with similar magnitudes of activation but whose activity is differentially synchronized with other brain systems across subject groups and/or types of stimuli. In a recent report, Finn et al. (2013) present the first whole-brain functional connectivity study of dyslexia. Results suggest that nonimpaired readers are better able to integrate visual information and modulate their attention to visual stimuli, thus

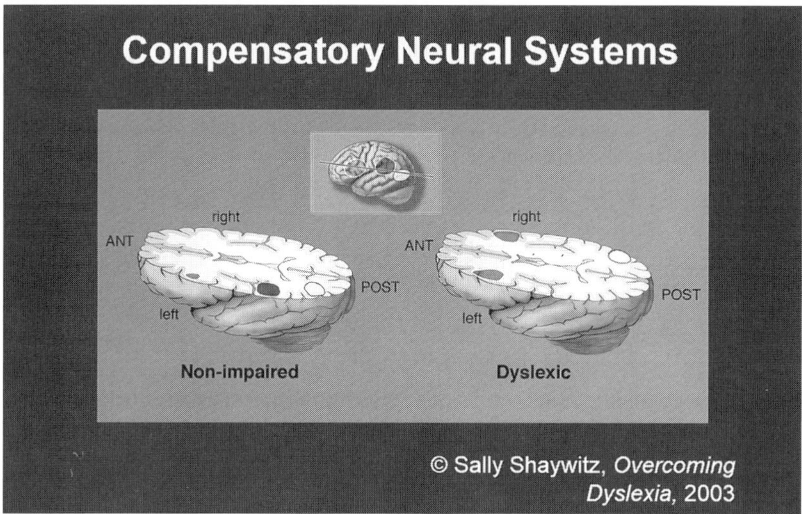

Figure 17.4. Compensatory neural systems and the neural basis for the requirement for extended time for dyslexic students on high-stakes testing. The image is a cutaway view of the brain showing the left and right hemispheres. Typical readers activate three left-hemisphere neural systems for reading: an anterior system and two posterior systems. Dyslexic readers have an inefficient functioning in the left-hemisphere posterior neural systems for reading but compensate by developing anterior systems in the left and right hemispheres and the posterior homolog of the visual word form area in the right hemisphere. Adapted from *Overcoming Dyslexia: A New and Complete Science-Based Program for Reading Problems at Any Level*, by S. Shaywitz, 2003, New York, NY: Knopf. Copyright 2003 by S. Shaywitz. Adapted with permission.

allowing them to recognize words on the basis of their visual properties, whereas dyslexic readers recruit altered reading circuits and rely on laborious phonology-based "sounding out" strategies into adulthood.

DIAGNOSIS

From the very first descriptions over a century ago, dyslexia has always been a paradox: a child or adult with problems in reading, yet smart in every other way. In *Overcoming Dyslexia*, Sally Shaywitz (2003) conceptualized this as a weakness in phonology (getting to the sounds of spoken words) surrounded by a sea of strengths in higher-order thinking. In younger children there is an encapsulated weakness in decoding surrounded by strengths in, for example, problem solving, critical thinking, concept formation, and reasoning. In older children, adolescents, and adults it may be thought of as an encapsulated weakness in fluent reading surrounded by these strengths in higher-order thinking.

Emphasizing the strengths, some have proposed that dyslexia is a gift. We believe it is best to conceptualize dyslexia as a paradox: individuals who have difficulty getting to the sounds of spoken language that is unexpected given the person's intelligence, age, and professional accomplishments. Considering what they have had to experience throughout school, for nearly everyone with dyslexia, having dyslexia can in no way be considered a gift or an advantage. Recently, lecturing at a dyslexia conference in New Jersey, one of the other speakers told the audience what her 10-year-old daughter with dyslexia told her: "If dyslexia is a gift, can I please give it back?"

The diagnosis of dyslexia is basically no different from that of any other disorder. Guided by knowledge of the presumed underlying pathophysiology, the clinician seeks to determine, through history, observation, and psychometric assessment, if there are (a) unexpected difficulties (for age, intelligence, or level of education) in reading and (b) associated linguistic problems at the level of phonologic processing. There is no one single test score that is pathognomonic of dyslexia. As with any other medical diagnosis, the diagnosis of dyslexia should reflect a thoughtful synthesis of all the clinical data available. What the clinician is seeking is converging evidence of a phonologically based reading disability as indicated by a disparity between the individual's reading and phonologic skills in contrast to his or her intellectual capabilities, age, or level of education. Dyslexia is distinguished from other disorders that may prominently feature reading difficulties by the unique, circumscribed nature of the phonologic deficit, one not intruding into other linguistic or cognitive domains. How reading and language are assessed will reflect the age and educational level of the patient (see Tables 17.1 and 17.2).

Diagnosis in Preschool and at School Entry

Currently, most children with a reading disability are not diagnosed until they are in third grade or about 9 years old. Good evidence indicates that it is possible to screen children as young as 4–5 years of age and identify those at risk for reading disability, an identification based on poor reading relative to chronological age, that is, poor reading defined solely on the basis of low reading achievement. A history of language delay or not attending to the sounds of words (e.g., trouble playing rhyming games with words, confusing words that sound alike), along with a positive family history, are significant risk factors for dyslexia. The most helpful measures in predicting reading difficulties are those designed to assess phonemic awareness and phonological skills.

Table 17.1
CLUES TO DYSLEXIA IN SCHOOL-AGE CHILDREN

History

- Delayed language
- Problems with the sounds of words (trouble rhyming words, confusion of words that sound alike)
- Expressive language difficulties (mispronunciations, hesitations, word-finding difficulties)
- Difficulty naming (difficulty learning letters of alphabet and the names of numbers)
- Difficulty learning to associate sounds with letters
- History of reading and spelling difficulties in parents and siblings

Reading

- Difficulty decoding single words
- Particular difficulty reading nonsense or unfamiliar words
- Inaccurate and labored oral reading
- Slow reading
- Comprehension often superior to isolated decoding skills
- Poor spelling

Language

- Relatively poor performance on tests of word retrieval (name the pictured item)
- Relatively superior performance on tests of word recognition (point to the pictured item)
- Poor performance on tests of phonological awareness

Clues most specific to young children at risk for dyslexia

- Difficulty on tests assessing: knowledge of the names of letters, the ability to associate sounds with letters and phonological awareness

Clues most specific to bright young adults with dyslexia

- Childhood history of reading and spelling difficulties
- Accurate but not automatic writing
- Very slow performance on timed reading tests (e.g., *Nelson-Denny Reading Test*)
- Penalized by multiple-choice tests

Note. Clues are based on history, observations, testing, or a combination of the three. From "Current Concepts: Dyslexia," by S. Shaywitz, 1998, *New England Journal of Medicine, 338*(5), pp. 307–312. Copyright 1998 by *New England Journal of Medicine.* Reprinted with permission.

Table 17.2

TYPES OF TESTS USEFUL IN IDENTIFYING CHILDREN AT RISK FOR DYSLEXIA AT TIME OF SCHOOL ENTRY

Letter identification (naming letters of the alphabet)
Letter–sound association (e.g., identifying words that begin with the same letter from a list: *doll, dog, boat*)
Phonological awareness (e.g., identifying the word that would remain if a particular sound was removed, such as if the /k/ sound was taken away from *cat*)
Verbal memory (e.g., recalling a sentence or a story that was just told)
Rapid naming (rapidly naming a continuous series of familiar objects, digits, letters, or colors)
Expressive vocabulary, or word retrieval (e.g., naming single-pictured objects)

Note. From "Current Concepts: Dyslexia," by S. Shaywitz, 1998, *New England Journal of Medicine, 338*(5), pp. 307–312. Copyright 1998 by *New England Journal of Medicine.* Reprinted with permission.

Tests of phonological capabilities and reading readiness are becoming increasingly available, for example, the *Comprehensive Test of Phonological Processing, Second Edition* (CTOPP-2; Wagner, Torgesen, Rashotte, & Pearson, 2013), which is normed from age 4 through adult.

Diagnosis at School Age

Presenting complaints most commonly center on school performance—"She's not doing well in school"—and often parents (and teachers) do not appreciate that the reason for this is a reading difficulty. Thus, an evaluation for dyslexia should be considered in all children presenting with school difficulties, even if reading difficulty is not the chief complaint. As with most other medical disorders, the history is critical to the diagnosis of dyslexia. Clinicians need to develop a sense of the developmental pattern demonstrated by children with dyslexia. Overall, the ontogeny of dyslexia is that of a child who may have had a delay in speaking, does not learn letters during kindergarten, and has not begun to learn to read by the completion of first grade. The child progressively falls behind, with teachers and parents puzzled as to why such an intelligent child may have difficulty learning to read. The reading difficulty is unexpected with respect to the child's ability, age, or grade. Even after acquiring decoding skills, the child generally remains a slow reader. When teachers are not informed, they may unnecessarily pressure or hurry the student. Dysgraphia is often present, and accompanied by laborious note taking. Self-esteem is frequently affected, particularly if the disorder has gone undetected for a long period of time. Dyslexic children are likely to have encountered negative test-taking experiences in which there was a disparity between their knowledge and their test scores, especially on timed tests, and thus they tend to exhibit more test anxiety than nondisabled peers. Test scores may thus be artificially depressed as a result of such anxiety. Adults with strong histories of dyslexia who have compensated for their reading disability demonstrate good accuracy in reading but are less automatic. Compensated dyslexics take longer to apply their decoding skills and thus are slower readers; however, given sufficient time, they score very well on tests of reading comprehension.

In the school-age child, reading is assessed by measuring accuracy, fluency, and comprehension. Specifically, in the school-age child, an important element of the evaluation is how accurately the child can decode words (i.e., read single words). This is measured with standardized tests of single real-word and pseudoword reading, such as the Woodcock-Johnson IV (WJ-IV) (Schrank, Mather, & Woodcock, 2014). Because pseudowords are unfamiliar and cannot be memorized, each nonsense word must be sounded out. Tests of nonsense word reading are referred to as "word attack." Reading (passage) comprehension is also assessed by the WJ-IV. Reading fluency, the ability to read accurately, rapidly, and with good prosody—an often-overlooked component of reading—is of critical importance because it allows for the automatic, attention-free recognition of words. Fluency is generally assessed by asking the child to read aloud using the *Gray Oral Reading Test, Fifth Edition* (GORT-5) (Wiederholt & Bryant, 2012). This test consists of increasingly difficult passages, each followed by comprehension questions; scores for accuracy, rate, fluency, and comprehension are provided. Such tests of oral reading are particularly helpful in identifying a child who is dyslexic; by its nature, oral reading forces a child to pronounce each word. Listening to a struggling reader attempt to pronounce each word leaves no doubt about the child's reading difficulty. In addition to reading passages aloud, single-word reading efficiency may be assessed using, for example, the *Test of Word Reading Efficiency, Second Edition* (TOWRE-2) (Torgesen, Wagner, & Rashotte, 2013), a test of speeded oral reading of individual words. Children who struggle with reading often have trouble spelling; spelling can be assessed with the WJ-IV spelling test (Schrank et al., 2014). Because dyslexia is defined as an unexpected difficulty in a child or adult, unexpected in relation to intelligence, it is not surprising that a measure of intelligence such as the *Wechsler Intelligence Scale for Children, Fifth Edition* (WISC-V) is an important component of a comprehensive assessment of the child or adult with dyslexia. Very often an IQ test can reveal areas of strength, particularly in areas of abstract thinking and reasoning, which are very reassuring to parents and especially, to the child him- or herself. They also indicate that the reading difficulty is isolated and not reflective of a general lack of learning ability.

Diagnosis in Adolescents and Young Adults

The developmental course of dyslexia has now been characterized. First, dyslexia is persistent, it does not go away; on a practical level, this means that once a person is diagnosed as dyslexic, there is no need for reexamination following high school to confirm the diagnosis. Second, over the course of development, skilled readers become more accurate and more automatic in decoding; they do not need to rely on context for word identification. Dyslexic readers, too, become more accurate over time, but they do not become automatic in their reading. Residua of the phonological deficit persist so that reading remains effortful and slow, even for the brightest of individuals with childhood histories of dyslexia. Failure to either recognize or measure the lack of automaticity in reading represents, perhaps, the most common error in the diagnosis of dyslexia in accomplished young adults. It is often not appreciated that tests measuring word accuracy are inadequate for the diagnosis of dyslexia in young adults at the level of college, graduate, or professional school and that, for these individuals, timed measures of reading must be employed in making the diagnosis.

Because they are able to read words accurately (albeit very slowly), dyslexic adolescents and young adults may mistakenly be assumed to have "outgrown" their dyslexia (Bruck, 1998; Lefly & Pennington, 1991; S. Shaywitz, 2003). Data from studies of children with dyslexia who have been followed prospectively support the notion that in adolescents, the rate of reading as well as facility with spelling may be most useful clinically in diagnosing dyslexia in students in secondary school, college, and even graduate school. It is important to remember that these older dyslexic students may be similar to their typically reading peers on untimed measures of word recognition yet continue to suffer from the phonologic deficit that makes reading less automatic, more effortful, and slow. Thus, the most consistent and telling sign of a reading disability in an accomplished young adult is slow and laborious reading and writing.

The failure either to recognize or to measure the lack of automaticity in reading is perhaps the most common error in the diagnosis of dyslexia in older children and in accomplished young adults. Tests relying on the accuracy of word identification alone are inappropriate to use to diagnose dyslexia in accomplished young adults; tests of word identification reveal little to nothing of his or her struggles to read. It is important to recognize that since they assess reading accuracy but not automaticity, the kinds of reading tests commonly used for school-age children may provide misleading data on bright adolescents and young adults. The most critical tests are those that are timed; they are the most sensitive to a phonologic deficit in a bright adult. However, there are very few standardized tests for young adult readers that are administered under timed and untimed conditions; the Nelson-Denny Reading Test (Brown, Fishco, & Hanna, 1993) is an exception. Any scores obtained on testing should be considered relative to those of peers with the same degree of education or professional training.

In bright young adults a history of phonologically based reading difficulties, requirements for extra time on tests, and current slow and effortful reading (i.e., signs of a lack of automaticity in reading) are the sine qua non of a diagnosis of dyslexia. At *all* ages, and especially in young adults, dyslexia is a *clinical diagnosis*.

HOW DOES RESPONSE TO INTERVENTION (RTI) FIT INTO THE PICTURE?

As *part* of an evaluation for dyslexia and other learning disabilities, the Individuals With Disabilities Education Act (IDEA, 2004) now allows states to use response to intervention (RTI), a process that theoretically examines whether or not a student responds to scientific, research-based interventions for reading. In principle, RTI involves the systematic use of data-based decision making to identify struggling readers in a school and then provide a series (in RTI parlance, "tiers") of increasingly more intensive interventions for those in need (VanDerHeyden & Burns, 2010). Many questions, issues, and concerns, however, have been raised regarding the use and implementation of RTI (for a review, see Reynolds & Shaywitz, 2009).

When viewed in the context of dyslexia evaluations, RTI has serious shortcomings as a means of diagnosis or determination of a disability. The RTI approach fosters the dangerous concept of relativity of a disability in the context of the individual classroom as opposed to the long-accepted concept of a disability as residing *within* the individual. The RTI model focuses on the failure of a child–school interaction that is complex and modified by the overall achievement level of an individual classroom that will vary within schools and across schools. Consequently, a child may be identified by RTI in one classroom and not found to require intervention in the classroom next door, depending on the makeup of each class.

Another serious concern is that RTI ignores bright struggling readers in the identification process. In the RTI process itself, consider the impact of so-called peer comparison to classmates if a specific child is highly intelligent or even gifted. What if such a child is in a class of "peers" who are functioning at lower cognitive levels? Such a bright student might be struggling and functioning well below his or her own capability but at an absolute level comparable to the class average of his or her less able peers. That struggling reader would be entirely invisible and overlooked in an RTI process. Most critically, such struggling readers would not receive helpful interventions or accommodations "despite the fact that their relative deficit in a particular domain could cause severe psychological distress as well as unexpected underachievement" (Boada, Riddle, & Pennington, 2008, p. 185), which could be ameliorated through interventions and accommodations. It would be no fairer to leave out these bright struggling readers than it would be to leave out their lower functioning classmates.

MANAGEMENT

The management of dyslexia demands a life-span perspective. Early on, the focus is on remediation of the reading problem. In fact, federal law, specifically the Individuals with Disabilities Education Act (IDEA), mandates "a free, appropriate, public education in the least restrictive environment" to dyslexic students attending public schools. As part of IDEA, students with dyslexia must receive services designed to meet their needs free of charge. It should be more widely known that the word "dyslexia" is mentioned specifically in IDEA.

Often students and their parents are caught up in ensuring that the child with dyslexia is considered eligible to receive interventions (services) that they need and are required by the law. In recent years there has developed what many believe to be a false dichotomy between dyslexic children diagnosed on the basis of a discrepancy compared to dyslexic children diagnosed as poor readers on the basis of low reading achievement for age, for example, defined on the basis of a reading score below a certain cut point (e.g., below a standard score of 90). Seventy-five percent of children identified by discrepancy criteria also meet low-achievement criteria in reading; the remaining 25% who meet only discrepancy criteria may fail to be identified and yet still be struggling to read (B. Shaywitz, Fletcher, Holahan, & Shaywitz, 1992). These findings have strong educational implications: It is not valid to deny the education services available for disabled or at-risk readers to either low-achieving, nondiscrepant children or to those children who are not low achieving but at the same time are reading below a level expected for their ability.

For more than a decade now, on the basis of a prior consensus report from the National Research Council (Snow, Burns, & Griffin, 1998) and the results of the National Reading Panel (2000), it has been well reported that five critical elements must be in place to effectively teach reading: phonemic awareness (i.e., ability to focus on and manipulate phonemes, speech sounds, in spoken syllables and words), phonics (i.e., understanding how letters are linked to sounds to form letter-sound correspondences and spelling patterns), fluency (i.e., ability to read accurately, rapidly, and with good intonation), vocabulary, and comprehension.

Teaching children to decode words is the first step in teaching children to read. Numerous studies over the past two decades have demonstrated that systematic, explicit instruction that focuses on the sound structure of words is more effective than "whole word" instruction, which teaches little or no phonics or teaches phonics haphazardly or in a "by-the-way" approach. Large-scale studies have focused on younger children, and there are few or no data available on the effect of these training programs on older children. The data on younger children are more encouraging (Foorman, Brier, & Fletcher, 2003; National Reading Panel, 2000; S. Shaywitz et al., 2003; Torgesen et al., 1999). Despite such successes, investigators have begun to question whether the current dogma needs to be reevaluated. As reviewed most recently by Compton, Miller, Elleman, and Steacy (2014), the plethora of intervention studies in dyslexic readers show "significant and lasting improvements in nonword decoding but much less so in real word identification" (p. 61).

Fluency represents the next developmental stage in the reading process and bridges word identification and reading comprehension (Zimmerman & Rasinski, 2012). It is considered to comprise three components: decoding words accurately, decoding words automatically (rapidly), and oral reading of connected text with appropriate prosody (appropriate expression). The critical importance of fluency is that it enables the reader to deploy attentional and other cognitive resources to comprehend what he or she has read. Encouraging children to read more seems to be the most critical element in improving reading fluency.

Teaching vocabulary, and especially teaching comprehension, has not been as easily implemented as teaching decoding skills and teaching fluency. But just what is reading comprehension? As quoted in Compton et al. (2014) and attributed to Kamhi (2009), reading comprehension is not a skill but rather "comprises a set of complex higher level mental processes that include thinking, reasoning, imagining, and interpreting" (p. 175).

Accommodations

As a child matures and enters the more time-demanding setting of secondary school, the emphasis shifts to incorporate the important role of providing accommodations. In fact, an essential component of the management of dyslexia in students in secondary school, college, and graduate school incorporates the provision of accommodations. And it is at this time that the student and his or her parents often call upon another federal law, Section 504 of the Rehabilitation Act of 1973, which entitles children with a disability such as dyslexia to a public education comparable to that provided to children who do not have a disability. In adolescents and young adults applying for high-stakes standardized tests for college or graduate or professional schools, the Americans with Disabilities Amendment Act of 2008 provides the legal protection for accommodations on these tests.

High school and college students with a history of childhood dyslexia often present a paradoxical picture; they may be similar to their unimpaired peers on measures of word recognition and comprehension, but they continue to suffer from the phonological deficit that makes reading less automatic, more effortful, and slow. Neurobiological data provide strong evidence for the necessity of extra time for readers with dyslexia (see Figure 17.4). Functional MRI data demonstrate that in the word-form area, the region supporting rapid reading functions inefficiently. Readers compensate by developing anterior systems bilaterally and the right homolog of the left word-form area. Such compensation allows for accurate reading, but it does not support fluent or rapid reading (B. Shaywitz et al., 2002). For these readers with dyslexia, the provision of extra time is an essential accommodation, particularly on high-stakes tests such as the SAT and ACT, as well as tests for professional schools, such as the LSAT, MCAT, and GRE. The accommodation of extra time allows the student time to decode each word and to apply his or her unimpaired higher-order cognitive and linguistic skills to the surrounding context to get at the meaning of words that he cannot entirely or rapidly decode. While readers who are dyslexic improve greatly with additional time, providing additional time to nondyslexic readers results in very minimal or no improvement in scores.

Although providing extra time for reading is by far the most common accommodation for people with dyslexia, other helpful accommodations include allowing the use of computers for writing essay answers on tests, access to recorded books (from organizations such as Learning Ally and Bookshare), and text-to-voice software from a number of vendors, including Kurzweil, apps such as Pdf to Speech, Go Read, and many others. Other helpful accommodations include providing access to syllabi and lecture notes, tutors to "talk through" and review the content of reading material, alternatives to multiple-choice tests (e.g., reports, projects), waivers of high-stakes oral exams, a separate, quiet room for taking tests, and a partial waiver of the foreign-language requirement (S. Shaywitz, 2003). Students with dyslexia who have difficulty accessing the sound system of their primary language will, almost invariably, have difficulties learning a foreign language. With such accommodations, many students with dyslexia are successfully completing studies in a range of disciplines, including science, law, medicine, and education.

REFERENCES

Americans With Disabilities Amendment Act of 2008, Pub. L. 110-325, (S 3406).

Bailet, L. (2001). Development and disorders of spelling in the beginning school years. In A. M. Bain, L. L. Bailet, & L. C. Moats (Eds.), *Written language disorders: Theory into practice* (2nd ed., pp. 1–41). Austin, TX: PRO-ED.

Boada, R., Riddle, M., & Pennington, B. (2008). Integrating science and practice in education. In E. Fletcher-Janzen & C. Reynolds (Eds.), *Neuropsychological perspectives on learning disabilities in the era of RTI: Recommendations for diagnosis and intervention* (pp. 179–191). New York, NY: Wiley.

Brambati, S., Termine, C., Ruffino, M., Danna, M., Lanzi, G., Stella, G., . . . Perani, D. (2006). Neuropsychological deficits and neural dysfunction in familial dyslexia. *Brain Research, 1113*(1), 174–185.

Brown, J., Fishco, V., & Hanna, G. (1993). *Nelson Denny Reading Test–Manual for Scoring and Interpretation (forms G and H).* Itasca, IL: Riverside.

Bruck, M. (1992). Persistence of dyslexics' phonological awareness deficits. *Developmental Psychology, 28*(5), 874–886.

Bruck, M. (1998). Outcomes of adults with childhood histories of dyslexia. In C. Hulme & R. Joshi (Eds.), *Reading and spelling: Development and disorders* (pp. 179–200). Mahwah, NJ: Erlbaum.

Clark, D., & Uhry, J. (1995). *Dyslexia: Theory and practice of remedial instruction* (2nd ed.). Timonium, MD: York Press.

Compton, D., Miller, A., Elleman, A., & Steacy, L. (2014). Have we forsaken reading theory in the name of "Quick Fix" interventions for children with reading disability? *Scientific Studies of Reading, 18*, 55–73.

Critchley, M. (1970). *The dyslexic child.* Springfield, IL: Thomas.

Dejerine, J. (1891). Sur un cas de cecite verbale avec agraphhie, suivi d'autopsie. *C. R. Societé du Biologie, 43,* 197–201.

Duncan, D. (2009, August 24). Scientist at work: Eric Shadt, enlisting computers to unravel the true complexity of disease. *New York Times.*

Felton, R., Naylor, C., & Wood, F. (1990). Neuropsychological profile of adult dyslexics. *Brain and Language, 39*(4), 485–497. http://dx.doi.org/10.1016/0093-934X%2890%2990157-C

Ferrer, E., Shaywitz, B., Holahan, J., Marchione, K., & Shaywitz, S. (2010). Uncoupling of reading and IQ over time: Empirical evidence for a definition of dyslexia. *Psychological Science, 21*(1), 93–101.

Finn, E., Shen, X., Holahan, J., Papdemetrix, X. Scheinost, D., Lacadie, C., . . . Constable, R. T. (2013). Disruption of functional networks in dyslexia: A whole-brain, data-driven approach to fMRI connectivity analysis. *Biological Psychiatry.* http://dx.doi.org/10.1016/j.biopsysch.2013.08.031

Fletcher, J., Shaywitz, S., Shankweiler, D., Katz, L., Liberman, I., & Stuebing, K. (1994). Cognitive profiles of reading disability: Comparisons of discrepancy and low achievement definitions. *Journal of Educational Psychology, 86*(1), 6–23.

Foorman, B., Brier, J., & Fletcher, J. (2003). Interventions aimed at improving reading success: An evidence-based approach. *Development Neuropsychology, 24,* 613–639.

Francis, D., Shaywitz, S., Stuebing, K., Shaywitz, B., & Fletcher, J. (1996). Developmental lag versus deficit models of reading disability: A longitudinal, individual growth curves analysis. *Journal of Educational Psychology, 88*(1), 3–17.

Gilger, J., Borecki, I., Smith, S., DeFries, J., & Pennington, B. (1996). The etiology of extreme scores for complex phenotypes: An illustration using reading performance. In C. H. Chase, G. D. Rosen, & G. F. Sherman (Eds.), *Developmental dyslexia: Neural, cognitive, and genetic mechanisms* (pp. 63–85). Baltimore, MD: York Press.

Hanley, S., & Vandenberg, B. (2010). Tip of the tongue and word retrieval deficits in dyslexia. *Journal of Learning Disability, 43,* 15–23.

Individuals With Disabilities Education Act, Pub. L. 101-476, 104 Stat. 1142 (1990).

Interagency Committee on Learning Disabilities. (1987). *Learning disabilities: A report to the U.S. Congress.* Washington, DC: Author.

Kamhi, A. (2009). The case for the narrow view of reading. *Language, Speech, and Hearing Services in Schools, 40,* 174–177.

Kirk, S., & Bateman, B. (1962). Diagnosis and remediation of learning disabilities. *Exceptional Children, 29*(2), 73–78.

Kronbichler, M., Hutzler, F., Staffen, W., Mair, A., Ladurner, G., & Wimmer, H. (2006). Evidence for a dysfunction of left posterior reading areas in German dyslexic readers. *Neuropsychologia, 44*(10), 1822–1832.

Lefly, D., & Pennington, B. (1991). Spelling errors and reading fluency in compensated adult dyslexics. *Annals of Dyslexia, 41,* 143–162.

Levelt, W. J., Roelofs, A., & Meyer, A. S. (1999). A theory of lexical access in speech production. *Behavioral and Brain Sciences, 22,* 1–75.

Liberman, I., & Shankweiler, D. (1991). Phonology and beginning to read: A tutorial. In L. Rieben & C. A. Perfetti (Eds.), *Learning to read: Basic research and its implications.* Hillsdale, NJ: Erlbaum.

Lyon, G. (1995). Toward a definition of dyslexia. *Annals of Dyslexia, 45*, 3–27.

Meaburn, E. (2008). Quantitative trait locus association scan of early reading disability and ability using pooled DNA and 100K SNP microarrays in a sample of 5760 children. *Molecular Psychiatry, 13*(7), 729.

Morgan, W. (1896). A case of congenital word blindness. *British Medical Journal*, 1378.

Morris, R., Stuebing, K., Fletcher, J., Shaywitz, S., Lyon, G., & Shankweiler, D. (1998). Subtypes of reading disability: Variability around a phonological core. *Journal of Educational Psychology, 90*, 347–373.

Myklebust, H. R. (1968). Learning disabilities: Definition and overview. In H. R. Myklebust (Ed.), *Progress in learning disabilities* (Vol. 1, pp. 1–15). New York, NY: Grune & Stratton.

National Reading Panel. (2000). *Teaching children to read: An evidence based assessment of the scientific research literature on reading and its implications for reading instruction*. Washington, DC: U.S. Department of Health and Human Services, National Institutes of Health, National Institute of Child Health and Human Development.

Pennington, B., & Gilger, J. (1996). How is dyslexia transmitted? In C. H. Chase, G. D. Rosen, & G. F. Sherman (Eds.), *Developmental dyslexia. Neural, cognitive, and genetic mechanisms* (pp. 41–61). Baltimore, MD: York Press.

Perfetti, C. A. (2011). Explaining individual differences in reading theory and evidence. In S. A. Brady, D. Braze, & C. A. Fowler (Eds.), *Explaining individual differences in reading theory and evidence* (pp. 137–152). New York, NY: Psychology Press.

Peterson, R., & Pennington, B. (2012). Developmental dyslexia. *Lancet, 379*(9830): 1997–2007. e-pub: 10.1016/S0140-6736(12)60198-6).

Price, C., & Devlin, J. (2011). The interactive account of ventral occipitotemporal contributions to reading. *Trends in Cognitive Sciences, 15*(6), 246–253.

Price, C., & Mechelli, A. (2005). Reading and reading disturbance. *Current Opinion in Neurobiology, 15*, 231–238.

Rehabilitation Act of 1973, Section 5, 29 U.S.C. 701 (1973).

Reynolds, C., & Shaywitz, S. (2009). Response to intervention: Ready or not? Or, From wait-to-fail to watch-them-fail. *School Psychology Quarterly, 24*(2), 130–145.

Richlan, F., Kronbichler, M., & Wimmer, H. (2009). Functional abnormalities in the dyslexic brain: A quantitative meta-analysis of neuroimaging studies. *Human Brain Mapping, 30*, 3299–3308.

Richlan, F., Kronbichler, M., & Wimmer, H. (2011). Meta-analyzing brain dysfunctions in dyslexic children and adults. *Neuroimage, 56*, 1735–1742.

Scarborough, H. (1990). Very early language deficits in dyslexic children. *Child Development, 61*, 1728–1743.

Schrank, F., Mather, N., & Woodcock, R. (2014). *Woodcock-Johnson-IV.* Rolling Meadows, IL: Riverside.

Shaywitz, B., Fletcher, J., Holahan, J., & Shaywitz, S. (1992). Discrepancy compared to low achievement definitions of reading disability: Results from the Connecticut Longitudinal Study. *Journal of Learning Disabilities, 25*, 639–648.

Shaywitz, B., Fletcher, J., Holahan, J., Shneider, A., Marchione, K., & Stuebing, K. (1995). Interrelationships between reading disability and attention-deficit/hyperactivity disorder. *Child Neuropsychology, 1*(3), 170–186.

Shaywitz, B., Shaywitz, S., Pugh, K., Mencl, W., Fulbright, R., & Skudlarski, P. (2002). Disruption of posterior brain systems for reading in children with developmental dyslexia. *Biological Psychiatry, 52*(2), 101–110.

Shaywitz, S. (1998). Current concepts: Dyslexia. *New England Journal of Medicine, 338*(5), 307–312.

Shaywitz, S. (2003). *Overcoming dyslexia: A new and complete science-based program for reading problems at any level.* New York, NY: Alfred A. Knopf.

Shaywitz, S., Escobar, M., Shaywitz, B., Fletcher, J., & Makuch, R. (1992). Evidence that dyslexia may represent the lower tail of a normal distribution of reading ability. *New England Journal of Medicine, 326*(3), 145–150.

Shaywitz, S., Fletcher, J., Holahan, J., Shneider, A., Marchine, K., & Stuebing, K. (1999). Persistence of dyslexia. The Connecticut Longitudinal Study at adolescence. *Pediatrics, 104*(6), 1351–1359.

Shaywitz, S., & Shaywitz, B. (2005). Dyslexia (specific reading disability). *Biological Psychiatry, 57,* 1301–1309.

Shaywitz, S. E., & Shaywitz, B. A. (2008). Paying attention to reading: The neurobiology of reading and dyslexia. *Development & Psychopathology, 20*(4), 1329–1349.

Shaywitz, S. E., & Shaywitz, B. A. (in press-a). Dyslexia. In R. G. Schwartz (Ed.), *Handbook of child language disorders* (2nd ed.). London, UK: Psychology Press.

Shaywitz, S. E., & Shaywitz, B. A. (in press-b). Dyslexia. In R. M. Kliegman, B. F. Stanton, J. W. St. Geme III, N. F. Schor, & R. E., Behrman (Eds.), *Kliegman: Nelson textbook of pediatrics* (20th ed.). Philadelphia, PA: Saunders Elsevier.

Shaywitz, S., Shaywitz, B., Fulbright, R., Skudlarski, P., Mencl, W., & Constable, R. (2003). Neural systems for compensation and persistence: Young adult outcome of childhood reading disability. *Biological Psychiatry, 54*(1), 25–33.

Snow, C., Burns, M., & Griffin, P. (Eds.). (1998). *Preventing reading difficulties in young children.* Washington, DC: National Academy Press.

Stanovich, K., & Siegel, L. (1994). Phenotypic performance profile of children with reading disabilities: A regression-based test of the phonological-core variable-difference model. *Journal of Educational Psychology, 86*(1), 24–53.

Torgesen, J., & Mathes, P. (2000). *A basic guide to understanding, assessing and teaching phonological awareness.* Austin, TX: PRO-ED.

Torgesen, J., Wagner, R., & Rashotte, C. (2013). *TOWRE-2: Test of word reading efficiency* (2nd ed.). Austin, TX: PRO-ED.

Torgesen, J., Wagner, R., Rashotte, C., Rose, E., Lindamood, P., & Conway, T. (1999). Preventing reading failure in young children with phonological processing disabilities. *Journal of Educational Psychology, 91*, 579–593.

U.S. Congress, H.R. Res. 456, 113th Cong. (2013–2014).

U.S. Department of Education, Institute of Education Sciences, National Center for Education Statistics, National Assessment of Education Progress (NAEP). (2013). *2013 mathematics and reading assessments.* Retrieved from http://nationsreportcard.gov/reading_math_2013

VanDerHeyden, A. M., & Burns, M. K. (2010). *Essentials of response to intervention.* New York, NY: Wiley.

Wagner, R., Torgesen, J., Rashotte, C., & Pearson, N. (2013). *CTOPP-2: Comprehensive test of phonological processing* (2nd ed.). Austin, TX: PRO-ED.

Wiederholt, J., & Bryant, B. (2012). *GORT-5 Examiner's Manual.* Austin, TX: PRO-ED.

Willcutt, E., Pennington, B., Olson, R., Chhabildas, N., & Hulslander, J. (2005). Neuropsychological analyses of comorbidity between reading disability and attention deficit hyperactivity disorder: In search of the common deficit. *Developmental Neuropsychology, 27,* 35–78.

Zimmerman, B., & Rasinski, T. (2012). The fluency development lesson: A model of authentic and effective fluency instruction. In T. Rasinski, C. Blachowica, & K. Lems (Eds.), *Fluency instruction: Research-based best practices* (2nd ed., pp. 172–184). New York, NY: Guilford Press.

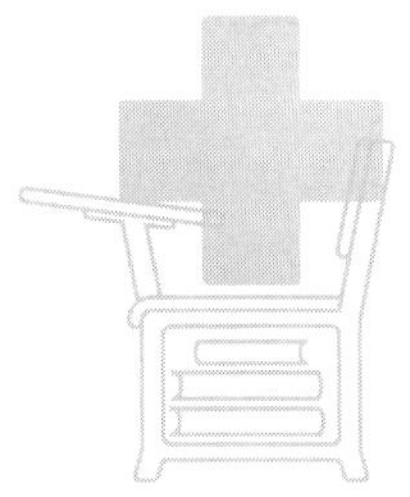

Chapter 18

The Short- and Long-Term Outcomes for Victims of Bullying

Implications for Educators and Clinicians[1]

Christina M. L. Beeson and Tracy Vaillancourt

Although not a new issue, bullying is potentially one of the biggest problems that many children and adolescents face on a regular basis. With outcomes extending beyond childhood and adolescence into adulthood, bullying is an ongoing issue with many ramifications for the individuals involved. It is for this reason that understanding the risk and protective factors, the numerous outcomes, and the specific roles that educators and clinicians may play in the intervention, prevention, and treatment of the outcomes of bullying is important.

Bullying is a complex relationship problem (Pepler, Craig, & O'Connell, 1999; Pepler et al., 2006) that extends beyond the aggressor and his or her victim, and includes bystanders who support the abuse, try to defend the victim, or simply do nothing. Although studies have shown that victims, bullies, and bystanders are each at risk for adverse outcomes (Janson & Hazler, 2004; McDougall & Vaillancourt, 2014), the focus of this chapter is on *victims* of bullying. Our attention to this group stems from the fact that studies suggest that victims of peer abuse are more likely to suffer poorer physical and mental health than those who bully (Wolke, Copeland, Angold, & Costello, 2013) and those who witness peer abuse (Janson & Hazler, 2004). We

[1]Funding support came from the Canadian Institutes of Health Research, Canada Research Chairs program.

also limit our discussion to bullying among children and adolescents in schools, with the recognition that bullying can involve adults and can take place in the workplace, in families, in community-based organizations, and the like.

DEFINITION OF BULLYING

Falling under the wider concept of aggression, *bullying* is defined as a systematic abuse of power involving intentional harmful acts that causes immediate or long-term distress to the victimized individual (Olweus, 1994, 2000; Smith & Sharp, 1994). There are three defining features of bullying that differentiate it from other forms of aggression: (a) intent to harm, (b) repeated behavior over time, and (c) an imbalance of power, whether physical or social, between the perpetrator and the victim (Olweus, 1994). It is important to bear in mind this operational definition when working with the general population because the term "bullying" can be overused by children and parents, who may attribute it to odd disagreements, occasional incivilities, or goodwill teasing between peers (Vaillancourt et al., 2008). Although these social experiences can be hurtful, they are not associated with the poor sequelae that bullying is associated with, precisely because bullying is repeated and severe in nature.[2] Moreover, with each repeated episode, the power dynamic between the victim and his or her abuser becomes consolidated (Lamb, Pepler, & Craig, 2009), which makes it difficult for the victim to stop the abuse.

TYPES OF BULLYING

Bullying takes many different forms. It can be direct, where the interaction between the perpetrator and the victim is face-to-face, or indirect, where the perpetrator uses social manipulation, such as spreading rumors or jeopardizing friendships, to hurt the victim mentally (relational bullying) (Björkqvist, Lagerspetz, & Kaukiainen, 1992). Typically, bullying manifests as physical, verbal, relational, or cyber.

Physical bullying is a form of direct bullying involving aggressive bodily contact between the perpetrator and the victim (e.g., hitting, pushing, pinching, kicking, scratching). Physical bullying is the most visible of all the types of bullying, and is the one most often noticed by adults in a school setting. Accordingly, examples of physical bullying

[2]One-off critical incidents can be considered bullying if the egregious act is coupled with the fear of re-occurrence.

are more often recalled by youth than are other forms of bullying (Yoon & Kerber, 2003).

Verbal bullying is another form of direct bullying involving spoken or written words (e.g., threatening, name-calling, yelling, racial or sexual harassment). Uttering verbal threats or hurtful words happens relatively quickly, and children who bully others verbally tend to wait until adults are out of earshot before acting, which makes verbal bullying difficult to detect; thus, adults are less likely to intervene (Smokowski & Kopasz, 2005).

Relational bullying (also called social bullying) is typically a form of indirect bullying involving the use of the victim's desire for inclusion and acceptance in the peer group to hurt him or her (e.g., spreading rumors or lies, social exclusion). Since relational bullying is less visible than physical bullying, adults tend to intervene less and do not consider it as serious as the other types of peer abuse (Blain-Arcaro, Smith, Cunningham, Vaillancourt, & Rimas, 2012; Duy, 2013).

Finally, cyberbullying occurs using some form of electronic device (e.g., computer, cell phone). Although traditional bullying and cyberbullying are both forms of aggression characterized by harassment or victimization of an individual (or group) in which there exists an imbalance of power, cyberbullying has unique qualities that make it different from traditional bullying. One especially troubling characteristic of cyberbullying is that it can be done any hour of the day and any day of the week, extending it well beyond the school environment and the school day (Mishna, Saini, & Solomon, 2009; Wong-Lo, Bullock, & Gable, 2011). This may lead the victim to feel unsafe in his or her own home. Another key factor unique to cyberbullying is the anonymity of the perpetrator, which creates a power imbalance between the bully and the victim (Çetin, Yaman, & Peker, 2011; Wong-Lo, Bullock, & Gable, 2011). This anonymity is also attractive to potential perpetrators who may not behave in this manner in person. Further to anonymity, cyberbullying also has a unique permanence, where the victim is able to see or read the attack over and over again (Wong-Lo, Bullock, & Gable, 2011), as well as a wider reach, with an ability to be viewed by an unlimited number of people in less time than traditional bullying (Çetin et al., 2011).

PREVALENCE

Bullying is prevalent among North American children and youth. Indeed, as many as 30% of students report being bullied at school within a two-month period, and 10% of those youth report being bullied on a daily basis (e.g., Nansel et al., 2001; Vaillancourt, Brittain, et al., 2010). Similar rates of persistent victimization have been found in studies in other countries, such as China (~25%; Cheng et al., 2010), Australia (~30%; Hemphill et al., 2011), Turkey (~35%; Piskin, 2010), and Egypt (~29%; Hussein, 2013).

The age at which peer victimization is most prevalent differs depending on the form of bullying taking place. For those who are victims of physical and verbal bullying, rates of victimization tend to decrease across adolescence, with the greatest amount occurring in late elementary school and the least in high school (Finkelhor, Ormrod, Turner, & Hamby, 2005; Nansel et al., 2001). Conversely, being a victim of cyberbullying tends to follow a parabolic curve, wherein it increases with age (Patchin & Hinduja, 2006; Vandebosch & Van Cleemput, 2009) and peaks at age 14, or Grade 8 (Cassidy, Jacson, & Brown, 2009), then declines after that (Wang, Iannotti, & Nansel, 2009), with older adolescents less likely to be victimized online (Sengupta & Chaudhuri, 2011).

A recent meta-analysis by Cook, Williams, Guerra, Kim, and Sadek (2010) reported that boys were more likely than girls to be involved in bullying as bullies, victims, and bully victims. Studies have also consistently found that boys are more likely to be victims of physical bullying, such as being threatened, physically assaulted, or having property stolen, whereas girls are more likely to be victims of relational aggression, including having rumors or lies spread about them, being socially excluded, or having sexual comments made about them (Bevans, Bradshaw, & Waasdorp, 2013; Nansel et al., 2001).

Most studies have also found that girls are more often victims of cyberbullying than are boys (Beckman, Hagquist, & Hellström, 2013; Devine & Lloyd, 2012; Dilmaç, 2009; Hinduja & Patchin, 2007; Perren, Dooley, Shaw, & Cross, 2010; Sengupta & Chaudhuri, 2011; Wang, Iannotti, & Nansel, 2009; Williford et al., 2013), with some exceptions (Fanti, Demetriou, & Hawa, 2012; Williams & Guerra, 2007). More research is required to establish whether there is a gender difference in cyberbullying, as well as other factors that may influence victimization rates.

TYPES AND CHARACTERISTICS OF VICTIMIZED CHILDREN AND YOUTH

There are two types of victims noted in the literature—(a) pure victims, also called passive victims in some literatures (and termed "victims" in this chapter), who do not retaliate when victimized, and

(b) aggressive victims, also termed bully victims, who are strongly reactive to being victimized (Hussein, 2013). Victims are more common, making up about two-thirds of all types of victims, with aggressive victims making up the remaining third (Brockenbrough, Cornell, & Loper, 2002). Aggressive victims have both the highest rates of bullying and the highest rates of victimization, due to their increased aggressive behavior (Yang & Salmivalli, 2013). They also use both proactive (i.e., goal-directed aggression) and reactive aggression toward their peers (Peeters, Cillessen, & Scholte, 2010).

Each type of victim has unique characteristics and suffers distinctive outcomes as a result of being on the receiving end of peer aggression (described below). However, it is important to note that aggressive victims are considered the most at risk for a varied range of adjustment problems, in large part because they have the symptoms of maladjustment that are associated with bullies and victims (Haltigan & Vaillancourt, 2014; for reviews, see Arseneault, Bowes, & Shakoor, 2010; Lereya, Samara, & Wolke, 2013).

There are a number of physical characteristics that make a person more at risk to be a victim of bullying. Victims of bullying tend to be physically smaller or weaker than their peers, which is especially true for boys (Olweus, 1993a). Further, having some sort of visible difference, such as being obese (Janssen et al., 2004; King, Puhl, Luedicke, & Peterson, 2013), having a physical disability such as cerebral palsy (Lindsay & McPherson, 2012), not being heterosexual (Berlan et al., 2010), or being less attractive, wealthy, athletic, or academically competent (Knack, Tsar, Vaillancourt, Hymel, & McDougall, 2012), is linked with increased peer victimization.

On a relational level, victims tend to have poorer social skills than bullies or those not involved in bullying behavior (Buhs, Ladd, & Herald, 2006; Crawford & Manassis, 2011), including being less able to use problem solving to resolve conflict with peers (Andreou, 2001). Additionally, victims tend to have deficits in emotional regulation and understanding, which is especially true for those who are victimized more frequently (Mahady-Wilton, Craig, & Pepler, 2000). For example, one study of students in Egyptian schools found that victims had a difficult time identifying the emotions they were feeling, and they were also more likely to hide or suppress their emotions from others (Hussein, 2013). Not surprisingly, this study also found that victims were less popular with their peers because of their difficulty in social situations (see also Knack et al., 2012).

When it comes to traditional bullying, aggressive victims have been found to be more immature than their peers, to be clumsier, and to have difficulty reading social cues (Kowalski, Limber, & Agatston,

2011). Aggressive victims are also characterized by restlessness, having difficulty concentrating, and being quick tempered (Olweus, 1993b). Similar to victims, aggressive victims also tend to have difficulty with emotional understanding and are unable to identify their own emotions and the causes for them; however, unique to aggressive victims is their difficulty in analyzing (i.e., trying to understand why they feel an emotion) their own emotions, as well as the emotions of others (Hussein, 2013). Like victims, aggressive victims have been shown to be less popular with their peers due to their lack of social skills (Hussein, 2013). They are also actively disliked by their peers, have very few friends, and experience less social support from their peers (Georgiou & Stavrinides, 2008).

Although there does not seem to be one clear profile for individuals who are victims of cyberbullying, there are factors that put certain people at higher risk of being cyberbullied than others. Adolescents who demonstrate more computer proficiency, such as through posting pictures, chatting, or flirting online (Hinduja & Patchin, 2007; Sengupta & Chaudhuri, 2011), or who are more dependent on the Internet (Vandebosch & Van Cleemput, 2009) are more likely to be victims of cyberbullying. Previous experience being a victim of traditional bullying (Hinduja & Patchin, 2007) or of cyberbullying (Wong-Lo, Bullock, & Gable, 2011) were found to be related to increased online victimization. Additionally, victims of cyberbullying are more likely to have depressive symptoms, to be victimized offline, and to demonstrate aggression (Wolak, Mitchell, & Finkelhor, 2007); however, because this study was cross-sectional in nature, it is impossible to determine the direction of causation (i.e., children who are depressed may more often be victims of cyberbullying, or they may develop depressive symptoms because they are victimized). Finally, one study by Kowalski and Fedina (2011) found that children who have special needs and who may lack social skills, such as those with autism-spectrum disorder or attention-deficit/hyperactivity disorder, were more likely to be victimized by cyberbullies.

Just as individual variables play a role in the occurrence of peer victimization, social and environmental factors also contribute to rates of peer abuse (Cook et al., 2010). There are a number of family variables that serve as risk factors for increased victimization. For example, having an insecure attachment relationship with parents is related to higher levels of peer victimization than those who have secure attachments (Kokkinos, 2013). Some studies have found that victimization is related to less parental warmth and greater parental rejection (Kokkinos, 2013), whereas others have found that children with overprotective parents (overly involved) are more likely to be victimized (Georgiou, 2008). Victims are more likely to come from lone-parent families (Nordhagen, Nielsen, Stigum, & Köhler, 2005). Interestingly, in one study, victims were more likely to come from families with incomes greater than $50,000 (Finkelhor et al., 2005), whereas in another study, victims of peer abuse were perceived by their peers as being poorer than their non-abused peers (Knack et al., 2012). Victims of cyberbullying are more likely to have more conflict with their parents, and they may be or have been physically or sexually abused (Wolak, Mitchell, & Finkelhor, 2007).

SHORT-TERM OUTCOMES

Victims of peer abuse have been found to have negative psychological, physical, and academic outcomes as a result of being bullied. Psychologically, victims tend to suffer from low self-esteem (Hawker & Boulton, 2000), increased rates of depression (Fekkes, Pijpers, & Verloove-VanHorick, 2004; Galand & Hospel, 2013; Hawker & Boulton, 2000), post-traumatic stress disorder (Idsoe, Dyregrov, & Idsoe, 2012), fear and anxiety, and suicidal ideation or self-harm (e.g., cutting, suicide attempts) (Cassidy, Jacson, & Brown, 2009; Fekkes et al., 2004; Hawker & Boulton, 2000; Hay & Meldrum, 2010; Hay, Meldrum, & Mann, 2010). Some studies have found that victims of cyberbullying are more stressed and have higher depressive symptoms than victims of traditional bullying (Perren, Dooley, Shaw, & Cross, 2010) and are more likely than perpetrators of cyberbullying to have low self-esteem and to feel socially isolated, anxious, and helpless (Wang, Nansel, & Iannotti, 2011; Williford et al., 2013). Often, victims end up expressing some of these psychological symptoms as physical or somatic ones, including bedwetting, headaches and stomachaches, trouble sleeping, and a poor appetite (Fekkes et al., 2004; Knack, Jensen-Campbell, & Baum, 2011; see also the meta-analysis by Gini & Pozzoli, 2013).

Victimization by cyberbullying has been linked not only to internalization problems but to a number of externalization problems in adolescents as well. Specifically, those who are victimized may have higher rates of substance use, such as alcohol or cigarettes (Perren et al., 2010), or delinquency (Sigfusdottir, Gudjonsson, & Sigurdsson, 2010), or they may use medications for anxiety and sleeplessness caused by bullying (Wang, Iannotti, Luk, & Nansel, 2010).

Academic achievement is another area negatively affected by peer victimization. As mentioned, although victimization is most common in late elementary or middle school (Finkelhor et al., 2005), children in younger grades are also victimized by peers, and the effects on academic success differ across grades (McDougall & Vaillancourt, 2014). In the early elementary grades, victims have been shown to be unhappy at school (Arseneault et al., 2006). As children enter late elementary and middle school, victimization is linked to school truancy and poor academic performance (Galand & Hospel, 2013; Hawker & Boulton, 2000). Cyberbullying can also have a detrimental effect on victims academically. Victims tend to skip school and get detentions, and some may even bring a weapon to school (Ybarra, Diener-West, & Leaf, 2007).

One study found an interaction between the way in which victims explained the reason for a bullying incident (i.e., attributional style) and the level of his or her psychological distress as a result of being bullied (Goldsmid & Howie, 2013). Specifically, victims who had a negative attributional style (i.e., attributed bullying to causes that are stable, internal, and global) were more likely to experience greater psychological distress after being victimized than those who had a positive attributional style.

Researchers have shown that aggressive victims have the most serious outcomes when compared to bullies and victims. Specifically, aggressive victims exhibit more problem behavior at school, lack self-control, lack social skills, are disliked by their peers, and may partake in self-harming behaviors (Kowalski, Limber, & Agatston, 2011). These outcomes are a combination of those seen in both bullies and victims.

LONG-TERM OUTCOMES

Longitudinal studies of children and youth involved in bullying suggest that the pain associated with these early peer experiences is long lasting. Meta-analytic work points to the fact that bullied children experience acute mental and physical health problems, as well as long-term problems in the areas of psychosomatic difficulties (Gini & Pozzoli, 2013); externalizing problems including hyperactivity, delinquency, and aggression (Reijntjes et al., 2011); internalizing problems such as loneliness, withdrawal, emotional problems, somatization, anxiety, and depression (Reijntjes, Kamphuis, Prinzie, & Telch, 2010; Ttofi, Farrington, Losel, & Loeber, 2011); and issues with academic achievement and attendance (Nakamoto & Schwartz, 2010). Again, those most at risk for these adverse outcomes are aggressive victims (e.g., Haltigan & Vaillancourt, 2014; for reviews, see Arseneault et al., 2010; Lereya, Samara, & Wolke, 2013).

Several recent studies have suggested that the poor sequelae associated with peer victimization extends well into adulthood. For example, controlling for known correlates of peer victimization, a recent 50-year British prospective birth-cohort study (Takizawa, Maughan, & Arseneault, 2014) showed that victims of childhood bullying had increased levels of psychological distress when they were 23 and 50 years old. Those who were frequently bullied as children were more likely to be depressed, anxious, and suicidal in adulthood than those who were not abused by their childhood peers. The authors suggested that these negative effects were similar to "those being placed in public or substitute care and an index of multiple childhood adversities" (Takizawa et al., 2014, p. 777). In another meta-analytic study, Ttofi et al. (2011) found that the probability of being depressed up to 36 years later was higher for bullied children than for children who were not bullied by their peers. These findings persisted even when controlling for major childhood risk factors.

BIOLOGICAL OUTCOMES

Vaillancourt and colleagues (e.g., Vaillancourt, Clinton, McDougall, Schmidt, & Hymel, 2010; Vaillancourt, Hymel, & McDougall, 2013) have suggested that the stress associated with peer victimization and the aftermath of these experiences parallel the experiences of children who have been abused or neglected by their caregivers. Indeed, like children abused by caregivers, bullied children suffer from a constellation of psychological, physical, and academic problems. Moreover, recent neurobiological data on bullied children are strikingly similar to those presented on neglected and abused children. Like maltreated and/or neglected children, bullied children show blunted hypothalamic–pituitary–adrenal axis activity that is consistent with stressors that are severe in nature (see Vaillancourt, Hymel, et al., 2013, for a review). Bullied children also have shorter telomeres (Shalev et al., 2012), the repetitive nucleotide sequence at the end of chromosomes that is involved in chromosomal stability and regulates the replicative life span of the cell (Kiecolt-Glaser et al., 2011). Telomere erosion is associated with normal progressions such as aging, but it has been linked to health behavior (e.g., smoking, obesity) and diseases (e.g., cancer, diabetes, cardiovascular problems; Kiecolt-Glaser et al., 2011; Vaillancourt, Hymel, et al., 2013, p. 244). Importantly, telomere erosion has also been linked to the psychological stress associated with early adversity such as child maltreatment (see Vaillancourt, Hymel, et al., 2013) and bullying (Shalev et al., 2012).

Consistent with the idea that peer victimization does "get under the skin" (Vaillancourt et al., 2013), a recent study of children followed prospectively from childhood to adulthood, which included nine waves of data, showed that high C-reactive protein levels in adulthood were linked to childhood experiences with being bullied (Copeland et al., 2014). This finding is noteworthy given that the anti-inflammatory effect of cortisol has been shown to be lower in bullied children and youth (e.g., Kliewer, 2006; Knack et al., 2011; Ouellet-Morin et al., 2011; Vaillancourt et al., 2008). Finally, studies examining the polymorphism in the promoter region of the serotonin transporter gene (5-HTTLPR) in relation to exposure to peer abuse and depression have replicated those found with maltreated children (e.g., Caspi et al., 2003). Specifically, those who had a short–short allele for 5-HTTLPR were far more likely to be depressed when bullied than those with a short–long or long–long allele (Banny, Cicchetti, Rogosch, Oshri, & Crick, 2013; Benjet, Thompson, & Gotlib, 2010; Iyer, Dougall, & Jensen-Campbell, 2013; Sugden et al., 2010). Taken together, these studies suggest that exposure to peer abuse is akin to the stress associated with another form of abuse—namely, child maltreatment by caregivers.

PROTECTIVE FACTORS

Studies are beginning to look at factors that predict why some bullied individuals fare better, or are more resilient, to being victimized than others. Victims with lower levels of behavioral issues, such as delinquency, are more likely to be girls (Bowes et al., 2010), whereas victims with lower levels of internalization issues, such as depression, are more likely to be boys (Sapouna & Wolke, 2013). Resilience is also related to victims who have higher self-esteem, less conflict in parental and sibling relationships, and, for girls, fewer close friendships (Sapouna & Wolke, 2013). Having a higher IQ, a higher socioeconomic status, and fewer emotional and behavioral problems as a preschooler also predict higher levels of resilience to peer victimization (Bowes et al., 2010).

There are a number of family variables that are related to children and adolescents being better able to cope with being a victim of bullying. Individuals with warm mothers, warm sibling interactions, and a positive home atmosphere showed more resilience to bullying than those who did not have these family characteristics (Bowes et al., 2010). Maternal warmth plays an especially protective role against victimization. Twin studies demonstrate that differences in maternal warmth for monozygotic twins were related to differences in resilience, with the twin who receives greater maternal warmth being more resilient to bullying than the twin receiving less maternal warmth (Bowes et al., 2010).

Victims with families who are more supportive, who have stronger communication skills, and who utilize more external resources to deal with bullying also tend to be more resilient to peer victimization (Greeff & Van den Berg, 2013). As well, adolescents who have more perceived family support are less likely to be victims of cyberbullying (Wang, Iannotti, & Nansel, 2009), especially when victims do not have supportive friendships (Fanti et al., 2012). In a recent longitudinal study, Brittain, Krygsman, and Vaillancourt (2014) found that in families with low levels of family functioning, peer-victimized children were at risk for lower grades than their nonvictimized peers, whereas at high levels of family functioning, peer victimization was not related to grades. These studies demonstrate that strong social support of any kind can protect against peer victimization and its negative outcomes.

IMPLICATIONS FOR EDUCATIONAL AND CLINICAL PRACTICE

The Role of the Teacher

Most bullying takes place at school (Vaillancourt, Brittain et al., 2010), with some schools providing more opportunities than others for victimization. One important school factor contributing to bullying is the amount of adult supervision, especially in locations other than the classroom. Bullying tends to occur most often when there is minimal adult supervision. Large areas that are less governed by rules and where there is a high student-to-teacher ratio (which compromises teachers' abilities to closely monitor the actions of the students) have been shown to be related to increased bullying rates (Craig, Pepler, & Atlas, 2000; Vaillancourt, Brittain, et al., 2010). There are also characteristics of schools that provide environments that promote or discourage bullying. For example, schools that have a positive school climate that includes *structure* (enforced school discipline) and *support* (caring and involved adults) have lower bullying rates than schools in which students' safety and well-being are less considered (e.g., Gregory et al., 2010; Konold et al., 2014; Olweus, 1994; Swearer et al., 2010; Wang, Vaillancourt, et al., 2014).

When it comes to the prevention of bullying, teachers play an important role in the success or failure of school-based programs

(Horne, Orpinas, Newman-Carlson, & Bartolomucci, 2004). The sensitivity of the teacher to incidents of bullying, and the way in which he or she deals with the problem, can reduce the occurrence of school bullying. For example, rates of bullying have been shown to decrease dramatically when a teacher intervenes directly in a bullying incident (Olweus, 1994). Unfortunately, studies have also shown that teachers often do not notice bullying taking place on the schoolyard and therefore intervene rarely (4% of the time) (Craig & Pepler, 1997; see also Fekkes, Pijpers, & Verloove-VanHorick, 2005). Moreover, when they do intervene, teachers are more likely to address physical or verbal incidents than relational ones, perhaps because they view relational bullying to be less serious than the other forms of bullying (Blain-Arcaro et al., 2012; Duy, 2013; Yoon & Kerber, 2003). This belief could potentially and inadvertently create a school environment that supports relational peer victimization.

Supportive teachers also play an important role in preventing and protecting against the adverse outcomes for victims of bullying. Students who perceive higher support from their teachers are less likely to be involved in bullying, as perpetrators or victims (Flaspohler, Elfstrom, Vanderzee, & Sink, 2009). Further, the role of teacher support has as strong an effect on lowering victims' depressive symptoms as family support or peer support, particularly for victims who lack social support in other areas of their lives (Galand & Hospel, 2013). Teachers can also play an indirect supportive role for victims. Teachers trained in the understanding of classroom social structure were better able to identify social groups within their class (Farmer, Hall, Petrin, Hamm, & Dadisman, 2010). Having this knowledge of peer relationships can help teachers to prevent bullying by understanding which groups do not get along; similarly, teachers are better able to create or strengthen peer support systems by understanding which groups and peers do get along (Farmer & Xie, 2007).

School-Based Interventions

Many schools are working to raise awareness and prevent peer victimization by implementing school-based anti-bullying programs. Anti-bullying programs tend to target the entire school population (i.e., universal programs) and involve active participation by educators (Horne et al., 2004; Swearer et al., 2010). The intention of these programs is to decrease bullying in the school; however, school-based programs have had varying success rates, which raised the question of which programs should be implemented in schools, and what constitutes a successful anti-bullying program.

A number of meta-analyses have been conducted to get a better understanding of the outcomes of school-based anti-bullying programs and which characteristics of a program provide the greatest decrease in bullying and victimization in schools (Ferguson et al., 2007; Lee, Kim, & Kim, 2013; Merrell, Gueldner, Ross, & Isava, 2008; Polanin, Espelage, & Pigott, 2012; Smith, Schneider, Smith, & Ananiadou, 2004; Ttofi & Farrington, 2011; Ttofi, Farrington, & Baldry, 2008; Vreeman & Carroll, 2007). Even among meta-analyses, results are conflicting regarding program success. Although some meta-analyses did not find a significant change in bullying behavior after intervention (Ferguson et al., 2007; Merrell et al., 2008), most concluded that there are small to moderate positive effects for change in bullying and victimization reports (Lee et al., 2013; Smith et al., 2004; Ttofi & Farrington, 2011; Ttofi et al., 2008), with programs targeted at high school students having greater rates of success than those directed at elementary school students (Lee et al., 2013; Polanin et al., 2012).

The programs that demonstrated the greatest success rates involved transparent schoolwide rules and consequences (Ttofi et al., 2008; Vreeman & Carroll, 2007), which include implementing a school policy on bullying (Lee et al., 2013), increased communication (Ttofi et al., 2008), and specific training for students, such as in emotional control (Lee et al., 2013) or on positive bystander behavior (Polanin et al., 2012). The most successful programs also provided training for a range of social support for victims, such as teachers (Vreeman & Carroll, 2007), parents (Ttofi et al., 2008), and in some cases, peers (Lee et al., 2013; Polanin et al., 2012). However, findings on the involvement of peers have been mixed and not always positive, with some indicating an increase in victimization when programs targeted peers (Ttofi & Farrington, 2011). Program success was also found to increase when they incorporated a greater number of these elements (Ttofi & Farrington, 2011; Ttofi et al., 2008).

It has been suggested that one way to ameliorate anti-bullying prevention and intervention efforts is to directly involve stakeholders such as educators, students, and parents in the design of programs (Cunningham, Cunningham, Ratcliff, & Vaillancourt, 2010; Cunningham, Vaillancourt et al., 2009; Cunningham, Vaillancourt, Cunningham, Chen, & Ratcliffe, 2011). Prevention science research from other areas such as children's mental health has shown that attending to the needs and preferences of end users is associated with increased program adoption, greater fidelity in implementation, and the long-term support needed to achieve meaningful changes (e.g., Cunningham et al., 2008). Educators exert a lot of influence on the adoption of prevention and intervention programs, and accordingly, program developers ought to consider the voice of this powerful ally, as well as the voice of students and parents when designing anti-bullying programs.

The Role of the Clinician

The World Health Organization has stated that "bullying is a major public health problem that demands the concerted and coordinated time and attention of health-care providers, policy-makers and families" (Srabstein & Leventhal, 2010, p. 403). To date, most anti-bullying efforts have been initiated and directed by the education system, largely, in part, because most bullying takes place in schools (Vaillancourt, Brittain et al., 2010). However, it is clear from our review of the literature that bullying is associated with significant *health* concerns, and thus, it behooves health-care providers to also prioritize the reduction of bullying. But how can this prioritization be achieved? In the absence of established guidelines on what health-care practitioners should do, we suggest the following (i.e., screening, validation, and advocacy), extended from our comprehensive knowledge of this issue.

Screening

Health-care practitioners should screen children and youth for involvement with bullying, and if present, they should work in partnership with the school and family to help promote positive social relationships (see Lamb et al., 2009; Vaillancourt, Hepditch et al., 2013). The screening for involvement with bullying should be incorporated into routine visits. Lamb et al. (2009) suggest that physicians ask four questions pertaining to bullying involvement: (a) "How often do you get bullied (or bully others)?" (b) "How long have you been bullied (or bullied others)?" (c) "Where are you bullied (or where do you bully others)?" and (d) "How are you bullied (or how do you bully others)?" These questions can also be used by educators to monitor students' involvement with bullying.

Validation

When the parents or children present with peer relationship difficulties, it would be helpful for health-care providers to validate the notion that such concerns "are legitimate, significant, and worthy of as much careful attention and necessary intervention as the biomedical impairments" (Vaillancourt, Hepditch et al., 2013, p. 98). Unfortunately, the social lives of children tend to be ignored by clinicians, who are more inclined to focus their attention on the physical and mental health aspects of the child. The current state of knowledge supports a causal link between poor peer treatment and poor physical and psychological health (for a review, see McDougall & Vaillancourt, 2015); thus, the social lives of children are not incidental.

Advocacy

Physician groups and organizations such as the American Academy of Pediatrics (AAP), the Canadian Pediatric Society, the American Academy of Family Physicians, the College of Family Physicians of Canada, the American Psychiatric Association, and the Canadian Psychiatric Association are powerful advocacy groups mandated to promote the health and well-being of children. Many of these organizations have a policy or position statement about the role of the physician in the prevention and intervention of youth violence. For example, the AAP has the program Connected Kids: Safe, Strong, Secure, designed to help pediatricians develop their role and skills in the prevention of youth violence. The AAP (2009) also argues for advocacy. Specifically, it states that "as advocates, pediatricians may bring newly developed information regarding key risk factors such as exposure to firearms, teen dating violence, and bullying to the attention of local and national policy makers" (p. 393). We agree. Physicians have a powerful activism voice that needs to be used to reduce the burden associated with bullying.

CONCLUSION

Peer victimization is clearly a problem with far-reaching consequences, tapping into every aspect of a victim's life. Research has consistently shown the negative effects on a victim's psychological health, physical health, academic achievement, and behavior, both as an immediate consequence of being victimized by peers and long-term, even decades into adulthood. A more recent concern that has emerged involves the neurobiological outcomes victims are susceptible to as a result of the stress caused by bullying. These widespread negative outcomes pose a challenge for educators and clinicians working with victimized individuals.

Although bullying does have serious negative consequences for those involved as victims, there are a number of protective factors that individuals may possess or acquire that increase their resilience against the negative outcomes of bullying. These protective factors can be intrinsic, such as higher IQ and higher self-esteem, or extrinsic, such as receiving social support. This knowledge can be especially useful for educators who provide emotional and academic guidance and support to their students on a daily basis, as well as for health-care practitioners because these are areas where focus can be placed during clinical visits, therapy, or treatment sessions. Building strength in these areas may promote resilience and, in turn, better health outcomes for victimized children and youth.

Because bullying is such a prevalent issue, educators and health-care practitioners are likely to work with individuals who are being bullied. By being able to identify risk factors and recognize symptoms, educators are able to intervene on behalf of victimized individuals and health-care practitioners are able to treat outcomes, thus both playing an important role in the reduction of bullying.

REFERENCES

American Academy of Pediatrics. (2009). Connected kids: Safe, strong, secure program. *Pediatrics, 124*, 393–402. doi:10.1542/peds.2009-0943

Andreou, E. (2001). Bully/victim problems and their association with coping behaviour in conflictual peer interactions among school-age children. *Educational Psychology, 21*, 59–66. doi:10.1080/01443410125042

Arseneault, L., Bowes, L., & Shakoor, S. (2010). Bullying victimization in youths and mental health problems: "Much ado about nothing"? *Psychological Medicine, 40*(5), 717–729. doi:10.1017/S0033291709991383

Arseneault, L., Walsh, E., Trzesniewski, K., Newcombe, R., Caspi, A., & Moffitt, T. E. (2006). Bullying victimization uniquely contributes to adjustment problems in young children: A nationally representative cohort study. *Pediatrics, 118*, 130–138. doi:10.1542/peds.2005-2388

Banny, A. M., Cicchetti, D., Rogosch, F. A., Oshri, A., & Crick, N. R. (2013). Vulnerability to depression: A moderated mediation model of the roles of child maltreatment, peer victimization, and serotonin transporter linked polymorphic region genetic variation among children from low socioeconomic status backgrounds. *Development and Psychopathology, 25*(3), 599–614. doi:10.1017/S0954579413000047

Beckman, L., Hagquist, C., & Hellström, L. (2013). Discrepant gender patterns for cyberbullying and traditional bullying: An analysis of Swedish adolescent data. *Computers in Human Behavior, 29*, 1896–1903. doi:10.1016/j.chb.2013.03.010

Benjet, C., Thompson, R. J., & Gotlib, I. H. (2010). 5-HTTLPR moderates the effect of relational peer victimization on depressive symptoms in adolescent girls. *Journal of Child Psychology and Psychiatry, 51*(2), 173–179. doi:10.1111/j.1469-7610.2009.02149.x

Berlan, E. D., Corliss, H. L., Field, A. E., Goodman, E., & Austin, S. B. (2010). Sexual orientation and bullying among adolescents in the Growing Up Today Study. *Journal of Adolescent Health, 46*, 366–371. doi:10.1016/j.adohealth.2009.10.015

Bevans, K. B., Bradshaw, C. P., & Waasdorp, T. E. (2013). Gender bias in the measurement of peer victimization: An application of item response theory. *Aggressive Behavior, 39*, 370–380. doi:10.1002/ab.21486

Björkqvist, K., Lagerspetz, K. M. J., & Kaukiainen, A. (1992). Do girls manipulate and boys fight? Developmental trends in regard to direct and indirect aggression. *Aggressive Behavior, 18*, 117–127. doi:10.1002/1098-2337(1992)18:2<117::AID-AB2480180205>3.0.CO;2-3

Blain-Arcaro, C., Smith, J. D., Cunningham, C., Vaillancourt, T., & Rimas, H. (2012). Contextual attributes of indirect bullying situations that influence teachers' decisions to intervene. *Journal of School Violence, 11*, 226–245. doi:10.1080/15388220.2012.682003

Bowes, L., Maughan, B., Caspi, A., Moffitt, T. E., & Arseneault, L. (2010). Families promote emotional and behavioural resilience to bullying: Evidence of an environmental effect. *Journal of Child Psychology and Psychiatry, 51*(7), 809–817. doi:10.1111/j.1469-7610.2010.02216.x

Brittain, H. L., Krygsman, A., & Vaillancourt, T. (2014). *A multi-informant longitudinal study of peer victimization and academic achievement: The moderating role of family functioning.* Poster presented at the XXI World Meeting for the International Society for Research on Aggression, Atlanta, Georgia.

Brockenbrough, K. K., Cornell, D. G., & Loper, A. B. (2002). Aggressive attitudes among victims of violence at school. *Education & Treatment of Children, 25*, 273–287.

Buhs, E. S., Ladd, G. W., & Herald, S. L. (2006). Peer exclusion and victimization: Processes that mediate the relation between peer group rejection and children's classroom engagement and achievement. *Journal of Educational Psychology, 98*, 1–13. doi:10.1037/0022-0663.98.1.1

Caspi, A., Sugden, K., Moffitt, T. E., Taylor, A., Craig, I. W., Harrington, H., . . . Poulton, R. (2003). Influence of life stress on depression: Moderation by a polymorphism in the 5-HTT gene. *Science, 301*(5631), 386–389. doi:10.1126/science.1083968

Cassidy, W., Jacson, M., & Brown, K. N. (2009). Sticks and stones can break my bones, but how can pixels hurt me? Students' experiences with cyber-bullying. *School Psychology International, 30*(4), 383–402. doi:10.1177/0143034309106948

Çetin, B., Yaman, E., & Peker, A. (2011). Cyber victim and bullying scale: A study of validity and reliability. *Computers & Education, 57*, 2261. doi:10.1016/j.compedu.2011.06.014

Cheng, Y., Newman, I. M., Qu, M., Mbulo, L., Chai, Y., Chen, Y., & Shell, D. F. (2010). Being bullied and psychosocial adjustment among middle school students in China. *Journal of School Health, 80*, 193–199. doi:10.1111/j.1746-1561.2009.00486.x

Cook, C. R., Williams, K. R., Guerra, N. G., Kim, T. E., & Sadek, S. (2010). Predictors of bullying and victimization in childhood and adolescence: A meta-analytic investigation. *School Psychology Quarterly, 25*(2), 65–83. doi:10.1037/a0020149

Copeland, W. E., Wolke, D., Lereya, S. T., Shanahan, L., Worthman, C., & Costello, E. J. (2014). Childhood bullying involvement predicts low-grade systemic inflammation into adulthood. *Proceedings of the National Academies of Sciences, 111*(21), 7570–7575. doi:10.1073/pnas.1323641111

Craig, W. M., & Pepler, D. J. (1997). Observations of bullying and victimization in the school yard. *Canadian Journal of School Psychology, 13*, 41–60. doi:10.1177/082957359801300205

Craig, W. M., Pepler, D., & Atlas, R. (2000). Observations of bullying in the playground and in the classroom. *School Psychology International, 21*(1), 22–36. doi:10.1177/0143034300211002

Crawford, A. M., & Manassis, K. (2011). Anxiety, social skills, friendship quality, and peer victimization: An integrated model. *Journal of Anxiety Disorders, 25,* 924–931. doi:10.1016/j.janxdis.2011.05.005

Cunningham, C. E., Cunningham, L. J., Ratcliffe, J., & Vaillancourt, T. (2010). A qualitative analysis of the bullying prevention and intervention recommendations of students in Grades 5 to 8, *Journal of School Violence, 9,* 321–338. doi: 10.1080/15388220.2010.507146

Cunningham, C. E., Deal, K., Rimas, H., Buchanan, D. H., Gold, M., Sdao-Jarvie, K., . . . Boyle, M. (2008). Modeling the information preferences of parents of children with mental health problems: A discrete choice conjoint experiment. *Journal of Abnormal Child Psychology, 7,* 1128–1138.

Cunningham, C. E., Vaillancourt, T., Cunningham, L. J., Chen, Y., & Ratcliffe, J. (2011). Modeling the bullying prevention design recommendations of students from grade five to eight: A discrete choice conjoint experiment. *Aggressive Behavior, 37,* 521–537. doi:10.1002/ab.20408

Cunningham, C. E., Vaillancourt, T., Rimas, H., Deal, K., Cunningham, L., Short, K., & Chen, Y. (2009). Modeling the bullying prevention program preferences of educators: A discrete choice conjoint experiment. *Journal of Abnormal Child Psychology, 37,* 929–943. doi:10.1007/s10802-009-9324-2

Devine, P., & Lloyd, K. (2012). Internet use and psychological well-being among 10-year-old and 11-year-old children. *Child Care in Practice, 18*(1), 5–22. doi:10.1080/13575279.2011.621888

Dilmaç, B. (2009). Psychological needs as a predictor of cyber bullying: A preliminary report on college students. *Educational Sciences: Theory & Practice,* 9(3), 1307–1325.

Duy, B. (2013). Teachers' attitudes toward different types of bullying and victimization in Turkey. *Psychology in the Schools, 50*(10), 987–1002. doi:10.1002/pits.21729

Fanti, K. A., Demetriou, A. G., & Hawa, V. V. (2012). A longitudinal study of cyberbullying: Examining risk and protective factors. *European Journal of Developmental Psychology, 9*(2), 168–181. doi:10.1080/17405629.2011.643169

Farmer, T. W., Hall, C. M., Petrin, R., Hamm, J. V., & Dadisman, K. (2010). Evaluating the impact of a multicomponent intervention model on teachers' awareness of social networks at the beginning of middle school in rural communities. *School Psychology Quarterly, 25*(2), 94–106. doi:10.1037/a0020147

Farmer, T. W., & Xie, H. (2007). Aggression and school social dynamics: The good, the bad, and the ordinary. *Journal of School Psychology, 45,* 461–478. doi:10.1016/j.jsp.2007.06.008

Fekkes, M., Pijpers, F. I. M., & Verloove-VanHorick, S. P. (2004). Bullying behavior and associations with psychosomatic complaints and depression in victims. *Journal of Pediatrics, 117,* 1568–1574. doi:10.1542/peds.2005-0187

Fekkes, M., Pijpers, F. I. M., & Verloove-VanHorick, S. P. (2005). Bullying: Who does what, when and where? Involvement of children, teachers and parents in bullying behavior. *Health Education Research, 20,* 81–91. doi:10.1093/her/cyg100

Ferguson, C. J., San Miguel, C., Kilburn, J. C., & Sanchez, P. (2007). The effectiveness of school-based anti-bullying programs: A meta-analytic review. *Criminal Justice Review, 32*(4). doi:10.1177/0734016807311712

Finkelhor, D., Ormrod, R., Turner, H., & Hamby, S. L. (2005). The victimization of children and youth: A comprehensive, national survey. *Child Maltreatment, 10*(1), 5–25. doi:1-.1177/1077559504271287

Flaspohler, P. D., Elfstrom, J. L., Vanderzee, K. L., & Sink, H. E. (2009). Stand by me: The effects of peer and teacher support in mitigating the impact of bullying on quality of life. *Psychology in the Schools, 46*(7), 636–649. doi:10.1002/pits.20404

Galand, B., & Hospel, V. (2013). Peer victimization and school disaffection: Exploring the moderation effect of social support and the mediation effect of depression. *British Journal of Educational Psychology, 83*, 569–590. doi:10.1111/j.2044-8279.2012.02077.x

Georgiou, S. (2008). Bullying and victimization at school: The role of mothers. *British Journal of Educational Psychology, 78*, 109–125. doi:10.1348/0000709907X204363

Georgiou, S., & Stavrinides, P. (2008). Bullies, victims and bully-victims: Psychosocial profiles and attribution styles. *School Psychology International, 29*, 574–589. doi:10.1177/0143034308099202

Gini, G., & Pozzoli, T. (2013). Bullied children and psychosomatic problems: A meta-analysis. *Pediatrics, 132*(4), 720–729. doi:10.1542/peds.2013-0614

Goldsmid, S., & Howie, P. (2013). Mediating and moderating role of attributional style in the association between victimisation and wellbeing. *Emotional and Behavioural Difficulties, 18*(4), 423–434. doi:10.1080/13632752.2013.803682

Greeff, A. P., & Van den Berg, E. (2013). Resilience in families in which a child is bullied. *British Journal of Guidance & Counselling, 41*(5), 504–517. doi:10.1080/03069885.2012.757692

Gregory, A., Cornell, D., Fan, X., Sheras, P., Shih, T.-H., & Huang, F. (2010). Authoritative school discipline: High school practices associated with lower bullying and victimization. *Journal of Educational Psychology, 102*(2), 483–496. doi:10.1037/a0018562

Haltigan, J. D., & Vaillancourt, T. (2014). Joint trajectories of bullying and peer victimization across elementary and middle school and associations with symptoms of psychopathology. *Developmental Psychology, 50*(11), 2426–2436. doi:10.1037/a00380301037

Hawker, D., & Boulton, M. (2000). Twenty years' research on peer victimization and psychosocial maladjustment: A meta-analytic review of cross-sectional studies. *Journal of Child Psychology and Psychiatry and Allied Disciplines, 41*(4), 441–455. doi:10.1111/1469-7610.00629

Hay, C., & Meldrum, R. (2010). Bullying victimization and adolescent self-harm: Testing hypotheses from general strain theory. *Journal of Youth and Adolescence, 39*, 446–459. doi:10.1007/s10964-009-9502-0

Hay, C., Meldrum, R., & Mann, K. (2010). Traditional bullying, cyber bullying, and deviance: A general strain theory approach. *Journal of Contemporary Criminal Justice, 26*(2), 130–147. doi:10.1177/1043986209359557

Hemphill, S. A., Kotevski, A., Herrenkohl, T. I., Bond, L., Jung Kim, M., Toumbourou, J. W., & Catalano, R. F. (2011). Longitudinal consequences of adolescent bullying perpetration and victimisation: A study of students in Victoria, Australia. *Criminal Behaviour and Mental Health, 21*, 107–116. doi:10.1002/cbm.802

Hinduja, S., & Patchin, J. W. (2007). Offline consequences of online victimization: School violence and delinquency. *Journal of School Violence, 6*(3), 89–112. doi:10.1300/J202v06n03_06

Horne, A., Orpinas, P., Newman-Carlson, D., & Bartolomucci, C. L. (2004). Elementary school bully buster program: Understanding why children bully, and what to do about it. In D. Espelage & S. M. Swearer (Eds.), *Bullying in American schools: A social-ecological perspective on prevention and intervention* (pp. 297–325). Mahwah, NJ: Erlbaum.

Hussein, M. H. (2013). The social and emotional skills of bullies, victims, and bully-victims of Egyptian primary school children. *International Journal of Psychology, 48*(5), 910–921. doi:10.1080/00207594.2012.702908

Idsoe, T., Dyregrov, A., & Idsoe, E. C. (2012). Bullying and PTSD symptoms. *Journal of Abnormal Child Psychology, 40*, 901–911. doi:10.1007/s10802-012-9620-0

Iyer, P. A., Dougall, A. L., & Jensen-Campbell, L. A. (2013). Are some adolescents differentially susceptible to the influence of bullying on depression? *Journal of Research in Personality, 47*(4), 272–281. doi:10.1016/j.jrp.2013.02.004

Janson, G. R., & Hazler, R. J. (2004). Trauma reactions of bystanders and victims to repetitive abuse experiences. *Violence and Victims, 19*(2), 239–255.

Janssen, I., Craig, W. M., Boyce, W. F., & Pickett, W. (2004). Associations between overweight and obesity with bullying behaviors in school-aged children. *Pediatrics, 113*(5), 1187–1194. doi:10.1542/peds.113.5.1187

Kiecolt-Glaser, J. K., Gouin, J.-P., Weng, N.-P., Malarkey, W. B., Beversdorf, D. Q., & Glaser, R. (2011). Childhood adversity heightens the impact of later-life caregiving stress on telomere length and inflammation. *Psychosomatic Medicine, 73*(1), 16–22. doi:10.1097/PSY.0b013e31820573b6

King, K. M., Puhl, R. M., Luedicke, J., & Peterson, J. L. (2013). Eating behaviors, victimization, and desire for supportive intervention among adolescents in weight-loss camps. *Eating Behaviors, 14*, 484–487. doi:10.1016/j.eatbeh.2013.080004.

Kliewer, W. (2006). Violence exposure and cortisol responses in urban youth. *International Journal of Behavioral Medicine, 13*(2), 109–120. doi:10.1207/s15327558ijbm1302_2

Knack, J. M., Jensen-Campbell, L. A., & Baum, A. (2011). Worse than sticks and stones? Bullying is associated with altered HPA axis functioning and poorer health. *Brain and Cognition, 77*(2), 183–190. doi:10.1016/j.bandc.2011.06.011

Knack, J., Tsar, V., Vaillancourt, T., Hymel, S., & McDougall, P. (2012). What protects rejected adolescents from also being bullied by their peers? The moderating role of peer-valued characteristics. *Journal of Research on Adolescence, 22*, 467–479. doi:10.1111/j.1532-7795.2012.00792.x

Kokkinos, C. M. (2013). Bullying and victimization in early adolescence: Associations with attachment style and perceived parenting. *Journal of School Violence, 12*, 174–192. doi:10.1080/15388220.2013.766134

Konold, T., Cornell, D., Huang, F., Meyer, P., Lacey, A., Nekvasil, E., . . . Shukla, K. (2014). Multilevel multi-informant structure of the authoritative school climate survey. *School Psychology Quarterly*. doi:10.1037/spq0000062

Kowalski, R. M., & Fedina, C. (2011). Cyber bullying in ADHD and Asperger syndrome populations. *Research in Autism Spectrum Disorders, 5*, 1201–1208. doi:10.1016/j.rasd.2011.01.007

Kowalski, R. M., Limber, S. P., & Agatston, P. W. (2011). *Cyber bullying: Bullying in the digital age.* Malden, MA: Blackwell.

Lamb, J., Pepler, D., & Craig, W. (2009). Approach to bullying and victimization. *Canadian Family Physician, 55*, 356–360.

Lee, S., Kim, C.-J., & Kim, D. H. (2013). A meta-analysis of the effect of school-based anti-bullying programs. *Journal of Child Health Care,* 1–18. doi:10.1177/1367493513503581

Lereya, S. T., Samara, M., & Wolke, D. (2013). Parenting behavior and the risk of becoming a victim and a bully/victim: A meta-analysis study. *Child Abuse & Neglect, 37*(12), 1091–1108. doi:10.1016/j.chiabu.2013.03.001

Lindsay, S., & McPherson, A. C. (2012). Experiences of social exclusion and bullying at school among children and youth with cerebral palsy. *Disability & Rehabilitation, 34*(2), 101–109. doi:10.3109/09638288.2011.587086

Mahady-Wilton, M., Craig, W. M., & Pepler, D. J. (2000). Emotional regulation and display in classroom victims of bullying: Characteristic expressions of affect, coping styles and relevant contextual factors. *Social Development, 9*, 226–245. doi:10.1111/1467-9507.00121

McDougall, P., & Vaillancourt, T. (2015). Long-term outcomes of peer victimization in childhood and adolescence: Pathways to adjustment and maladjustment. *American Psychologist.*

Merrell, K. W., Gueldner, B. A., Ross, S. W., & Isava, D. M. (2008). How effective are school bullying intervention programs? A meta-analysis of intervention research. *School Psychology Quarterly, 23*, 26–42. doi:10.1037/1045-3830.231.26

Mishna, F., Saini, M., & Solomon, S. (2009). Ongoing and online: Children and youth's perceptions of cyber bullying. *Children and Youth Services Review, 31*, 1222–1228. doi:10.1016/j.childyouth.2009.05.004

Nakamoto, J., & Schwartz, D. (2010). Is peer victimization associated with academic achievement? A meta-analytic review. *Social Development, 19*(2), 221–242. doi:10.1111/j.1467-9507.2009.00539.x

Nansel, T. R., Overpeck, M., Pilla, R. S., Ruan, W. J., Simons-Morton, B., & Scheidt, P. (2001). Bullying behaviors among US youth: Prevalence and association with psychosocial adjustment. *Journal of the American Medical Association, 285*(16), 2094–2100. doi:10.1001/jama.285.16.2094

Nordhagen, R., Nielsen, A., Stigum, H., & Köhler, L. (2005). Parental reported bullying among Nordic children: A population-based study. *Child: Care, Health and Development, 31*(6), 693–701. doi:10.1111/j.1365-2214.2005.00559.x

Olweus, D. (1993a). *Bullying at school: What we know and what we can do.* New York, NY: Blackwell.

Olweus, D. (1993b). Victimization by peers: Antecedents and long-term outcomes. In K. H. Rubin & J. H. B. Asendort (Eds.), *Social withdrawal, inhibition, and shyness* (pp. 315–341). Hillsdale, NJ: Erlbaum.

Olweus, D. (1994). Bullying at school: Basic facts and effects of a school based intervention program. *Journal of Child Psychology and Psychiatry, 35*(7), 1171–1190. doi:10.1111/j.1469-7610.1994.tb01229.x

Olweus, D. (2000). Sweden. In P. K. Smith, Y. Morita, J. Junger-Tas, D. Olweus, R. Catalano, & P. Slee (Eds.), *The nature of bullying: A cross-national perspective* (pp. 7–27). New York, NY: Routledge.

Ouellet-Morin, I., Danese, A., Bowes, L., Shakoor, S., Ambler, A., Pariante, C. M., . . . Arseneault, L. (2011). A discordant monozygotic twin design shows blunted cortisol reactivity among bullied children. *Journal of the American Academy of Child & Adolescent Psychiatry, 50*(6), 574–582. doi:10.1016/j.jaac.2011.02.015

Patchin, J. W., & Hinduja, S. (2006). Bullies move beyond the schoolyard: A preliminary look at cyberbullying. *Youth Violence and Juvenile Justice, 4*(2), 123–147. doi:10.1177/1541204006286288

Peeters, M., Cillessen, A., & Scholte, R. (2010). Clueless or powerful? Identifying subtypes of bullies in adolescence. *Journal of Youth and Adolescence, 39*, 1041–1052. doi:10.1007/s10964-009-9478-9

Perren, S., Dooley, J., Shaw, T., & Cross, D. (2010). Bullying in school and cyberspace: Associations with depressive symptoms in Swiss and Australian adolescents. *Child and Adolescent Psychiatry and Mental Health, 4*(28), 1–10.

Pepler, D. J., Craig, W. M., Connolly, J. A., Yuile, A., McMaster, L., & Jiang, D. (2006). A developmental perspective on bullying. *Aggressive Behavior, 32*, 376–384. doi:10.1002/ab.20136

Pepler, D. J., Craig, W., & O'Connell, P. (1999). Understanding bullying from a dynamic systems perspective. In A. Slater & D. Muir (Eds.), *Developmental psychology: An advanced reader.* Malden, MA: Blackwell.

Piskin, M. (2010). Examination of peer bullying among primary and middle school children in Ankara. *Education and Science, 35(*156), 175–189.

Polanin, J. R., Espelage, D. L., & Pigott, T. D. (2012). A meta-analysis of school-based bullying prevention programs' effects on bystander intervention behavior. *School Psychology Review, 41(*1), 47–65.

Reijntjes, A., Kamphuis, J. H., Prinzie, P., Boelen, P. A., van der Schoot, M., & Telch, M. J. (2011). Prospective linkages between peer victimization and externalizing problems in children: A meta-analysis. *Aggressive Behavior, 37*(3), 215–222. doi:10.1002/ab.20374

Reijntjes, A., Kamphuis, J. H., Prinzie, P., & Telch, M. J. (2010). Peer victimization and internalizing problems in children: A meta-analysis of longitudinal studies. *Child Abuse & Neglect, 34*(4), 244–252. doi:10.1016/j.chiabu.2009.07.009

Sapouna, M., & Wolke, D. (2013). Resilience to bullying victimization: The role of individual, family and peer characteristics. *Child Abuse & Neglect, 37*, 997–1006. doi:10.1016/j.chiabu.2013.05.009

Sengupta, A., & Chaudhuri, A. (2011). Are social networking sites a source of online harassment for teens? Evidence from survey data. *Children and Youth Services Review, 33*, 284–290. doi:10.1016/j.childyouth.2010.09.011

Shalev, I., Moffitt, T. E., Sugden, K., Williams, B., Houts, R. M., Danese, A., . . . Caspi, A. (2012). Exposure to violence during childhood is associated with telomere erosion from 5 to 10 years of age: A longitudinal study. *Molecular Psychiatry, 18*, 576–581. doi:10.1038/mp.2012.32

Sigfusdottir, I. D., Gudjonsson, G. H., & Sigurdsson, J. F. (2010). Bullying and delinquency: The mediating role of anger. *Personality and Individual Differences, 48*, 391–396. doi:10.1016/j.paid.2009.10.034

Smith, J. D., Schneider, B. H., Smith, P. K., & Ananiadou, K. (2004). The effectiveness of whole-school antibullying programs: A synthesis of evaluation research. *School Psychology Review, 33*, 547–560.

Smith, P. K., & Sharp, S. (1994). *School bullying: Insights and perspectives.* New York, NY: Routledge. doi:10.4324/9780203425497

Smokowski, P. R., & Kopasz, K. H. (2005). Bullying in school: An overview of types, effects, family characteristics, and intervention strategies. *Children & Schools, 27*(2), 101–110. doi:10.1093/cs/27.2.101

Srabstein, J. C., & Leventhal, B. L. (2010). Prevention of bullying-related morbidity and mortality: A call for public health policies. *Bulletin of the World Health Organization, 88*(6), 403–404. doi:10.1590/S0042-96862010000600003

Sugden, K., Arseneault, L., Harrington, H., Moffitt, T. E., Williams, B., & Caspi, A. (2010). Serotonin transporter gene moderates the development of emotional problems among children following bullying victimization. *Journal of the American Academy of Child & Adolescent Psychiatry, 49*(8), 830–840. doi:10.1016/j.jaac.2010.01.024

Swearer, S. M., Espelage, D. L., Vaillancourt, T., & Hymel, S. (2010). What can be done about school bullying? Linking research to educational practice. *Educational Researcher, 39*(1), 38–47. doi:10.3102/0013189X09357622

Takizawa, R., Maughan, B., & Arseneault, L. (2014). Adult health outcomes of childhood bullying victimization: Evidence from a five-decade longitudinal British birth cohort. *American Journal of Psychiatry, 171*, 777–784. doi:10.1176/appi.ajp.2014.13101401

Ttofi, M. M., & Farrington, D. P. (2011). Effectiveness of school-based programs to reduce bullying: A systematic and meta-analytic review. *Journal of Experimental Criminology, 7*, 27–56. doi:10.1007/s11292-010-9109-1

Ttofi, M. M., Farrington, D. P., & Baldry, A. C. (2008). *Effectiveness of programmes to reduce school bullying.* Stockholm, Sweden: Swedish Council for Crime Prevention, Information, and Publications.

Ttofi, M. M., Farrington, D. P., Losel, F., & Loeber, R. (2011). Do the victims of school bullies tend to become depressed later in life? A systematic review and meta-analysis of longitudinal studies. *Journal of Aggression, Conflict and Peace Research, 3*(2), 63–73. doi:10.1108/17596591111132873

Vaillancourt, T., Brittain, H., Bennett, L., Arnocky, S., McDougall, P., Hymel, S., . . . Short, K. (2010). Places to avoid: Population-based study of student reports of unsafe and high bullying areas at school. *Canadian Journal of School Psychology, 25*(1), 40–54.

Vaillancourt, T., Clinton, J., McDougall, P., Schmidt, L., & Hymel, S. (2010). The neurobiology of peer victimization and rejection. In S. R. Jimerson, S. M. Swearer, & D. L. Espelage (Eds.), *The handbook of bullying in schools: An international perspective* (pp. 293–327). New York, NY: Routledge.

Vaillancourt, T., Hepditch, J., Vitoroulis, I., Krygsman, A., Blain-Arcaro, C., & McDougall, P. (2013). The characteristics of peer relations among children with neurological and developmental conditions. In G. Ronen & P. Rosenbaum (Eds.), *Life quality outcomes in children and young people with neurological and developmental conditions: Concepts, evidence and practice: Clinics in Developmental Medicine* (pp. 87–106). Oxford, UK: Mac Keith Press.

Vaillancourt, T., Hymel, S., & McDougall, P. (2013). The biological underpinnings of peer victimization: Understanding why and how the effects of bullying can last a lifetime. *Theory Into Practice, 52*, 241–248. doi:10.1080/00405841.2013.829726

Vaillancourt, T., McDougall, P., Hymel, S., Krygsman, A., Miller, J., Stiver, K., & Davis, C. (2008). Bullying: Are researchers and children/youth talking about the same thing? *International Journal of Behavioral Development, 32*(6), 486–495. doi:10.1177/0165025408095553

Vandebosch, H., & Van Cleemput, K. (2009). Cyberbullying among youngsters: Profiles of bullies and victims. *New Media & Society, 11*(8), 1349–1371. doi:10.1177/1461444809341263

Vreeman, R. C., & Carroll, A. E. (2007). A systematic review of school-based interventions to prevent bullying. *Archives of Pediatric and Adolescent Medicine, 161*, 78–88.

Wang, J., Iannotti, R. J., Luk, J. W., & Nansel, T. R. (2010). Co-occurrence of victimization from five subtypes of bullying: Physical, verbal, social exclusion, spreading rumors, and cyber. *Journal of Pediatric Psychology, 35*(10), 1103–1112. doi:10.1093/jpepsy/jsq048

Wang, J., Iannotti, R. J., & Nansel, T. R. (2009). School bullying among adolescents in the United States: Physical, verbal, relational, and cyber. *Journal of Adolescent Health, 25*, 268–275. doi:10.1016/j.jadohealth.2009.03.021

Wang, J., Nansel, T. R., & Iannotti, R. J. (2011). Cyber and traditional bullying: Differential association with depression. *Journal of Adolescent Health, 48*, 415–417. doi:10.1016/j.jadhealth.2010.07.012

Wang, W., Vaillancourt, T., Brittain, H. L., McDougall, P., Krygsman, A., Smith, D., . . . , Hymel, S. (2014). School climate, peer victimization, and academic achievement: Results from a multi-informant study. *School Psychology Quarterly.* doi:10.1037/spq0000084

Williams, K. R., & Guerra, N. G. (2007). Prevalence and predictors of Internet bullying. *Journal of Adolescent Health, 41*, S14–S21. doi:10.1016/j.jadohealth.2007.08.018

Williford, A., Elledge, L. C., Boulton, A. J., DePaolis, K. J., Little, T. D., & Salmivalli, C. (2013). Effects of the KiVa antibullying program on cyberbullying and cybervictimization frequency among Finnish youth. *Journal of Clinical Child & Adolescent Psychology, 42*(6), 820–833. doi:10.1080/15374416.2013.787623

Wolak, J., Mitchell, K. J., & Finkelhor, D. (2007). Does online harassment constitute bullying? An exploration of online harassment by known peers and online-only contacts. *Journal of Adolescent Health, 41*, S51–S58. doi:10.1016/j.jadohealth.2007.08.019

Wolke, D., Copeland, W. E., Angold, A., & Costello, E. J. (2013). Impact of bullying in childhood on adult health, wealth, crime, and social outcomes. *Psychological Science, 24*(10), 1958–1970. doi:10.1177/0956797613481608

Wong-Lo, M., Bullock, L. M., & Gable, R. A. (2011). Cyber bullying: Practices to face digital aggression. *Emotional and Behavioural Difficulties, 16*(3), 317–325. doi:10.1080/13632752.2011.595098

Yang, A., & Salmivalli, C. (2013). Different forms of bullying and victimization: Bully-victims versus bullies and victims. *European Journal of Developmental Psychology, 10*(6), 723–738. doi:10.1080/17405629.2013.793596

Ybarra, M. L., Diener-West, M., & Leaf, P. J. (2007). Examining the overlap in Internet harassment and school bullying: Implications for school intervention. *Journal of Adolescent Health, 41*, S42–S50. doi:10.1016/j.jadohealth.2007.09.004

Yoon, J. S., & Kerber, K. (2003). Bullying: Elementary teachers' attitudes and intervention strategies. *Research in Education, 69*, 27–34. doi:10.7227/RIE.69.3

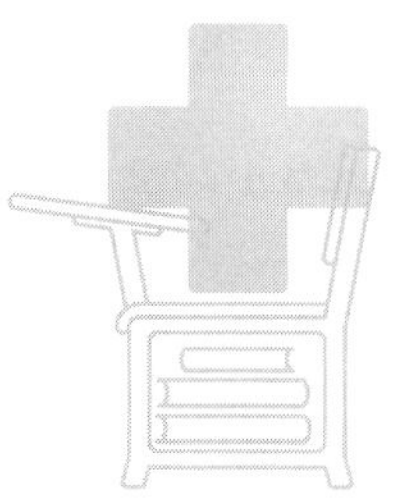

Chapter 19
Antisocial Behavior and School Violence

Understanding and Preventing Destructive Outcomes

Hill M. Walker, Jeffrey R. Sprague,
and Herbert H. Severson

This chapter addresses issues associated with the destructive pathways that increasing numbers of behaviorally at-risk children and youth are following toward later health-risk outcomes in adolescence and young adulthood (Hawkins, Catalano, Kosterman, Abbott, & Hill, 1999; Reid, Patterson, & Snyder, 2002; Walker, Ramsey, & Gresham, 2004). This well-traveled road, sometimes called the path to prison or the school-to-prison pipeline (Christle, Jolivette, & Nelson, 2005), usually begins early in a child's life and often ends tragically in long-term incarceration, mental and physical health problems, and early death (Anda, Felitti, & Bremner, 2006). This pathway is sometimes associated with violent acts, but more often it results from exposure to a host of risk factors, primarily occurring within nonschool settings, and it results in dysfunctional outcomes, such as school failure, delinquency, substance abuse, frequent bullying, peer harassment, and aggression toward others. In addition, it often produces active rejection by peers, teachers, and even primary caregivers during adolescence (see Loeber & Farrington, 1998; Patterson, Reid, & Dishion, 1992).

The social and economic costs of these preventable outcomes are extraordinary, and society increasingly views them as unacceptable. Ironically, we have developed the intervention methods, parent and teacher support systems, and behavioral technologies needed to prevent and reduce the vast majority of these destructive behavior patterns (Reid et al., 2002; Robinson, 2004; Shinn & Walker, 2010; Walker & Gresham, 2014). Yet at best, we continue as a society to be engaged in a holding pattern of action that suggests little in the way of future improvements in addressing these challenges because we seem unable to broadly implement, and to do so well, the practices that can potentially solve them (Biglan, 2013).

This chapter describes essential information that educators need for regarding these problems. The topics dealt with herein include definitions of violence, school violence as a form of terrorism, behavioral characteristics of at-risk youth, causal factors and influences on violent behavior, developmental pathways, trends in youth violence, and solutions that can be implemented primarily within school contexts but in collaboration with families, law enforcement, courts, and social service agencies (i.e. mental health), as appropriate. We believe schools and school personnel can and should be major players in the development of solutions to youth violence and the antisocial behavior patterns that provide a fertile breeding ground for violent acts.

During the past decade, schools have become tragic targets for the rage of some very disturbed students and adults who seek to redress their grievances and register their social impact through acts of violence directed against innocent students and educators (Cornell, 2006). Preventing and coping with these tragedies, once they occur, remains one of the most excruciating situations our society must deal with. We conclude the chapter with commentary about the changing landscape of school violence and its social impact, resulting from such factors as (a) media coverage of school shootings and copycat tragedies, (b)) the role of mental health problems in school shootings and rampage killings, and (c) violence against teachers by today's students.

VIOLENCE DEFINED

Youth violence and violence generally have emerged as among our society's most pressing public health problems (American Psychological Association, APA, 1993; Report on rampage killings, 2013; Satcher, 2001). Violence has spilled over into our school systems in the most unfortunate manner imaginable and now ranks as a social toxin that poisons school cultures and the atmosphere of the larger society. Violent acts are similar to sudden natural disasters (e.g., earthquakes, tsunamis), which cannot be easily predicted given their extremely low base rate, appear to come out of nowhere, account for incredible damage in a matter of minutes, and require long periods for recovery. Individuals and society are victimized not only by the actual occurrence of violent acts but also, and especially, by the fear of them. The threat of violence requires enhanced vigilance and can reduce our overall quality of life.

The definitions of violence promoted by numerous experts, including academics and social commentators, are often polarizing and have the effect of diluting the meaning of this concept. For example, some argue that if individuals are required to alter their routines or lifestyle because of the possibility of violence, then they have experienced violence already and victimization is palpable and real (Crowe, 1995). While this observation may be partially true, it occurs thousands of times daily in our society (especially with females), is a functional survival skill in high-risk areas, and is a fact of life. Vigilance in this context strikes us as a valued attribute. In a similar vein, Henry (2009) has presented a very broad-based, complex, and multiply determined definition of violence that incorporates the perception of violent behavior directed toward oneself and consists of acts that range from physical violence to relatively innocuous forms of misbehavior, such as being a target of an insult or a negative verbal characterization. It is unlikely that individuals who are charged with preventing violence, especially school administrators, find such formulations helpful in making schools safer and more secure. It is now no longer an option for schools not to plan accommodations and protective strategies that can make the setting more secure (Sprague & Walker, 2010).

In the legal system, *violence* is defined as involving one or more of the following acts: (a) robbery, (b) rape, (c) aggravated assault, or (d) murder (Dinkes, Cataldi, & Lin-Kelly, 2007). We believe that school violence should be based on this legal definition and that lesser forms of aggressive behavior or attempts at assault should be classified as destructive but not as violence. Although a broad range of acts are referred to in the media and popular culture as violent, they do not represent actual violence in most cases but rather are often associated with violence or are the precursors or antecedents of violent behavior. Among children and youth, the precursors of violence are expressed through antisocial acts that can involve extreme forms of aggression, bullying, threats, intimidation, and/or harassment directed toward others, especially peers and, on occasion, school staff (Farrington, 1998; Patterson, Reid, & Dishion, 1992; Walker, Colvin, & Ramsey, 1995). It should be noted that, for youth who are the most severely at risk, it is not all that unusual for other adults to be targets of their antisocial acts as well (Thompson, 2013).

VIOLENCE AS A FORM OF DOMESTIC TERRORISM

As the public's willingness to tolerate the risk of potential mass school shootings has declined precipitously, school violence has emerged as a form of domestic terrorism. Symbolically, the U.S. Office of Safe and Drug Free Schools has been assigned to the Department of Homeland Security (Sprague, Close, & Walker, 2014). Nothing terrorizes parents quite like the specter of a disturbed student unleashing violence on fellow students and school staff—or even worse, a deranged adult who invades the school and tries to wound, kill, and maim as many as possible, as happened in 2012 at Sandy Hook Elementary in Newtown, Connecticut. Parents and the larger society have demanded that schools become palpably more secure, as many have lost their sense that schools are a safe environment in which children and youth are free to learn absent the risk of potential violence. Even though we are constantly reassured that the odds of such an event happening are extremely remote and that schools are one of the safest places for our children, parents have every right to insist that school leaders make safety a very high priority and take concrete steps to accomplish that.

This widespread psychological fear, or "terror," according to Henry (2009) and Muschert and Peguero (2010), results from the trauma induced by such tragedies as the 1998 Thurston High School shooting and the 1999 shooting at Columbine High School, and their extensive media coverage. According to these experts, this phenomenon has transformed schools into fortress-like structures that are driven by security practices and policies that are intrusive, overly restrictive, and not effective. They refer to this broad-based psychological trauma and fear as "the Columbine effect" and advocate resistance to efforts by schools to address it through enhanced school security. In the absence of compelling evidence to the contrary, we would argue that schools' responses to these pressures are logical and fall within the purview of what schools can actually do and control. There is no central database tracking the extent and nature of school security practices in U.S. schools. The Readiness and Emergency Management for Schools Technical Assistance Center (http://rems.ed.gov), operated by the Department of Education, provides written resources on school security and development for emergency operations plans, but no inventory of school security measures is mentioned or provided.

The horrific tragedy at Sandy Hook has produced a strong surge in the use of technology and architectural design to enhance school security and safety across the country. In a December 9, 2013, report for the *Columbian* titled *Schools Strive for Safety in Designing New Buildings*, Susan Parish describes the impact of the Newtown tragedy on the architectural design of new buildings and the retrofitting of older buildings to maximize their security and safety along with the use of commonsense, protective methods to make it difficult for someone to invade the school. These latter techniques range from classroom doors that can lock from the inside, entrance and exit doors that can be opened only electronically by a staff member, and the sophisticated use of video surveillance (more than 450 cameras are used to monitor the school grounds and settings in schools in Vancouver, Washington). Architects are rapidly embracing the knowledge base provided by the Crime Prevention Through Environmental Design (CPTED) model of securing public spaces through structural design, redesign, and retrofitting techniques (see Crowe, 1995; Schneider, Walker, & Sprague, 2000). CPTED is a highly respected and widely adopted model that can make public spaces much more secure. It has been adopted by a broad range of public agencies and is highly recommended for adoption by schools.

The impact of these scaled-up measures and policies should be assessed not only in terms of their possible impact in reducing the likelihood of school shootings but also according to the extent to which they (a) reduce pervasive psychological fears of school violence among families, policy makers, and the larger society and (b) help restore a sense of school security and safety among students. Reformulating school safety and security and the development of new metrics to assess and monitor it would be useful contributions in addressing this concern.

One of the discouraging and oft-repeated responses to the justifiable outrage about rampage shootings, such as those that have occurred at Sandy Hook Elementary, a U.S. Navy Yard, and a Colorado movie house, is the inevitable expert commentary that the frequency of such episodes has not increased appreciably in several decades. The effect of this commentary often places a damper on renewed efforts to address the proximal root causes and by implication to sustain current levels of risk tolerance for potential violence in the search for society-based causal factors of a more distal nature (see Muschert, Henry, Bracy, & Peguero, 2014). As the number of individuals killed and wounded in these rampage shootings escalates, the public's tolerance for risk correspondingly declines and calls for more direct protective actions increase. *CBS Evening News* reported in November 2013 that in a 12-month period in 2012 and 2013, 85 individuals were killed in 11 rampage shootings in the United States. Americans find such statistics appalling, making prompt calls for new methods to prevent these acts. Until we as a society can gain control over these events and reduce their likelihood of occurrence in school and societal contexts, school protective actions (e.g., use of school resource officers, retrofitting of school buildings, installation of metal detectors, use of nonobvious video surveillance, a push button to lock down the school and dial 911 simultaneously, zero-tolerance policies) seem reasonable even though their social costs can be measured in such outcomes as loss of privacy and confidentiality, the option to refuse treatment for severe mental health problems, and more restrictive and intrusive social control procedures adopted by institutions such as schools, courtrooms, and legislatures.

BEHAVIORAL CHARACTERISTICS OF AT-RISK AND ANTISOCIAL YOUTH

At-risk and antisocial youth, many of whom engage in the precursors of violence and ultimately become violent, are very challenging to their families, teachers, and social networks given the highly aversive, confronting, and intimidating nature of their behavioral styles. They can be demanding, impulsive, coercive, oppositional–defiant, disruptive, and extremely aggressive. These youth are generally successful in resisting adult influence strategies designed to change their behavior but are often open to the negative influences of deviant peers, which further socializes them toward delinquent and violent lifestyles (Patterson et al., 1992). The two following brief cases illustrate how antisocial youth are often socialized to view their social environs and their respective role(s) in them.

Some years ago, the senior author and his colleagues were developing an intervention for dealing with aggressive K–3 children (Walker, Hops, & Greenwood, 1988) who teased and bullied others during school recess (Walker & Sprague, 1999a). Ritchie, a second-grader, was referred by his school counselor and homeroom teacher for possible inclusion in the intervention. During a playground recess period, Ritchie's social behavior was observed and recorded to determine whether he was an appropriate candidate for the program. Ritchie impulsively attacked a kindergarten boy in the presence of the observer, playground supervisor, and program consultant. He knocked the smaller boy to the ground and was choking him, with an apparent attempt to cause bodily harm and to inflict pain. The playground supervisor intervened and called the principal and school counselor who escorted Ritchie into the school to call his parents. Ritchie was asked what prompted him to make the attack. "Can you tell us why you were choking Jason like that?" Ritchie seemed surprised and responded, "Well, it was recess!"

Sarah was a fourth-grader who was commonly regarded as a holy terror by her teachers and peers. Sarah was passively aggressive, smart, a natural leader, and skilled in manipulating others. Ms. Billie Webb was a school psychologist who served Sarah's school part-time, along with two others, and visited her school several times weekly. As a general rule, Sarah was a regular visitor of Billie's each time she visited the school; Billie and Sarah were on a first-name basis. During one of Billie's visits, the school's principal and counselor were waiting for Billie to tell her the latest things Sarah had done on the playground. Billie called Sarah into a conference to hear her side of things.

Billie started, "Sarah, I understand you've been having problems on the playground, again!" Sarah just stared at Billie and said nothing. While attempting to engage Sarah in a problem-solving process, Billie asked another question. "What do you think people will say about that, Sarah?" Sarah thought a minute, looked at Billie, and said, "Well Billie, some people might say *you're* not doing your job!"

These actual scenarios illustrate how many antisocial youth see themselves and the world they live in. These youth are frequently egotistical, self-absorbed, and insensitive to the feelings and needs of others. The behavioral standards they have developed are qualitatively divergent from those of others. Children like Ritchie and Sarah are heavily into denial and often refuse to assume responsibility for their actions (Walker & Sprague, 1999a; Walker et al., 1995). By adolescence, approximately half of antisocial youth are also committing covert acts of stealth, such as vandalism, fire setting, shoplifting, property destruction, and/or substance abuse (Patterson et al., 1992). In the classroom setting, covert antisocial behavior is usually expressed as lying, cheating, and stealing, which are three forms of student behavior that teachers broadly view as among the most objectionable (see Walker, 1986).

These behavioral characteristics are dysfunctional in the extreme and set up behaviorally at-risk youth for destructive outcomes and health-risk behaviors over the long term. Longitudinal studies conducted over the past four decades in Australia, New Zealand, Canada, the United States, the British Isles, and Western Europe converge in documenting these outcomes in late adolescence and young adulthood for this population. They include the following: substance abuse, heavy drinking, delinquency, severe depression, school failure, chronic disciplinary problems, dependence on welfare and social service systems, dishonorable military discharges, criminal offenses and arrests, and higher hospitalization and mortality rates (see Kazdin, 1985; Loeber & Farrington, 1998; Patterson et al., 1992; Walker et al., 1995).

COMORBIDITY AND THE SEVERITY OF DESTRUCTIVE OUTCOMES

The issue of comorbidity, or "mixed syndromes," has emerged in the past decade as a most important development in defining the severity and long-term developmental course of behaviorally at-risk youth (see Gresham, Lane, & Lambros, 2000). For example, Seeley, Rohde, Lewinsohn, and Clarke (2002) noted that when conduct disorder (CD) is combined or mixed with severe depression among at-risk youth, the adolescent suicide-attempt rate increases from approximately 13% for adolescents in general to about 40% for this subpopulation. Similarly, Lynam (1996) has reviewed extensive research on the relationship between attention-deficit/hyperactivity disorder (ADHD) and conduct disorder. Lynam has developed a compelling and elegant conceptual model regarding the comorbidity of ADHD and CD, arguing that this "mixture" provides the foundation for the later development of severe psychopathology. Significant numbers of antisocial youth may be vulnerable to these two forms of elevated risk as well as other possibilities (e.g., conduct disorder, severe learning disabilities). It is essential that behaviorally at-risk youth be assessed for the presence of comorbid conditions, and that attempts are made to divert them from this developmental pathway as early as possible in their lives and school careers.

CAUSAL FACTORS AND INFLUENCES

The toxic conditions and negative forces of our society are producing thousands of children like Ritchie and Sarah who come from backgrounds and environmental conditions that put them at high risk. Dysfunctional families, drug and alcohol abuse by caregivers, poverty, neglect, weak parenting skills, deteriorating neighborhoods, association with deviant peers, and portrayals of media violence are but a few of the risks to which increasing numbers of children and youth are exposed on a daily basis. Reid (1993) has noted that the more of these risks to which one is exposed and the longer such exposure lasts, the greater the likelihood that destructive outcomes will occur in the lives of behaviorally at-risk youth.

In its seminal report on youth violence, the APA (1993) identified four causal factors for youth violence that act as accelerators along the pathway that propels at-risk youth toward destructive outcomes: (a) early involvement with drugs and alcohol, (b) easy access to weapons, especially handguns, (c) depiction of violent acts in media and interactive games, (d) and association with antisocial groups. These risk factors form a toxic mixture and are more likely to come into play in preadolescence and adolescence than earlier in a child's development. At-risk children are commonly made vulnerable to these causal influences through the risks they have previously experienced (e.g., weak parenting, dysfunctional families).

Moffitt (1994) has made an important distinction between early and later starters in the development of antisocial behavior patterns. Early starters are socialized to this lifestyle by their family situations, whereas later starters are socialized to it by peers. Early starters experience a host of risk factors, and few protective factors, from the moment of birth, and they are likely to manifest antisocial forms of behavior over their life course. Later starters, in contrast, have many more advantages and generally engage in "adolescent limited" antisocial behavior that often reduces after several years and typically does not emerge until the late elementary grades. It is essential that early starters receive appropriate screening, evaluation, and interventions as soon as possible in their lives and school careers (Severson, Walker, Hope-Doolittle, Kratochwill, & Gresham, 2007).

It is important to note herein that predicting future acts of violence on a case-by-case basis ranges from difficult in the extreme to impossible given the state of our current knowledge and the limited tools available to us for this purpose. The U.S. Surgeon General's 2001 *Report on Youth Violence*, for example, correctly notes that it is nearly impossible to predict which highly aggressive young children (i.e., early starters) will become violent in adolescence. That said, however, we can identify groups of individuals who have a much higher likelihood of committing later violent acts—*as a group*. Patterson, Reid, and Dishion (1992), for example, found that the following profile of antisocial youth was predictive of later, violent acts among a sample of severely at-risk adolescents: (a) the first arrest occurred early in the youth's life (i.e., age 10 years or younger), (b) the first arrest was for a serious offense, and (c) by age 12, the youth had three or more arrests and was considered a chronic offender. It is important to note, however, that although it is possible to identify and profile such high-risk groups, determining in advance *which* individual group member(s) will commit a later violent act is still extremely difficult. Thus, prediction of future violent acts at the individual child or youth level remains extremely problematic.

THE ROLE OF RISK AND PROTECTIVE FACTORS

In the psychological literature on antisocial behavior and youth violence, it is quite common to see causal factors and influences arrayed in terms of risk and protective factors. Risk factors are identifiable conditions and influences that increase the likelihood of destructive outcomes; protective factors are positive influences operating in a youth's life that can buffer or offset the negative impact of risk exposure. For example, a dysfunctional family is a commonly occurring risk factor, but having access to a caring adult in one's life is a protective factor that can attenuate the damaging impact of such a family environment. Both risk and protective factors have been shown to operate at five different levels: individual, family, school, peer group, and societal (Bronfenbrenner, 1979). Two of the strongest risk factors for youth violence early on in a child's life are (a) an early pattern of general, repeat offending and (b) substance use and abuse. In adolescence, the most powerful risks in this regard are having weak social ties, having antisocial and/or delinquent peers, and gang membership. Protective factors that can buffer and offset these risks are having an intolerant attitude toward deviance, having a high IQ, being female, having a positive social orientation, and understanding the relationship between transgressions and sanctions (see Satcher, 2001). Table 19.1 contains a more elaborate listing of risk and protective factors related to shared vulnerability for both delinquency and violence.

It is very difficult for schools and educators to affect many of the risk factors (e.g., poverty, dysfunctional families, weak parenting, neglect, abuse) that impinge directly on children's lives and impair their school performance. However, it is possible to enhance and develop offsetting protective factors that will have a positive influence in their lives. Typically, school personnel do not investigate or assess the types of risk and protective factors that operate in a student's life. We think this practice is a shortcoming and that educators would be better able both to understand problematic student behavior in the school setting and to reduce and/or replace it if such information were available on a systematic basis (Metzler et al., 2008).

The adoption of the functional behavior assessment (FBA) approach to assessment by many school personnel (e.g., behavioral

Table 19.1

RISK-PROTECTIVE FACTORS ASSOCIATED WITH YOUTH VIOLENCE AND DELINQUENCY

Factors associated with elevated risk for violence and delinquency

1. Poor social skills
2. Poor school engagement
3. Family with one or more of the following characteristics: lack of parental supervision, mother or father ever arrested, evidence of child abuse or neglect, at least one family transition such as divorce or remarriage
4. Predelinquent problem behaviors, such as bullying and annoying others, fighting, being stubborn and defiant, and telling lies
5. Early drug and alcohol use
6. Early age of onset of delinquent activity
7. A high level of "daily hassles" (minor stressors)
8. Attention-deficit/hyperactivity disorder
9. Learning disabilities
10. Low IQ, especially verbal ability
11. Poor school performance, especially poor grades in high school
12. Delinquent peers
13. Having multiple risk factors (the cumulative effect of several family and child risk variables has been found to be a better predictor of delinquency than any single variable alone)

Factors that buffer against the risk of developing violent or destructive behavior

1. Family stability
2. Positive temperament
3. Academic success
4. Positive school experiences
5. Positive work or work training experiences
6. High self-esteem
7. Structure in the environment (school and home)
8. A good relationship with a parent or other adult
9. Advanced self-help and problem-solving skills
10. Internal locus of control (e.g., anger management, limit setting, goal setting)
11. Identified network of family and friends who are available for support in times of crisis
12. High engagement in positive activities (e.g., sports, hobbies, art, community service)

specialists, school psychologists) is an attempt to understand and identify the causal factors that account for a student's problem behavior in school contexts (O'Neill, Albin, Storey, Horner, & Sprague, 2014; O'Neill, Horner, Albin, Sprague, Storey, & Newton, 1997; O'Neill & Stephenson, 2010; Van Acker, Boreson, Gable, & Potterton, 2005). In this method, hypotheses or notions are developed that may help explain what accounts for the student's motivation to perform problem behavior (e.g., seeking attention, avoiding aversive tasks, seeking to establish dominance or control). The immediate causes or antecedents of the behaviors are also identified, along with more acceptable replacement behaviors (Dunlap, Iovannone, Wilson, Kincaid, & Strain, 2010). Assessments (typically direct observations) are then conducted to verify or reject these "hunches" or behavioral hypotheses. However, although FBA approaches are useful in better understanding a student's behavior within a specific school setting such as the classroom or playground, to more fully understand and account for a student's overall school behavior patterns, it is also necessary to conduct a thorough risk and protective factor analysis (for a discussion of FBA versus risk and protective assessment issues, see Walker & Sprague, 1999b).

ASSESSING RISK AND PROTECTIVE FACTORS IN THE SCHOOL SETTING

Along with the work of Najaka, Gottfredson, and Wilson (2001), the research of Vance, Fernandez, and colleagues ranks as some of the most important research conducted to date on assessing and analyzing risk-protective factors as they impact educational achievement and behavioral adjustment within school settings (see Vance, Fernandez & Biber, 1998). Recently, Vance, Bowen, Fernandez, and Thompson, (2002) reported a predictive study of the role of risk and protective factors as predictors of longitudinal outcomes among adolescents having serious psychiatric disorders and aggression. The study involved 337 adolescents enrolled in a treatment program for youth with severe aggression and emotional disturbance in North Carolina. Historical and current psychosocial risk-protective factors, along with ratings of the severity of psychiatric symptoms recorded at time 1, were used to predict problematic outcomes (e.g., risk-taking, self-injurious, threatening, assaultive behavior) at time 2 one year later. These authors reported that 11 risk and protective factors predicted the time 2 outcomes, whereas none of the psychiatric symptom ratings did. These findings are important in documenting the invaluable role that the assessment and analysis of risk-protective factors can play in understanding and accounting for problematic youth behavior in the context of schooling.

Gottfredson and Gottfredson (1999) have developed a number of measures and batteries to assess the social ecology of school settings including risk-protective factors. Their self-report measure of risk and resiliency factors is a highly recommended tool for educators in assessing student characteristics. This instrument, What About You? (WAY), has three different forms that also take into account student reading levels. The WAY spans Grades 5–12 and provides a standardized and validated method of gathering information to identify problems, set goals and objectives, plan interventions, and evaluate progress. WAY also provides objective measures of risk factors for problem behavior and drug use as well as protective factors for social integration and self-esteem (see Gottfredson & Gottfredson, 1999, for a description of the psychometric features and technical development of the instrument). Information about WAY and related school assessments can be obtained by writing to Gottfredson Associates Inc., 3239 B Corporate Court, Ellicott City, MD, 21042.

DEVELOPMENTAL PATHWAYS

Walker and Sprague (1999a) and Walker and Severson (2002) have previously discussed the developmental pathways through which behaviorally at-risk children and youth come to acquire violent and delinquent lifestyles. The classic research of Patterson, Reid, and Dishion (1992), Eddy, Reid, and Curry (2002), and Loeber and Farrington (1998) has been instrumental in illuminating the nature and etiology of these pathways as well as the behavioral processes that operate across developmental stages within them. Through longitudinal studies of antisocial children, youth, and their families, there are now strong and clearly established links between exposure to the previously mentioned risk factors; the maladaptive behavioral manifestations that result from them; the short-term negative outcomes that accrue to the at-risk child associated with these behavioral manifestations over time; and finally the costly and socially destructive long-term outcomes that (a) typically complete this developmental progression and (b) prove very destructive to the at-risk child or youth, family members, friends, peers, and, finally, the larger society (see Vance et al., 2002).

Figure 19.1 shows the connecting links in this developmental trajectory that defines a well-traveled pathway from early exposure to experiencing serious conditions of risk, and the later development of destructive outcomes and health-risk behaviors that can reduce dramatically one's life chances and quality of life (Hawkins et al., 1999).

More and more young children are experiencing a plethora of risk factors from the moment of birth with few offsetting protective factors. As a consequence, we are seeing many youth who are following this unfortunate path that too often ends in school failure and dropout, delinquency, adult crime, and sometimes violence. Hawkins et al. (1999) reported a widely cited and impressive 12-year longitudinal intervention study in which the role of school bonding, engagement, and attachment was examined as a protective factor in preventing health-risk outcomes for an at-risk sample in adolescence. These researchers found that through early intervention in Grades 1–4 with the target child, teachers and parents had a powerful impact in preventing health-risk outcomes at age 18. They concluded that the key prevention variable in their study was the protective influence of school engagement, bonding, and attachment, which was targeted by their intervention at the point of school entry. School bonding seems to be emerging in a number of experimental studies and reviews as a strong factor in predicting adolescent outcomes of this nature (see Najaka et al., 2002). We believe that assisting behaviorally at-risk children in getting off to the best start possible in their school careers enhances school bonding and attachment, and thus engages the protective influences of the schooling process (Shinn, Walker, & Stoner, 2002).

TRENDS IN YOUTH VIOLENCE

In the 1990s, the United States and its public schools were shocked by a series of school shootings that changed the landscape of school security and shattered the sense of relative safety that students, families, and educators traditionally held about our buildings and campuses. All concerned with the schooling and protection of vulnerable children and youth were traumatized by these terrible events (Sprague & Walker, 2010). Even though schools statistically are the *least likely* places for children and youth to be killed, compared with other social settings, Americans stopped regarding school settings as safe havens in which students are free to develop academically and socially, unburdened by concern for their personal safety.

The publication *Indicators of School Crime and Safety* (Robers, Kemp, & Truman, 2013) presents data on crime and safety at school from the perspectives of students, teachers, and principals. This annual report, a joint effort by the Bureau of Justice Statistics and the

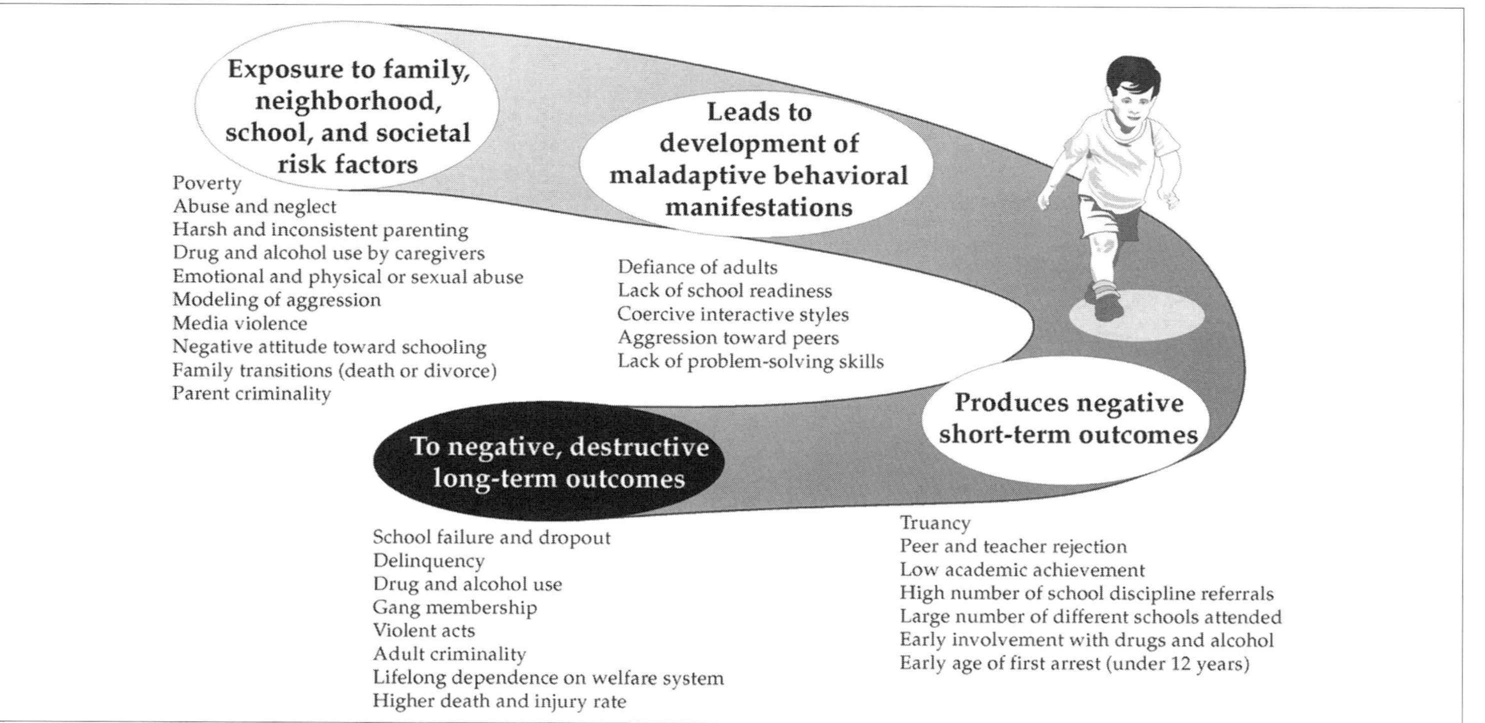

Figure 19.1. The path to long-term negative outcomes for at-risk children and youth. From "The Path to School Failure, Delinquency, and Violence: Causal Factors and Some Potential Solutions," by H. M. Walker and J. R. Sprague, 1999, *Intervention in School and Clinic, 35*, 68. Copyright 1999 by PRO-ED, Inc. Reprinted with permission.

National Center for Education Statistics (NCES), provides detailed statistical information on the nature of crime in schools. This report contains 21 indicators of crime at school from a number of sources, including the National Crime Victimization Survey (NCVS), the School Crime Supplement to the NCVS, the Youth Risk Behavior Survey, the School Survey on Crime and Safety, and the School and Staffing Survey. Topics covered include victimization at school, teacher injury, bullying and cyberbullying, school conditions, fights, weapons, availability and student use of drugs and alcohol, and student perceptions of personal safety at school.

Data on school-associated violent deaths are collected using the School-Associated Violent Deaths Study (SAVD). School-associated violent deaths include those that occurred while the victim was on the way to or returning from regular sessions at school or while the victim was attending or traveling to or from an official school-sponsored event. Victims of school-associated violent deaths include not only students and staff members but also others who are not students or staff members, such as parents.

From 1992 to 1999, a consistent pattern was observed in the number of homicides at school (Dinkes et al., 2007). During this period, between 28 and 34 homicides of school-age youth occurred at school in each school year. The number of school-associated homicides declined between the 1998–1999 and 1999–2000 school years, from 33 to 13 homicides. This pattern of school shootings continued into the 21st century, punctuated by the 2005 incident in Red Lake, Minnesota, where a 16-year-old killed his grandfather and a companion, then went to school, where he killed a teacher, a security guard, five students, and finally himself, leaving a total of 10 people dead. In addition, school shootings occurred that involved adults as perpetrators, including the 2006 incident in Nickel Mines, Pennsylvania, where a man entered the one-room West Nickel Mines Amish School and shot 10 schoolgirls, ranging in age from 6 to 13 years, and then himself. Five of the girls and the shooter died. This phenomenon of large-scale, rampage shootings has also spread to college campuses, including the 2007 incident at Virginia Tech, where a student killed two other students in a dorm, then killed 30 more two hours later in a classroom building. His suicide brought the death toll to 33, making this shooting rampage the most deadly in U.S. history. Homicides at school increased from 11 to 21 between the 2000–2001 and 2004–2005 school years, and dropped to 14 in 2005–2006. The 2007–2010 school years showed a decline in school-related homicides from 21 to 11.

The most recent data collected from this survey cover the period from July 1, 2010, through June 30, 2011. During this period, there were 31 school-associated violent deaths in elementary and secondary schools in the United States. Of the 31 student, staff, and nonstudent school-associated violent deaths occurring between July 1, 2010, and June 30, 2011, 25 were homicides and 6 were suicides. The 2011 data are considered preliminary until police interviews are conducted to fully document them. The percentage of youth homicides occurring at school remains at less than 2% of the total number of youth homicides, even though the absolute number of homicides of school-age youth at school varies across the years. Figure 19.2 illustrates this multiyear pattern (Robers et al., 2013).

It should be noted that a true picture of a youth's criminal behavior is not provided by arrest indices alone. Youth self-reports of illegal activities, which do not result in arrests, are also an important index of criminal behavior, and they do not always agree with arrest data. This is true in the case of youth violence. Numerous experts in the justice system agree that there is approximately one arrest for every ten arrestable offenses committed. Around 1983, arrests for both violent acts and youth self-reports of violent behavior showed acceleration. However, even though youth violence arrests dropped off in the mid-1990s, youth self-reports of violent activity in annual confidential reports continued at high levels through 1999. This development is of concern to policy makers, legislators, and law enforcement personnel, since confidential annual surveys of adolescent, self-reported activities consistently show that (a) many youth hold attitudes and beliefs that support aggressive, violent behavior and (b) relatively large proportions (i.e., 30% and up) of responding youth report committing violent acts that could have resulted in serious injury or even death.

These findings call for systematic actions to teach all children and youth the attitudes, beliefs, positive values, and skills that support nonviolent behavior and the peaceful resolution of interpersonal conflicts, which often escalate into destructive and sometimes dangerous situations. Schools have a key role to play in addressing this problem and are ideally positioned to do so effectively; the schools' role in this regard is discussed in the following section.

THE SCHOOL'S ROLE IN ADDRESSING YOUTH VIOLENCE AND SCHOOL SAFETY

In the face of the toxic changes that have occurred in U.S. society over the past three to four decades, policy makers and legislators are confronted with the critical question of how to reduce and offset the damaging effects of the conditions of risk to which more and more of our

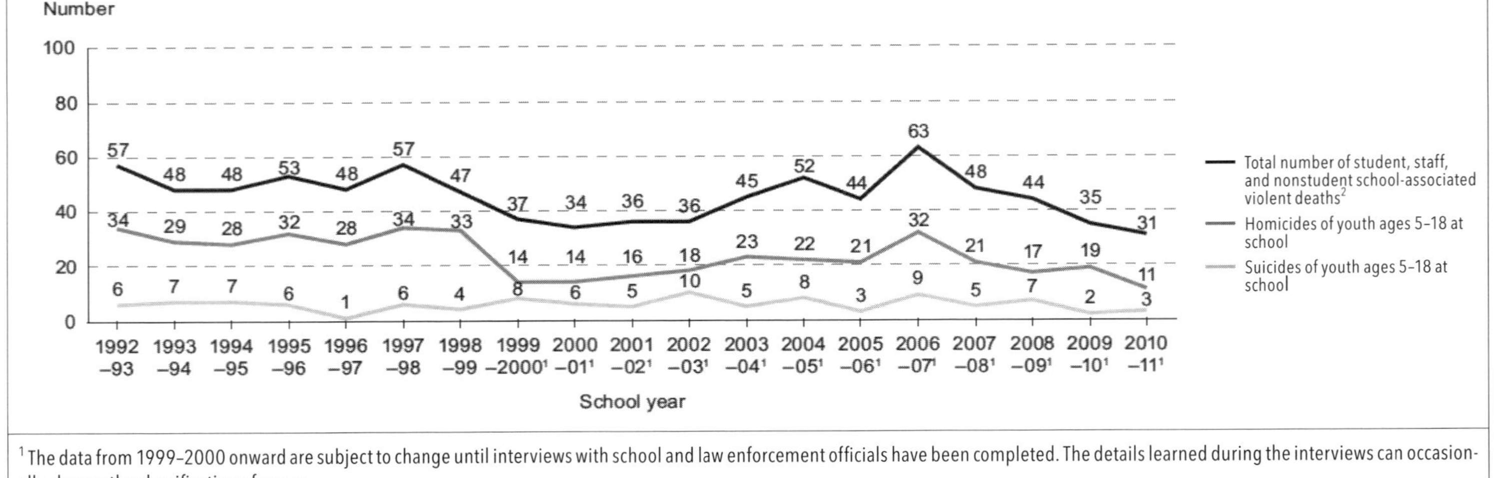

[1] The data from 1999–2000 onward are subject to change until interviews with school and law enforcement officials have been completed. The details learned during the interviews can occasionally change the classification of a case.

[2] A school-associated violent death is defined as "a homicide, suicide, or legal intervention (involving a law enforcement officer), in which the fatal injury occurred on the campus of a functioning elementary or secondary school in the United States" while the victim was on the way to or from regular sessions at school or while the victim was attending or traveling to or from an official school-sponsored event. Victims include students, staff members, and others who are not students, from July 1, 1992, through June 30, 2011.

Figure 19.2. Number of student, staff, and nonstudent school-associated violent deaths, and number of homicides and suicides of youth ages 5–18 at school: School years 1992–93 to 2010–11. From *Indicators of School Crime and Safety: 2012* (p. 7), by S. Robers, J. Kemp, and J. Truman (NCES 2013-036/NCJ 241446), Washington, DC: National Center for Education Statistics, U.S. Department of Education, and Bureau of Justice Statistics, Office of Justice Programs, U.S. Department of Justice.

youth are being subjected. As a starting point, we believe there is an urgent need to target and address as many of these risks as possible. Thousands of families are currently in crisis because of the stressors to which they are exposed daily (e.g., domestic violence, unemployment, poverty, divorce, abuse in emotional, sexual, and drug forms). In a real sense, the problems our society has experienced in this domain begin and end with the family. As a society, we must recommit ourselves to raising our children safely and effectively. We seem to have lost our capacity to do so on a broad scale (Walker et al., 1995; Walker & Sprague, 1999a).

Next to families, perhaps the most important institutional influence on child and youth development is the school and the socializing experiences and skill development opportunities it provides. As noted earlier, *effective* schooling along with students' experience of school success is likely one of the most important protective influences in the lives of youth, but only *if* the student fully engages and bonds with the schooling experience (see Hawkins et al., 1999). The school is also a major source of mental health support for school-age students. Hoagwood and Erwin (1997), for example, indicate that approximately 75% of all mental health services are typically delivered within the context of schooling.

If schools are to be significant players in developing solutions to the youth violence problems of U.S. society, some key assumptions, in our view, must be in evidence for them to be effective:

1. School systems must become far more collaborative with families and other agencies in forging and implementing promising strategies.
2. School personnel from the top down must own the problem of youth violence and resist the temptation to displace it to other sectors of our society.
3. Schools must engage *all* students and ensure that they are connected to and bonded with the schooling process.

Public schools have an unfortunate history of making themselves unwelcoming to marginalized students and their families. For instance, the common practice of pressuring at-risk students, who do not easily accommodate the demands of schooling, to leave school early is one of the worst strategies imaginable and merely displaces this social problem to other sectors of our society, where it is even more difficult to solve (Fabelo et al., 2011). At-risk youth who leave school early and join the street culture have their overall risk status literally skyrocket. Many such youth then come into contact with social forces that rapidly propel them toward delinquency, violence, and other toxic conditions (Dishion, Dodge, & Lansford, 2006). Schools and school systems need to increase their holding power for all students and reduce the unacceptably high dropout rates (25% and higher) that result in future generations of unskilled workers who must struggle to earn a living wage. In her classic investigation of this issue, *Within Our Reach,* Lizbeth Schorr (1988) notes that the three most important risk outcomes confronting adolescents, their families, and our society are (a) school failure often associated with early school leaving, (b) too-early parenthood, and (c) committing delinquent acts—all factors that can be addressed and prevented with early and comprehensive societal investments (Lynch, 2004).

We believe there are three groups of at-risk students that schools are responsible for and who can benefit from the services, supports, opportunities, and experiences that effective schooling offers. These groups are early starters, later starters, and school violence perpetrators. Early starters bring a well-developed pattern of antisocial behavior to the process of schooling and are desperately in need of interventions and supports provided at the point of school entry and that continue as needed throughout their school careers. Later starters, in contrast, begin their antisocial careers later on in the schooling process (usually around fourth or fifth grade) and engage in a period of adolescent limited delinquency that lasts three to five years (see Moffitt, 1994). The student who commits violent acts against students or school staff can be characterized as *internalizing aggressors* who, as a rule, tend to internalize their problems and direct them inwardly rather than outwardly toward the social environment (Note: numerous rampage shooters and perpetrators of school violence seem to fit this profile to some degree). As we have seen, some at-risk internalizing students are capable of extraordinary aggression in the process of settling their grievances against others—real or imagined. Kip Kinkle, Eric Harris, and Dylan Klebold are classic examples of such students. These three individuals are responsible for the deaths of 15 fellow students and three adults (two parents and a teacher) plus injuries to more than 30 other students.

The U.S. Secret Service (Stephens, 2000) and the Federal Bureau of Investigation (O'Toole, 2000) have conducted exhaustive analyses of the histories and characteristics of the school shooters of the past decade. Their research finds two common themes among these students as follows: fully two-thirds were bullied, teased, and/or harassed by their fellow students, and they did not feel connected to school and saw no one in the school who they believed actually cared about them. These findings speak volumes about the need to address the often coarse, cruel nature of the peer culture in schools and the importance of taking concrete steps to assist students in fully engaging schooling and to help them be successful in the process of bonding and attaching to it.

The remainder of this chapter is focused on solutions and describes proven and promising strategies for enhancing the safety and security of the school setting, integrating and coordinating prevention-based interventions that address the needs of *all* students in the school setting, and improving the classroom teacher's ability to teach and manage all students, including those with very antisocial tendencies. As noted earlier, the chapter concludes with some commentary and analysis of key emerging issues and problems relating to violence (i.e., violence against teachers, media coverage of school and rampage shootings, and the role of mental health in school and rampage shootings).

Enhancing School Security

In the 1990s, the landscape of school safety and the behavioral expression of youth violence changed substantially—for the worse. Some assumptions about the associated characteristics of this unfortunate trend and some potential causal factors associated with it are listed here:

1. Although the prevalence of school tragedies has declined, the number of deaths and injuries per tragedy has increased substantially.
2. Much larger numbers of planned school tragedies have been detected and averted in recent years primarily because peers have revealed their knowledge of these plans to school authorities and parents in advance of their planned occurrence. Peers are perhaps the best information source about a school shooting conspiracy planned by a disturbed student.
3. Each school tragedy now tends to produce a number of copycat incidents following soon after, which raises the possibility that such events may have been in the planning stages or contemplated for some time rather than spontaneously arising in connection with a tragedy.
4. The public and parents generally have now moved beyond expressing concern for troubled youth who commit these tragedies to outrage about them and making demands for ensuring that schools become safer for all children and youth.
5. Schools, students, and parents are increasingly victimized by fears about the possibility of a tragedy occurring in their particular

setting, which lowers everyone's overall quality of life and reduces a student's ability to get the most out of the schooling process.

6. Our society has to assume ownership of the spate of school-shooting tragedies that have occurred during the past two decades, as the societal forces that spill over into the schooling process and are associated with these tragedies include dysfunctional families, incivility, substance abuse, child neglect and abuse, the coarsening of our culture, the flood of media violence, the anger and social fragmentation that is pervasive in our society, and so on. These forces have been at play for a long time, and they will not change or go away in the near term.
7. A major concern relating to school tragedies is today's peer culture, which has absorbed the darker sides of our society's unfortunate changes of the past three decades; increasingly, our youth are immersed in a peer culture that is coarse, crude, cruel, uncaring, and often destructive to an individual's self-esteem and is expressed most destructively via intimidation of vulnerable students through harassment, relational aggression, and cyberbullying.
8. In vivo bullying, cyberbullying, mean-spirited teasing, and the humiliation of certain peers are normative processes in many school settings and poison their climates; these destructive processes are often encouraged and supported by the presence and attention of peer bystanders (Nishioka, Coe, Burke, Hanita, & Sprague, 2011; Sprague & Nishioka, 2012). Approximately 160,000 students miss school every day in the United States because of bullying and threats of intimidation.
9. It is remarkable that so many of today's youth are willing to write off the rest of their lives as a consequence of settling their grievances through violence against their peers and adults in the school setting; many of these same youth are very likely suicidal, extremely depressed, and in urgent need of mental health services and care.

Recommended School-Safety Response Strategies

We believe the following strategic approaches, when used in combination, can move schools in the direction of greater safety and will reduce the likelihood over time of a school tragedy occurring: (a) secure the school; (b) address the peer culture and its problems; (c) involve parents in making the school safer; (d) create a positive, inclusive school culture; and (e) develop a written school-safety and crisis-response plan. The more at-risk a school is judged to be, the more important it is that these priority areas for ensuring school safety and security be systematically addressed.

Secure the School

The most immediate and direct method of addressing school safety needs is to secure the school to the extent possible. The three primary approaches to seriously consider in this regard are (a) the appropriate use of school-security technology, (b) employment of school resource officers, and (c) use of Crime Prevention Through Environmental Design (CPTED) principles and techniques (see Additional Resources at the end to this chapter for more information on school safety). When used in combination, these three approaches can be effective in reducing the likelihood or probability of a school-shooting tragedy.

Considerable progress has been made in the development and appropriate use of security technology to make schools safer while preserving their effectiveness and positive climate. This technology is being used increasingly within schools across the country. An excellent resource on this topic has been developed and published by the U.S. Office of Juvenile Justice and Delinquency Prevention (see Green, 1999; see also Additional Resources). School administrators should be aware of the status, advantages, and limitations of this technology when considering implementation of school-safety options and strategies.

Address the Peer Culture and Its Problems

A primary target for our prevention and safer-schools efforts should be the peer culture. The normative behavior and actions, beliefs, and values existing in broad sectors of today's peer culture are socially destructive and demeaning. Many youth experience a trial by fire in negotiating the complex and difficult social tasks involved in finding one's place in this peer culture. Far too many fail this critical test, become lost within it, and wander aimlessly while seeking acceptance that is generally not forthcoming. They become homeless individuals within the larger peer group, and their lack of fit is well known among peers. This process forces many marginalized youth to affiliate with atypical or deviant peer groups, which can prove destructive for them. Too often, media reports of school-shooting tragedies show clearly that many of the perpetrators are alienated from their peers and have been cruelly tormented by them.

Transforming this destructive peer culture is perhaps our most formidable task in the area of school safety. This culture is not of the schools' making, but schools are perhaps the only social institution, excluding the family, capable of addressing it effectively. Five strategies are recommended for consideration in this regard.

1. *Involve students as key partners in making schools safe and free of violence.* Encouraging students' school engagement and commitment to conventional pursuits is increasingly recognized as essential to promoting academic achievement and preventing antisocial and violent behavior (Blum, 2005; Gottfredson, 2001). One example of such a program is Students Against Violence Everywhere (SAVE; Riley & Segal, 2002). SAVE is a student-initiated program that promotes nonviolence within schools and communities. The program teaches about the effects and consequences of violence and helps provide safe activities for students, parents, and communities. As reported by students and advisers, SAVE improves school environments by teaching students how to manage and resolve conflict, reduces violence, and helps more students get involved. Students report that they joined SAVE to improve the school environment by making the school a safer place, and students who participate in SAVE demonstrate increased self-esteem and confidence, conflict resolution skills, presentation and public speaking skills, and knowledge about different violence-prevention strategies.

The Safe School Ambassadors program (http://community-matters.org/programs-and-services/safe-school-ambassadors) relies on social norms change and the power of students to help stop bullying and violence. The developers assert that student bystanders see, hear, and know things adults do not; can intervene in ways adults cannot; and are often on the scene of an incident before an adult. The Safe School Ambassadors program engages and mobilizes these bystanders, socially influential leaders of a school's diverse cliques, the ones who shape the social norms that govern other students' behavior. These "alpha" leaders are carefully identified through student and staff member surveys. They are selected on the basis of specific criteria, such as strong position and influence in their peer group, good communication skills, and a history of standing up for friends.

The recruited students participate in a two-day interactive training along with several adults who serve as program mentors. The training aims to give student ambassadors the motivation and skills to resolve conflicts, defuse incidents, and support isolated and excluded students. After the training, small-group meetings of ambassadors are held every few weeks. These meetings, led by the adult mentors, provide time for strengthening skills, support data collection and analysis of ambassador interventions, and help sustain student and adult commitment to the program. The program is shown to reduce school suspensions by up to 33% compared to control schools, which show an increase in suspensions of 10% (White, Raczynski, Pack, & Wang, 2011).

Programs like SAVE and Safe School Ambassadors are designed to transform peer attitudes and beliefs about the risks to school safety that emerge from their culture. The programs promote peer ownership of the tasks involved in preventing school tragedies and are highly recommended as a first strategy for enlisting a school's peer culture in this effort.

These programs are designed to transform peer attitudes and beliefs about the risks to school safety represented by the peer culture. They promote ownership by peers of the tasks involved in preventing school tragedies and are highly recommended as a first strategy for enlisting a school's peer culture in this effort. As a rule, the peers of potential school shooters are the best information source for the prevention of a tragedy. Schools need to make the reporting of suspicious behavior or knowledge of a conspiracy easy to report and confidential. The Ribbon of Promise videos have been widely distributed nationally and are now available to educators (see Additional Resources).

2. Bully-proof the school setting by adopting effective anti-bullying/harassment programs, such as Bully Proofing PBIS, the Olweus Bullying Prevention Program, and Steps to Respect. The best disinfectant for bullying, mean-spirited teasing, and harassment is sunlight. These events need to be defined as clearly unacceptable in the school by everyone (administrators, teachers, other school staff, students, and parents) and made public when they do occur. Students should be given strategies for reporting and resisting them in an adaptive, confidential manner. The reporting to school authorities of those who commit these acts should be made normative and widely acceptable. The above-cited programs incorporate these principles and strategies (see Additional Resources). The best work to date on bullying and peer harassment in school contexts has been conducted by Espelage and Swearer (2010); their writings and products on bullying are highly respected and highly recommended.

3. Teach anger management and conflict-resolution techniques as part of regular curricular content. The Second Step Violence Prevention Program, developed by the Committee for Children in Seattle, is one of the best means available for creating a peaceful peer culture of caring and civility and for teaching specific strategies that work in controlling or managing one's anger and resolving conflicts without resorting to coercion or violence (see Additional Resources). This program has been rated as the most effective of all those currently available for creating safe and positive schools by an expert panel of the Safe and Drug Free Schools Division of the U.S. Department of Education.

Muschert and Peguero (2010), in their review of strategies for ensuring school safety, singled out approaches that establish positive school climates as effective and recommended. A highly recommended and effective resource in creating and sustaining positive peer cultures, as well as a positive school climate, is the School-Wide Positive Behavior Support Program (Horner, Sugai, & Anderson, 2010). SWPBS systematically teaches three core values that infuse and permeate the school setting and are designed to foster a positive school climate. These values are be safe, be respectful, and be responsible. They are taught and reviewed regularly, using an instructional model, with all students, teachers, and support staff. Implementation of SWPBS involves five steps as follows: (a) set and promote schoolwide expectations, (b) recognize expected behavior and actively supervise students, (c) define and effectively correct problem behaviors and their consequences for students and staff members, (d) report and use data for problem solving and decision making, and (e) implement for sustainability (Sprague et al., 2014). The SWPBS approach has been adopted by more than 20,000 U.S. schools and is judged to be highly effective in addressing this important issue. A major strength in accounting for SWPBS's phenomenal success is the manner in which it fits seamlessly within school routines and operations.

4. *Refer troubled, agitated, and depressed youth to mental health services and ensure that they receive the professional attention they need.* Youth with serious mental health problems and disorders, who are alienated, socially rejected, and taunted by peers, can be dangerous to themselves and others. These students are often known to peers and staff in the school and should be given the appropriate professional and parental attention, access to services, and social supports. When mental health problems, such as depression, schizophrenia, and paranoia, are combined with being the target of severe bullying and taunting by peers, the result is often a dangerous combination in the context of school safety (Blaber & Bershad, 2011). These problems call for a universal screening and early-intervention approach to detect and treat them successfully.

5. *Ask students to sign a pledge not to tease, bully, or put down others.* Reports from schools that have tried this tactic indicate that it makes a difference in the number of incidents that occur and in the overall school climate.

Involve Parents in Making the School Safer

With each new school-shooting tragedy, parents of school-age children and youth seek greater assurances that their child's school is safe and, increasingly, are asking for a voice and role in helping the school attain this goal. Recently, a prosecuting attorney, the mother of four children, described a plan for creating a parent-based advocacy group on school safety that would rate the safety of schools and make this information broadly available to all parents. Parents have much to offer schools as a resource in this regard and can be a powerful force in creating greater safety and a sense of security in the school setting.

We recommend four strategies for facilitating such parent involvement:

1. *Create a parent-advisory planning group at each school that is devoted to school safety issues for that school.* Such an advisory group would bring invaluable knowledge, experience, and advocacy to the process of dealing with local school-safety challenges. It could also serve as a forum for reacting to district- and state-level policy directives in this area.
2. *Advocate for parents to teach their children adaptive, nonviolent methods of responding to bullying, teasing, and harassment at school and to avoid encouraging them to fight back.* In the vast majority of cases, fighting back will not be effective and may escalate the situation to dangerous levels. It will more likely increase the likelihood of the offensive behavior occurring again—rather than reducing it. An anti-bullying program at school with parent–educator support and active involvement will be much more effective.
3. *Advocate for the securing of weapons at home and to access gun safety instruction for all family members.* Given the society we live in and the number of guns in U.S. homes, it is becoming imperative that everyone have some understanding of the dangers involved in handling guns and being in proximity to those who are doing so. Trigger locks and secured gun cases are essential elements for storing weapons in the home where the keys to same are also secured. The National Rifle Association has developed some excellent information on gun safety that can be accessed by anyone. In connection with these efforts, young children need to be taught a golden rule about the sanctity of life and that guns are deadly, life-ending instruments.
4. *Make available to parents solid information on effective parenting practices and provide access to those parents who seek training and*

> *support in more effective parenting.* There are five generic parenting practices that are instrumental in determining how children develop (see Table 19.2): discipline, monitoring and supervision, parent involvement in children's lives, positive family-management techniques, and crisis intervention and problem solving. Table 19.2 explains these techniques in some detail, and this information can be shared with parents as a handout or included in a school's newsletter. A large number of available parent-training programs address these parenting practices.

Create a Positive, Inclusive School Climate and Culture

There is solid evidence that effective schools are safer schools and vice versa. The research of Gottfredson and colleagues (Najaka et al., 2002), along with that of others, shows that a school climate that is positive, inclusive, and accepting is a key component of an effective school. Three recommended strategies are provided here for addressing this component of school safety.

1. Create and promote a set of school-based positive values about how we treat others that include civility, caring, and respect for the rights of others. It is unfortunate that schools have to teach civility in addition to everything else they do but such is now the case. Children and youth are daily exposed to very poor models of incivility toward others by adult society. The partisanship and vitriolic treatment of members within the U.S. Congress is a case in point and provides an unfortunate example for our youth and larger society. Making civility a core value of the school's culture may help reduce some of the coarseness of the peer culture that has become such a problem in our schools and society.

2. Teach all students how to separate from their own lives the exaggerated media images of interpersonal violence, disrespect, and incivility to which they are exposed daily. School curricula exist that teach media literacy relative to interpersonal violence. It is especially important that young children learn how to make the disconnect between media displays of violence and their own behavior and actions.

3. Establish schoolwide rules and behavioral expectations, and set specific applications of same. Universal intervention programs designed for schoolwide application are an excellent and proven vehicle for accomplishing this goal. Examples of such intervention programs are Best Behavior: Building Positive Behavior Supports in Schools, and Peacebuilders (see Additional Resources) along with SWPBS. These are highly recommended approaches for schools to use in creating orderly, positive, well-managed school environments.

Table 19.2

TIPS FOR PARENTS ON EFFECTIVE FAMILY MANAGEMENT TECHNIQUES

Tips

1. **Discipline.** Parental discipline needs to be fair, consistent, and predictable. It should *never* be harsh or punitive. There should be a logical relationship between child behavior and the consequences that are applied to it.
2. **Monitoring.** Careful parental monitoring of a child's activities, whereabouts, and friendships and peer associations is one of the single most important things that parents can do to ensure that their children grow up healthy, well adjusted, and safe.
3. **Parent involvement.** Involvement means simply spending time with the child in either structured or unstructured activities. The parent–child contact is the important thing, and the activity chosen is usually incidental to the time spent together and the positive interactions that occur.
4. **Positive parenting techniques.** Positive parenting means being supportive and encouraging of one's child. It is important to establish a warm, caring relationship between parent and child that involves mutual respect and affection. In this way, parents will be better able to influence their child in the right directions using techniques like social interest, praise and approval, persuasion, and logical thinking, without resorting to punishment and other negative methods of behavioral control.
5. **Problem solving, conflict resolution, and crisis intervention.** During their upbringing, children experience many minor crises that, nevertheless, loom very large in their lives. When they bring problems to their parents for assistance, it is very important that parents respond immediately and completely. Alternatives should be developed for them to consider in solving the problem and they should be encouraged to choose one that is acceptable and that works for them. Children should always have the confidence that such problems will receive a fair hearing and that they will have access to parental assistance as needed.

Rules for Parenting

1. Set up a daily debriefing time for reviewing the child's day. To encourage the child to talk, ask questions such as "What did you do today?" "What did you do that was fun or interesting?" "Who did you play or talk with?" or "Did anything happen that was a problem or that you didn't like?" Debriefing tells the child that the parent cares for him or her and is concerned about what happens in the child's life. Also, it is an excellent method for screening to detect problems in the child's life that parents might not discover otherwise. Once the child starts schooling, it is extremely important to conduct a daily debriefing of this type.

Table 19.2 *(continued)*

2. Monitor the child's activities, behavior, schedules, whereabouts, friendships, and associations very carefully. It is important to provide such monitoring in a positive, caring manner, and in a way that is not smothering or unpleasant. Careful monitoring of this type can be a very powerful protective factor in the child's life. As a child grows and matures, such monitoring may have to change form and become more subtle and less direct. However, it is extremely important that it occur, especially as the child enters adolescence, when the potential for problems is so much greater.
3. Children should be taught positive attitudes toward school and shown that their parents consider schooling a highly valued activity. A pattern of cooperative, prosocial behavior will do a great deal to foster a good start in school that will ensure both academic achievement and social development over the long term.
4. The most important skill parents can teach their child before entering school is to listen as they read to him or her. The child should see the material the parent is reading and associate the sounds of the words with their symbols on the page. This activity is an important precondition for developing a child who is a good reader and who is interested in reading. It is one of the best things that can be done to prevent later school failure and to help ensure academic success.

Note. Research has identified five key parenting practices that are very important in the upbringing of well-adjusted children.

Develop a Written School-Safety and Crisis-Response Plan

The state of Oregon recently enacted a new law requiring each school to develop a written school-safety and crisis-response plan. In today's environment, it is essential that each school go through a planning process designed to reduce the likelihood of a school tragedy and to manage a crisis when it occurs. The key elements that should be addressed in a comprehensive school-safety plan are as follows:

- School-safety audits that evaluate school safety and violence vulnerabilities due to structural characteristics of the building and patterns of building usage.
- A crisis-intervention plan that allows school personnel to respond to and control crises that carry potential implications for violence or reduced school safety.
- A schoolwide curricular program that teaches social skills instrumental in violence prevention (anger management, conflict resolution, empathy, and impulse control).

- A well-established communication plan that provides interactive linkages between school personnel, public safety, and parents.

These four elements are essential to improving the safety and security of any school building and surrounding grounds. Well-developed procedures exist for assessing a school's degree of risk and for implementing each of the components listed above.

School-Based Prevention Applications

We need to make the school's role in the prevention of disruptive, antisocial behavior patterns an effective reality. Educators tend to give lip service to prevention strategies, but they are often unwilling to invest in them at the necessary levels because of suspicions about their effectiveness and worries about their long-term costs. However, the trauma of school-shooting tragedies has shocked a majority of school personnel into advocating a prevention agenda and searching for intervention approaches that are proven and promising. Table 19.3 provides some general guidelines about what does and does not work in the area of school crime prevention based on the work of Gottfredson and Gottfredson (1999).

These guidelines and recommendations should be considered carefully by school administrators, as they are derived from numerous and comprehensive analyses of school environments as developed through the seminal work of these investigators.

Walker and Sprague (1999a) described the key elements and components of a comprehensive approach for use by schools in addressing the mental health and behavioral needs of *all* students within a school. This approach is based on an integrated service-delivery model contributed originally by Walker et al. (1996) for the prevention of antisocial behavior patterns. It relies upon the foundation of the U.S. Public Health Service's classification system, which involves primary, secondary, and tertiary forms of prevention. For example, primary prevention strategies rely on universal interventions, such as schoolwide discipline and behavior management systems, grade-level teaching of violence prevention skills, and effective instruction, which are designed to keep problems from emerging. Secondary prevention strategies are more complex, costly, and intensive, and they are designed for addressing the problems and skill deficits of children and youth who already show clear signs of being at risk. Primary prevention strategies are not of sufficient intensity or strength to effectively solve the problems of children and youth who require secondary prevention strategies because of the intractability or severity of their problems. Finally, tertiary prevention strategies are designed for the most severely at-risk children and youth whom schools must attempt to accommodate. In general, their problems demand resources, supports, interventions, and services that cannot be provided by schools alone (i.e., wraparound services and interagency partnerships are

Table 19.3

SCIENTIFIC CONCLUSIONS REGARDING WHAT'S EFFECTIVE IN SCHOOL CRIME PREVENTION

What Works?

- Programs aimed at building school capacity to initiate and sustain innovation
- Programs aimed at clarifying and communicating norms about behaviors–by establishing school rules, improving the consistency of their enforcement (particularly when they emphasize positive reinforcement of appropriate behavior), or communicating norms through schoolwide campaigns (e.g., anti-bullying campaigns) or ceremonies
- Comprehensive instructional programs that focus on a range of social competency skills (e.g., developing self-control, stress-management, responsible decision-making, social problem-solving, and communication skills) and that are delivered over a long period of time to continually reinforce skills

What Does Not Work?

- Counseling students, particularly in a peer-group context
- Offering youths alternative activities such as recreation and community service activities in the absence of more potent prevention programming
- Instructional programs focused on information dissemination, fear arousal, moral appeal, and affective education

What Is Promising?

- Programs that group youth into smaller "schools within schools" to create smaller units, more supportive interactions, or greater flexibility in instruction
- Behavior modification programs that teach "thinking skills" to high-risk youths
- Programs aimed at building school capacity to initiate and sustain innovation
- Programs that improve classroom management and that use effective instructional techniques

Note. Based on "School-Based Crime Prevention," by D. C. Gottfredson, 1997, in *Preventing Crime: What Works, What Doesn't, What's Promising: A Report to the United States Congress* (pp. 5-1 to 5-74), by L. Sherman et al. (Eds.), Washington, DC: US Department of Justice, Office of Justice Programs; and on "School-Based Crime Prevention," by D. C. Gottfredson, D. B. Wilson, and S. S. Najaka, 2002, in *Evidence-Based Crime Prevention,* L. W. Sherman, D. P. Farrington, B. C. Welsh, and D. L. MacKenzie (Eds.), London: Routledge.

necessary). Figure 19.3 illustrates these three prevention approaches and the approximate proportion of the general K–3 student population that will require and likely respond to each type of prevention.

We currently have a school-to-prison pipeline that is filled with at-risk students who are experiencing traumatic behavioral events and outcomes as they progress through it. If we respond only reactively to their challenges and rely exclusively on secondary and tertiary strategies, applied after these destructive events and outcomes are in evidence, we will continue to invest larger and larger amounts of resources in return for weaker and weaker therapeutic effects and outcomes. There will always be students who come to school with such severe behavioral involvements that secondary and even tertiary supports and interventions will be necessary from the first day of their school careers. That said, however, we can make much greater and more effective use of primary prevention strategies in the school setting than we traditionally have.

As noted above, universal interventions are used for achieving primary prevention goals. It is estimated that 80%–90% of a school's student population will respond positively, at some level, to these universal intervention strategies. Those who do not respond to primary prevention approaches, anywhere from 5%–15% of the school's

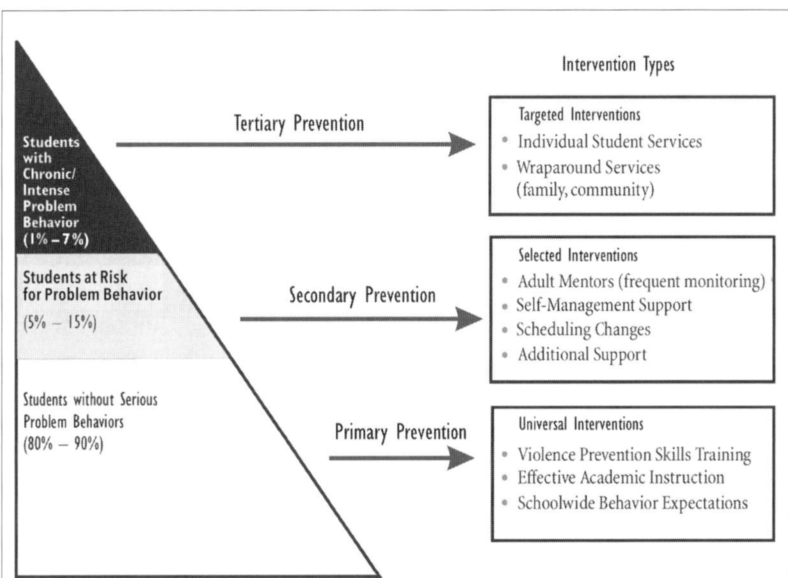

Figure 19.3. Preventing violent and destructive behavior in schools using primary, secondary, and tertiary systems of intervention. From "The Path to School Failure, Delinquency, and Violence: Causal Factors and Some Potential Solutions," by H. M. Walker and J. R. Sprague, 1999, *Intervention in School and Clinic, 35*, 71. Copyright 1999 by PRO-ED, Inc. Reprinted with permission.

population, select themselves out as candidates needing additional secondary and/or tertiary prevention strategies and approaches. However, for those students who require the most intensive, individualized interventions, approximately 1%–7% of all students, the existence of a well-designed and carefully implemented primary prevention base in the school setting provides a powerful context for their effective application. This approach is ideally suited for schools' use in allocating resources for student groups that are differentiated on the basis of problem severity.

Developing Academic Competence

Academic failure and especially difficulties in reading are strong correlates of delinquency in adolescence (Maguin & Loeber, 1996). The evidence is powerful as to the existence and consistency of this relationship. An intense focus on developing the academic skills of at-risk youth is an essential part of any comprehensive strategy to address their needs and to divert them from the path that leads to antisocial behavior, school failure and dropout, and often later delinquency. All students and especially at-risk students should be taught to read as well as they possibly can in the primary grades. It is difficult to underestimate its importance in forging a successful school career.

Collaborative Interagency Prevention Approaches

In our view, an important component of interagency collaborations focused on prevention is to create full service schools that (a) have an expanded capacity to address the complex needs of today's school population and (b) that can address true prevention goals through effective collaborations forged between schools, families, and communities. Such schools could easily and effectively accommodate school mental health approaches and professionals. We know the key elements that are necessary to create such full service schools and to address prevention goals, strategies, and outcomes in a manner that will be sufficient to arrest and turn around the rising tide of at-risk children and youth we see at the schoolhouse door. They include the following critical elements: early intervention services, proactive family support systems, mental health, public health, social services, and transition supports and services to post-schooling environs. We need to build effective partnerships between families, schools, social service systems, public safety, churches, and other agencies to create the socializing experiences that will give all youth a chance to develop along positive lines.

Metzler et al. (1998) have described the elements of a comprehensive approach to the prevention of child and adolescent behavior problems that integrates family and community-based approaches to strengthening the application of universal as well as individually targeted behavior management programs in schools. We need to carefully research prevention models of this type and learn how to scale them up so they can be adopted and implemented on a broad basis in a cost-effective manner by school systems.

Managing Interactions With Difficult Students at the Classroom Level

Teachers today are confronted with more challenges in teaching and managing students than at any point in our history. Today's students are more diverse, ever more challenging, and powerfully influenced by negative social forces (e.g., media violence, societal fragmentation, poor anger control by adult models) that negatively affect their school performance and behavior. Teachers at all levels are more likely to encounter antisocial students in their normal teaching routines who are disrespectful and unresponsive to traditional behavior management strategies and tactics of adult social influence. Many of these students are early starters who come to the schooling experience from highly chaotic and dysfunctional family situations. They typically have developed coercive behavioral repertoires that are based upon confrontation and escalation as generic strategies for dealing with interpersonal processes and negotiating social tasks. Teachers find them to be highly agitated, difficult in the extreme, and frequently become engaged in hostile exchanges with them. Figure 19.4 contains a conceptual model developed by Colvin (1993) that illustrates the escalating and destructive properties of these unfortunate interactions.

Teachers inadvertently become locked into hostile, escalating interactions with antisocial students that are very public, extremely damaging to the teacher–student relationship, and difficult to withdraw from. These students are masters at engaging teachers both prior to and during this hostile interactive process. As long as the teacher is willing to keep responding to the student's questions and provocations, the teacher is not in control of the interaction—the student is! The longer the interaction goes on and the more hostile it becomes, the greater the likelihood of an undesirable ending and ensuing damage to the teacher's ability to teach and manage all students in the class. In this scenario, the student is generally the professional and the teacher is the amateur!

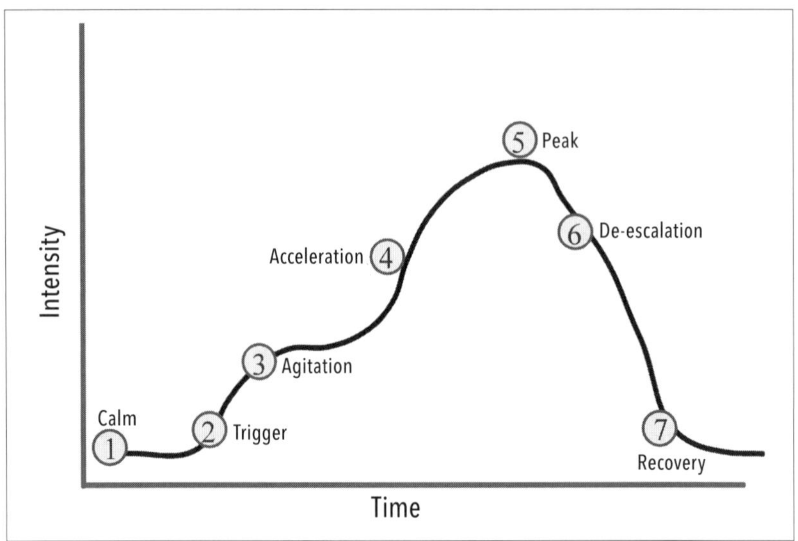

Figure 19.4. Phases of escalating behavior. *Note.* From *Managing Acting-Out Behavior: A Staff Development Program To Prevent and Manage Acting-Out Behavior* (p. 4), by Colvin, 1992, Eugene, OR: Behavior Associates. Copyright 1992 by Behavior Associates. Reprinted with permission.

The answer is not to play the escalation game in which the antisocial student is so accomplished. These interactions should be avoided and stopped soon after they begin, to prevent the resulting damage that is inevitable. The teacher stops these interactions by refusing to continue the interaction and answer the student's queries. It may be necessary to prearrange the front office support necessary to remove and discipline the antisocial student whenever these events occur. After the student has settled down, the teacher can quietly approach him or her and debrief about how the situation that prompted the hostile exchange could have been handled differently and avoided.

The senior author has written extensively on the issues of managing difficult students, on classroom ecology, and on preventing behavioral episodes through the judicious use of teacher requests, demands, and commands. Perhaps a majority of hostile exchanges and difficult situations with behaviorally at-risk students could be avoided through the careful application of known behavioral principles in this context. Table 19.4 contains a listing of general principles for the teacher's use in preventing and defusing oppositional–aggressive student behavior among at-risk student populations. See Walker (1995) for a thorough treatment of this topic and for detailed information on how to apply these principles.

Teaching today is qualitatively different from heretofore due primarily to sharp changes in the student population and to our society's

Table 19.4

SUGGESTIONS FOR PREVENTING AND DEFUSING OPPOSITIONAL–AGGRESSIVE STUDENT BEHAVIOR

1. Establish an ecology for the classroom setting that is positive, inclusive, and supportive of *all* students, regardless of their behavioral and academic characteristics.
2. Be aware that adults can unconsciously form and behaviorally express negative impressions of low-performing, uncooperative students, and students are quite sensitive to these. Teachers should carefully monitor their impressions, keep them as neutral as possible, communicate a positive regard for students, and give them the benefit of the doubt whenever possible.
3. Establish and communicate high expectations in achievement and behavior for *all* students.
4. Create a structured learning environment in which students know what is expected of them and where they can access needed assistance in completing academic tasks.
5. Allow sharp demarcation to occur between academic periods, but hold transition times between periods to a minimum.
6. Consider using cooperative learning strategies that allow diverse groups of students to interact, problem solve, and develop skills in working together.
7. Systematically teach social skills curricula that incorporate instruction in anger management and conflict resolution strategies.
8. Be sure that academic programming and task difficulty are commensurate with the skill levels of low-performing students. Students who act out, in particular, tend to have weak academic skills and may react negatively to academic tasks or demands that they feel are too difficult for them. These situations very often lead to hostile teacher–student interactions.
9. Teach students how to be assertive in an appropriate manner (e.g., to disagree or resist the demands of others without being hostile).
10. Use difficult situations as "teaching opportunities" for developing student skills in responding to such situations without being angry, aggressive, or coercive.
11. Be sure to find ways to praise and encourage low-performing students at the same or a higher rate than that for higher performing students.
12. Find ways to communicate a genuine interest in the progress of low-performing students and support them as they struggle to meet the complex demands of schooling.
13. Maximize the performance of low-performing students through the use of individualized instruction, cues, prompting, breakdown of academic tasks, debriefing, coaching, and providing positive incentives (e.g., praise, free time, home privileges).
14. Try to avoid criticizing, ridiculing, verbally punishing, or arguing with any student, especially students who are low performing or who act out.

disinvestment in its children and youth—particularly in the realm of schooling. Teachers need strong administrative support and access to mental health specialists for managing severely involved students. The threat of school violence is always present but teachers can play critical roles in (a) referring troubled students promptly to appropriate mental health support systems, (b) teaching all students the violence prevention skills, such as empathy, conflict resolution, impulse control, and anger management, that will assist them in avoiding violent solutions to interpersonal conflicts, and (c) demonstrating a sense of caring and concern for each and every student. If applied with conviction, these actions can be effective in helping students bond with and connect to the schooling process.

CRITICAL ISSUES AND DEVELOPMENTS RELATING TO SCHOOL AND YOUTH VIOLENCE

Media Coverage of School Shootings and Copycat Tragedies

It is very often the case that a major, well-publicized school shooting is followed within several weeks by what appears to be a copycat school shooting and, if not, at least a conspiracy to do so. It is difficult to believe that the glare of national or international media attention is so powerful as to stimulate or prompt disturbed youth to contemplate and carry out school tragedies—but such seems to be the case.

Intense media coverage of a tragic event tends to galvanize some individuals into a state where they identify with perpetrators and seek to duplicate their actions in some way. Research has long documented such replications of events, particularly of well-known individuals, like celebrities. When Marilyn Monroe committed suicide, for example, there was a 12% spike in suicides during the month immediately following her tragic death at age 36. Similarly, spikes occurred in 26 of 33 suicides that were reported on the front page of the *New York Times* between 1948 and 1967, resulting in an increase of 2,000 cases of "excess" deaths. Saturation-level media coverage of mass murder leads to one additional murder in the next two weeks, according to Dr. Paul Dietz, who is a nationally known criminal profiler. He argues that agitated, disturbed individuals often perceive a commonalty and identification with the perpetrator who is profiled in the media and seek to replicate or exceed his actions. This phenomenon is known as the Werther effect and was discovered in 1974 by David Phillips, who has systematically tracked copycat suicides (Greenfield,

2012). Phillips makes the case that coverage of such events, depending upon how they are portrayed, can produce a form of media contagion, which gives the impression that the tragedy or traumatic event is an epidemic and occurs at a much higher rate and is more pervasive than is actually the case.

The media does have a choice in how such events are covered and that choice is controlled, to a large extent, by producers, news directors, and reporters. In perhaps most cases, the choice is to focus on details of the event that galvanize the public's attention and imagination in a way that maximizes viewer interest and also maximizes revenues. In any school-shooting event, there are three elements: the shooter, the victim(s), and the actual event. News media entities have to decide how to frame coverage of the event and they often do so in a way that leads to "mediatization" of the event, which has the effect of blurring the lines between the actual event and media portrayals and viewer perceptions of it. In school shootings and rampage killings, this often involves focusing on the shooter and profiling minute details of his life and also sensationalizing the egregious nature of the event as opposed to a more factual reporting of the tragedy.

Increasingly we are dependent on the media to forge and construct our understanding of reality (Muschert & Ragnedda, 2010), and it often does so in a way that distorts events in terms of their impact, severity, and pervasiveness. Some experts have even argued that the media is complicit in exacerbating the phenomenon of school shootings. While urging more responsible media reportage so as not to stimulate copycat phenomena in the realm of school shootings, we recognize the possibility of infringement on the free speech protections of the press. Nevertheless, the media has and continues to come under intense scrutiny for the way it covers such events and its possible destructive impact (Muschert & Carr, 2006; Pollack & Kubrin, 2007). In the case of school and rampage shootings, the media would do well to (a) carefully consider how framing the coverage will affect public perception of the event, (b) focus on more factual reporting of the event, and (c) avoid reportage that sensationalizes the event, stimulates mediatization, and leads to media contagion.

The Role of Mental Health in School and Rampage Shootings

Each time there is an egregious school-shooting tragedy or a rampage killing, we revisit past arguments in our collective rhetoric about the responsible factors and conditions. Commentary about the role of distal causal agents has tended to dominate this discussion among many experts (Muschert et al., 2014). The breakdown of the family, child neglect and abuse, deteriorations in our cultural cohesion, adverse social and economic conditions, the widespread availability of guns, the unresponsiveness of our governing institutions, and so on have frequently been offered as possible contributors. Though these factors doubtless exert some influence at some level over these events, there is very little that our society can do collectively to address them in a way that will make any difference in the short term.

However, two of the more proximal, likely contributors have to do with how alienated students are from other students and the schools they attend and the mental health status of shooters. A significant number of today's students are depressed and alienated from their peers and become targets for peer harassment, bullying, and cruel taunting. When school shooters emerge with this profile, it is assumed they are settling grievances against peers and/or staff for real or imagined slights. Recent rampage shooters have been documented as having significant mental health challenges. Media reports of the shooters involved in rampage killings at Newtown, Virginia Tech, the U.S. Navy Yard, Thurston, Columbine, Arizona, and Colorado all fit this profile. In some of these cases, repeated attempts were made to seek out mental health treatment before the killings, either by relatives or by the perpetrator, but without success (Thurston school shooter, U.S. Navy Yard shooter).

It appears that individuals involved in rampage killings often fluctuate between being suicidal and homicidal. Unfortunately, many of them ultimately end up choosing both paths. In one follow-up study of 62 rampage shooters, 36 committed suicide either during or immediately after the event and another seven died in later shootouts with police. In a recent review of rampage shooting incidents, Faria (2013) described a 2000 *New York Times* study in which 100 rampage incidents were reviewed. Sixty-three of the shooters had made potentially credible threats of violence prior to the event, and half of those had overt behavioral signs of mental illness that had gone untreated. Although there is a convergence of expert opinion that individuals with mental health diagnoses who avoid drugs and alcohol, stay in treatment, and take their medication(s) on schedule have a violence perpetration rate that is no different from normal, it is difficult to know how many shooters without a diagnosis have significant mental health issues and how many of those with a diagnosis have adhered consistently to a medically prescribed regimen as per above (e.g., avoid drugs and alcohol).

So the question remains: How do we cope with the mental health crisis that seems to be driving many rampage killings in the face of massive cuts to the mental health system of the past four years or so?

Approximately $5 million has been removed from this system in the past several decades, and we have far fewer mental health beds today than in the past. A number of states, however, are restoring or adding to their mental health agency budgets in the wake of the Newtown tragedy. On the basis of recommendations from the FBI, the school-shooting literature, and the mental health field, we suggest the following steps for addressing this issue:

1. Develop the institutional capacity for individuals, who are agitated and perceive themselves in crisis and in need of mental health supports or treatment, to access mental health services via an on-demand basis or through prompt referral.
2. Develop protocols for use by schools, law enforcement, and mental health professionals to assess and investigate credible threats against persons that are made by alienated individuals.
3. Establish a thorough background vetting process for all individuals who seek to purchase guns and especially for those suffering from mental health problems. (However, it should be noted that the parents of Kip Kinkle, the Thurston shooter, and Adam Lanza, the Newtown shooter, purchased guns for them that they used in their rampages).
4. Create legislation and develop the infrastructure that would allow a meaningful infusion of mental health services and expertise into the public school system.
5. Investigate ways individuals who are close to a potential shooter (e.g., relatives, family members, peers, coworkers) can easily report suspicious or threatening behavior to responsible authorities in a timely manner.
6. Establish interagency communication capacity and practices that provide for the immediate sharing of information about mental health patients who are suspected of having violent tendencies or who make threats regarding violence.

Violence Against Teachers by Today's Students

Physical violence against teachers by students is a growing problem in U.S. schools that is not well understood and is poorly researched. Just recently, two popular teachers—one in Danvers, Massachusetts, and one in Sparks, Nevada, were brutally murdered on school grounds by a student attending the school. The principal of Sandy Hook Elementary in Newtown was killed along with five other school staff in a rampage shooting that occurred approximately two and a half years ago. Although it is rare for school staff to lose their lives to school shooters, teacher-directed violence is a problem that seems to be growing in frequency and severity. In the 2007–2008 school year, for example, 4% of public school teachers reported they had been physically attacked at some point; and a 2011 survey found that 80% of teachers reported they had been harassed, intimidated, assaulted, or otherwise victimized (Thompson, 2013). Tiesman, Konda, Hendricks, Mercer, and Amadus (2013) recently reported that 30% of school staff had experienced at least one nonphysical, violent event in the workplace during the past year. Their research showed that special education teachers were at substantially greater risk of physical violence than general education teachers, that urban teachers were more at risk than rural, and that males were at greater risk than females.

The American Psychological Association created the national Taskforce on Violence Directed Toward Teachers, chaired by Dorothy Espelage of the University of Illinois, to investigate this issue and to make recommendations for addressing it. As part of its work, the taskforce conducted an online survey of 3,000 teachers involving schools and teachers in 48 states. Key findings from this study are listed here and are available in Espelage et al. (2013):

- 44% of survey respondents reported physical offenses including thrown objects, student attacks, and weapons shown.
- 6% reported being the target of verbal abuse by their students.
- 7% reported being threatened with actual physical injury by students.
- Half of victimized teachers reported they had experienced offenses by two or more different perpetrators (e.g., student and parent).
- 72.5% reported receiving one harassment offense.
- 50% experienced property offenses (e.g., theft, property damage).
- Being male and working in an urban setting was associated with a greater likelihood of victimization.

The APA taskforce recommended that a national registry be created to track the nature and frequency of incidents in order to serve as a basis for schools' policy development efforts regarding prevention and intervention. It also recommended that all educators be required to master effective classroom management strategies before they are licensed to teach (see Walker & Gresham, 2014). It is likely that a substantial portion of the teacher–student interactions ending in teacher-directed aggression and violent behavior are due to escalations in conflict intensity and student anger that teachers need to manage better than they typically do (see Figure 19.4). This recommendation no doubt stems from the taskforce's conclusion that teachers need to become more skilled in preventing and coping with escalated interactions that involve students who carry high levels of agitation with limited ability to regulate their emotions. The APA taskforce also recommended that teacher preparation programs make teacher-directed violence a priority, which is typically not the case. Finally, the taskforce produced a number of practice recommendations aimed at student, teacher, classroom, and school levels of implementation. This is an invaluable survey and compilation of essential knowledge that can transform school responses in coping with violence against teachers by students. It should form a blueprint for policy development at the highest levels of the education profession.

CONCLUSION

The United States has a violent history as a country, and many experts argue that we are a violent culture as well. Far more children and youth die each year in America through gun violence than in any other developed country (see Osofsky, 1997). The number of guns estimated to exist in the U.S. population is approximately 300 million and nearly equals the current U.S. population of 330 million. The tragic spate of school shootings that has continued since the decade of the 1990s, the rising level of assault and violence against teachers, and the escalation in rampage shootings in schools and the larger society since 2009 offer grim testimony as to how the destructive influences and violent images that pervade our daily lives are registering their negative effects upon our children and youth (Walker, Ramsey, & Gresham, 2004; Walker & Sprague, 1999a).

We have also become a highly punitive and fearful society; the United States has 5% of the world's population but approximately 25% of the world's total incarcerated population. As a society, we should hold up a mirror and examine ourselves in the light of this fact and so many other indicators that we are failing our children and youth on a massive scale. We need to take a close look at what we have become, how we got here, and how we might change for the better. Numerous experts believe that we have now become the most violent developed society in the world.

Policy generally lags well behind the research that validates evidence-based approaches that can inform and guide policy decisions and practices based on them (Kauffman, 2014). This is especially true in the area of school safety and youth violence prevention. The pressures and demands of the moment force school administrators into making decisions about school-safety strategy and tactics that may appear promising but are not, as yet, proven through the research process. However, this is a luxury (waiting for validation of such techniques) of which we are not able to avail ourselves. Thus, we have been left with the option of basing many of our decisions about school safety upon practices that appear promising while relying on our experience and using our best judgment.

However, the scientific and empirical knowledge base on school safety is rapidly expanding, and some promising approaches are now becoming available for adoption (e.g., thoroughly investigating credible threats). It is incumbent on school leaders and administrators to stay on top of this emerging body of knowledge. The action recommendations contained herein represent much of what we seem to know about these complex issues at present. Schools can be made safer and behaviorally at-risk youth can be far better served by implementing well that which we currently know. As Huffman (2013) recently noted, we need to make it measurably more difficult for school-shooting tragedies to occur. We believe it is within our grasp to do so.

ADDITIONAL RESOURCES

Crowe, T. (2000). *Crime prevention through environmental design.* Lexington, KY: Tim Crowe & Associates.

Gottfredson, D. (1997). School-based crime prevention. In L. Sherman, D. Gottfredson, D. MacKenzie, J. Eck, P. Ruter, & S. Bushway (Eds.), *Preventing crime: What works, what doesn't, what's promising: A report to the U.S. Congress* (pp. 1–74). Washington, DC: U.S. Department of Justice, Office of Justice Programs.

Green, M. (1999). *The appropriate and effective use of security technologies in U.S. schools.* Washington, DC: U.S. Department of Justice, Office of Justice Programs.

Miller, T. (2008). *School violence and primary prevention.* New York, NY: Springer.

Trump, K. (2011). *Proactive school security and emergency preparedness planning.* Thousand Oaks, CA: Corwin Press.

Walker, H. M., & Gresham, F. M. (2014). *Handbook of evidence-based practices for emotional and behavioral disorders: Applications in schools.* New York, NY: Guilford.

Walker, H. M., Ramsey, E., & Gresham, F. M. (2004). *Antisocial behavior in school: Evidence-based practices.* New York, NY: Cengage.

Weist, M., Lever, N., Bradshaw, C., & Owens, J. (2014). *Handbook of school mental health.* New York, NY: Springer.

REPORTS

Early warning/timely response: A guide to safe schools. Retrieved from http://www.ed.gov/offices/OSERS/OSEP/earlywrn.html

Safeguarding our children: An action guide. Retrieved from http://www.ed.gov/offices/OSERS/OSEP/ActionGuide

ARTICLES AND CHAPTERS

Espelage, D. (2013, January 7). Violence against teachers spurs call to action. *APA Newsletter.*

Hawkins, D., Catalano, R., Kosterman, R., Abbott, R., & Hill, K. (1999, March). Preventing adolescent health-risk behaviors by strengthening protection during childhood. *Archives of Pediatrics & Adolescent Medicine, 153,* 226–234.

Walker, H., & Shinn, M. (2010). Systemic, evidence-based approaches for promoting positive student outcomes within a multitier framework: Moving from efficacy to effectiveness. In M. Shinn & H. Walker (Eds.), *Interventions for achievement and behavior problems in a three-tier model including RTI* (pp. 1–26). Bethesda, MD: National Association of School Psychologists.

RECOMMENDED PROGRAMS AND APPROACHES FOR PREVENTING VIOLENCE AND BULLYING OR HARASSMENT

Bully proofing your school. (Available from Sopris West, Inc., P.O. Box 1890, Longmont, CO, 80502-1809; 800/547-6747).

Second Step Violence Prevention Program. (Available from the Committee for Children, Seattle, WA; 800/634-4449; http://www.cfchildren.org).

Steps to Respect (anti-bullying program). (Available from the Committee for Children, Seattle, WA; 800/634-4449; http://www.cfchildren.org).

Positive Behavior Interventions and Supports (PBIS). http://www.pbis.org; University of Oregon.

SAFE SCHOOLS ORGANIZATIONAL RESOURCES

Department of Homeland Security (School Safety Planning, Training & Resources). http://www.dhs.gov/school-safety

NASP School Safety Resources. http://nasponliine.org/resources/crisis_safety/schoolsafety.aspx

National Association of School Principals (School Safety Resources & Initiatives). http://www.naesp.org/school-safety-resources

National School Safety Center—Ron Stephens, director; 141 Duesenberg Drive, Suite 11, Westlake Village, CA 91362

NATIONAL EXPERTS ON SCHOOL SAFETY

Kenneth Trump (School Safety Expert Leadership). http://schoolsecurity.org.
Ron Stephens (director, National School Safety Center). www.schoolsafety.us.

REFERENCES

American Psychological Association. (1993). *Violence and youth: Psychology's response. Volume I: Summary report of the American Psychological Association Commission on Violence and Youth.* Washington, DC: Author.

Anda, R. F., Felitti, V. J., & Bremner, J. D. (2006). The enduring effects of abuse and related adverse experiences in childhood: A convergence of evidence from neurobiology and epidemiology. *European Archives of Psychiatry and Clinical Neuroscience*, 256, 174–186.

Biglan, A. (2013, July 28). Nurturing schools. [Op-ed commentary]. *Eugene Register Guard.*

Blaber, C., & Bershad, C. (2011). *Realizing the promise of the whole-school approach to children's mental health: A practical guide for schools.* Washington, DC: American Institutes for Research, National Center for Mental Health Promotion and Youth Violence Prevention Education Development Center, Health and Human Development Division.

Bronfenbrenner, U. (1979). *The ecology of human development: Experiments by nature and design.* Cambridge, MA: Harvard University Press.

CBS Evening News. (2013, November). Report on rampage shootings in 2012–2013.

Christle, A. C., Jolivette, K., & Nelson, C. M. (2005). Breaking the school to prison pipeline: Identifying school risk and protective factors for youth delinquency. *Exceptionality, 13*, 69–88.

Cornell, D. (2006). *School violence: Fears versus facts.* Mahwah, NJ: Erlbaum.

Crowe, T. (1995, January). *Youth crime and community safety.* Keynote address to the Eugene City Club, Eugene, OR.

Dinkes, R., Cataldi, E. F., & Lin-Kelly, W. (2007). *Indicators of school crime and safety: 2007* (NCES 2008-021/NCJ 219553). Washington, DC: National Center for Education Statistics.

Dishion, T. J., Dodge, K. A., & Lansford, J. E. (2006). Findings and recommendations: A blueprint to minimize deviant peer influence in youth interventions and programs. In *Deviant peer influences in programs for youth: Problems and solutions* (pp. 366–394). New York, NY: Guilford.

Dunlap, G., Iovannone, R., Wilson, K. J., Kincaid, D. K., & Strain, P. (2010). Prevent-teach-reinforce: A standardized model of school-based behavioral intervention. *Journal of Positive Behavior Interventions, 12*(1), 9–22. doi:10.1177/1098300708330880

Eddy, M., Reid, J., & Curry, V. (2002). The etiology of youth antisocial behavior, delinquency, and violence and a public health approach to prevention. In M. Shinn, H. M. Walker, & G. Stoner (Eds.), *Interventions for academic and behavior problems: II. Preventive and remedial approaches* (pp. 27–52). Bethesda, MD: National Association of School Psychologists.

Espelage, D., Anderson, E., Brown, V., Jones, A., Lane, K., McMahon, S., . . . Reynolds, C. (2013). Understanding and preventing violence directed against teachers: Recommendations for a national research, practice, and policy agenda. *American Psychologist, 68*(2), 75–87.

Fabelo, T., Thompson, M. D., Plotkin, M., Carmichael, D., Marchbanks, M. P., & Booth, E. A. (2011). *Breaking schools' rules: A statewide study of how school discipline relates to students' success and juvenile justice involvement.* New York, NY: Council of State Governments Justice Center; Public Policy Research Institute at Texas A&M University.

Faria, M. A. (2013). Shooting rampages, mental health, and the sensationalization of violence. *Surgical Neurology International, 4,* 16.

Gottfredson, G., & Gottfredson, D. (1999). *Development and applications of theoretical measures for evaluating drug and delinquency prevention programs* (Technical Manual for Research Editions of What About You? WAY). Elliott City, MD: Gottfredson Associates.

Green, M. (1999). *The appropriate and effective use of security technologies in U.S. schools: A guide for schools and law enforcement agencies.* Washington, DC: U.S. Department of Justice, Office of Justice Programs.

Greenfield, D. (2012, December). America's foremost criminal profiler warns media coverage causes school shootings. *Psychology Today.*

Gresham, F. M., Lane, K. L., & Lambros, K. L. (2002). Comorbidity of conduct problems and ADHD: Identification of "fledging psychopaths." *Journal of Emotional and Behavioral Disorders, 8,* 83–93.

Hawkins, D., Catalano, R., Kosterman, R., Abbott, R., & Hill, K. (1999). Preventing adolescent health-risk behaviors by strengthening protection during childhood. *Archives of Pediatrics and Adolescent Medicine, 153,* 226–234.

Henry, S. (2009). School violence beyond Columbine: A complex problem in need of an interdisciplinary analysis. *American Behavioral Scientist, 52*(9), 1246–1265.

Hoagwood, K., & Erwin, H. (1997). Effectiveness of school-based mental health services for children: A 10 year research review. *Journal of Child and Family Studies, 1,* 129–140.

Horner, R., Sugai, G., & Anderson, C. (2010). Examining the evidence base for school-wide positive behavior support. *Focus on Exceptional Children, 42*(8), 1–15.

Huffman, T. (2013, December 10). Op-ed commentary. *Eugene Register Guard.*

Kauffman, J. (2014). Prologue: On following the scientific evidence. In H. M. Walker & F. M. Gresham (Eds.), *Handbook of evidence-based practices for emotional and behavioral disorders: Applications in schools* (pp. 1–5). New York, NY: Guilford.

Kazdin, A. E. (Ed.). (1985). *Treatment of antisocial behavior in children and adolescents.* Homewood, IL: Dorsey Press.

Loeber, R., & Farrington, D. P. (Eds.). (1998). *Serious and violent juvenile offenders: Risk factors and successful interventions.* Thousand Oaks, CA: Sage.

Lynam, D. (1996). Early identification of chronic offenders: Who is the fledgling psychopath? *Psychological Bulletin, 120,* 209–234.

Lynch, R. (2004). *Exceptional returns: Economic, fiscal and social benefits of investment in early childhood development.* Washington, DC: Economic Policy Institute.

Maguin, E., & Loeber, R. (1996). Academic performance and delinquency. In M. Tonry (Ed.), *Crime and justice: A review of research* (Vol. 20, pp. 145–264). Chicago, IL: University of Chicago Press.

Metzler, C. W., Biglan, A., Rusby, J., & Sprague, J. (2001). Evaluation of a comprehensive behavior management program to improve school-wide positive behavior support. *Education and Treatment of Children, 24*(4), 448–479.

Moffitt, T. (1994). Adolescence-limited and life-course-persistent antisocial behavior: A developmental taxonomy. *Psychological Review, 100*(4), 674–701.

Muschert, G., & Carr, D. (2006). Media salience and frame changing across events: Coverage of nine school shootings, 1997–2001. *Journalism and Mass Communication Quarterly, 83*(4), 747–766.

Muschert, G., Henry, S., Bracy, N., & Peguero, A. (2014). *Responding to school violence: Confronting the Columbine effect.* London, UK: Lynne Rienner.

Muschert, G., & Peguero, A. (2010). The Columbine effect and school anti-violence policy. *Research in Social Problems and Public Policy, 17,* 117–148.

Muschert, G., & Ragnedda, M. (2010). Media and violence control: The framing of school shootings. In W. Heitmeyer, H. G. Haupt, S. Malthaner, & A. Kirschner (Eds.), *The control of violence in modern society: Multidisciplinary perspectives, from school shootings to ethnic violence* (pp. 345–361). New York, NY: Springer.

Najaka, S., Gottfredson, D. C., & Wilson, D. (2001). A meta-analytic inquiry into the relationship between selected risk factors and problem behavior. *Prevention Science, 2*(4), 257–271.

Nishioka, V., Coe, M., Burke, A., Hanita, M., & Sprague, J. (2011). *Student-reported overt and relational aggression and victimization in grades 3–8.* (Issues & Answers Report, REL 2011, No. 114). Washington, DC: U.S. Department of Education, Institute of Education Sciences, National Center for Education Evaluation and Regional Assistance, Regional Educational Laboratory Northwest. Retrieved from http://ies.ed.gov/ncee/edlabs

O'Neill, R. E., Albin, R. W., Storey, K., Horner, R. H., & Sprague, J. R. (2014). *Functional assessment and program development for problem behavior* (3rd ed.). Independence, KY: Cengage Learning.

O'Neill, R., Horner, R. H., Albin, R. W., Sprague, J. R., Newton, S., & Storey, K. (1997). *Functional assessment and program development for problem behavior: A practical handbook* (2nd ed.). Pacific Grove, CA: Brooks/Cole.

O'Neill, S., & Stephenson, J. (2010). The use of functional behavioral assessment for students with challenging behaviours: Current patterns and experience of Australian practitioners. *Australian Journal of Educational and Developmental Psychology, 10,* 65–82.

Osofsky, J. D. (1997). *Children in a violent society.* New York, NY: Guilford Press.

O'Toole, M. E. (2000). *The school shooter: A threat assessment perspective.* Quantico, VA: National Center for the Analysis of Violent Crime, FBI Academy.

Patterson, G. R., Reid, J. B., & Dishion, T. J. (1992). *Antisocial boys.* Eugene, OR: Castalia Press.

Pollack, J., & Kubrin, C. (2007). Crime in the news: How crimes, offenders, & victims are portrayed in the media. *Journal of Criminal Justice and Popular Culture, 14*(1), 59–83.

Reid, J. (1993). Prevention of conduct disorder before and after school entry: Relating interventions to developmental findings. *Development and Psychopathology, 5*(1–2), 243–262.

Reid, J., Patterson, G. R., & Snyder, J. (2002). *Antisocial behavior in children and adolescents: A developmental analysis and the Oregon Model for Intervention.* Washington, DC: American Psychological Association.

Robers, S., Kemp, J., & Truman, J. (2013). *Indicators of School Crime and Safety: 2012* (NCES 2013-036/NCJ 241446). Washington, DC: National Center for Education Statistics, U.S. Department of Education, and Bureau of Justice Statistics, Office of Justice Programs, U.S. Department of Justice.

Robinson, K. (2004). *Advances in school-based mental health interventions: Best practices and program models.* New York, NY: Civic Research Institute.

Satcher, D. (2001). *Youth violence: A report of the surgeon general.* Washington, DC: Department of Health and Human Services, U.S. Public Health Service.

Schneider, T., Walker, H. M., & Sprague, J. R. (2000). *Safe school design.* Eugene, OR: Educational Resources Information Clearinghouse (ERIC), University of Oregon.

Schorr, L. (1988). *Within our reach: Breaking the cycle of disadvantage.* New York, NY: Doubleday.

Seeley, J., Rohde, P., Lewinsohn, P., & Clarke, G. (2002). Depression in youth: Epidemiology, identification, and intervention. In M. Shinn, H. M. Walker, & G. Stoner (Eds.), *Interventions for academic and behavior problems. II: Preventive and remedial approaches* (pp. 885–912). Bethesda, MD: National Association of School Psychologists.

Severson, H., Walker, H., Hope-Doolittle, J., Kratochwill, R., & Gresham, F. (2007). Proactive, early screening to detect behaviorally at-risk students: Issues, approaches, emerging innovations, and professional practices. *Journal of School Psychology, 45*, 193–223.

Shinn, M., & Walker, H. M. (2010). *Interventions for achievement and behavior problems in a three-tier model including RTI.* Bethesda, MD: National Association of School Psychologists.

Shinn, M., Walker, H. M., & Stoner, G. (2002). *Interventions for academic and behavior problems. II: Preventive and remedial approaches.* Bethesda, MD: National Association of School Psychologists.

Sprague, J., & Nishioka, V. (2012). Preventing and responding to bullying and harassment in schools: What we know and what can be done. In B. G. Cook, M. Tankersley, & T. J. Landrum (Eds.), *Classroom behavior, contexts, and interventions: Advances in learning and behavioral disabilities* (Vol. 25, pp. 217–245). Bingley, UK: Emerald.

Sprague, J. R., & Walker, H. M. (2010). Building safe and healthy schools to promote school success: Critical issues, current challenges, and promising approaches. In M. R. Shinn, H. M. Walker, & G. Stoner (Eds.), *Interventions for achievement and behavior problems in a three-tier model including RTI* (pp. 225–258). Bethesda, MD: National Association of School Psychologists.

Stephens, R. (2000) School safety update: Secret service study of school shootings focuses on "targeted violence." *Newsletter of the National School Safety Center* (Westlake Village, CA), 1–4.

Thompson, C. (2013, November 18). Teacher killings bring profession's risks to light. *Eugene Register Guard.*

Tiesman, H., Konda, S., Hendricks, S., Mercer, D., & Amadus, H. (2013). Workplace violence among Pennsylvania education workers: Differences among occupations. *Journal of Safety Research, 44,* 65–71.

Van Acker, R., Boreson, L., Gable, R., & Potterton, T. (2005). Are we on the right course? Lessons learned about current FBA/BIP practices in schools. *Journal of Behavioral Education, 14,* 35–56.

Vance, J., Bowen, N., Fernandez, G., & Thompson, S. (2002). Risk and protective factors as predictors of outcome in adolescents with psychiatric disorder and aggression. *Journal of the American Academy of Child and Adolescent Psychiatry, 41*(1), 36–43.

Vance, J., Fernandez, G., & Biber, M. (1998). Educational progress in a population of youth with aggression and emotional disturbance: The role of risk and protective factors. *Journal of Emotional and Behavioral Disorders,* 6(4), 214–221.

Walker, H. M. (1986). The AIMS (Assessments for Integration into Mainstream Settings) assessment system: Rationale, instruments, procedures and outcomes. *Journal of Clinical Child Psychology, 15*(1), 55–63.

Walker, H. M. (1995). *The acting out child.* Longmont, CO: Sopris West.

Walker, H. M., Colvin, G., & Ramsey, E. (1995). *Antisocial behavior in schools: Strategies and best practices.* Pacific Grove, CA: Brooks/Cole.

Walker, H. M., & Gresham, F. M. (2014). *Handbook of evidence-based practices for emotional and behavioral disorders: Applications in schools.* New York, NY: Guilford.

Walker, H. M., Hops, H., & Greenwood, C. R. (1988). *RECESS: Reprogramming environmental contingencies for effective social skills.* Seattle, WA: Educational Achievement Systems.

Walker, H. M., Horner, R. H., Sugai, G., Bullis, M., Sprague, J. R., Bricker, D., & Kaufman, M. (1996). Integrated approaches to preventing antisocial behavior patterns among school-age children and youth. *Journal of Emotional and Behavioral Disorders,* 4(4), 194–209.

Walker, H. M., Ramsey, E., & Gresham, F. M. (2004). *Antisocial behavior in school: Evidence-based practices* (2nd ed.). Belmont, CA: Wadsworth.

Walker, H. M., & Severson, H. H. (2002). Developmental prevention of at-risk outcomes for vulnerable antisocial children and youth. In F. M. Gresham, K. L. Lane, & T. E. O'Shaughnessy (Eds.), *Interventions for academic and behavior problems. II: Preventive and remedial approaches.* Silver Spring, MD: National Association of School Psychologists.

Walker, H. M., & Sprague, J. R. (1999a). The path to school failure, delinquency, and violence: Causal factors and some potential solutions. *Intervention in School and Clinic, 35*(2), 67–73.

Walker, H. M., & Sprague, J. R. (1999b). Longitudinal research and functional behavioral assessment issues. *Behavioral Disorders, 24*(4), 335–337.

White, A., Raczynski, K., Pack, C., & Wang, A. (2011). *The Safe School Ambassadors Program: A student led approach to reducing mistreatment and bullying in schools.* San Marcos, TX: Texas State University.

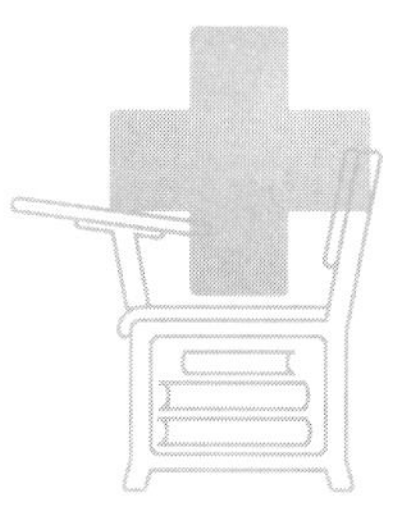

Chapter 20
Child and Youth Maltreatment

Lana Dépatie, Laila Nurmohamed,
and Michelle Shouldice

The teachers at school are concerned about Billy, a 6-year-old boy in first grade. He misses at least two days of school per week. He comes to school dirty and inadequately dressed for the weather on a regular basis. He never has lunch or snacks with him. His language is delayed, and he doesn't reliably know the alphabet. He often falls asleep in class. When he is not asleep, he is difficult to manage, often swearing and hitting other kids. He appears hyperactive and has trouble following class instructions.

A gym teacher at school notices bruises on 10-year-old Susan's back when she is changing for gym class and asks her about it. She says that her father hit her the night before because she got a C on her report card. She says that he hits her regularly using spoons, sticks, and a belt, and that he puts her in an ice bath as punishment. Her older brother is also being hit regularly. She is often afraid to go home.

The police arrive at school to investigate a reported sexual assault. They are preparing to arrest a 15-year-old tenth-grader, Jack, who is alleged to have raped his 14-year-old girlfriend Samantha, taken naked pictures of her, and sent them to two of his friends, who then posted them on Facebook. Both adolescents are students in the school. The parents of the girl are now calling the school principal.

HOW DO YOU RESPOND?

Child maltreatment is common. As an educator, you have likely encountered cases similar to these. If you have not been involved in a child abuse case involving a student, the reality is that you most likely will be. Given the amount of time that children spend in school, and the close and trusting relationships they develop with their teachers, it is not a surprise that school staff are the predominant source of recognizing and reporting child maltreatment concerns. In Canada and the United States, educators report 25%–50% of all child maltreatment cases investigated by child protection authorities (Public Health Agency of Canada, 2010; Sedlak et al., 2010). It is essential for school personnel to understand when and how to report child maltreatment, and how to respond when child abuse and neglect issues arise in the school setting.

WHAT IS CHILD MALTREATMENT?

Child maltreatment encompasses "the physical and emotional maltreatment, sexual abuse, neglect and negligent treatment of children, as well as their commercial or other exploitation" (World Health Organization, WHO, 2006). Although child maltreatment often refers to inappropriate actions or care provided by a child's parent or guardian, we have included sexual assault (by a stranger, acquaintance, or peer) in this chapter. In many jurisdictions, legal definitions of the various forms of maltreatment include harm that has occurred to a child and likely or potential harm resulting from the actions of another individual.

WHAT IS PHYSICAL ABUSE?

Physical abuse is the use of physical force against a child that results in harm (or risk of harm) to the child's health, survival, development, or dignity (Myers, Berliner, Briere, Hendrix, & Reid, 2002; WHO, 2006). Physical abuse can take the form of hitting, kicking, shaking, strangling, burning, poisoning, and suffocating, among other forms of physical violence (WHO, 2006). The boundary between physical discipline and physical abuse is defined by the criminal code of each jurisdiction. In general, in Canada and the United States, the law permits parents "reasonable force" in disciplining children. This has often been interpreted as the use of force with children who are able to understand the basis of that force (i.e., not in infants and toddlers), which does not involve the use of implements or result in physical injuries (i.e., does not leave marks or bruises) or occur to body locations where physical harm is more likely (i.e., not on face, abdomen, genitals). Although reasonable force in applying discipline is described under the law, studies have repeatedly indicated that physical discipline is not as effective as behavior management approaches are and is associated with increased childhood aggression, teen delinquency and antisocial behaviors, poorer parent–child relationships, mental health difficulties (e.g., depression), and increased risk of physical abuse. The impacts of physical discipline in childhood continue into adulthood, with increased aggression, poorer mental health outcomes, and an increased risk of abusing one's own children and/or spouse (Thompson-Gershoff, 2002). Physical force as a form of discipline is therefore not recommended (Canadian Pediatric Society, 2004; Gershoff, 2008), and in general, health-care professionals and child protection systems encourage nonphysical forms of discipline.

When to Be Concerned About Physical Abuse

Physical abuse is identified in schools through recognition of concerning physical injuries (most frequently bruises) or when a child reports physical force applied by an adult (e.g., being hit). The case vignette of Susan illustrates a common presentation of physical abuse in school:

> Susan shows her gym teacher her back. There are long, linear, curved bruises running diagonally across her lower back.

Bruising is normal in an active school-age child. Common accidental bruises are typically small, oval, or round shaped without clear borders, located on the front of the body, and over bone prominences such as the forehead, knees, shins, and forearms. Some characteristics of bruises are more common in physical abuse injuries and less likely to occur in typical childhood activity, including bruises on the ears, neck, feet, buttocks, or torso; on the back of the body; over cushioned areas (e.g., the cheeks and abdomen); and those with specific patterns (rectangular, looped, parallel linear bruises) (Ward, Ornstein, Niec, Murray, & Canadian Pediatric Society, 2013). In addition to bruising, other signs of physical abuse can include bite marks, frequent fractures, burns, or signs of pain such as a limp. Susan's story continues:

> Susan's bruises are unusual and unlikely to result from common household or playground bumps and falls because of their location on her back, their linear pattern, and their size. These bruises are concerning for physical abuse and fit with Susan's explanation of being hit with sticks and a belt.

WHAT IS SEXUAL ABUSE?

Sexual abuse encompasses any sexual activity involving a child or youth where consent is not or cannot be given or that violates the laws or social taboos of society (Myers et al., 2002; Kellogg, 2005). Sexual abuse includes sexual contact (e.g., touching, orogenital contact, penetration) and noncontact sexual acts (e.g., child pornography, exposure to pornography, exposure to sexual violence, luring) (Myers et al., 2002). The age of consent for sexual activity is defined by the criminal code of each jurisdiction.

When to Be Concerned About Sexual Abuse/Assault

Sexual abuse or assault comes to the attention of school personnel most commonly when a student tells someone about something that has happened. Sometimes, the police are notified directly by a youth or family and arrive at the school to begin the investigation. The case of Jack and Samantha is one such example:

> Samantha was distraught when she found nude pictures of her posted on Facebook. She told her mother about it, and the police were called.

In Samantha's case, both sexual contact (rape) and noncontact (sharing of naked pictures) were reported. Both of these are forms of sexual assault.

Concerns of sexual abuse may also arise on the basis of interactions of a sexual nature by a child or between children. Children's normal sexual development includes a range of sexual behaviors that can at times include the participation of other children. Sexual behaviors that are less common and require further evaluation involve children of different ages, disparities in development, or dissimilar size. Other concerning features include accompanying coercion, threats, and/or use of weapons. Both children involved in atypical sexual behavior need help, and any concerns are reportable to child protection agencies (Myers et al., 2002).

WHAT IS NEGLECT?

Neglect can refer to an isolated incident or the failure of a caregiver over time to provide for the health, development, and well-being of a child (WHO, 2006). Neglect occurs when there is a failure to meet the standard of acceptable care, as determined by society, specific to a time and place. Several subtypes of neglect have been identified including physical neglect (e.g., inadequate food, clothing, or housing), emotional neglect (e.g., inadequate nurturing), medical neglect (e.g., inadequate health care), mental health neglect (e.g., failure to seek help for significant emotional, behavioral, or psychiatric issues), and educational neglect. In each of these subtypes, caregivers fail to provide the necessities in a child's life for which the child depends on the caregiver's support (Myers et al., 2002). The vignette describing Billy illustrates this form of child maltreatment:

> Billy appears to be suffering from a pattern of physical neglect (e.g., dirty, not wearing clothing appropriate for the weather, inadequate food) and educational neglect (e.g., frequently missing school) that is affecting his behavior and ability to function in the classroom.

WHAT IS EMOTIONAL ABUSE?

Emotional abuse, also referred to as psychological maltreatment, includes specific concerning interactions between a caregiver and child, or the more generalized failure of a parent or caregiver to provide an appropriate and supportive environment for a child (WHO, 2006). This is often the most difficult type of maltreatment to recognize, investigate, and prove, but it has significant and lasting detrimental effects on a child's functioning. Emotional abuse takes many forms, including threatening, belittling, terrorizing, frightening, and rejecting. Exposure to domestic violence is a form of terrorizing and is considered a form of emotional abuse (Myers et al., 2002). Psychological maltreatment conveys to children that they are worthless, flawed, unloved, unwanted, endangered, or of value only in meeting another's needs (Myers et al., 2002). Emotional abuse commonly occurs in association with other forms of maltreatment, but it may also occur in isolation (Myers et al., 2002). In Susan's vignette, the use of the ice bath for punishment and her expression of fear illustrate emotional abuse that accompanies the physical abuse she has sustained.

HOW BIG IS THE PROBLEM?

Child maltreatment is a widespread problem. More than 1.25 million children (1 in 58) in the United States experienced maltreatment, substantiated by a child protection investigation, between 2005 and 2006 (Sedlak et al., 2010). This is comparable to other jurisdictions that have defined and studied this issue (Finkelhor, Vanderminden, Turner, Hamby, & Shattuck, 2014; MacMillan, Tanaka, Duku, & Vaillancourt, 2013).

Neglect is the most common form of child maltreatment (Myers et al., 2002). Of the 1.25 million children with substantiated child maltreatment, 61% were found to be neglected and 44% of those had been abused sexually, physically, and/or emotionally (NIS, 2010). Of the children who were abused, physical abuse was the most common form of abuse (58%), followed by emotional abuse (27%) and sexual abuse (24%) (NIS, 2010).

The extent of the problem, however, is even larger than these statistics illustrate. Nearly 3 million children in the United States were felt to be at risk of child maltreatment over the course of a year from 2005 to 2006. This equates to 1 in every 25 children feeling at risk for some form of child maltreatment. More than 75% of cases were concerns regarding neglect (NIS, 2010).

In addition, a limitation to incidence and prevalence data regarding child maltreatment is that national statistics measure only those cases that are reported to a child protection authority. It is clear that such data results in underestimations, as many situations of abuse and neglect go unrecognized and unreported. Anonymous surveys of adults on experiences of abuse during childhood can be helpful in this regard. In 2011, a US national household survey was conducted of more than 4,000 youth and their caregivers. Physical abuse was reported by 4% of the children and caregivers, emotional abuse was reported by 5.6% of children, sexual abuse was reported by 2.2% of children, and neglect was reported in 4.7% of cases. Overall, 12.1% of the sample had experienced at least one form of maltreatment, and 2.8% of the sample had experienced more than one type of abuse (Finkelhor et al., 2014). These studies demonstrate the true magnitude of the problem.

SHOULD I REPORT, AND TO WHOM?

The rules and regulations regarding school personnel's mandate to report suspected child maltreatment vary by jurisdiction. Within a particular country, the obligations may vary by province or state. Most states and provinces in North America mandate that teachers report any suspicion of child maltreatment to a child protection agency. The majority of these jurisdictions are in agreement that a *reasonable* ground for suspecting abuse is sufficient for reporting, and certainty is not required. It is prudent for teachers to become familiar with relevant laws and regulations regarding child maltreatment reporting, and local school board policies and procedures in cases of suspected maltreatment. Ideally, each school should have a policy in place that outlines the details regarding child maltreatment reporting. It should outline who is mandated to report, whom to report to, and what information may be transmitted. If an educator believes that a child may be a victim of maltreatment, he or she should identify the appropriate agency to which to report these concerns. In most cases, child protection services will take such calls; however, this can vary from region to region. In all three of the described vignettes here, a report to child protection services is indicated.

WHO GETS INVOLVED, AND WHAT ARE THEIR ROLES IN THE SYSTEM?

School

Teachers and school personnel play an important role in the identification, prevention, and management of child maltreatment. More than half of abuse cases reported to child protection agencies are initiated by teachers. Teachers are often the first to notice the signs of abuse or neglect, given their close relationship to students. Children also often entrust teachers with disclosures. Teachers are tasked with the important role of providing ongoing support for students after a disclosure is made, as an investigation proceeds, and afterward.

Police

The police are not involved in all cases, although they may be the first responders in cases of abuse, and often in cases of sexual assault. In many jurisdictions, there are protocols for joint investigation of physical and sexual abuse concerns by child protection services and police. Child protection services often receive the initial report and determine the need for police involvement. The police become involved when there is the potential for criminal charges. The police work with the child protection agency to interview the victim (if possible), as well as potential offenders and others who may be helpful in the case. The police also organize and facilitate witnesses in court proceedings and act as a link between the child and the court. In most situations, physicians and teachers are bound by confidentiality clauses and therefore may be unable to share information with police without consent. It is important, however, to document conversations or observations clearly, as these details could be helpful to the investigation.

Child Protection Services

Many child protection service responders are trained as social workers. The mandate of the child protection system is to assess the risk of harm to children and make protection decisions on the basis of those risks. They help clarify child maltreatment concerns by interviewing children and their families and gaining a better understanding of the home environment. Child protection services often seek to keep families together and to provide supportive interventions when possible. They may take over custody of a child in cases where the danger to the child is clear and significant.

Courts

The role of the court is to make decisions as required in child custody situations arising from child protection involvement and when criminal charges have been laid. Overall, a small proportion of child maltreatment cases result in criminal charges and proceed to a formal hearing, such as a trial. When a case does go to a formal child protection or criminal trial, witnesses with direct involvement in the case can be called to court to testify, and teachers may be called to court as part of this process (although this is uncommon).

Physicians

Physicians may be involved in the identification, prevention, or treatment of child maltreatment. The first physician to evaluate a patient who has experienced abuse or neglect is often an emergency room doctor, family doctor, or pediatrician. Concerns of maltreatment may arise during any type of medical or mental health evaluation. Pediatricians with special training in child maltreatment may be consulted to provide opinions regarding injuries or assessments of children who may have experienced child maltreatment. These pediatricians are trained to work with other health-care professionals and with the child protection and law enforcement or criminal justice systems in responding to child maltreatment concerns.

Mental Health Professionals

Mental health professionals such as psychiatrists, psychologists, social workers, nurses, and victim services workers are an integral part of the team in child maltreatment cases. Children who have suffered from abuse or been witness to abuse may suffer from trauma reactions (see section Trauma Reactions) and can receive therapeutic intervention targeting symptom relief. Medical centers or child and youth advocacy centers often offer these services to children and to nonoffending parents and caregivers.

RESPONDING TO A DISCLOSURE OF ABUSE

The response of an adult to a child at the time of disclosure of abuse is critical to the child's outcome. Research has consistently shown that victims who receive a positive or supportive (e.g., believing and protective) response from adults they tell about the abuse have a better prognosis, with fewer negative psychological and physiological health consequences, than victims who do not receive a supportive response (Kendall-Tackett, Williams, & Finkelhor, 1993; Ullman, 2003). Teachers, coaches, and other school staff play a crucial role in this regard. However, individuals in contact with children and adolescents can feel uncertain about how they should respond to the victims of abuse. For example, a teacher may be unsure of what to say or do after a child has disclosed being abused. Others who suspect that a child may be abused often wonder whether they should talk with the child, or whether they should contact the caregivers to discuss their concerns.

The following steps are recommended in response to a direct disclosure of maltreatment to a teacher or other school personnel: First and foremost, listen to the child, and maintain a calm, supportive reaction. Next, the child's disclosure should be immediately and clearly documented in written form and reported to the appropriate authorities without delay. Ensuring the child's safety and preventing further harm is crucial. Child protection authorities will respond to reported abuse or neglect according to local protocols, which may include attending the school and interviewing the child in the school setting. In this event, steps should be taken to ensure that the child's privacy is protected and to minimize secondary harm to the child related to other children hearing or noticing that a child protection worker or police officer came to meet them at school. Child protection authorities are responsible for decision making regarding how safety is best ensured.

Following the initial response by child protection authorities and/or police, in most cases, the child will remain in the same school. School personnel need to be aware of the possible impact of abuse, disclosure, various stressors (possible involvement of the authorities and court process), and possible unsettling changes (e.g., breakdown of family relationships, the child may be apprehended and placed into foster care) that the child may experience in the days, weeks, and months that will follow. The child may experience symptoms that impair functioning in the school environment (for more information about specific symptoms, see Trauma Reactions section). The child is likely to need support from adults in his or her life. Supportive and understanding adults in the school setting are likely to make a significant difference for the child. Ensuring that the child has a "safe" adult at school that he or she can talk to when in need or when experiencing challenges in coping is often beneficial. The routines, structures, and predictability of the school environment are usually helpful in assisting the child in coping with stressors and changes in other areas of life. School personnel may also be in a good position to identify a need for emotional support or therapeutic intervention, and they may be able to facilitate access to such support.

In general, it would be helpful to work with a supportive, nonabusive caregiver in planning around how to best support a child who has experienced maltreatment. However, this may not always be possible. In some cases, a teenager may not wish for his or her parents to know about a sexual assault. It may be helpful to explore the reasons for this decision and work with the teen to identify other supports, such as extended family members, friends, or other adults who could provide support.

Responding When One Suspects Child Abuse (Before or Without a Direct Disclosure)

In some instances, concerns of abuse arise because of a child's presentation, behavior, or changes in functioning rather than a direct disclosure of victimization. It is important to know that there is no specific psychological, social, or emotional profile for children who have experienced abuse or neglect, and most symptoms these children experience are also observed among children exposed to other types of adversity (e.g., parental separation and divorce, bullying).

The approach of an adult to a child in the case of suspected abuse, where no disclosure of abuse has yet occurred, requires an atmosphere of trust and support, as well as recognition that, if abuse has occurred, the child may not be ready or feel safe to report what has happened. It is very common for children who have experienced abuse to disclose it long after the events or not at all (e.g., Smith et al., 2000). Factors such as age at the time of abuse, multiple incidents of abuse, and closeness of relationship between the victim and perpetrator (i.e., family member) have all been found to affect delay and/or rates of disclosure. Gentle exploration of how things are going at home, in school, and with friends may provide an opening to discuss stressors, including abuse. It is often helpful to have one school staff (most likely a school social worker, but it could be a coach, teacher, principal, or vice principal) meet with the child on a regular basis to build rapport and trust, such that he or she eventually may feel more comfortable disclosing any difficulties, including abuse. An assessment of the child's functioning may be of assistance in identifying the child's specific needs for socioemotional or academic difficulties, regardless of whether concerns of abuse are confirmed. Further, teachers and other school staff can ensure the children's safety while they are in the school environment, which is an important component to enhancing functioning and minimizing symptoms related to trauma and stress.

Trauma Reactions (Possible Signs of Abuse and Impact of Abuse on Functioning)

Not all children react to abuse in a similar fashion. Although some children are greatly affected, others do not appear to show any significant distress. Although a child may not appear to be symptomatic, some children "compartmentalize" different aspects of their lives, allowing them to function despite horrific abuse histories. As such, for some children, school performance plummets following a recent incident; others thrive academically in spite of the stress associated with abuse. This can reflect a coping mechanism whereby the child has "separated" the abuse from the rest of his or her life and focuses attention and energies on schoolwork, attempting to avoid thinking about the abuse. Various factors affect a child's resiliency to adversity. These include abuse-related factors (e.g., chronicity, severity of abuse and neglect), relational factors with others (e.g., response to abuse by the system and caregiver, having close friendships), and child-focused factors (e.g., self-regulation skills, attributions made regarding the abuse) (Barker-Collo & Read, 2003; Haskett, Nears, Sabourin Ward, & McPherson, 2006). These factors interact in a complex fashion and affect a child's prognosis relative to the experience of abuse (Barker-Collo & Read, 2003). Nevertheless, most children with a history of abuse will be affected in some way by their experience (Haskett et al., 2006). It is therefore important to be aware of what type of symptoms children with histories of abuse may exhibit.

A child's experience of abuse must be considered in the context of the child's developmental stage. Some symptoms are more commonly experienced in younger children, but others tend to be more frequently observed among teenagers. As children develop, their increasingly sophisticated ability to process information, the evolving complexity of their thinking, and their growing understanding of feeling states all affect their understanding of abuse experiences. Furthermore, the process of maturation allows for an increased repertoire of coping strategies to manage feelings of distress. As such, children at different stages of development can be expected to manifest their distress to abuse in varying ways and access different coping resources.

In young children (approximately age 4–6 years), regressive behavior and loss of previously achieved developmental milestones may be observed. For example, incidents of enuresis (inability to control urination) and encopresis (fecal soiling) when the child had previously been toilet trained, difficulty sleeping (e.g., decreased sleep and nightmares), and changes in feeding have been observed. Exhibiting behaviors more typical of younger children, being clingier, and having difficulty separating from caregivers are also commonly reported. Ability to regulate emotions (e.g., temper tantrums, increased anger and irritability) and behaviors (e.g., provocation, demanding and challenging behaviors toward adults and peers) can be affected. These children might also experience increased fears and anxiety. Children in this age group have limited cognitive abilities, life experiences, and knowledge. As such, they may have difficulty understanding various aspects of the abuse. They can be confused by what occurred and develop explanations for the events that may be frightening and contribute to the distress associated with the abuse.

Children age 7–12 years may engage in various disruptive behaviors. For example, some engage in lying, stealing, or fighting. There can be increased conflicts over the limits set by adults, agreed-on household chores, or hygiene tasks. Similar to younger children, they may experience enuresis or encopresis and/or changes in sleep and feeding. They may also alternate between their need for separation–individuation from their caregivers and increased reliance on them, becoming anxious at the thought of separation. Some children have trouble getting along with their peers or experience challenges in developing and maintaining positive peer relationships.

Teens can also experience many different symptoms following abuse. Attachment and interpersonal relationships can become challenging (e.g., increased conflicts with peers, caregivers, and other adults). Further, experiences of abuse can have an impact on how the teen perceives him- or herself and can affect the process of developing one's identity, which is among the most important developmental tasks at this stage of development. Depression, suicidality, self-harm, low self-esteem, anxiety, post-traumatic stress, dissociation, and somatic complaints have all been reported among teens with a history of abuse. Further, high-risk behaviors such as promiscuous sexuality, substance abuse, and illegal activities, as well as anger and physical aggression toward others have also been reported. Teens can put themselves in risky situations, have behaviors characterized as self-destructive, or show behavior consistent with conduct disorder.

In some instances, such behaviors represent the teen's adaptation to a long-standing history of victimization (Briere & Lanktree, 2012; Singer, Menden Anglin, Yu Song, & Lunghofer, 1995). These behaviors in turn can lead to increased risk for revictimization and further trauma. It is therefore important to provide intervention targeting such symptoms.

Although the symptoms here are listed according to developmental stages, they are by no means exclusively seen within that specific age group. For example, it is possible for a teenager to experience enuresis and/or encopresis. Similarly, a young child may experience symptoms of depression, anxiety, post-traumatic stress, and/or dissociation associated with abuse. School personnel should keep this in mind if they suspect that a child or teenager may be the victim of abuse.

Trauma reactions as described here are broad and encompass more than the traditional understanding of trauma as post-traumatic stress disorder (PTSD). Nevertheless, PTSD symptoms are found at increased rates among children with such histories (Copeland, Keeler, Angold, & Costello, 2007). The disorder is characterized by symptoms such as recurrent intrusive distressing memories of a traumatic event (in this case abuse), avoidance of trauma reminders, negative alterations in cognitions (e.g., inability to recall aspects of traumatic events, self-blame), and changes in arousal and reactivity (e.g., increased irritability). Dissociative symptoms can also be involved. Such symptoms are characterized by a sense of detachment from reality or altered states of consciousness. A child experiencing such symptoms can seem as though he or she is daydreaming in the classroom. Such symptoms can be mistaken for the child experiencing inattention issues or absence seizures, when in fact they reflect a symptom associated with trauma.

Symptoms such as inattention, impulsivity, and motor hyperactivity are not uncommon among victims of abuse. These are criterial symptoms of attention-deficit/hyperactivity disorder (ADHD) (American Psychiatric Association, APA, 2013), and ADHD is a common diagnosis among children with abuse histories. However, in the context of abuse, such symptoms (e.g., inattention, impulsivity, hyperactivity) can represent anxiety associated with the trauma of the abusive environment (Famularo, Kinscherff, & Fenton 1992), and as such they need to be understood in that context so that the appropriate intervention can be provided. In contrast, ADHD and trauma can co-occur, and whether the symptoms represent ADHD, a traumatic reaction to abuse, or both needs to be assessed by a professional such that the child may receive the appropriate treatment.

There may be differences in the clinical presentation of victims of one or a few recent acute incidents of abuse compared to children who have been victimized over many years and have encountered several traumatic events. In the case of a child who has been victimized on one occasion, the adults in the child's life may be able to readily identify changes in functioning across various domains. For example, the child who was previously compliant and attentive, got along well with peers, and showed effective emotional regulation is now, seemingly inexplicably, breaking rules, being inattentive in class, getting into quarrels with peers and teachers, easily becoming angry, and lacking involvement in previously enjoyed extracurricular activities. The recent changes in functioning may raise suspicion among teachers and caregivers regarding what may have triggered the difficulties. In contrast, in many instances, there is a pattern of long-term and repetitive abuse involving children's key relationships (i.e., relationship with caregivers). These children may not show sudden changes. Rather, the impact of the abuse in these cases may be more substantial and difficulties may be long-standing, affecting how the child is perceived through his or her academic life. For example, a child with a long history of abuse may have appeared inattentive, hyperactive, oppositional, and/or difficult to manage in the classroom for years, with the link between the abuse and the difficulties not having been identified and therefore no appropriate supports having been provided.

SEXUAL BEHAVIORS IN CHILDREN AND ADOLESCENTS

Sexual behaviors are commonly exhibited (e.g., 88% of children, according to Larsson & Svedin, 2002) in children younger than age 13 years, although the extent to which children engage in such behaviors varies, and the behaviors can range from healthy to problematic throughout development. It is currently believed that while a history of sexual abuse can be a contributor to sexual behavior problems in children (e.g., Silovsky & Niec, 2002), several other factors can influence the development of such behaviors (e.g., child characteristics, social competence, family adversity) (Friedrich, Davies, Feher, & Wright, 2003).

It can be difficult for individuals to determine whether a sexual behavior is healthy or cause for concern. There are several signs that may suggest that sexual behaviors are problematic. Table 20.1 provides examples of indicators that would suggest that seeking consultation, having a professional evaluation of the child, and/or reporting to the authorities may be appropriate.

Table 20.1

CHARACTERISTICS SUGGESTING POSSIBLE PROFESSIONAL EVALUATION AND/OR REPORTING TO AUTHORITIES

1. The children participating in sexual behaviors do not have an equal and reciprocal relationship.
2. There is a discrepancy in age and/or developmental levels between the children engaged in the behaviors.
3. The behaviors are inconsistent with other facets of the child's existence and activities.
4. The child appears to have knowledge about sexuality that exceeds what would be expected given the age and developmental level.
5. The sexual behaviors persist in spite of repeated instructions that they must stop.
6. There is an increase in the rate, intensity, or invasiveness of the behavior over time.
7. The behaviors cause distress (physical or emotional) to the child and/or others.

Note. The characteristics listed here are examples only and do not constitute an exhaustive list. For more information about healthy and problematic sexual behaviors, see *Understanding Children's Sexual Behaviors: What's Natural and Healthy*, by T. Cavanagh-Johnson, 2011, San Diego, CA: Institute on Violence, Abuse and Trauma.

School personnel, like many other individuals, can feel uncomfortable addressing sexual behaviors with a child. Obtaining some understanding of the nature of the behavior and factors contributing to the maintenance of the problematic sexual behavior is an important component of addressing the issue. At times, one's discomfort around sexuality and discussing topics of a sexual nature can prevent an appropriate intervention from taking place in a timely manner and contribute to the continuation of the behavior. This is illustrated in this example: A 9-year-old boy observed to repeatedly pull at other students' clothing to look at their genitals was referred to a mental health professional. The behavior continued in spite of his repeatedly being told by school staff that it was not appropriate and that the behavior needed to stop. When the psychologist explored the behavior with the child, it became apparent that the child was confused as to whether all boys "looked the same" and all girls "look the same" and that the boy had decided to collect data to answer the question for himself. Once the psychologist reassured the boy that indeed all boys have similar genitalia and all girls have similar genitalia, the behavior stopped.

Although parents and school personnel had thought of discussing the inappropriate nature of the behavior, no one had thought to discuss the possible motivation behind the behavior.

It is important for families and school personnel to meet a victim's needs for protection in the case of sexual behaviors between children. A primary focus should be the victim's sense of safety while in the school environment. It is unlikely that a teacher could meet such needs appropriately on his or her own. It is suggested that a team be organized, and it could include the principal, vice principal, teachers for both the instigator of the behavior and the victim, and the parents of the victim (in ideal cases, the parents of the perpetrator of the behavior would also be included in the dialogue, although we recognize that this is not always feasible). Further, a victim may have opinions and ideas as to what might increase his or her own sense of safety. It is important to take such ideas into account in building a safety plan, as they give the child an increased sense of control. It may be very valuable to consult with a representative from child protection authorities in order to guide safety planning.

When a child exhibits sexual behavior problems at school, it is important to provide adequate supervision so that other children are protected from victimization. It is suggested that the supervision of the child exhibiting problematic sexual behaviors be consistent with the child's need for assistance in regulating the behavior, as well as with the level of risk associated with the likelihood that other students will be victimized. In some situations, organizing regular check-ins between a teacher and the youth to discuss whether the youth has difficulties preventing the behavior will be sufficient. At other times, it may mean that there is increased supervision (e.g., increased staff-to-student ratio) during recess and lunch. Yet in other situations, the risk may be such that it is necessary for school personnel to thoroughly monitor the youth exhibiting the behaviors at all times during school hours (e.g., monitoring hallways, stairwells, and washrooms in addition to supervision during recess, lunch, and as students are getting on and off the school bus). School boards may have policies regarding how to approach such situations.

Children who exhibit sexual behaviors may be treated differently than others. For example, others may be reluctant to touch them and intensively watch the child, with the expectation that he or she will express negative behaviors. This can have negative consequences on a child's sense of self and can increase the child's sense that he or she is "bad." In general, we advocate for adequate and thorough supervision while being the least intrusive possible (although, as stated earlier, in some situations intruding cannot be avoided given the level of risk to others). It goes without saying that children who engage in problematic sexual behaviors need to be treated respectfully, be provided therapeutic support when in need, and have access to a nurturing and healthy environment.

Adolescence is a period of development when sexual assaults (e.g., teen sexual violence, date rape) occur, and the victim and alleged assailant may attend the same school. A victim and perpetrator in that case are likely to come into contact, which can pose further challenges. It is not uncommon for victims not to disclose the assault out of fear of retaliation from perpetrators and their social network. Teenagers are also often concerned about the social impact that can be associated with information of a sexual assault being leaked around school. The stress related to such concerns, combined with the stress of the sexual assault itself, can lead to difficulty coping and can affect the victim's functioning. In addition, further emotional, academic, and social difficulties for the victim can arise over time, as rumors around the sexual assault may surface and as the social impact of the disclosure persists. Access to social media and having information or rumors of a sexual assault involving two students circulate can be difficult to manage and can contribute to a youth's further victimization. Many teens are unaware that accessing and sending compromising pictures of a victim or other sexual images involving a minor can lead to criminal charges associated with making and/or distributing child pornographic images. As such, teens can fail to realize that the viewing and distributing of compromising images of a classmate not only victimizes or revictimizes that classmate but also can lead to involvement with the legal system. Teachers can bring awareness about these issues to their students as a form of prevention. Further, we suggest that school personnel be prepared to ensure students' safety and protect the victim from revictimization. How to achieve that may vary depending on the nature of the assault being disclosed, the needs of the victim, and his or her ability to cope, as well as the extent of the perpetrator's difficulties. As such, gathering information about the incident and involving different staff, the victim, and his or her caregivers, the perpetrator and caregivers, as well as the appropriate authorities, may be appropriate in developing a response to the situation.

CONCLUSION

School personnel should be able to define and identify various forms of abuse and neglect, know which systems to engage to assess and maintain safety for victims of abuse, know how to respond to optimize outcomes for children who have been subjected to maltreatment, and have an understanding of common reactions to abuse to watch out for in the school setting.

ADDITIONAL RESOURCES

Child Welfare Information Gateway (http://www.childwelfare.gov): Information and resources to help protect children and strengthen families

National Children's Alliance (http://www.nca-online.org): Information on state statutes

REFERENCES

American Psychiatric Association. (2013). *Diagnostic and statistical manual of mental disorders* (5th ed.). Arlington, VA: Author.

Barker-Collo, S., & Read, J. (2003). Models of response to childhood sexual abuse: Their implications for treatment. *Trauma, Violence & Abuse, 4*, 95–111.

Briere, J. N., & Lanktree, C. B. (2012). *Treating complex trauma in adolescents and young adults.* Thousand Oaks, CA: Sage.

Canadian Pediatric Society, Psychosocial Pediatrics Committee. (2004). Effective discipline for children. *Paediatrics & Child Health,* 9(1), 37–41.

Copeland, W. E., Keeler, G., Angold, A., & Costello, E. J. (2007). Traumatic events and posttraumatic stress in childhood. *Archives of General Psychiatry, 64*, 577–584.

Famularo, R., Kinscherff, R., & Fenton, T. (1992). Psychiatric diagnoses of maltreated children: Preliminary findings. *Journal of the American Academy of Child and Adolescent Psychiatry, 31*(5), 863–867.

Finkelhor, D., Vanderminden, J., Turner, H., Hamby, S., & Shattuck, A. (2014). Child maltreatment rates assessed in a national household survey of caregivers and youth. *Child Abuse & Neglect, 38*, 1421–1435.

Friedrich, W. N., Davies, W., Feher, E., & Wright, J. (2003). Sexual behavior problems in preteen children: Developmental, ecological, and behavioral correlates. *Annals of the New York Academy of Sciences, 989*, 95–104.

Gershoff, E. T. (2008). *Report on physical punishment in the United States: What research tells us about its effects on children.* Columbus, OH: Center for Effective Discipline.

Haskett, M. E., Nears, K., Sabourin Ward, C., & McPherson, A. V. (2006). Diversity in adjustment of maltreated children: Factors associated with resilient functioning. *Clinical Psychology Review, 26*, 796–812.

Kellogg, N. (2005). The evaluation of sexual abuse in children. *Pediatrics, 116*(2), 506–512.

Kendall-Tackett, K. A., Williams, L. M., & Finkelhor, D. (1993). Impact of sexual abuse on children: A review and synthesis of recent empirical studies. *Psychological Bulletin, 113*, 164–180.

Larsson, I., & Svedin, C.-G. (2002). Sexual experiences in childhood: Young adults' recollections. *Archives of Sexual Behavior, 31*(3), 263–273.

MacMillan, H. L., Tanaka, M., Duku, E., & Vaillancourt, T. (2013). Child physical and sexual abuse in a community sample of young adults: Results from the Ontario Child Health Study. *Child Abuse & Neglect, 37,* 14–21.

Myers, J. E. B., Berliner, L., Briere, J., Hendrix, C. T., & Reid T. A. (Eds.) (2002). *The APSAC handbook on child maltreatment* (2nd ed.). Thousand Oaks, CA: Sage.

Public Health Agency of Canada. (2010). *Canadian Incidence Study of Reported Child Abuse and Neglect—2008: Major Findings.* Ottawa, ON: Author.

Sedlak, A. J., Mettenburg, J., Basena, M., Petta, I., McPherson, K., Greene, A., & Li, S. (2010). *Fourth National Incidence Study of Child Abuse and Neglect* (NIS-4): Report to Congress, Executive Summary. Washington, DC: U.S. Department of Health and Human Services, Administration for Children and Families.

Silovsky, J. F., & Niec, L. (2002). Characteristics of young children with sexual behavior problems: A pilot study. *Child Maltreatment, 7,* 187–197.

Singer, M. I., Menden Anglin, T., Yu Song, L., & Lunghofer, L. (1995). Adolescents' exposure to violence and associated symptoms of psychological trauma. *Journal of the American Medical Association, 273,* 477–482.

Smith, D. W., Letourneau, E. J., Saunders, B. E., Kilpatrick, D. G., Resnick, H. S., & Best, C. L. (2000). Delay in disclosure in childhood rape: Results from a national survey. *Child Abuse & Neglect, 24*(2), 273–287.

Thompson Gershoff, E. (2002). Corporal punishment by parents and associated child behaviors and experiences: A meta-analytic and theoretical review. *Psychological Bulletin, 128*(4), 539–579.

Ullman, S. E. (2003). Social reactions to child sexual abuse disclosures: A critical review. *Journal of Child Sexual Abuse, 12*(1), 89–121.

Ward, M. G. K., Ornstein, A., Niec, A., Murray, C. L., & Canadian Pediatric Society Child and Youth Maltreatment Section. (2013). The medical assessment of bruising in suspected child maltreatment cases: A clinical perspective. P*ediatrics and Child Health, 18*(8), 433–437.

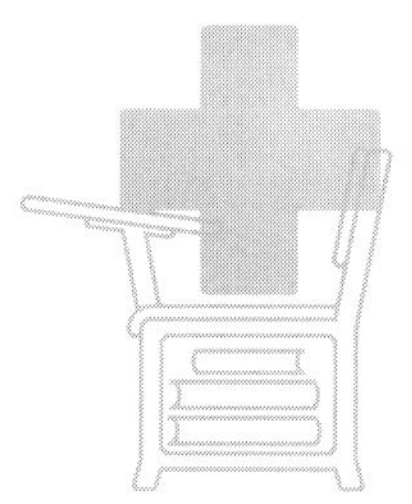

Chapter 21
Youth Suicide

The Role of the School System With At-Risk Youth

Antonio F. Cianflone, Jitender Sareen, Sarah Fotti, and Laurence Y. Katz

Among the problems faced in schools today, there are few, if any, more urgent than that of suicidal behavior in youth (Miller & Eckert, 2009). The third-leading cause of death in youth and young adults worldwide, suicide results in approximately 1 million fatalities each year (Gould & Kramer, 2001; Szumilas & Kutcher, 2008). In the United States suicide accounts for more deaths than all natural causes combined for youths and young adults between 15 and 24 years old, a demographic in which, alarmingly, rates of suicide have tripled in the past 50 years, even as rates in adult and elderly suicide have declined (Clore et al., 2003; Cutler, Glaeser, & Norberg, 2000; Gould & Kramer, 2001; Gutierrez & Osman, 2008; Weber, 2000). Among youths aged 10–14, most suicides occur between the ages of 12 and 14 (although still less frequently than those aged 15–24), while it is relatively uncommon younger than age 10 (Gould & Kramer, 2001). The number of children aged 10–14 dying by suicide also spiked 51% between 1981 and 2004, and although rates seem to fluctuate marginally, the general trend has been an increase in occurrence (Miller & Eckert, 2009). Although between 1991 and 2000 the rate of youth suicides in the United States did decline, the trend reversed from 2001 to 2009, which was again marked by a near continuous increase in youth suicide fatalities (Centers for Disease Control and Prevention, CDC, 2014).

Investigation into potential risk factors for youth suicide reveals several highly correlated associations. These include a variety of family factors (e.g., history of suicide, impaired parent–child relationships), cognitive and personal factors (e.g., the "genetics" of suicide, psychopathology, prior suicidal ideation and attempts), and life circumstances (e.g., interpersonal loss, physical and sexual abuse, difficulty in school and work). There also, however, seems to be a number of "protective" factors that are correlated with youths who appear less likely to attempt or die by suicide. The two most highly observed, which are discussed in this chapter, are family cohesion and religiosity.

The purpose of this chapter is to familiarize teachers and school administrators with the issue of youth suicide and to identify ways that educators can both directly and indirectly help at-risk youth. Prevalence, epidemiology, and a summation of characteristics, conditions, and behaviors that seem to be most highly correlated with youth suicide are discussed, as are factors that seem to be "protective" or preventative against suicide. The unique platform afforded to teachers and administrators in schools for monitoring youth and their mental well-being is further examined, as are the roles of teachers and school administrators working with youths believed to be at risk of suicide. Finally, the chapter concludes with a summation of some of the various programs that have been implemented in schools by administrators.

EPIDEMIOLOGY

Examination into the epidemiology of youth suicide reveals the severity of the issue. As already mentioned, the consistently high prevalence of suicide in youth aged 12 and older is both clear and concerning. Thus it is interesting to note that suicide younger than age 10, or before the onset of puberty, is very rare, so much so as to be described as a "universal phenomenon" by the World Health Organization (WHO) in 2002 (Gould, Greenberg, Velting, & Shaffer, 2003). Although there are many theories as to why this may be, the most commonly accepted, proposed by Shaffer et al. in 1996, suggests that exposure to and abuse of substances (drugs and alcohol) and depression are not commonly experienced in prepubescent youths. As those are two seemingly large risk factors for suicide, it is logical that youth unexposed to these problems would have lower rates of suicide as a result.

Examination of death by suicide according to sex also reveals trends. In the United States, in the 15- to 19-year-old demographic, boys are significantly more likely to die by suicide than girls, although ideation and suicide attempts are more common among females (Berman, Jobes, & Silverman, 2006; CDC, 2014; Clore et al., 2003; Miller & Eckert, 2009). This trend is also noted in Canada, Western Europe, New Zealand, and Australia; however, in some Asian countries (e.g., Singapore) suicide rates are equal among the sexes. Conversely, in China, females tend to die by suicide more than males (Gould et al., 2003). Although the noted discrepancy between suicide rates among females versus males is not fully understood, it is believed that potential reasons are that males are less likely to engage in protective behaviors (e.g., seeking help, having and using coping skills) and are more often associated with various risk factors (e.g., firearm access, alcohol or other substance abuse) than females are; this is further discussed later in the chapter. It is also important to note that statistics on recent rates of youth suicide show a decline in suicide rates for males (much larger in the age group 15–19 years) and an increase in rates for females (Skinner & McFaull, 2012).

Variation is also found in the race and ethnicity of youth with suicide attempts. Research seems to verify that ethnic groups differ in rates of suicide, the pattern of seeking help, and the context in which suicide occurs (Langhinrichsen-Rohling, Friend, & Powell, 2009). In the United States, the highest youth suicide rate is among Caucasians, followed by African Americans and then Latinos (Berman et al., 2006). While African American suicide rates have traditionally been lower than those of Caucasians, among the 15- to 19-year-olds an increase of 234% has been noted in recent decades (Berman et al., 2006). As well, when considering proportion of suicides to total ethnic population, the highest rates are found among Native American youth. Hypotheses for this include the proportionally higher use of alcohol and firearms in this group, as well as a lack of social integration between clans in terms of band-level organization within the communities (Miller & Eckert, 2009). It is important to note, however, that relatively little research has been conducted on the suicidal behavior of adolescents in different cultural groups (Langhinrichsen-Rohling et al., 2009).

One of the most discussed factors in suicidal behavior is socioeconomic status, believed by many to be one of the greatest indicators of suicidal risk. It has not, however, been found to be a positive epidemiological indicator of youth suicide. A Danish study composed of 20,000 youth who died by suicide found that those in the lowest socioeconomic class were at roughly five times greater risk of suicide, and an inverse relationship between higher socioeconomic class and death by suicide was generally found. However, thus far, attempts at empirical investigation into the influence of this factor have been inconclusive and mixed (Berman et al., 2006).

Another important epidemiological component is geography. Although it is commonly believed that suicide is an issue predominantly in urban centers, this has been proved false in recent years. In the United States it was found that the states with the largest increases in youth suicide between 1950 and 1990 were rural (e.g., Wyoming, South Dakota, Montana), whereas those with troubled inner cities (e.g., New York, New Jersey, District of Columbia) had the smallest increase (Cutler et al., 2000). Since 1990 this trend toward more rural suicides has continued, and today rural areas have higher suicide rates than urban areas (Berman et al., 2006). This is potentially explained by the relative isolation of rural youth and sparser population, which might lead to the experience of greater social disconnect, which can lead to depression, suicide, and other noted risk factors for suicide (Berman et al., 2006).

Increasing the magnitude of the issue of youth suicide is the strikingly high number of suicide attempts, with estimates of attempted suicides versus death by suicide varying from 25:1 to 400:1 (CDC, 2009; Crosby, Han, Ortega, Parks, & Gfroerer, 2011; Cutler et al., 2000). According to the 2007 Youth Risk Behavior Surveillance in the United States, of high school students surveyed across 39 states, within 12 months prior to the survey, roughly 14.5% (10.3% for males, 18.7% for females) had seriously considered suicide; 11.3% (13.4% for females, 9.2% for males) had gone so far as to make a plan for completion. Furthermore, 6.9% (9.3% for females, 4.6% for males) had attempted suicide at least once, and 2.0% of teens surveyed (2.4% for females, 1.5% for males) had made attempts that required treatment by a doctor or nurse (because of physical injury, poisoning, or overdose) (Langhinrichsen-Rohling et al., 2009). When put into proportion, these findings indicate that in US high school students, approximately 1 out of every 7 students has seriously considered suicide, 1 out of every 10 to the point of making a plan, and 1 out of every 14 have made a suicide attempt (Miller, Eckert, & Mazza, 2009). It is clear from these statistics that suicidal behaviors are of paramount concern to all school personnel and a significant public health issue (Miller et al., 2009).

Risk Associations

Although there are many commonalities among youth who have attempted suicide or died by suicide, it is important to note that nothing has been or can be conclusively deemed to be a "cause" (DiCara, O'Halloran, Williams, & Brooks, 2009). Epidemiologically, Caucasian males are the most common group to die by suicide (Cash &

Bridge, 2009; Gould & Kramer, 2001; Miller & Eckert, 2009). This, however, does not justify the conclusion that all Caucasian males should be considered at high risk of suicide. This difference between correlation (or association) and causality is of critical importance when assessing the various factors mentioned in this chapter. Particularly, that correlation does not equal causation when trying to apply the data shared in this chapter, and that issues as complicated as suicide in youths are often the result of an amalgamation of many causes and stresses built up over extended periods of time (DiCara et al., 2009). It is the goal of this part of the chapter to share a collection of the most highly statistically correlated factors that have been associated with youth suicide, so as to educate teachers and administrators in their prevalence and appearance.

A quickly emerging area of research in youth suicide is that of the effects of its increased coverage by media, with theories of a possible media-contagion effect being hypothesized. A summation of the many variants of this is explained by Cutler et al. (2000) as the following: "Exposure to suicide in the community or social setting may serve as a 'multiplier' to amplify the effects of stressors leading to, through a variety of means, an end result of suicide" (p. 233; see also Nepon, Fotti, Katz, Sareen, & Swampy Cree Suicide Prevention Team, 2009). There have been a number of studies that argue that social contagion serves as a strong factor among all age groups, and even more so for children and adolescents, who are more susceptible to imitating other suicidal youth (Wyman et al., 2010). In 2014, Gould, Kleinman, Lake, Forman, and Midle conducted a study of the correlation between newspaper coverage of suicide and suicide clusters in American teenagers and found what they believe to be an empirical basis to support this hypothesis. Alternatively, there are those in media and other areas who argue that the news is merely better reporting a traditionally underreported occurrence and has no effect on the fluctuation of the actual rates of suicide. It is the opinion of these authors that the most reasonable theory lies between both sides of the debate. While data seem to support youth suicide contagion in public or group settings (e.g., speaking about suicide in education classes, reporting details of suicides in mass media formats), there is no observable increase in likelihood of suicide attempt or completion when talking to an already-suicidal youth on an individual basis (i.e., asking a suicidal youth about the nature of his or her suicidality does not increase his or her risk). In other words, while talking about suicide with a group of youth who may or may not be feeling suicidal is not recommended, it is highly unlikely that speaking individually to a youth who is already feeling suicidal will have any negative effects (DiCara et al., 2009). According to the World Health Organization (2000), it is unwise to teach young people about suicide explicitly; rather, it is better to replace the issues of suicide with positive topics related to stronger mental health. The issue of suicidal contagion in youth, and how large of a "multiplier" it can serve as, has been brought into renewed focus, particularly with the advent of social media and the journalistic coverage of school shootings, bullying-related suicide, and other such tragedies, and it has the potential to help our understanding of youth suicide in the future.

Possibly the strongest correlation to be found in studying youth suicide is that of previous suicide attempts (Alexandria City Public Schools, 2013; Canadian Mental Health Association, 2012; DiCara et al., 2009; WHO, 2000). The correlation is so high, in fact, that boys who have previously attempted suicide are believed to be 30 times more likely to die by suicide, and girls 3 times more likely (Shaffer et al., 1996). Youth who have died by suicide have been noted to experience more interpersonal life events than others, with the number of these events in many cases being highest in the weeks before the date of death (Cooper, Appleby, & Amos, 2002). High correlations have also been made with having difficulty in school, not attending school, and not working; however, further research is needed to control for possible concurrent factors, such as mental health and whether poor attendance and/or performance in school could be the result of a more complex issue rather than the school issue itself (Gould et al., 2003).

In addition to the increased previous suicide attempts by youth, their family life and family psychiatric history seem to offer many significant correlations (American Foundation for Suicide Prevention, 2009; DiCara et al., 2009; WHO, 2000). The greatest risk factor relating to the family is that of a history of suicide among relatives, which is believed to substantially increase a child's or adolescent's risk of dying by suicide (Agerbo, Nordentoft, & Mortensen, 2002; Alexandria City Public Schools, 2013). Adjusting for parental psychiatric history, the Danish Registry study found youth suicide to be twice as common in the children of fathers who died by suicide and five times as common in the children of mothers who died by suicide as in children without a history of parental suicide (Gould et al., 2003). Although it is not fully understood whether this pattern is a result of the psychologically damaging effects of losing a parent by suicide or a heritable psychiatric illness or heritable vulnerability to suicide, current data seem to indicate the latter. In the Missouri Adolescent Twin Study, conducted by Heath et al. (2002), 3,416 female twins were picked, with 130 pairs of them having been exposed to and affected by suicide. The study found odds ratios of 5.6 and 4.0 for monozygotic and dizygotic twins, respectively, which indicates a potential degree of suicidality inheritance. McGuffin, Marušic, and Farmer (2001) reported further support for this in their finding that first-degree relatives of someone who has died by suicide are more than twice as likely to themselves die similarly, with said risk increasing to about 11 times if the relatives are co-twins. Through estimation from this meta-analysis, McGuffin et al. (2001) found heritability for dying by suicide of about 43%.

Another factor believed to increase the risk of suicide in youth is that of parental divorce (Gould et al., 2003). While a correlation between youth suicide and families affected by divorce can be made, the correlation is heavily attenuated once parental psychopathology is taken into account (Gould et al., 2003). Fergusson, Boden, and Horwood (2007) argue that even though, after the age of 16, living in a single-parent household for an increasing duration results in higher rates of anxiety, there is no significant association with suicidal ideation or attempt. Factoring in psychopathology also appears to inhibit the association between challenged parent–child relationships and death by suicide (Gould et al., 2003). Thus, it is not clear if family relational stresses like divorce, poor relationships, or strained communication between child and parent are drivers in youth suicide or rather a by-product of mental disorders in parents and/or youth. The correlation does, however, remain that youth who have died by suicide are more often noted to have much less satisfying communication with their parents (Gould et al., 2001). Unlike family relationships, other stressful life events are correlated with both suicide and suicide attempts (Gould et al., 2003). These events include interpersonal loss (e.g., breaking up with partner, death of partner or family member) or disciplinary or legal problems, and they vary in prevalence depending on age (Lahti, Rasanen, Riala, Keranen, & Hakko, 2011).

Another significant correlation of note in both suicide and attempted suicide is abuse, which can be separated into physical and sexual abuse (American Foundation for Suicide Prevention, 2009; Canadian Mental Health Association, 2012). Studies investigating the extent of suicidality in youth who have been sexually abused are difficult to interpret, as increased risk of suicide may be accounted for by other concurrent factors. The correlation, however, does remain, which suggests that sexual abuse as a youth and traumatic recall of the events later on is at least partly responsible for increased suicidality (Gould et al., 2003). Furthermore, it has been found that those exposed to sexual abuse as youth have poorer mental health than those exposed only to physical abuse (Cash & Bridge, 2009). Conversely, unlike sexual abuse, even after controlling for other potentially confounding factors (e.g., psychiatric disorders, demographics), physical abuse remains highly correlated with youth suicidality. Some studies assert that in the mid-puberty age range, frequent arguments with others coupled with a lack of close friendships could be responsible for more suicide attempts and death by suicide, as these are frequent correlates of physical abuse and many account for the association to physical abuse. This is qualified by Johnson et al. (2002), who hypothesized that children who had been physically abused could have difficulty developing the necessary social skills to maintain healthy relationships, thus causing the aforementioned situation and increased suicidality.

Sexual orientation of youth is also linked to suicide and attempted suicide, with youth who self-identify as homosexual or ambivalent about their sexuality at greater risk than heterosexual youth (Canadian Mental Health Association, 2012; Cash & Bridge, 2009; DiCara et al., 2009). After controlling for factors such as family history, depression, and alcohol abuse, this correlation remains; however, it is heavily attenuated when psychiatric disorders are taken into account (Cash & Bridge, 2009; Gould et al., 2003).

Psychopathology seems to play a role, not only in the case of sexual orientation but in all risk factors for suicide, if not as the underlying cause, then as a significant comorbid stressor (American Foundation for Suicide Prevention, 2009; Cash & Bridge, 2009; DiCara et al., 2009; New Zealand Ministry of Education, 2013). In 2006, Mazza hypothesized that suicide does not occur in isolation but as the byproduct of mental health problems. It is believed that of all risk factors identified for suicide attempts and youth suicide, psychopathology is the most reliable and robust, with at least 90% of youth who have died by suicide having suffered from at a minimum one mental disorder at time of death (Miller & Eckert, 2009). Furthermore, most youth suicides are marked by multiple comorbid psychiatric disorders and/or psychological problems (Miller & Taylor, 2005). It is also important to note that psychiatric disorders experienced by youth who die by suicide are very similar to those who attempt it (Gould et al., 2003). The most common psychiatric conditions present in suicidal youth are anxiety (including panic disorder and post-traumatic stress disorder), mood, conduct, and substance abuse disorders (American Foundation for Suicide Prevention, 2009; Cash & Bridge, 2009; Social Planning & Research Council of Hamilton, 2012). As well, a diagnosis of depression is correlated with up to 60% of youth who die by suicide and up to 80% of youth suicide attempts (Cash & Bridge, 2009). Depression is also considered the leading predictor of suicidal ideation; up to 85% of people with a diagnosis of depression will have suicidal ideation. Of this percentage, 2.5%–7% will eventually die by suicide (Cash & Bridge, 2009). Substance abuse (alcohol and/or drugs) is also substantially correlated with suicide in youth, most notably in older adolescent males (Cash & Bridge, 2009; Clore et al., 2003; New Zealand Ministry of Education, 2013). It is also of interest that substance abuse and dependence are more closely associated with attempted suicide than with suicidal ideation (Gould et al., 2003). Studies have found that youth who participated in heavy episodic drinking (i.e., binge drinking) when younger than age 13 years were 2.6 times more likely to attempt suicide than those who did not binge drink, and that drinking when feeling sad or down tripled the rate of self-reported suicide attempts (Cash & Bridge, 2009). Other psychiatric disorders linked to suicide and suicide attempts in youth include schizophrenia, borderline personality disorder, bipolar disorder, and adjustment disorder (Gould et al., 2003). Varying rates of suicidal behaviors have been found for each of these disorders, though studies on some of these behaviors, bipolar disorder in particular, have been inconclusive. While some investigations into suicide in bipolar youths have shown high rates of occurrence, others have shown few or none (Gould et al., 2003). Schizophrenia generally serves as a high risk for suicide in youth; however, comparatively it contributes to a very low number of total youth suicides (Gould et al., 2003; Shaffer et al., 1996). There is also some evidence to support the theory that panic attacks may increase risk of suicide in the general population, but further research specifically into prevalence in youth is needed (Gould et al., 2003; Rappaport, Moskowitz, Galynker, & Yaseen, 2014).

Often paired with psychopathology when trying to understand the motives of suicide in youth are biological risk factors believed to have their own role. The most notable and well researched of these biological factors is that of a deficit in serotonin functioning in people who are suicidal as well as impulsive and aggressive (American Foundation for Suicide Prevention, 2009; Miller & Eckert, 2009). This trend was noted across all populations, regardless of any psychiatric diagnoses, and it is best explained by Mann (1999), who proposes a stress–diathesis model in which those who are mentally ill and suffer from decreased serotonin functioning are more likely to respond to stress or traumatic experiences with impulsivity, including attempting and dying by suicide (Gould et al., 2003; Portzky, Audenaert, & van Heeringen, 2009). A family of antidepressant drugs (selective serotonin reuptake inhibitors, SSRIs) act by inhibiting the neuronal uptake of serotonin, thus correcting the decrease in serotonin function noted earlier, and they therefore may be beneficial in the prevention of suicide. Research on the effects of decreased serotonin uptake has led to significant controversy in the administration of antidepressants to youth (Miller & Eckert, 2009). The concern of increased suicidality from antidepressant use was furthered in 2004 when the U.S. Food and Drug Administration issued a warning regarding the use of antidepressants in youth, which resulted in significant decreases in prescription rates for the drugs in children and adolescents (Katz et al., 2008). While some, including Bostwick (2006), have hypothesized that the risk of suicidality with antidepressant use is not clear, the concern gave rise to a new risk (Miller & Eckert, 2009). With so much controversy surrounding antidepressants, decreased prescriptions of them may be responsible for an increase in youth suicide, as these children and adolescents are not getting the medication that they may need (Katz et al., 2008; Lu et al., 2014; Miller & Eckert, 2009).

PROTECTIVE FACTORS

Although there are many factors that are believed to increase a youth's risk for attempting and dying by suicide, there are also some, albeit fewer, that are believed to counteract suicidality in youth. These are known as "protective" factors, the two chief ones being religiosity and family cohesion (DiCara et al., 2009; Gould et al., 2003). There has been significantly less research done on protective factors and their effect on preventing or counteracting suicidality than on risk factors, and more studies must be undertaken before we can properly understand just how, and even if, these factors truly alleviate the various risks aforementioned (Gould et al., 2003). Religiosity has been a focus of examination for years, and it has often been ascribed as the main reason behind the historically lower rates of suicide in African Americans than in Caucasians (Gould et al., 2003). It was relatively recently, however, that religious protective factors were first applied specifically to youth, and many of the studies that have been conducted have not taken enough care to adequately control for potential cofounders (most notably substance abuse) (Gould et al., 2003). Unlike religiosity, however, family cohesion has been better studied, with more quantifiable links having been made between it and its protective benefits (Canadian Mental Health Association, 2012). Both longitudinal and cross-sectional community studies in students ranging from middle school to college found that those who self-reported strong emotional support, shared interests, and high degree of mutual involvement in their family life were 3.5–5.5 times less likely to be suicidal than youth with the same levels of depression or stress but less cohesive families (Blum, McNeely, & Rinehart, 2002; Gould et al., 2003). Other protective factors include having a sense of personal control, plans and hope for the future, strong anger management, conflict resolution, as well as problem-solving and decision-making abilities (DiCara et al., 2009).

ROLE OF TEACHERS AND ADMINISTRATORS

Youth suicide is influenced, as aforementioned, by a variety of factors that stem from both the individual and the environment the youth are in (Young, Sweeting, & Ellaway, 2011). Schools, where youth spend an average 33% of their day, can have a strong effect on the lives of students (King, 2001; Young et al., 2011). Thus, the school faculty and staff have a near unprecedented level of interaction with youth and can develop strong relationships with them, and by doing so, they create an opportunity to monitor students and intervene when necessary (Domitrovich et al., 2008; Johnson & Parsons, 2012; King, 2001; Whitney, Renner, Pate, & Jacobs, 2011). In this way teachers, administrators, and other faculty members serve as gatekeepers in their school community, uniquely positioned to recognize suicidal risk factors and suicidal behaviors and facilitate access to the care and support necessary for the well-being of the students (American Foundation for Suicide Prevention, 2009; Johnson & Parsons, 2012; Nadeem et al., 2011; Tompkins, Witt, & Abraibesh, 2010). The rationale behind the importance of gatekeepers is that because people who are suicidal do not usually seek help independently, and because youth are often particularly hesitant to approach adults, people in the community must be able to recognize warning signs and take action so as to prevent harm to those at risk (Reis & Cornell, 2008). In this role teachers and other school personnel are critical (American Foundation for Suicide Prevention, 2009; Reis & Cornell, 2008).

While each school, school board, and jurisdiction has independent expectations and policies of their teaching staff on how they should act and behave when dealing with suicidal or believed-to-be-suicidal youth, there are a collection of actions that could be universally understood. The most important action a teacher can take, as alluded to in the earlier discussion of teachers' role as gatekeepers, is to notify a qualified professional (e.g., school nurse, counselor, psychologist, social worker) when suspicion arises that a student has contemplated or attempted suicide (Alexandria City Public Schools, 2013; American Foundation for Suicide Prevention, 2009; Nova Scotia Education, 2012; WHO, 2000). Of utmost importance is that each and every threat or indication of self-harm or suicide is taken seriously and investigation is followed through (DiCara et al., 2009; Toronto

Catholic District School Board, 2013). Some examples of indicators in the classroom that could be a sign of suicidal ideation include (but are not limited to) sudden drop in grades, lack of completion of assignments, depressive themes or fixation with suicide in writing or creative outlets, social isolation, and complaints of malaise or illness causing absence (Alexandria City Public Schools, 2013; American Foundation for Suicide Prevention, 2009; New Zealand Ministry of Education, 2013; WHO, 2000; Wolfe, 2004). It is important to note also that it is not necessary for there to be a corresponding action with ideation; probability of a student thinking about suicide is enough to warrant relaying that information to a qualified professional (Alexandria City Public Schools, 2013). It is the responsibility of the professional to then take further action, usually involving an informal interview to estimate suicide risk, consultation with other professionals to verify estimated risk, notification of the school administrator(s), and contacting of the parent(s) or caregiver(s) of the student, unless the situation warrants complete confidentiality (as in cases of domestic abuse or neglect) (Alexandria City Public Schools, 2013; DiCara et al., 2009; Toronto Catholic District School Board, 2013). When teachers become aware of an imminent suicide attempt or a student who has just attempted suicide, either by verification from the student or by a secondary source, the teacher takes on the additional function of crisis management (Main Youth Suicide Prevention Program, 2004; Toronto Catholic District School Board, 2013). School administrators must still be immediately notified; however, in these cases it is of paramount importance to remain with the student until adequate support has arrived (Alexandria City Public Schools, 2013; DiCara et al., 2009). Until help arrives, the priority is to calm the student down, attempt to engage him or her in conversation, and if necessary mediate and calm the environment by evacuating bystanders (Alexandria City Public Schools, 2013). Under no circumstances should the student be left unsupervised or sent home alone (DiCara et al., 2009; Social Planning & Research Council of Hamilton, 2012; Toronto Catholic District School Board, 2013). When speaking with the student in crisis, it is important not to act shocked, patronizing, embarrassed, sententious, dismissive, or challenging (DiCara et al., 2009; Social Planning & Research Council of Hamilton, 2012). It is also important that the teacher not promise to keep anything shared a secret, as breaching trust later could be damaging to the youth, but passing the information shared to qualified professionals will be necessary (DiCara et al., 2009).

In their classrooms teachers can take certain preventative measures aimed at improving the mental health of students so as to try to proactively prevent suicidal ideation. These include strengthening students' self-esteem, promoting emotional expression, preventing bullying and violence, and allowing for trustful, confidential communication (Blum et al., 2002; WHO, 2000).

The role of a school administrator parallels that of teachers and extends further, as administrators not only serve as gatekeepers but also must implement policies and programs to best serve and protect their students (New Zealand Ministry of Education, 2013). It is the role of the administrator to create the two protocols essential for proper suicide risk management: protocols for helping students at risk of suicide and protocols for responding to a death by suicide (Center for Mental Health Services, 2012). It is also the role of the school administrator to implement programs aimed at preventing suicide and limiting the potential ramifications of suicidal ideation in students.

One such method that has been implemented is a suicide awareness curriculum, aimed to educate students about suicide (Doan, Roggenbaum, Lazear, & LeBlanc, 2012; Gould et al., 2003; Whitney et al., 2011). While the curriculums may vary, they tend to focus most on warning signs and risk factors for suicide, statistics, and community resources available to students who feel they need them (Doan et al., 2012). The rationale behind suicide awareness curriculums is that by educating youths they become more comfortable with expressing when they have had suicidal thoughts and may be able to better identify other at-risk youths and refer them to the appropriate adults (Doan et al., 2012; Katz et al., 2013). The additional benefit of training youth in recognizing suicidality is that youth are more likely to approach other youth when feeling suicidal as opposed to seeking help from an adult (Doan et al., 2012; Gould et al., 2003; Katz et al., 2013). Although many studies have found positive results with the use of this method, there is, however, some hesitation in using a curriculum approach to curb suicide, as some suggest that further research is needed to fine-tune the approach before its safety can be conclusively proved (Gould et al., 2003; Katz et al., 2013). Findings have been mixed on the efficacy of modifying curriculums: Some studies have found that some students who had previously attempted suicide, when exposed to the curriculum, became unsettled and potentially slipped back into a suicidal state (Doan et al., 2012; Gould et al., 2003; Katz et al., 2013). Furthermore, boys were noted to exhibit increased hopelessness and dysfunctional coping mechanisms after being exposed to the curriculum, and youth of both sexes were sometimes noted to be less likely to recommend seeking help to a friend who expressed suicidal ideation (possibly because of the increased confidence in their own abilities to aid them) (Doan et al., 2012; Gould et al., 2003; Katz et al., 2013). Another significant risk of suicide curriculum programs is that they may offer youth examples of how to die by suicide and incite imagination; they inadvertently present the idea of suicide as a solution to stresses to youth who may not have considered it before (Gould et al., 2003).

Contrary to the focus on suicide in curriculum programs, skills training offers an alternate approach to the issue that focuses instead on teaching life skills such as coping, problem solving, cognitive skills, and decision making (Gould et al., 2003; Katz et al., 2013). The underlying belief of skills training is that, by targeting the risk factors behind suicide and teaching youth ways to better deal with stress and adversity, suicidal behavior can be stopped before it manifests (Katz et al., 2013). Many skills-training programs exist for a variety of age groups and cultural subpopulations. Some of the best developed of these programs include CARE (Care, Assess, Respond, Empower), CAST (Coping and Support Training), AILSD (American Indian Life Skills Development), and GBG (the Good Behavior Game) (Hooven, Herting, & Snedker, 2010; Katz et al., 2013). A study on the effectiveness of the Good Behavior Game was conducted with first-graders over a two-year period. Teams were made in the classrooms—all with equal boys and girls, as well as shy, aggressive, and disruptive children—and a set of rules for the games was made, along with a clear time window for when the game was active (usually during less structured periods of activity throughout the day) (Kellam et al., 2012). If any team made four or fewer infractions during these periods, they were rewarded (Kellam et al., 2012). Through these games aggressive and disruptive behaviors were targeted, and it was found that when the students who partook in these activities were studied again later as young adults, there was a present, though slight, correlation with reduced drug abuse, dependence, and dangerous sexual behaviors (Kellam et al., 2012). First- and second-grade participants in the Good Behavior Game were also shown to have reduced impulse-control problems and antisocial personality disorder, all of these positive correlations resulting in reduced suicide risk factors (Katz et al., 2013). Unlike many of the other programs, skills-training approaches such as the Good Behavior Game have not been associated with any significant negative results as of yet (Gould et al., 2003). Further investigation is, however, still needed, as it is unclear what in the training actually has a positive effect on youth versus a neutral effect or noneffect (Gould et al., 2003). Increased refinement of these programs would be beneficial for schools, as it would alleviate the stress on resources, both human and financial, and yield the same benefits in decreasing suicidality.

Another type of training employed in schools is peer leadership, aimed at reducing suicide in youth through the propagation of positive socioecological interactions in the community (Wyman et al., 2010). Sources of Strength is one such program, the first of its kind, which aims to identify youth leaders in various cliques and social circles and then train them in what is normal versus abnormal behavior (when dealing with stress, adversity, or other crises) (Katz et al., 2013; Wyman et al., 2010). These leaders are also taught to promote communication with trusted adults to friends who may be feeling suicidal and are educated on various coping resources (Wyman et al. 2010). It has been demonstrated that youth are more likely to talk to other youth than adults when feeling suicidal, a fact that is fundamental to the success of Sources of Strength as the hope is that through these methods suicidal youths will be connected with appropriate adults via the selected peer leaders, thereby helping them to combat their suicidality and avoiding possible suicide contagion to lower-risk youth in the same cliques (Katz et al., 2013; Wyman et al., 2010). This program is still very new, and at present has been evaluated only by one study, a randomized control trial, conducted by Wyman et al. in 2010. The study found that trained youth leaders showed improvement in their connectedness to adults, school engagement, and adaptive norms, and among other students in school showed a more positive view of adult support when dealing with suicidal thoughts or ideation (Katz et al., 2013; Wyman et al., 2010). This study did not, however, show whether or not Sources of Strength was effective in lowering the occurrence of suicide ideation or attempts, an area where further research must be conducted if the program is to be implemented as an effective method to curb suicidality in youth. There is currently a study under way to help identify these factors; however, at this time no data from that study are available (Katz et al., 2013).

Another method that has been investigated as a viable means of preventing suicide is that of screening, a method involving sourcing out potentially suicidal youth through often multistage assessments and recommending further treatment to help them (Gould et al., 2003; Katz et al., 2013). Screening can be done on any sample of the school or the student population in its entirety, and it searches for common suicide risk factors such as substance abuse, previous suicide attempts, recent suicidal ideation, and depression (Gould et al., 2003; Katz et al., 2013). It is, however, vital that there are adequate referral options ready for the youth who screen positively for suicidality before commencement of the screening process (Katz et al., 2013). The screening process is in actuality only the first step in treatment, as it merely identifies those who are at risk. It does not treat those youth who screen positive, and thus significant effort and resources must be allocated to the treatment programs that must follow (Gould et al.,

2003). While this method offers promising results, it is not without faults. One of the main problems with screening is the issue of false results, mostly false-positives (while false-negatives do occur, they are much less common) (Gould et al., 2003; Katz et al., 2013). It is difficult to modify the screening process to account for false-positives, as doing so increases the risk of missing a genuinely suicidal individual (Gould et al., 2003). The only viable means of accounting for false-positives seems to be employing an additional round of clinical tests on all those who report positively to try to filter out the false results. As well, false-negatives can be accounted for by multiple rounds of screening over extended periods of time, so as to account for variation in suicide risk (Gould et al., 2003). Although there was some concern of potential iatrogenic effects from screening programs in schools, studies like Gould et al.'s (2005) randomized controlled trial have not shown evidence to suggest that such concern is warranted.

The program that is perhaps most naturally able to be implemented in the school setting is gatekeeper training, which many principals and school psychologists view as significantly more acceptable than alternative programs (Eckert, Miller, DuPaul, & Riley-Tillman, 2003; Gould et al., 2003; Nadeem et al., 2011). The most common of these gatekeeper programs in school settings is the Question, Persuade, Refer (QPR) program (Katz et al., 2013; Tompkins et al., 2010). As previously mentioned, teachers and administrators already serve as natural gatekeepers in schools. This fact, coupled with the belief that suicidal youths are under-identified, creates a natural area of improvement, as training of adults about suicide and its risk factors could allow for increased identification of at-risk youth (Gould et al., 2003; Katz et al., 2013). A study conducted by King, Price, Telljohann, and Wahl (1999) found that only 9% of high school teachers in a sample population identified themselves as comfortable in recognizing an at-risk student. While, like screening programs, the ultimate effectiveness of QPR gatekeeper training depends on the services that the at-risk youth receive, studies into the benefits of this training tend to show a more positive attitude and increased knowledge toward suicide by teachers (Katz et al., 2013; Stuart, Waalen, & Haelstromm, 2003; Tompkins et al., 2010). Studies do not, however, show an increased level of comfort with approaching students believed to be at risk, except by those staff who normally approach youth to offer help, nor do they show improvement in subsequent mental health service use (Katz et al., 2013; Tompkins et al., 2010; Wyman et al., 2010). Perhaps the biggest benefit of using the gatekeeper program is the relatively small change that must be made to the school to implement it. While screening requires extensive input of resources to properly coordinate and facilitate the measurement and assessment, and skills training and curriculum changes require modification of teaching curriculums and flexibility in scheduling to account for such, gatekeepers utilize an already-integral part of the school system, the staff, and train them to better observe their students while maintaining their usual roles in the school setting. Using gatekeeper training, youth are effectively being monitored for suicidality any time a faculty member is with them, and this constant monitoring may serve as a means of catching suicidal ideation before it escalates to attempted suicide or death by suicide of a troubled student.

CONCLUSION

To date, no school-based suicide prevention approach has been found to reduce death by suicide. With the growing issue of youth suicide has come a consolidated effort to identify and execute ways to limit and reverse this problem. The programs, measures, risk factors, and protective factors mentioned in this chapter offer a summary of some of the ways that have been tested thus far; however, our current level of success in dealing with youth suicide is insufficient. Suicide is a problem affecting youth across the board (Social Planning & Research Council of Hamilton, 2012). All ethnicities, ages, genders, and social classes face this issue (Mott, 2011). While some of the studies and programs aforementioned are promising, much more research is needed before their efficacy can be truly understood. Part of the issue perhaps lies in the nature of suicide, a large, multidimensional aggregation of stressors that culminates in the ending of one's own life. Suicide cannot be treated as a single cause–effect issue, nor can proposed solutions be a single program or effort (White & Morris, 2010). It is unlikely that youth who are suicidal are that way due to only a problem at school, or only at home. It is more likely that the problem is a result of a combination of stressors in various aspects of the youth's life. Thus to curb suicide greater understanding of the complete life of suicidal youth must be obtained so that multiple programs offering a holistic approach to dealing with the issue can be implemented (White & Morris, 2010). A more integrated understanding of the various risk factors and their compounding effects on one another would serve as an invaluable tool in combating youth suicide. Ways to do this include having more studies that focus specifically on youth and using larger sample populations. Designing longer studies would also aid in our understanding of suicide, which could offer new awareness into potential issues or successes otherwise unknown in shorter trials.

Further insight may also come with greater understanding of the biology of suicide. Knowledge of the physiological mechanisms involved in causing suicidal ideation may allow us the ability to investigate predispositions to suicide and how to best deal with those predispositions before they result in full suicidality, thus stopping a potentially fatal problem in its infancy on a case-by-case basis. Greater research into protective factors, perhaps the least documented aspect of suicide to date, could also offer new areas of research in the future. Solidifying our understanding of the effects of protective factors would offer us a direction for future research and program implementation, as new programs aimed at combating youth suicide could incorporate these factors, presumably resulting in greater preventative success.

At present, however, teachers and administrators in our schools have nearly unprecedented insight into the lives and minds of young students, and with that insight comes the opportunity to recognize the risk factors for suicide that we do know about and facilitate proper treatment more quickly and effectively than might be otherwise achieved, in doing so saving the lives of youth and, hopefully, helping to turn the tables on this epidemic. It is the goal of this chapter to educate teachers and administrators on suicide, its risk factors, protective factors, epidemiology, and preventative programs, with the hope that increased awareness and understanding of this problem may help reverse the trends of suicidality in our youth.

REFERENCES

Agerbo, E., Nordentoft, M., & Mortensen, P. B. (2002). Familial, psychiatric, and socioeconomic risk factors for suicide in young people: Nested case-control study. *British Medical Journal, 325*, 74.

Alexandria City Public Schools. (2013). *Suicide prevention/intervention guidelines.* Alexandria, VA: Author.

American Foundation for Suicide Prevention. (2009). *More than sad (Suicide prevention education for teachers and other school personnel).* New York, NY: Author.

Berman, A. L., Jobes, D. A., & Silverman, M. M. (2006). *Adolescent suicide: Assessment and intervention.* Washington, DC: American Psychological Association.

Blum, R. W., McNeely, C. A., & Rinehart, P. M. (2002). *Improving the odds: The untapped power of schools to improve the health of teens.* Minneapolis, MN: Center for Adolescent Health and Development, University of Minnesota.

Bostwick, J. M. (2006). Do SSRIs cause suicide in children? The evidence is underwhelming. *Journal of Clinical Psychology, 62*(2), 235–241.

Canadian Mental Health Association. (2012). *Teen suicide resource toolkit.* Author.

Cash, S. J., & Bridge, J. A. (2009). Epidemiology of youth suicide and suicidal behavior. *National Institutes of Health, 21*(5), 613–619. http://dx.doi.org/10.1097/MOP.0b013e32833063e1

Center for Mental Health Services, Substance Abuse and Mental Health Services Administration. (2012). *Preventing suicide: A toolkit for high schools.* Rockville, MD: Author.

Centers for Disease Control and Prevention. (2012). *Suicide datasheet.* Washington, DC: Author.

Centers for Disease Control and Prevention. (2014, January 2). *Trends in suicide rates among persons ages 10 years and older, by sex, United States, 1991–2009.* Retrieved from http://www.cdc.gov/violenceprevention/suicide/statistics/trends01.html

Clore, J., Galloway, A., Miles, S., Swan, M., Coleman, S., Haskins, C., & Zarris, B. J. (2003). *Suicide prevention guidelines §22.1–272.1 Code of Virginia.* Richmond, VA: Board of Education, Commonwealth of Virginia, Richmond.

Cooper, J., Appleby, L., & Amos, T. (2002). Life events preceding suicide by young people. *Social Psychiatry Psychiatric Epidemiology, 37,* 271–275.

Crosby, A. E., Han, B., Ortega, L. A. G., Parks, S. E., & Gfroerer, J. (2011). Suicidal thoughts and behaviors among adults aged ≥18 years: United States, 2008–2009. *Centers for Disease Control and Prevention Morbidity and Mortality Weekly Report, 60*(13), 1–28.

Cutler, D. M., Glaeser, E. L., & Norberg, K. E. (2000). Explaining the rise in youth suicide. In *Risky behavior among youths: An economic analysis* (pp. 1–68). Chicago, IL: University of Chicago Press.

DiCara, C., O'Halloran, S., Williams, L., & Brooks, C. C. (2009). *Youth suicide prevention, intervention & postvention guidelines: A resource for school personnel* (4th ed.). Augusta, ME: Maine Youth Suicide Prevention Program.

Doan, J., Roggenbaum, S., Lazear, K. J., & LeBlanc, A. (2012). *Risk factors: How can a school identify a student at risk for suicide* (Research Report No. 3b). Tampa, FL: University of South Florida College of Behavioral & Community Sciences.

Domitrovich, C. E., Bradshaw, C. P., Poduska, J. M., Hoagwood, K., Buckley, J. A., Olin, S., & Ialongo, N. S. (2008). Maximizing the implementation quality of evidence-based preventative interventions in schools: A conceptual framework. *Advances in School Mental Health Promotion, 1*(3), 6–28. http://dx.doi.org/10.1080/1754730X.2008.9715730

Eckert, T. L., Miller, D. N., DuPaul, G. J., & Riley-Tillman, T. C. (2003). Adolescent suicide prevention: School psychologists' acceptability of school-based programs. *School Psychology Review, 32*(1), 57–76.

Fergusson, D. M., Boden, J. M., & Horwood, L. J. (2007). Recurrence of major depression in adolescence and early adulthood, and later mental health, educational and economic outcomes. *British Journal of Psychiatry, 191,* 335–342.

Gould, M. S., Greenberg, T., Velting, D. M., & Shaffer, D. (2003). Youth suicide risk and preventive interventions: A review of the past 10 years. *Journal of the American Academy of Child and Adolescent Psychiatry, 42*(4), 386–405. http://dx.doi.org/10.1097/01.CHI.0000046821.95464.CF

Gould, M. S., Kleinman, M. H., Lake, A. M., Forman, J., & Midle, J. B. (2014). Newspaper coverage of suicide and initiation of suicide clusters in teenagers in the USA, 1988–96: A retrospective, population-based, case-control study. *Lancet Psychiatry, 1*, 34–43. http://dx.doi.org/10.1016/

Gould, M. S., & Kramer, R. A. (2001). Youth suicide prevention. *Suicide and Life-Threatening Behavior, 31*, 6–31.

Gould, M. S., Marrocco, F. A., Kleinman, M., Thomas, J. G., Mostkoff, K., Cote, J., & Davies, M. (2005). Evaluating iatrogenic risk of youth suicide screening programs. *Journal of the American Medical Association, 293*(13), 1635–1643.

Gutierrez, P. M., & Osman, A. (2008). *Adolescent suicide: An integrated approach to the assessment of risk and protective factors.* DeKalb, IL: Northern Illinois University Press.

Heath, A. C., Howells, W., Bucholz, K. K., Glowinski, A. L., Nelson, E. C., & Madden, P. A. (2002). Ascertainment of a mid-western US female adolescent twin cohort for alcohol studies: Assessment of sample representativeness using birth record data. *Twin Research and Human Genetics, 5*, 107–112.

Hooven, C., Herting, J. R., & Snedker, K. A. (2010). Long-term outcomes for the promoting CARE suicide prevention program. *American Journal of Health Behavior, 34*(6), 721–736.

Johnson, J. G., Cohen, P., Gould, M. S., Kasen, S., Brown, J., & Brook, J. S. (2002). Childhood adversities, interpersonal difficulties, and risk for suicide attempts during late adolescence and early adulthood. *Archives of General Psychiatry, 59*, 741–749.

Johnson, L. A., & Parsons, M. E. (2012). Adolescent suicide prevention in a school setting. *National Association of School Nurses*, 313–317.

Katz, C., Bolton, S.-L., Katz, L. Y., Isaak, C., Tilston-Jones, T., Sareen, J., & Swampy Cree Suicide Prevention Team. (2013). A systematic review of school-based suicide prevention programs. *Depression and Anxiety, 30*, 1030–1045. http://dx.doi.org/10.1002/da.22114

Katz, L. Y., Kozyrskyj, A. L., Prior, H. J., Enns, M. W., Cox, B. J., & Sareen, J. (2008). Effect of regulatory body warnings on antidepressant prescription rates, use of health services, and outcomes among children, adolescents and young adults. *Canadian Medical Association Journal, 178*(8), 1005–1011.

Kellam, S. G., Wang, W., Mackenzie, A. C. L., Brown, C. H., Ompad, D. C., Or, F., & Windham, A. (2012). The impact of the Good Behavior Game, a universal classroom-based preventive intervention in first and second grades, on high-risk sexual behaviors and drug abuse and dependence disorders into young adulthood. *Prevention Science, 15*(1), S6–S18. http://dx.doi.org/10.1007/s11121-012-0296-z

King, K. A. (2001). Developing a comprehensive school suicide prevention program. *Journal of School Health, 71*(4), 132–137.

King, K. A., Price, J. H., Telljohann, S. K., & Wahl, J. (1999). High school health teachers' perceived self-efficacy in identifying students at risk for suicide. *Journal of School Health, 69*(5), 202–207.

Lahti, A., Rasanen, P., Riala, K., Keranen, S., & Hakko, H. (2011). Youth suicide trends in Finland, 1969–2008. *Journal of Child Psychology and Psychiatry, 52*(9), 984–991. http://dx.doi.org/10.1111/j.1469-7610.2011.02369.x

Langhinrichsen-Rohling, J., Friend, J., & Powell, A. (2009). Adolescent suicide, gender, and culture: A rate and risk factor analysis. *Aggression and Violent Behavior, 14*, 402–414. http://dx.doi.org/10.1016/j.avb.2009.06.010

Lu, C. Y., Zhang, F., Lakoma, M. D., Madden, J. M., Rusinak, D., Penfold, R. B., . . . Soumerai, S. B. (2014). Changes in antidepressant use by young people and suicidal behavior after FDA warnings and media coverage: Quasi-experimental study. *British Medical Journal,* 348, 1–11. http://dx.doi.org/10.1136/bmj.g3596

Mann, J. J. (1999). Role of the serotonergic system in the pathogenesis of major depression and suicidal behavior. *Neuropsychopharmacology, 21*(2), S99–S105.

Mazza, J. J. (2006). Youth suicidal behavior: A crisis in need of attention. In F. A. Villarruel & T. Luster (Eds.), *The crisis in youth mental health: Critical issues and effective programs* (Vol. 2, pp. 155–177). Westport, CT: Praeger/Greenwood.

McGuffin, P., Marušic, A., & Farmer, A. (2001). What can psychiatric genetics offer suicidology? *Crisis: The Journal of Crisis Intervention and Suicide Prevention, 22*(2), 61–65. http://dx.doi.org/10.1027//0227-5910.22.2.61

Miller, D. N., & Eckert, T. L. (2009). Youth suicidal behavior: An introduction and overview. *School Psychology Review, 38*(2), 153–167.

Miller, D., Eckert, T. L., & Mazza, J. J. (2009). Suicide prevention programs in the schools: A review and public health perspective. *School Psychology Review, 38*(2), 168–188.

Miller, T. R., & Taylor, D. M. (2005). Adolescent suicidality: Who will ideate, who will act? *Suicide and Life-Threatening Behavior, 35*(4), 425–435.

Mott, J. (2011). Suicide assessment in the school setting. *National Association of School Nurses*, 103–108. http://dx.doi.org/10.1177/1942602X10397664

Nadeem, E., Kataoka, S. H., Chang, V. Y., Vona, P., Wong, M., & Stein, B. D. (2011). The role of teachers in school-based suicide prevention: A qualitative study of school staff perspectives. *School Mental Health, 3*, 209–221. http://dx.doi.org/10.1007/s12310-011-9056-7

Nepon, J., Fotti, S., Katz, L. Y., Sareen, J., & Swampy Cree Suicide Prevention Team. (2009). *Media guidelines for reporting suicide* (Canadian Psychiatric Association Policy Paper). Ottawa, ON: Canadian Psychiatric Association.

New Zealand Ministry of Education. (2013). *Preventing and responding to suicide: Resource kit for schools.* Auckland, New Zealand: Author.

Portzky, G., Audenaert, K., & van Heeringen, K. (2009). Psychosocial and psychiatric factors associated with adolescent suicide: A case control psychological autopsy study. *Journal of Adolescence, 32*, 849–862. http://dx.doi.org/10.1016/j.adolescence.2008.10.007

Rappaport, L. M., Moskowitz, D. S., Galynker, I., & Yaseen, Z. S. (2014). Panic symptom clusters differentially predict suicide ideation and attempt. *Comprehensive Psychiatry,* 55, 762–769. http://dx.doi.org/10.1016/j.comppsych.2013.10.017

Reis, C., & Cornell, D. (2008). An evaluation of suicide gatekeeper training for school counselors and teachers. *Professional School Counseling Journal, 11*(6), 386–394.

Shaffer, D., Gould, M. S., Fisher, P., Trautman, P., Moreau, D., Kleinman, M., & Flory, M. (1996). Psychiatric diagnosis in child and adolescent suicide. *Archives of General Psychiatry, 53*(4), 339–348.

Skinner, R., & McFaull, S. (2012). Suicide among children and adolescents in Canada: Trends and sex differences, 1980–2008. *Canadian Medical Association Journal, 184*(9), 1029–1034. http://dx.doi.org/10.1503/cmaj.111867

Social Planning & Research Council of Hamilton. (2012, September). *The role of high school teachers in preventing suicide.* Hamilton, ON: Author.

Stuart, C., Waalen, J. K., & Haelstromm, E. (2003). Many helping hearts: An evaluation of peer gatekeeper training in suicide risk assessment. *Death Studies, 27*(4), 321–333. http://dx.doi.org/10.1080/07481180302906

Szumilas, M., & Kutcher, S. P. (2008). Youth suicide prevention. *Canadian Medical Association Journal, 178*(3), 282–286.

Tompkins, T. L., Witt, J., & Abraibesh, N. (2010). Does a gatekeeper suicide prevention program work in a school setting? Evaluating training outcome and moderators of effectiveness. *Suicide and Life-Threatening Behavior, 40*(5), 506–515.

Toronto Catholic District School Board. (2013). *TCDSB suicide intervention guidelines.* Toronto, ON: Author.

Weber, W. (2000). EU calls for action to prevent youth suicide. *Lancet, 356,* 1092.

White, J., & Morris, J. (2010). Precarious spaces: Risk, responsibility and uncertainty in school-based suicide prevention programs. *Social Science and Medicine, 71,* 2187–2194.

Whitney, S. D., Renner, L. M., Pate, C. M., & Jacobs, K. A. (2011). Principals' perceptions of benefits and barriers to school-based suicide prevention programs. *Children and Youth Services Review, 33,* 869–877. http://dx.doi.org/10.1016/j.childyouth.2010.12.015

Wolfe, K. D. (2004). *What every teacher should know about preventing youth suicide.* [Brochure]. Seattle, WA: Washington State Youth Suicide Prevention Program.

World Health Organization, Department of Mental Health. (2000). *Preventing suicide: A resource for teachers and other school staff.* Geneva, Switzerland: Author.

Wyman, P. A., Brown, H., LoMurray, M., Schmeelk-Cone, K., Petrova, M., Walsh, E., . . . Wang, W. (2010). An outcome evaluation of the Sources of Strength suicide prevention program delivered by adolescent peer leaders in high schools. *American Journal of Public Health, 100*(9), 1653–1661. http://dx.doi.org/doi:10.2105/AJPH.2009.190025

Young, R., Sweeting, H., & Ellaway, A. (2011). Do schools differ in suicide risk? The influence of school and neighbourhood on attempted suicide, suicidal ideation and self-harm among secondary school pupils. *BioMedical Central, 11*(874), 1–15. Retrieved from http://www.biomedcentral.com/1471-2458/11/874

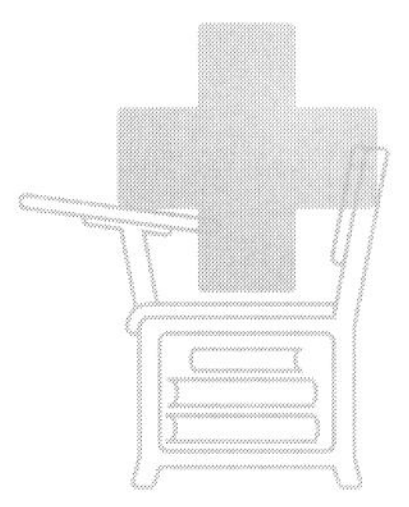

Chapter 22
Emotional and Behavioral Disorders in the Classroom

Regina M. Oliver, J. Ron Nelson,
and J. E. Gonzalez

Emotional disturbance (ED) as defined by the Individuals with Disabilities Education Act (IDEA) refers to various disorders in learning, interpersonal relationships, behaviors or feelings, moods, or physical symptoms or fears that persist over long periods of time, are of a marked degree, and adversely affect school performance. In 2006, 448,998 students age 6–21 in the United States were identified as ED and provided special education or related services in the public schools (U.S. Department of Education, 2012). Although this represents less than 1% of school-age children, epidemiological research suggests that the actual prevalence of ED may be much greater, ranging from 3% to 6% (Kauffman & Landrum, 2013). Disparities in the identification of ED also exist across states, with rates varying from 0.2% to more than 2% (U.S. Department of Education, 2012). Moreover, research on point prevalence (i.e., identified at any one point in time) versus cumulative prevalence (i.e., ever identified at some point in time) of ED suggests a point prevalence of 12% compared to cumulative prevalence estimates of 37%–39% (Forness, Freeman, Paparella, Kauffman, & Walker, 2012). Thus, it is not unreasonable to conclude that many children with ED remain underidentified, and thereby underserved, by schools (Kauffman & Landrum, 2013). Unfortunately, as the need for services for children with ED grows, the nation continues to fail in developing a cohesive and unified infrastructure to assist these children and their families. Too often, these children and families miss opportunities for early intervention and receive fragmented or low resource priority services (U.S. Department of Health and Human Services, 2000). In this chapter, we first ask who children are with ED. Second, we describe the status and scope of this population, a probable path to ED, and major underlying disorders. Third, we discuss federal eligibility criteria for inclusion into special education, along with screening procedures, assessment strategies, and sources of data. Finally, we conclude with some final thoughts.

WHO ARE CHILDREN WITH EMOTIONAL DISTURBANCE?

Children with ED are overwhelmingly white, male, behaviorally disruptive, noncompliant, verbally abusive, and aggressive. Because their behaviors are so disruptive and irritating, these children often arouse negative feelings in others, thus alienating schoolmates and adults, and ultimately robbing these children of the benefits of learning opportunities. Moreover, they often experience social rejection or alienation by peers, parents, and teachers (Quinn & Epstein, 1998). When these children do make friends, it does not take them long to alienate those friends, as they do not know how to foster, nurture, and maintain friendships. When they do obtain status among peers, it is usually among deviant groups who reinforce antisocial behavior. Finally, children with ED experience significant educational deficits across numerous academic domains (Reid, Gonzalez, Nordness, Trout, & Epstein, 2004).

STATUS AND SCOPE OF CHILDREN WITH ED

Data on identification, academic outcomes, graduation rates, absenteeism, employment status, and criminality among children with ED suggest that educating them is a complex, confusing, and often daunting task for educators, related service professionals, and family members alike (Smith & Coutinho, 1997). Perhaps the most disturbing finding is that it may take about five or more years before school personnel formally identify the need for special education services, despite the fact that a child's problems are noticed at a very early age (usually prior to age 4). To make matters worse, virtually no educational, mental health, or related services are provided between the time problems are first noticed and official identification (Forness et al., 2012; Wagner, Kutash, Duchnowski, Epstein, & Sumi, 2005).

Data from the *30th Annual Report to Congress on the Implementation of IDEA 2008* (U.S. Department of Education, 2012), the National Longitudinal Transition Study 2 and Special Education Elementary Longitudinal Study (Wagner et al., 2005), and other research (e.g., Landrum, Tankersley, & Kauffman, 2003) present a rather sobering and challenging picture of the status, scope, and outcomes for children with ED. The following conditions characterize the status of individuals with ED:

- According to the *30th Annual Report to Congress,* the percentage of youth with ED graduating with a regular high school diploma was 43.4%, higher only than youth with intellectual disabilities (36.7%), with a dropout rate of 44.9%, the highest for any disability category.
- The percentage of children and youth with ED living in poverty is significantly greater than for their general education peers as well as children and youth with other disabilities (Wagner et al., 2005).
- When considering students with disabilities, children with ED earn lower grades and fail more courses than any other disability category (Landrum et al., 2003).
- According to the *30th Annual Report to Congress,* students who are Black are 2.3 times more likely to be identified as ED than students in all other racial/ethnic groups combined.
- Research indicates a large proportion of children and youth with ED also have identified or unidentified language disorders (Hollo, Wehby, & Oliver, 2014).
- After graduating from high school, approximately one-third of children with ED were unemployed, not in school, or not receiving any training (Neel, Meadows, Levine, & Edgar, 1988).

THE PATH TO EMOTIONAL DISTURBANCE

ED begins early in life and is evident in some young children by the preschool years (Beare & Lynch, 1986; Campbell, 1990; Patterson,

De Baryshe, & Ramsey, 1989). Data from various sources indicate that children diagnosed with ED come from backgrounds in which they are exposed to myriad risk factors that over time foster damaging negative experiences with parents, teachers, and peers alike (Wagner et al., 2005; Walker & Sprague, 1999; Wehby, Symons, & Hollo, 1997). These risk factors may collectively include long-term residential instability, contact with numerous service agencies, mental illness, poverty, abuse, neglect, harsh and inconsistent parenting, high stress, parental psychopathology, criminality, and drug or alcohol abuse (Quinn & Epstein, 1998). With each negative experience encountered, children become at greater risk of developing chronic social adjustment problems, increasing the probability of special education referral (Walker & Sprague, 1999).

Unfortunately, the prognosis for young children with ED is bleak. Less than half of young children with early signs of maladjusted behavior show remission by the time they reach adolescence (Shaw, Gilliom, & Giovannelli, 2000). Moreover, as adolescents, it becomes increasingly difficult to intervene (Kazdin, 1985; Robbins, 1966). These adolescents often grow up to evince numerous forms of adult maladjustment at a significant cost to society in terms of loss of productivity and continued need for special services.

While debate continues about the dominant causes of ED, the emerging perspective is that individual child characteristics interact with family and environmental factors to place some children at high risk for ED by the time they reach school (Farrington, 1989; Garmezy & Masten, 1994; Kauffman & Landrum, 2013; Singh, Landrum, Donatelli, Hampton, & Ellis, 1994; Walker & Sprague, 1999). Syntheses of the research have identified major factors that contribute to the development of disruptive behavioral disorders—the most frequently identified disorders among children with ED (Duncan, Forness, & Hartsough, 1995). Among the global factors are family characteristics, child characteristics, and sociological characteristics (Farmer, Quinn, Hussey, & Holahan, 2001; Kauffman & Landrum, 2013).

Family Characteristics

Parent–Child Relationships

Parent–child relationships among children identified as ED are frequently governed by coercive and reciprocal interaction styles. Using harsh, inconsistent, or erratic discipline practices, parents simultaneously provoke and teach children to escape negative consequences by escalating their problem behaviors (Dishion, French, & Patterson,

1995). In a model outlining the development of disruptive behavioral patterns, Walker and Sprague (1999) demonstrated the connecting links in a chain that underlie a clear path from early exposure to risk factors and later development of maladjustment.

The family initially experiences severe stress caused by exposure to one of many risk factors (e.g., poverty, unemployment, family upheaval, neglect, abuse, substance abuse). These stressors subsequently disrupt normal parenting practices, which in turn yields high rates of negative interactions among family members. These negative interactions often develop into coercive processes and aversive control strategies aimed at controlling one another's behavior. This powerful set of circumstances often provides a context for inadvertently teaching antisocial behavior patterns that are virtually impervious to intervention and resistant to change (Walker & Sprague, 1999).

Child Characteristics

Hyperactivity and Attention

Externalizing behavioral problems are often associated with attention and hyperactivity (Farmer et al., 2001). Evidence reveals that the two most frequently co-occurring psychiatric disorders are attention-deficit/hyperactivity disorder (ADHD) and conduct disorder (CD). According to the American Psychiatric Association (APA, 2013), the combined presentation of ADHD and CD occurs in approximately half of children diagnosed with ADHD. The high comorbidity rate for ADHD and CD is problematic given that these children often possess the most deviant features of both disturbances, effectively interfering with appropriate social and academic development (APA, 2013; Wenar, Kerig, & Ludlow, 2012). When these disorders co-occur, they tend to be a precursor for adult aggression, substance use, violence, and criminality (APA, 2013; Brier, 1995; Farrington, 1989; Zuckerman, 1999).

Temperament

In studies examining the relationship between early temperament characteristics and conduct problems, researchers have found that infant and child negative emotionality is modestly related to later oppositional and aggressive behavior through its indirect effect on parenting (Shaw et al., 2000). According to this research, mothers who perceive their infants as high on negativity display less responsiveness to infant or child requests for attention and resort to harsher discipline strategies in response to those requests. Moreover, these researchers found that infants or children who respond with intense, sustained, and prolonged anger to goal attainment frustration are at a higher risk of developing aggressive behavioral problems. It is important to note, however, that although temperament may play an important role in heightening the risk of developing emotional and behavioral problems, it does so only as it interacts with the child's proximal environment (e.g., parent, caregivers)—either placing them at increased risk or making them resilient (Crockenberg & Leekes, 2000; Kauffman & Landrum 2013).

Attachment

Evidence has accumulated that specific patterns of infant–primary caregiver relationships determine the quality of the relationship as manifested by the security of the infant or child's attachment (Crockenberg & Leekes, 2000). Research suggests (e.g., U.S. Department of Health and Human Services, 2000) that the relationship between maternal problems (e.g., maternal depression) and family risk factors (e.g., abuse) often predisposes children to form insecure or disorganized attachments, particularly in the young. In fact, investigators now believe that the nature and the outcome of the caretaker–child attachment process often predicts later depression and conduct disorders among these infants and children (U.S. Department of Health and Human Services, 2000).

Academic Difficulties

As risk factors, low academic performance and maladaptive behavior patterns are highly related. Although the mechanism of the relationship is unknown, evidence suggests that an association exists between academic and conduct problems that emerges early in a child's development (Brier, 1995; Farrington, 1989). Compared to their classmates, students with ED tend to be academically deficient, often functioning a year or more below expected grade level across most academic areas (Kauffman & Landrum, 2013; Reid et al., 2004; Trout, Nordness, Pierce, & Epstein, 2003). Studies addressing the academic characteristics of youth with ED have found that large numbers of these students meet at least one learning disability definition (Greenbaum et al., 1998). While there remains speculation on prevalence estimates, Ruhl and Berlinghoff (1992) suggest that between 33% and 81% of children with behavioral disorders have academic difficulties. Finally, as they get older, academic problems appear to worsen, as evidenced by the lower-than-expected graduation rates for ED youth in comparison to general education students and students with other disabilities (Oswald & Coutinho, 1996).

Sociological Characteristics

Peer Relationships

The peer group can be a mechanism that contributes to development of ED in two ways. First, establishing positive and reciprocal peer interactions is critical for normal social development. Children who are unable to foster such positive exchanges are at high risk because the social peer group provides an important link to social learning. Second, socially skilled and adept children can become embedded in undesirable peer groups who promote maladaptive social response patterns (Kauffman & Landrum, 2013). Antisocial children who bring this behavior pattern to school are most likely to experience peer rejection, to affiliate with deviant peers, and possibly to adopt a delinquent or violent lifestyle (Walker, Ramsey, & Gresham, 2004). Their antisocial behavior interferes with the formation of positive peer relations, depriving them of the benefits of peer learning. Rejected by their peers (and teachers), these children become embedded in social networks that reinforce, promote, enhance, and maintain their maladaptive behavior patterns. Over time, antisocial children tend to develop affiliations toward other youth who value their disruptive behavior, increasing the likelihood of lifelong antisocial behavioral patterns (Farmer et al., 2001; Wehby et al., 1997).

Economic Disadvantage

Children from low socioeconomic status families often demonstrate higher levels of both externalizing and internalizing behavioral problems (Greenberg, Lengua, Coie, & Pinderhughes, 1999). Many of the conditions associated with poverty (e.g., chaotic living conditions, family psychological distress, lack of food, lack of opportunity to learn, violence, school failure), especially extreme poverty, have been linked to the development of ED (Aber, Jones, & Cohen, 2000; Kauffman & Landrum, 2013) by way of rearing practices. Often these children come from families in which poverty has taken a considerable toll on parents and other caregivers, who are left with little or no energy or skill to foster nurturance or stimulation in their children. As infants or toddlers, these children frequently demonstrate signs of attachment disorders well into middle childhood (Knitzer, 2000).

MAJOR DISORDERS ASSOCIATED WITH EMOTIONAL DISTURBANCE

Several diagnostic categories are subsumed under the general term "emotional disturbance." These disorders can be organized into two broad dimensions of disorders: externalizing or internalizing (Achenbach, 1991). *Externalizing disorders* refers to a distinct group of behaviors reflecting conflicts with other individuals and their behavioral expectations. In general, these disorders are directed outwardly and viewed as undercontrolled. *Internalizing disorders* generally refers to disorders that are directed toward the self (e.g., anxiety, depression, withdrawal from social contact; Achenbach & Rescorla, 2001). They are generally inner directed, such that the core symptoms are often related to the overcontrol of behavior (Reynolds, 1992b). While a complete description of all the externalizing and internalizing disorders is beyond the scope of this chapter, interested readers may consult the *Diagnostic and Statistical Manual of Mental Disorders,* 5th edition (APA, 2013) for more information.

Externalizing Disorders

Externalizing disorders generally are disruptive and outer directed in nature. They represent a domain of disorders characterized by the undercontrol of behavioral impulses (Reynolds, 1992b). Externalizing problems in the schools are often manifested as conflicted relationships with peers, teachers, and other school-related individuals (House, 1999).

Conduct Disorder (CD)

According to the DSM-V (APA, 2013), the qualifying feature of CD is "a repetitive and persistent pattern of behavior in which the rights of others or major age-appropriate societal norms or rules are violated" (p. 469). The disorder may manifest itself in aggression toward people or animals, property destruction, theft or deceit, or serious rule violations. These behavioral manifestations often result in difficulties with social, academic, or occupational functioning. Prevalence estimates suggest that among males, rates range from 6% to 16% and among females from 2% to 9% (Kauffman & Landrum, 2013). The prognosis for child-onset CD is not encouraging. Children diagnosed with CD often show behavioral patterns that meet criteria for later adult antisocial personality disorder (House, 1999). High comorbidity rates are also reported where CD may co-occur with oppositional disorders, affective disorders, anxiety disorders, and attention-deficit disorders (House, 1999; McConaughy & Skiba, 1994).

Oppositional–Defiant Disorder (ODD)

In ODD there is an ongoing pattern of uncooperative, defiant, and hostile behavior. These behaviors are directed toward authority figures or others and seriously interfere with a child's daily academic, social, or occupational functioning (APA, 2013). Children with ODD tend to be argumentative with adults, often lose their temper, appear angry, are prone to spite and vindictiveness, and are easily annoyed by others (APA, 2013; Goldstein, 1995). Prevalence rates of ODD range from 2% to 16%. The outcomes for ODD vary. In some children the disorder evolves into a conduct disorder or other mood disorder. As adults, oppositional ODD can develop into passive aggressive personality disorder or antisocial personality disorder (Goldstein, 1995).

Attention-Deficit/Hyperactivity Disorder (ADHD)

The diagnostic and treatment questions most frequently asked of school psychologists and other service-related personnel refer to problems of poor impulse control, overactivity, and distractibility (House, 1999). Because of the impact on others, since 1984, ADHD has been classified as a disruptive behavior disorder (Goldstein, 1995). ADHD involves two classic symptoms: inattention and hyperactivity or impulsivity. Children with ADHD display these characteristics significantly far more than their peers do and to a marked degree. Prevalence rates for ADHD among children are 3%–5%. The course of ADHD appears stable through early adolescence. Prognosis for children with ADHD is not encouraging. Research (APA, 2013) has suggested that ADHD in children may be a precursor to adult psychopathology. Follow-up studies have shown that between 25% and 33% of children diagnosed with ADHD develop antisocial and conduct disorders, leading to much higher arrest records in adulthood (Zuckerman, 1999).

Internalizing Disorders

Internalizing disorders subsume a wide array of inner-directed, self-related disorders. While teachers have no problem spotting children who act out, they often overlook those who may have internalizing disorders (e.g., depression, anxiety; Kauffman & Landrum, 2013). The school "problem child" is easily identified because he or she is unruly, draws attention, and is often scolded for his or her actions. Teachers, paraprofessionals, and other service-related personnel often devote significant amounts of time to dealing with these students. While teachers and others attend to the externalizing child, the internalizing child who suffers from a potentially serious problem, such as depression or anxiety, may go unnoticed.

Social Phobia

Children with social phobia (also known as social anxiety disorder) demonstrate extreme anxiety in age-appropriate performance situations where they believe they are being evaluated and fear embarrassment, humiliation, or being thought poorly of by peers (House, 1999). These situations are usually avoided or endured with extreme anxiety. Epidemiological studies have revealed the prevalence of social phobia in the range of 3% to 13%. Although it may diminish during adulthood, the course of social phobia is usually continuous, often being exacerbated or attenuated by stressors (APA, 2013).

Obsessive–Compulsive Disorder (OCD)

OCD is a debilitating disorder that can have a profoundly negative effect on the individual, family, and peer relationships as well as academic performance. The obsessive or compulsive behaviors (e.g., hand washing, counting, repeating words silently) are intrusive, recurrent, and time consuming, and they lead to elevated distress or impairment in the affected child. Because they fear ridicule, children with OCD often perform their compulsive behaviors in secret, which results in underidentification of this disorder. Recent epidemiological studies suggest that 1 in every 200 children is affected by OCD, which makes it relatively rare (Albano, Chorpita, & Barlow, 2003). Furthermore, the majority of OCD cases are commonly misdiagnosed as depression or anxiety disorder (APA, 2013; House, 1999; Walters, Barrett, & March, 2001). The prognosis for OCD is mixed, with affected children showing periods of elevated disturbance and periods of diminished symptoms (APA, 2013).

Generalized Anxiety Disorder (GAD)

With children, GAD typically involves excessive and persistent worries about their performance in school and/or social activities. Often, the worries are unrealistic, usually not under their control, and distressing. In response to the distress, children with GAD frequently engage in approval-seeking behaviors, perfectionism, intolerance for substandard performance, and they constantly seek reassurance on their performance. In addition, children with GAD frequently complain of headaches, difficulty sleeping, restlessness, or concentration problems (APA, 2013; UCLA-Neuropsychiatric Institute, 1999). Approximately 17% or more of children diagnosed with some type of anxiety disorder have concurrent diagnoses (e.g., depression; Goldstein, 1995; Zuckerman, 1999). Estimates put the prevalence of GAD at 3%. GAD tends to be chronic with the course of GAD waxing and waning as a function of stressors (APA, 2013).

Post-Traumatic Stress Disorder (PTSD)

Perhaps the most controversial of the anxiety disorders is PTSD. Researchers have, however, come to realize that it is far more frequent than previously thought (Goldstein, 1995). A child or adolescent who experiences or is exposed to a catastrophic event may develop PTSD. The traumatic event may involve a situation where someone's life has been threatened (e.g., school shooting, sexual or physical abuse, war), or a natural disaster (e.g., tornado) or severe injury has occurred or been witnessed (e.g., seeing another person killed, car accident). The probability of developing PTSD relates to the magnitude of the trauma, whether the event is repeated, the child's proximity to the stressor, or their affiliation to the victim(s). Often, the stressful event is reexperienced in numerous ways such as intrusive recollections, flashbacks, dreams, or feeling like the event is recurring. Shortly after the event, children may appear agitated, confused, or disorganized. They may demonstrate extreme fear, helplessness, anger, melancholy, horror, or denial. Some children may even disassociate from the stressful event by demonstrating emotional deadening. Depending on the population sampled, prevalence estimates for PTSD range from 1% to 14% with some estimates being much higher (e.g., Bosnian refugees exposed to "ethnic cleansing" by Serbians; Hawkins & Radcliffe, 2006; Zuckerman, 1999). With treatment, the prognosis for PTSD is good with most symptoms not persisting beyond 12 months.

Separation Anxiety Disorder

Children who suffer from separation anxiety disorder often experience intense developmentally inappropriate anxiety when separated from significant attachment figures (usually the mother). These children often avoid any situation that takes them away from home or other familiar surroundings (e.g., going to school). They tend to cling to parents or other attachment figures. When separated, these children often cry uncontrollably, fear being abandoned or not being reunited with parents, or experience distress over the possibility that some catastrophe will befall loved ones. It is also common for children with separation anxiety disorder to have difficulty sleeping or nightmares, and to complain of physical symptoms (APA, 2013; House, 1999; Huberty, 1987). The prevalence of separation anxiety disorder among children and adolescents is approximately 4%, with the course of separation anxiety disorder waxing and waning and decreasing through adolescence (APA, 2013).

Childhood and Adolescent Depression

Depressive disorders are quite rare in the preschool period, but are more common in middle childhood and adolescence. Moreover, they bear a striking similarity to adulthood manifestations (Kendall, 1991; Reynolds, 1992a; Wenar et al., 2012). Depressed children often report feeling down and out about themselves. The most common symptom is dysphoria or a feeling of melancholy. Associated features and symptoms include irritability, tiredness, moodiness, negativism, hostility, anger, aggressive and antisocial behavior, difficulty sleeping, low energy, and appetite disturbances. It is not uncommon for attention, concentration, and memory to be negatively affected as well (Kendall, 1991). Some researchers have posited that academic and behavioral performances can be very sensitive indicators of the sudden onset of depression in children (Goldstein, 1995).

Depending on the age of onset as well as the diagnostic method used, estimates of childhood depression range from a low of 1.9% to a high of 13.9%, with actual prevalence in the range of 3%–5% (Bhatia & Bhatia, 2007). Higher prevalence rates are, however, commonly found among special populations such as children referred for diagnostic assessment relating to academic or behavior problems. Studies show rates as high as 34% to 49% for these populations, with parental psychopathology (e.g., maternal depression) representing one of the most significant risk factors (Goldstein, 1995; Kendall, 1991; Seeley, Rohde, Lewinsohn, & Clarke, 2002). There is also a growing recognition that comorbidity exists between depression and other disorders such as CD and ADHD (Papolos, 2003). Unfortunately, many children with depression remain untreated (Seeley et al., 2002). The prognosis for depression among treated children is unequivocal. Large-scale studies have, however, emphasized that all treatments for depression, even psychological ones, do not permanently diminish or reduce the chances of relapsing into depression but must be maintained at some level to influence the course (Zuckerman, 1999).

Summary

In summary, given the persistent nature of and negative outcomes associated with ED, educating these children is a complex and overwhelming task. While the debate continues on the etiology of ED, emerging perspectives suggest that child characteristics interact with family and environmental factors to place some children at higher risk for developing ED. As the previous section outlined, there are numerous disorders subsumed under the term "emotional disturbance" with most disorders falling along externalizing and internalizing dimensions.

ELIGIBILITY FOR EMOTIONAL DISTURBANCE

The reauthorization of IDEA in 2004 added a provision for states to use a response to intervention process when making eligibility decisions. Response to intervention (RTI) is premised on the use of pre-referral interventions to address student needs prior to making eligibility determinations. RTI is defined as "an inadequate change in target behaviors as a function of intervention" (Gresham, 2005, p. 331). In other words, if students do not respond to evidence-based interventions implemented with fidelity, it is an indication that the student may have a disability. Before declaring that a student is eligible for special education services, the student must be shown to possess a disability (e.g., ED) either through an RTI process or through the more traditional psychometric eligibility framework. Moreover, the student must also demonstrate an educational or academic problem necessitating the need for special services (e.g., inadequate response to intervention). Along with federal guidelines, each state has an education code that determines under which conditions a student is considered disabled. Specifically, for children to receive special education services they must (a) be diagnosed with a disability, (b) possess special learning needs, and (c) require special educational services to promote better educational outcomes (McLoughlin & Lewis, 1994; Salvia, Ysseldyke, & Bolt, 2013). Readers wishing to learn more about the specific application of RTI for students with ED are referred to Gresham (2005). In the following section we discuss (a) the definition of ED, (b) screening for ED, (c) assessment for ED, and (d) sources of assessment data in an ED evaluation.

Definition

Emotional disturbance, as defined in IDEA, refers to "a condition exhibiting one or more of the following characteristics over a long period of time and to a marked degree that adversely affects a child's educational performance: (a) an inability to learn that cannot be explained by intellectual, sensory, or health factors; (b) an inability to build or maintain satisfactory interpersonal relationships with peers and teachers; (c) inappropriate types of behavior or feelings under normal circumstances; (d) a general pervasive mood of unhappiness or depression; or (e) a tendency to develop physical symptoms or fears associated with personal or school problems. The term includes schizophrenia. The term does not apply to children who are socially maladjusted, unless it is determined that they have an emotional disturbance" (Federal Register, 2006, p. 46756).

As described in the definition, children who possess one or more of the five characteristics of ED must also meet three conditions to qualify for special education services, namely, long period of time, marked degree, and adverse educational effects. To meet the qualifying condition of "long period of time," the identified difficulty must have existed much longer than would be expected of reactions to stressful events. Similarly, to meet the marked-degree requirement, a child's behavior must be more severe than would be expected for similar-age and -sex peers. Finally, adverse educational effects require demonstrating low scores on standardized tests and/or some other overall measure of school functioning (McConaughy, 1993).

The federal definition of children with ED has always and continues to be problematic because of issues of difficulty in operationalizing the definition, misinterpretation, stigma, and a lack of consensus about the nature of the disorders underlying ED (Forness et al., 2000). Although the qualifier "seriously" was removed in the 1997 reauthorization of IDEA, the definition remains neither clear nor comprehensive enough to determine appropriate eligibility as a special education category for several reasons. First, the five ED criteria are not supported by previous research on various subtypes of children with emotional or behavioral disorders. Second, the notion of adverse educational performance has been literally interpreted to pertain only to "academic" performance, thus effectively excluding "social" and "behavioral" performance as indicators. Finally, and arguably the most problematic feature, is the total exclusion of youth with social maladjustment, especially with regard to conduct disorders. This exclusion virtually ignores the possibility of comorbidity of mental disorders among youth identified as emotionally disturbed (Cullinan & Epstein, 2001). Indeed, the second emotional disturbance criterion (i.e., inability to build or maintain satisfactory relationships with peers and teachers) practically defines the behavioral repertoire of social maladjustment (Forness, Kavale, & Lopez, 1993; Walker, Ramsey, & Gresham, 2004).

Despite these definitional concerns, IDEA continues to guide the provision of educational services for children diagnosed with ED (Kauffman & Landrum, 2013). A clear definition of ED is important because it influences the criteria that students must satisfy to be identified and subsequently receive special education services. Consequently, the definition also influences prevalence estimates for ED. Moreover, the definition influences decisions on such issues as services and research, as well as funding by policy makers, administrators, and advocacy groups. Intra- and interdisciplinary communication and discussion about ED is also shaped by the definition used (Epstein & Walker, 2001).

Screening for Emotional Disorders

Given that many children with ED remain underidentified and underserved by the schools (Walker & Sprague, 1999), systematic screening of all children is recommended and should be part of any RTI system. The *Systematic Screening for Behavior Disorders* (SSBD; Walker & Severson, 1990) is a multigate system that provides an equal opportunity for all students in a class to be considered and be identified as at risk of ED. The SSBD provides a solution to the problems of underreferral by providing teachers uniform behavioral standards for use in identifying candidates for differing levels of pre-referral intervention. The screening occurs in three stages, namely (a) general education teachers rank order all children on their class roster to identify the three students who present with externalizing (e.g., oppositional) or internalizing (e.g., withdrawn) behavior problems; (b) teachers rate the top-ranked externalizers ($n = 3$) and internalizers ($n = 3$) on three scales that assess children's critical events (adaptive and maladaptive behaviors); and (c) for students who exceed criteria at Step 2, direct observation of attention to task and social interaction behaviors in classroom and playground settings is conducted. The SSBD has been shown to meet acceptable levels of reliability, validity, cost efficiency, and consumer satisfaction (Phillips, Nelson, & McLaughlin, 1993; Walker & Severson, 1990; Walker et al., 1994).

Another screening instrument is the *Student Risk Screening Scale* (SRSS; Drummond, 1994). The SRSS is a screening tool used to identify the strengths and deficits of students aged 3–17 years in the areas of social behavior. Raters (i.e., teacher, parent, and self-report for ages 11–17 only) score items across the factors of (a) emotional symptoms, (b) conduct problems, (c) hyperactivity, (d) peer problems, and (e) prosocial behavior. The 25-item teacher-completed form is most commonly used. Teachers complete the one-page measure for each student on their roster by rating each item using a four-point, Likert scale ranging from 0 (never) to 3 (frequently). The ratings are summed (range 0–21), and students are placed into one of three levels of risk: low (0–3), moderate (4–8), and high (9–21; Drummond, 1994). The SRSS is a no-cost screener noted for its ease of use and scoring and only requires approximately 10 minutes to screen an entire class (Lane, Kalberg, Bruhn, Mahoney, & Driscoll, 2008; Oakes et al., 2010). Psychometric studies of the SRSS have shown acceptable levels of reliability and validity, as well as convergent validity with the SSBD (Lane, Kalberg, Lambert, Crnobori, & Bruhn, 2010; Lane et al., 2009; Menzies & Lane, 2012; Oakes et al., 2010).

ASSESSMENT FOR EMOTIONAL DISTURBANCE

School-based assessment typically serves the following purposes: (a) pre-referral classroom decisions, (b) entitlement decisions, (c) post-entitlement decisions, and (d) accountability or outcome decisions (Salvia et al., 2013). In pre-referral classroom decisions, assessment seeks to assist in the provision of special help or enrichment, referral to a teacher assistance team, or provision of intervention assistance as in the case of schools using an RTI model (Gresham, 2005; Kauffman, Bruce, & Lloyd, 2012). Assessment for entitlement decisions assists in screening, referral, identifying the disability, documenting special learning needs, and determination for special education or related services eligibility. Post-entitlement classroom assessment includes testing for instructional planning, determining best instructional setting, and monitoring progress evaluation. Finally, assessment with regard to accountability and outcomes for individuals assists in program evaluation.

To meet IDEA eligibility criteria for ED, assessment should be guided by a multidimensional (i.e., multimethod, multitrait, multisource, multisetting) approach (Landrum, 2011; McConaughy & Ritter, 1995). The multimethod component relies on self-reports, teacher reports, parent reports, behavior rating scales, interviews with the child or adolescent, direct observation, standardized inventories, and projective techniques. The multitrait component relies on assessing interpersonal skills, personal coping methods, behavior types and magnitude, affect or mood and states, and academic performance. The multisource component relies on obtaining information from the child, parents, teachers, other school personnel, health professionals, mental health professionals, and family members. Finally, assessment should be conducted across multiple settings, to include the home, the school, different classes, different activities in the same room, structured versus unstructured settings, and different teachers in the same and different settings. Overall, to conduct a thorough assessment, a multimethod, trait, source, and setting assessment should be conducted.

Although the process varies from setting to setting, a multidimensional assessment of ED relies on both low and high inference and objectivity strategies. While all assessment techniques make a unique contribution, surveys of school psychologists reveal that not all methods possess utility in guiding intervention practices. In a survey, researchers found that interviews (child, teacher, and parent) were rated highest in terms of guiding classification practices, whereas direct observation was most useful for intervention purposes (Cheramie, Griffin, & Morgan, 2000).

SOURCES OF DATA COLLECTION

Functional Behavioral Assessment

In recent years, behavioral researchers and practitioners have developed and used functional behavioral assessment procedures in an attempt to improve decision making in the development of treatment plans. The assumption underlying functional behavioral assessment is that treatment effectiveness is enhanced if the treatment matches the function of behavior. The goal of a functional behavioral assessment is to identify relationships between person–environment events and the occurrence and nonoccurrence of a target behavior (Fox & Gable, 2004). If performed accurately, a functional assessment allows an interventionist (e.g., teacher, psychologist) to develop a specific description of the problem behavior, identify the factors that contribute to the occurrence of the behavior, and establish a link between the behavior and a treatment (Smith, 2001).

Functional behavioral assessment is designed to (a) promote hypotheses-driven treatment, (b) place more emphasis on skill building rather than punishment, (c) increase the prospect of a positive treatment outcome, (d) increase the chance of maintenance and generalization of treatment effects, and (e) contribute to the scientific advancement of treatment efforts (Blakeslee, Sugai, & Grub, 1994). Although the specific procedures used by researchers vary, they tend to use a combination of indirect and direct methods when conducting a functional behavioral assessment. The assumption is that compiling information from a variety of sources can create a more accurate picture of the problem behavior, including its function.

Standardized Behavior Rating Scales

Rating scales provide an index of various individuals' (e.g., teacher, parent) perception of a student's behavioral patterns. Respondents are asked to assess the presence or absence of a behavior and to gauge the amount, intensity, or frequency of that behavior (Salvia et al., 2013). Examples of rating scales include the Child Behavior Checklist (CBCL) for parents or caregivers, the Teacher Report Form (TRF), and the Youth Self-Report (YSR; Achenbach, 1991). For preschool children companion forms are also available (Achenbach & Rescorla, 2001). Another example that also includes teacher, parent, and self-report is the *Behavior Assessment System for Children* (BASC; Reynolds & Kamphaus, 1992). Because it operationally defines the federal definition of ED, the *Scale for Assessing Emotional Disturbance* (SAED; Epstein & Cullinan, 2010) is especially important in helping identify children who qualify for special education services under IDEA's category of ED. In general, rating scales provide a more reliable measure of a child's externalizing and internalizing functioning (McConaughy, 1993).

Clinical Interview

Parent, child, and teacher interviews should all be routinely obtained when conducting an evaluation for ED. These interviews provide valuable information that is not as readily obtained or less accessible to other procedures. Most interviews should be focused on eliciting information on medical and developmental history, social–emotional functioning, educational and academic progress, and level of community involvement (Salvia et al., 2013). Examples of interview questions are "Have there been any hospitalizations in the past?" "Does your child play well with his/her brother and sisters?" and "Do you have any academic concerns?"

Information derived from interviews is used for clarifying information as well as in deciding which additional assessment procedures to pursue (McConaughy & Ritter, 1995). In general, several principles for conducting interviews should be used as guidelines (Lentz & Wehmann, 1995). First, an ecological framework should always underlie the interview. Questions should be directed at the natural and observable constellation of variables surrounding the problem situation, the referring agent, and beliefs and perceptions of the interviewee. Second, explicitly stated outcomes should, prior to beginning the interview, be clearly articulated. Third, because of time limitations, interviews should always be focused and economical. Fourth, once objectives for the interview are established, questions and responses should be structured for purposes of achieving those objectives. Finally, a plan should be in place for connecting the interview information with decisions about subsequent professional practices (Lentz & Wehmann, 1995).

Behavioral Observation

When conducting an evaluation for ED, behavioral observation yields the most useful data and, more than any other method of assessment, represents the most direct and desirable approach to data collection (Goldstein, 1995). In behavioral observations, the observer (a) has a goal of measuring a specific behavior (e.g., counting noncompliant episodes), (b) has previously defined the behavior of interest, (c) uses procedures for objectively gathering information about the behavior (e.g., frequency count chart), (d) specifically knows when and where the behavior will be observed, and (e) knows how the behaviors will be quantified (e.g., percentage of time noncompliant). Measuring behavior typically relies on four fundamental characteristics: duration (i.e., beginning and end of behavior), latency (i.e., the length of time between a prompt to begin a behavior and actual beginning), frequency (i.e., how often the behavior occurs), and amplitude (i.e., intensity of behavior). In determining which behavior to assess, observers should pick the most salient aspect of the behavior in the most relevant situation (Salvia et al., 2013).

Personality Assessment

Because of its subjective nature, personality is a complex concept and somewhat difficult to accurately assess. More important, the choice of instruments used to assess personality depends by and large on the theoretical orientation of the assessment personnel. For example, one might expect a psychoanalytic evaluator to focus on an individual's personality traits, whereas a behaviorally oriented evaluator might consider the manner in which someone behaves as a function of situational specificity.

In general, there are three types of personality assessment tools, namely, self-report inventories, projective techniques, and behavioral rating assessments (Ludy, Hopkins, & Nation, 1994). For example, the *Children's Depression Inventory* (Kovacs, 1982) is a self-report, symptom-oriented scale that is designed for all school-age children and adolescents suspected of depression. Personality assessment also includes strategies that focus on projective techniques. One popular projective technique is the *Roberts Apperception Test for Children* (McArthur & Roberts, 1994), which is used to subjectively assess and evaluate children's and adolescents' perceptions of common interpersonal situations. Many school psychologists also use projective drawing approaches. One popular instrument is the *Draw a Person: Screening Procedure for Emotional Disturbance* (Naglieri, McNeish, & Bardos, 1991). As the name implies, this instrument is used to screen children who may show signs of ED requiring further evaluation. Finally, many evaluators use behavioral rating scales such as the CBCL or SAED, described earlier.

From a behavioral perspective, projective evaluation techniques represent an ambiguous task at best (Knoff, 1990). While many tests have objective scoring procedures (e.g., *Draw a Person*), the interpretation of these results relies quite heavily on subjective judgment. Personality assessment procedures that use projective techniques should be conducted only by trained psychologists, should never be the primary source of data, and should be interpreted with great caution (McConaughy & Ritter, 1995).

Achievement and Educational Performance

As with all referrals for school-based diagnostic comprehensive psychological evaluations, assessment of ED must include information about current levels of academic achievement and performance. Information derived from achievement and performance evaluations is required to assess whether the identified behavioral or emotional difficulty adversely affects educational performance, one of the qualifying conditions for ED as stated in IDEA. Academic assessment generally involves the use of standardized tests such as the *Woodcock-Johnson III Tests of Achievement* (Woodcock, McGrew, & Mather, 2000), curriculum-based assessment (CBA; Gickling & Rosenfield, 1995), report cards, and work samples. CBA refers to a group of assessment techniques that serve multiple purposes but primarily are used for instructional planning and progress monitoring in tandem with what is being taught in the classroom. Over time, CBA permits continuous and direct assessment of student progress (Gickling & Rosenfield, 1995).

Strength-Based Assessment

Up to this point, the focus of all previously discussed models, procedures, instruments, and protocols for the collection of assessment data on children suspected of, diagnosed, or identified with ED has been deficit based. Although these data may be necessary for decision-making purposes (e.g., special education placement), they unduly limit the scope and range of information gathered and, in the process, stress the negatives at the expense of the positives in a child's functioning (Epstein, 1999). According to Epstein and Sharma (1998), "Strength-based assessment is defined as the measurement of those emotional and behavioral skills, competencies, and characteristics that create a sense of personal accomplishment; contribute to satisfying relationships with family members, peers, and adults; enhances one's ability to deal with adversity and stress; and promotes one's personal, social, and academic development" (p. 3). For these reasons, Epstein and Sharma developed the *Behavioral and Emotional Rating Scale-2: A Strength-Based Approach to Assessment* (Epstein & Sharma, 2004). Another strength-based assessment instrument is the *Devereux Early Childhood Assessment* (DECA; Lebuffe & Naglieri, 1999). The DECA is designed to evaluate within-child protective factors in children in an effort to generate information about the strengths and areas of need in a child's protective factors (e.g., attachment, self-control, initiative). More recent scales also incorporate the concept of resilience (i.e., an individual's ability to cope and adapt to major life stressors and trauma). The *Social Emotional Assets and Resilience Scale's* (Merrell, 2011) is a comprehensive, cross-informant measure to assess the social strengths and resilience of school-age children and adolescents (ages 5–18).

INTERVENTION STRATEGIES FOR CHILDREN WITH ED

Students with ED represent significant challenges to schools. Often these students are the most difficult to teach and manage in the classroom. It is not uncommon for these students to present with a wide range of social and emotional adjustment problems (e.g., conduct disorder, depression, anxiety) that impair their ability to form appropriate relationships and experience academic success. Three-tiered schoolwide prevention models (i.e., primary, secondary, and tertiary prevention programs) have been recommended to assist schools in creating more positive teaching and learning environments for these students (Sugai, Sprague, Horner, & Walker, 2000; Walker et al., 1996; Walker & Sprague, 1999). Three-tiered schoolwide prevention models represent the application of risk-factor causal theory (Hawkins, Von Cleve, & Catalano, 1991; Lynam, 1996) in the schools. Risk-factor theory is rooted in the notion that prolonged and pervasive exposure to one or more key risk factors (e.g., poverty, neglect, abuse) is associated with negative, destructive, and long-term outcomes (Patterson,

Reid, & Dishion, 1992). The longer a child is exposed and the greater the number of risks involved, the greater the likelihood the child will develop and sustain a dysfunctional and maladaptive behavioral repertoire (Walker & Sprague, 1999).

Three-tiered schoolwide prevention models are premised on the view that in any school setting, three types of youth can be seen: (a) typical children not at risk for problems, (b) children at risk (i.e., evince one or more risk factors) for developing maladaptive behavior repertoires, and (c) children who show signs of pervasive life-course and persistent maladaptive behavioral repertoires (Moffitt, 1993). Children in each category represent candidates for various levels of programs or interventions that provide greater specificity, intensity, comprehensiveness, and costliness (Reid, 1993). Primary, secondary, and tertiary forms of prevention are appropriate for each identified child and adolescent group, respectively. School and community approaches that encourage all three of these prevention levels are necessary to maintain the health of children, schools, and communities.

Primary prevention services are aimed at enhancing protective factors (e.g., discipline practices) on a schoolwide basis so that students exposed to this level of intervention do not become at risk for developing problematic and maladaptive behavior patterns. Interventions used for primary prevention are universal in their focus (i.e., all students are exposed to the services). As an example of primary-level prevention strategy, Nelson (1996) developed one of the few empirically validated schoolwide prevention programs. In systematic fashion, this program addresses (a) adjusting the school's ecological arrangements (e.g., scheduling and use of space in common areas), (b) clearly stated and consistent behavioral expectations, (c) active supervision of students in common areas (e.g., hallways), (d) a consistent classroom disciplinary response connected to a continuum of disciplinary responses, and (e) functional behavioral assessment, along with concomitant behavioral intervention plans to students' curricular and behavioral difficulties. According to the U.S. Department of Health and Human Services (2001) Surgeon General's report on violence, other examples of promising primary prevention programs include Life Skills Training (Botvin, Mihalic, & Grotpeter, 1998) and the Montreal Longitudinal Study/Preventative Treatment Program (Tremblay et al., 1992).

Secondary prevention programs are more intensive and costly. These programs are directed at providing behavioral, social, or academic support and skills development to children who already demonstrate signs of their at-risk status (Walker & Sprague, 1999). Secondary prevention programs are designed to positively address one or a combination of risk factors before they grow into significant maladaptive behavioral repertoires. First Step to Success (Walker et al., 1998) is a secondary-level early intervention program that targets primary-grade children who show clear signs of emerging antisocial behavior patterns (e.g., aggression toward others, oppositional–defiant behavior, tantrums, rule infractions, escalating confrontations with peers and adults). Teachers and/or parents or caregivers participate in the intervention as implementation agents, under the direction and supervision of a school consultant who has primary responsibility for coordinating the intervention. The intervention specifies clear roles and duties for each social agent. First Step to Success incorporates many of the strategies, principles, and practices recommended in a comprehensive program. These include continuous assessment and monitoring of progress, provision for the practice of newly learned skills, treatment matched to presenting problems, multicomponent treatment strategies, programming for transfer and maintenance of new skills, commitment to sustaining the intervention, and family involvement (Epstein & Walker, 2001). Other examples of secondary prevention programs include functional family therapy (Alexander et al., 1998) and Second Step (Beland, 1988).

Tertiary prevention programs are directed to children who evince severe involvement in life-course persistent maladaptive behavioral repertoires. In general, these youth require services interventions and supports that very likely exceed the capacity of the school alone. Successful tertiary programs for youth involved in tertiary-level programs are likely to be intensive, comprehensive, and long term; to include parental involvement, siblings, and peers; and to involve interagency collaboration. Multisystemic therapy (MST; Henggeler & Borduin, 1990) is a family- and home-based tertiary-level treatment that strives to change how children function in their natural settings—home, school, and neighborhood—in ways that promote positive social behavior while decreasing antisocial behavior. This "multisystemic" approach characterizes individuals as embedded within a network of interconnected systems that encompass individual, family, and extrafamilial (e.g., peer, school, neighborhood) factors and recognizes that intervention involves a combination of these systems. Most significant, the conceptual framework of MST fits closely with the known causes of mental health problems, delinquency, and substance abuse. MST addresses these factors in an individualized, comprehensive, and integrated manner.

Based on the belief that the most effective and ethical route to helping children is through helping their families, MST views parent(s) or guardians as valuable resources, even when they have serious and multiple needs of their own. The primary goals of MST are

(a) to reduce the frequency and severity of mental health problems, (b) to reduce other types of antisocial behavior, and (c) to achieve these outcomes at a cost savings by decreasing rates of incarceration and out-of-home placements. MST achieves these goals through adherence to the nine MST treatment principles. Other examples of tertiary programs include multidimensional treatment foster care (Chamberlain & Mihalic, 1998) and the Intensive Protective Supervision Project (Land, McCall, & Williams, 1992).

In summary, children with ED represent a significant challenge to schools. To create sustained positive teaching and learning environments, three-tiered (i.e., primary, secondary, tertiary) schoolwide prevention models along with suggested programs have been outlined. Each of the highlighted programs has the potential to reduce the risk of ED among children and has been identified as either model or promising by the Surgeon General's report on youth violence (U.S. Department of Health and Human Services, 2001).

CONCLUSION

The United States is facing a health crisis in the mental well-being and care of children. Many children enter and remain in schools with mental health problems that interfere with social and academic development. Evidence from the World Health Organization suggests that by 2020, childhood neuropsychiatric disorders will rise proportionately by more than 50%, effectively becoming one of the top five reasons for childhood morbidity, mortality, and disability (U.S. Department of Health and Human Services, 2000). To date, research in the area of ED continues to report a chronic problem of under-referral and underidentification of children, thus creating growing numbers of children at risk of persistent, chronic, and lifelong emotional and behavioral maladjustment. Despite the significant challenges to families, schools, and society that these children present, recent evidence suggests that there is hope. Schoolwide three-tiered prevention programs have shown promise by taking an ecological approach to service delivery that involves multiple systems interacting in synergistic ways to bring about positive outcomes for children at risk or already diagnosed with ED. Moreover, the Surgeon General in a report on children's mental health (U.S. Department of Health and Human Services, 2000) focused attention on evidence-based treatments (i.e., systematically tested treatments). These treatments have been shown to yield positive treatment effects, often comparable to those found in adult outcome research. Unlike untested treatments, these interventions are manualized, specific to the identified problems, and durable, and they often show maintenance six months or more beyond the initial treatment. With continued focus on early identification and intervention through screening and RTI, as well as implementation of evidence-based treatments, the sobering statistics presented at the beginning of this chapter can be altered—thus leading to increased success for children with ED.

REFERENCES

Aber, J. L., Jones, S., & Cohen, J. (2000). The impact of poverty on the mental health and development of very young children. In C. H. Zeanah (Ed.), *Handbook of infant mental health* (2nd ed., pp. 113–128). New York, NY: Guilford Press.

Achenbach, T. M. (1991). *Manual for the youth self-report and 1991 Profile.* Burlington, VT: University of Vermont Department of Psychiatry.

Achenbach, T. M., & Rescorla, L. A. (2001). *Manual for ASEBA school-age forms and profiles.* Burlington, VT: University of Vermont, Research Center for Children, Youth and Families.

Albano, A. M., Chorpita, B. F., & Barlow, D. H. (2003). Childhood anxiety disorders. In E. J. Mash & R. A. Barkley (Eds.), *Child psychopathology* (2nd ed., pp. 279–329). New York, NY: Guilford Press.

Alexander, J., Pugh, C., Parsons, B., Barton, C., Gordon, D., Grotpeter, J., . . . Sexton, J. (1998). *Functional family therapy: Blueprints for violence prevention* (Blueprints for Violence Prevention Series 3). Boulder, CO: Center for the Study and Prevention of Violence, Institute of Behavioral Science, University of Colorado.

American Psychiatric Association. (2013). *Diagnostic and statistical manual of mental disorders* (5th ed.). Washington, DC: Author.

Beare, P. L., & Lynch, E. C. (1986). Underidentification of preschool children at risk of behavioral disorders. *Behavioral Disorders, 15,* 177–183.

Beland, K. (1988). Second Step, grades 1–3: *Pilot project 1987–1988 summary report.* Seattle, WA: Committee for Children.

Bhatia, S. K., & Bhatia, S. C. (2007). Childhood and adolescent depression. *American Family Physician, 75,* 73–80.

Blakeslee, T., Sugai, G., & Grub, J. (1994). A review of functional assessment use in data-based intervention studies. *Journal of Behavioral Education, 4,* 397–413.

Botvin, G. J., Mihalic, S. F., & Grotpeter, J. K. (1998). *Life skills training* (Blueprints for Violence Prevention Series 5). Boulder, CO: Center for the Study and Prevention of Violence, Institute of Behavioral Science, University of Colorado.

Brier, N. (1995). Predicting antisocial behavior in youngsters displaying poor academic achievement: A review of risk factors. *Developmental and Behavioral Pediatrics, 16,* 271–276.

Campbell, S. B. (1990). *Behavior problems in school children.* Baltimore, MD: Guilford Press.

Chamberlain, P., & Mihalic, S. F. (1998). *Blueprints for violence prevention, book 8: Multidimensional treatment foster care.* Boulder, CO: Center for the Study and Prevention of Violence.

Cheramie, G. M., Griffin, K. M., & Morgan, T. (2000). Usefulness of assessment techniques in assessing classification for emotional disturbance and generating classroom interventions. *Perceptual and Motor Skills, 90*, 250–252.

Crockenberg, S., & Leekes, E. (2000). Infant social and emotional development in family context. In C. H. Zeanah (Ed.), *Handbook of infant mental health* (pp. 60–90). New York, NY: Guilford Press.

Cullinan, D., & Epstein, M. H. (2001). Comorbidity among students with emotional disturbance. *Behavioral Disorders, 26*, 200–213.

Dishion, T. J., French, D. C., & Patterson, G. R. (1995). The development and ecology of antisocial behavior. In D. Cicchetti & D. J. Cohen (Eds.), *Developmental psychopathology: Risk, disorder, and adaptation* (Vol. 2, pp. 421–471). New York, NY: Wiley.

Drummond, T. (1994). *The student risk screening scale* (SRSS). Grants Pass, OR: Josephine County Mental Health Program.

Duncan, B. B., Forness, S. R., & Hartsough, C. (1995). Students identified as seriously emotionally disturbed in school-based day treatment: Cognitive, psychiatric, and special education characteristics. *Behavioral Disorders, 20*, 238–252.

Epstein, M. H. (1999). The development and validation of a scale to assess the emotional and behavioral strengths of children and adolescents. *Remedial & Special Education, 20*, 258–268.

Epstein, M. H. (2004). *Behavioral and Emotional Rating Scale 2nd edition: A strength-based approach to assessment.* Austin, TX: PRO-ED.

Epstein, M. H., & Cullinan, D. (2010). *Scales for assessing emotional disturbances.* Austin, TX: PRO-ED.

Epstein, M. H., & Sharma, H. M. (1998). *Behavioral and Emotional Rating Scale: A strength-based approach to assessment.* Austin, TX: PRO-ED.

Epstein, M. H., & Walker, H. M. (2001). *Special education: Best practices and First Step to Success.* Unpublished manuscript.

Farmer, T. W., Quinn, M. M., Hussey, W., & Holahan, T. (2001). The development of disruptive behavioral disorders and correlated constraints: Implications for intervention. *Behavioral Disorders, 26*, 117–130.

Farrington, D. P. (1989). Early predictors of adolescent aggression and adult violence. *Violence and Victims, 4*, 79–100.

Federal Register. (2006, August). Assistance to states for the education of children with disabilities and preschool grants for children with disabilities; Final Rule 34. CFR Parts 300 & 301, 71 Fed. Reg. 46540.

Forness, S. R., Freeman, S. F., Paparella, T., Kauffman, J., & Walker, H. M. (2012). Special education implications of point and cumulative prevalence for children with emotional and behavioral disorders. *Journal of Emotional and Behavioral Disorders, 20*, 4–18.

Forness, S. R., Kavale, K. A., & Lopez, M. (1993). Conduct disorders in school: Special education eligibility and comorbidity. *Journal of Emotional and Behavioral Disorders, 1*(2), 101–108.

Forness, S. R., Serna, L. A., Nielsen, E., Lambros, K., Hale, M. J., & Kavale, K. A. (2000). A model for early detection and primary prevention of emotional and behavioral disorders. *Education and Treatment of Children, 23*, 325–345.

Fox, J., & Gable, R. A. (2004). Functional behavioral assessment. In R. B. Rutherford, M. M. Quinn, & S. R. Mathur (Eds.), *Handbook of research in emotional and behavioral disorders* (pp. 143–162). New York, NY: Guilford.

Garmezy, N., & Masten, A. S. (1994). Chronic adversities. In M. Rutter & E. Taylor (Eds.), *Child and adolescent psychiatry* (pp. 191–208). Oxford, UK: Blackwell Scientific.

Gickling, E. E., & Rosenfield, S. (1995). Best practices in curriculum-based assessment. In A. Thomas & J. Grimes (Eds.), *Best practices in school psychology II* (pp. 587–607). Washington, DC: National Association of School Psychologists.

Goldstein, S. (1995). *Understanding and managing children's classroom behavior.* New York, NY: Wiley.

Greenbaum, P. E., Dedrick, R. F., Friedman, R. M., Kutash, K., Brown, E., Lardieri, S. P., & Pugh, A. M. (1998). National Adolescent and Child Treatment Study (NACTS): Outcomes for children with serious emotional and behavioral disturbance. In M. H. Epstein, K. Kutash, & A. Duchnowski (Eds.), *Outcomes for children and youth with behavioral and emotional disorders and their families: Programs and evaluation best practices* (pp. 21–54). Austin, TX: PRO-ED.

Greenberg, M. T., Lengua, L., Coie, J. D., & Pinderhughes, E. E. (1999). Predicting developmental outcomes at school entry using a multiple-risk model: Four American communities. *Developmental Psychology, 35*, 403–417.

Gresham, F. (2005). Response to intervention: An alternative means of identifying students as emotionally disturbed. *Education and Treatment of Children, 28*, 328–344.

Hawkins, J. D., Von Cleve, E., & Catalano, R. F. (1991). Reducing early childhood aggression: Results of a primary prevention program. *Journal of the American Academy of Child and Adolescent Psychiatry, 30*, 208–217.

Hawkins, S., & Radcliffe, J. (2006). Current measures of PTSD for children and adolescents. *Journal of Pediatric Psychology, 31*, 420–430.

Henggeler, S. W., & Borduin, C. M. (1990). *Family therapy and beyond: A multisystemic approach to treating the behavior problems of children and adolescents.* Pacific Grove, CA: Brooks/Cole.

Hollo, A., Wehby, J. H., & Oliver, R. M. (2014). Unidentified language deficits in children with emotional and behavioral disorders: A meta-analysis. *Exceptional Children, 80*, 169–186.

House, A. E. (1999). *DSM-IV diagnosis in the schools.* New York, NY: Guildford Press.

Huberty, T. J. (1987). Children and anxiety. In A. Thomas & J. Grimes (Eds.), *Children's needs: Psychological perspectives* (pp. 45–51). Washington, DC: National Association of School Psychologists.

Individuals with Disabilities Improvement Act of 2004. Pub. L. 108-466.

Kauffman, J. M., Bruce, A., & Lloyd, J. W. (2012). Response to intervention (RtI) and students with EBD. In J. P. Bakken, F. E. Obiakor, & A. Rotatori (Eds.), *Advances in special education. Vol. 22: Behavioral disorders: Current perspective and issues* (pp. 107–127). Bingley, UK: Emerald.

Kauffman, J. M., & Landrum, T. J. (2013). *Characteristics of emotional and behavioral disorders of children and youth* (10th ed.). Upper Saddle River, NJ: Pearson.

Kazdin, A. E. (1985). Selection of target behaviors: The relationship of the treatment focus to clinical dysfunction. *Behavioral Assessment, 7*, 33–47.

Kendall, P. C. (1991). *Child and adolescent therapy.* New York, NY: Guildford Press.

Knitzer, J. (2000). *Promoting resilience: Helping young children and parents affected by substance abuse, domestic violence, and depression in the context of welfare reform.* New York, NY: National Center for Children in Poverty.

Knoff, H. (1990). Best practices in personality assessment. In A. Thomas & J. Grimes (Eds.), *Best practices in school psychology II*. Washington, DC: National Association of School Psychologists.

Kovacs, M. (1982). *Children's depression inventory*. Washington, DC: Multi-Health Systems.

Land, K. C., McCall, P. L., & Williams, J. R. (1992). Intensive supervision of status offenders: Evidence of continuity of treatment effects for juveniles and a "Hawthorne Effect" for counselors. In J. McCord & R. Tremblay (Eds.), *Preventing antisocial behavior: Interventions from birth through adolescence*. New York, NY: Guilford Press.

Landrum, T. J. (2011). Emotional and behavioral disorders. In J. M. Kauffman & D. P. Hallahan (Eds.), *Handbook of special education* (pp. 209–220). New York, NY: Taylor & Francis.

Landrum, T. J., Tankersley, M., & Kauffman, J. M. (2003). What is special about special education for students with emotional or behavioral disorders? *Journal of Special Education, 37*, 148–156.

Lane, K. L., Kalberg, J. R., Bruhn, A. L., Mahoney, M. E., & Driscoll, S. A. (2008). Primary prevention programs at the elementary level: Issues of treatment integrity, systematic screening, and reinforcement. *Education and Treatment of Children, 31*, 465–494.

Lane, K. L., Kalberg, J. R., Lambert, W., Crnobori, M. E., & Bruhn, A. L. (2010). A comparison of systematic screening tools for emotional and behavioral disorders: A replication. *Journal of Emotional and Behavioral Disorders, 18*, 100–113.

Lane, K. L., Little, M. A., Casey, A. M., Lambert, W., Wehby, J. H., Weisenbach, J. L., & Phillips, A. (2009). A comparison of systematic screening tools for emotional and behavioral disorders: How do they compare? *Journal of Emotional and Behavioral Disorders, 17*, 93–105.

Lebuffe, P. A., & Naglieri, J. A. (1999). *Devereux Early Childhood Assessment user's guide*. Lewisville, NC: Kaplan.

Lentz, F. E., & Wehmann, B. A. (1995). Best practices in interviewing. In A. Thomas & J. Grimes (Eds.), *Best practices in school psychology III* (pp. 637–650). Washington, DC: National Association of School Psychologists.

Ludy, B. T., Hopkins, R., & Nation, J. R. (1994). *Psychology* (3rd ed.). New York, NY: Macmillan.

Lynam, D. R. (1996). Early identification of chronic offenders: Who is a fledgling psychopath? *Psychological Bulletin, 120*, 209–234.

McArthur, D. S., & Roberts, G. E. (1994). *Roberts apperception test for children*. Los Angeles, CA: Western Psychological Services.

McConaughy, S. H. (1993). Evaluating behavioral and emotional disorders with CBCL, TRF, and YSR cross-informant scales. *Journal of Emotional and Behavioral Disorders, 1*, 40–52.

McConaughy, S. H., & Ritter, D. R. (1995). Best practices in multidimensional assessment of emotional or behavioral disorders. In A. Thomas & J. Grimes (Eds.), *Best practices in school psychology III* (pp. 1303–1320). Washington, DC: National Association of School Psychologists.

McConaughy, S. H., & Skiba, R. J. (1994). Comorbidity of externalizing and internalizing problems. *School Psychology Review, 22*, 421–436.

McLoughlin, J. A., & Lewis, R. B. (1994). *Assessing special students.* New York, NY: Macmillan College.

Menzies, H. M., & Lane, K. L. (2012). Validity of the Student Risk Screening Scale: Evidence of predictive validity in a diverse, suburban elementary setting. *Journal of Emotional and Behavioral Disorders, 20,* 82–91.

Merrell, K. W. (2011). *Social and emotional assets and resilience scales* (SEARS). Lutz, FL: Psychological Assessment Resources.

Moffitt, T. E. (1993). Adolescence-limited and life-course-persistent antisocial behavior: A developmental taxonomy. *Psychological Review, 100,* 674–701.

Naglieri, J. A., McNeish, T. J., & Bardos, A. N. (1991). *Draw a Person: Screening procedure for emotional disturbance.* Austin, TX: PRO-ED.

Neel, R. S., Meadows, N., Levine, P., & Edgar, E. B. (1988). What happens after special education: A statewide follow-up study of secondary students who have behavioral disorders. *Behavioral Disorders, 13,* 209–216.

Nelson, J. R. (1996). Designing schools to meet the needs of students who exhibit disruptive behavior. *Journal of Emotional and Behavioral Disorders, 4,* 147–161.

Oakes, W. P., Wilder, K., Lane, K. L., Powers, L., Yokoyama, L., O'Hare, M. E., & Jenkins, A. B. (2010). Psychometric properties of the Student Risk Screening Scale: An effective tool for use in diverse urban elementary schools. *Assessment for Effective Intervention, 35,* 231–239.

Oswald, D. P., & Coutinho, M. J. (1996). Leaving school: The impact of state economic and demographic factors for students with serious emotional disturbance. *Journal of Emotional and Behavioral Disorders, 4,* 114–125.

Papolos, D. F. (2003). Bipolar disorder and comorbid disorders: The case for a dimensional nosology. In B. Geller & M. P. DelBello (Eds.), *Bipolar disorder in childhood and early adolescence* (pp. 76–106). New York, NY: Guilford Press.

Patterson, G., De Baryshe, B. D., & Ramsey, E. (1989). A developmental perspective on antisocial behavior. *American Psychologist, 44,* 329–335.

Patterson, G., Reid, J., & Dishion, T. (1992). *Antisocial boys.* Eugene, OR: Castalia.

Phillips, V., Nelson, C. M., & McLaughlin, J. R. (1993). Systems change and services for students with emotional/behavioral disorders in Kentucky. *Journal of Emotional and Behavioral Disorders, 1,* 155–164.

Quinn, K. P., & Epstein, M. H. (1998). Characteristics of children, youth, and families served by local interagency systems of care. In M. H. Epstein, K. Kutash, & A. Duchnowski (Eds.), *Outcomes for children and youth with emotional and behavioral disorders and their families.* Austin, TX: PRO-ED.

Reid, R. (1993). Implementing self-monitoring interventions in the classroom: Lessons from research. *Monograph in Behavior Disorders: Severe Behavior Disorders in Youth, 16,* 43–54.

Reid, R., Gonzalez, J., Nordness, P., Trout, A., & Epstein, M. (2004). A meta-analysis of the academic status of students with emotional/behavioral disturbance. *Journal of Special Education, 38,* 130–143.

Reynolds, C. R., & Kamphaus, R. W. (1992). *Behavior assessment system for children.* Circle Pines, MN: American Guidance Service.

Reynolds, W. M. (1992a). Depression in children and adolescents. In W. M. Reynolds (Ed.), *Internalizing disorders in children and adolescents* (pp. 150–253). New York, NY: Wiley.

Reynolds, W. M. (1992b). The study of internalizing disorders in children and adolescents. In W. M. Reynolds (Ed.), *Internalizing disorders in children and adolescents* (pp. 1–18). New York: Wiley.

Robbins, L. N. (1966). *Deviant children grown up: A sociologic and psychiatric study of sociopathic personality.* Baltimore, MA: Williams & Wilkins.

Ruhl, K. L., & Berlinghoff, D. H. (1992). Research on improving behaviorally disordered students' academic performance: A review of the literature. *Behavioral Disorders, 17,* 178–190.

Salvia, J., Ysseldyke, J. E., & Bolt, S. (2013). *Assessment* (12th ed.). Belmont, CA: Wadsworth.

Seeley, J. R., Rohde, P., Lewinsohn, P. M., & Clarke, G. N. (2002). Depression in youth: Epidemiology, identification, and intervention. In M. R. Shinn, H. M. Walker, & G. Stoner (Eds.), *Interventions for academic and behavior problems II: Preventive and remedial approaches* (pp. 885–911). Bethesda, MD: National Association of School Psychologists.

Shaw, D. S., Gilliom, M., & Giovannelli, J. (2000). Aggressive behavior disorders. In C. H. Z. Jr. (Ed.), *Handbook of infant mental health* (2nd ed., pp. 397–411). New York, NY: Guilford Press.

Singh, N. N., Landrum, T. J., Donatelli, L. S., Hampton, C., & Ellis, C. R. (1994). Characteristics of children and adolescents with serious emotional disturbance in systems of care. Part I: Partial hospitalization and inpatient psychiatric services. *Journal of Emotional and Behavioral Disorders, 2,* 13–20.

Smith, M. A. (2001). Functional assessment of challenging behaviors. In S. Alper, D. L. Ryndak, & C. N. Schloss (Eds.), *Alternative assessment of students with disabilities in inclusive settings* (pp. 256–272). Boston, MA: Allyn and Bacon.

Smith, S. W., & Coutinho, M. J. (1997). Achieving the goals of the national agenda: Progress and prospects. *Journal of Emotional and Behavioral Disorders, 5,* 2–5.

Sugai, G., Sprague, J. R., Horner, R. H., & Walker, H. (2000). Preventing school violence: The use of office discipline referrals to assess and monitor schoolwide discipline interventions. *Journal of Emotional and Behavioral Disorders, 8,* 94–101.

Tremblay, R. E., Vitaro, F., Bertrand, L., LeBlanc, M., Benchesne, H., Boileau, H., & David, L. (1992). Parent and child training to prevent early onset of delinquency: The Montreal Longitudinal Experimental Study. In J. McCorea & R. Tremblay (Eds.), *Preventing antisocial behavior: Interventions from birth through adolescence.* New York, NY: Guilford Press.

Trout, A., Nordness, P., Pierce, C., & Epstein, M. (2003). The academic status of children with emotional and behavioral disorders: A review of the literature from 1961 to 2000. *Journal of Emotional and Behavioral Disorders, 11,* 198–210.

U.S. Department of Education. (2012). *Thirtieth annual report to Congress on the implementation of the Individuals with Disabilities Improvement Act 2008.* Washington, DC: Author.

U.S. Department of Health and Human Services. (2000). *Report of the Surgeon General's conference on children's mental health: A national action agenda.* Washington, DC: Author.

U.S. Department of Health and Human Services. (2001). *Youth violence: A report of the Surgeon General.* Washington, DC: Office of the Surgeon General.

UCLA-Neuropsychiatric Institute. (1999). *Generalized anxiety disorder in children.* Retrieved from http://www.semel.ucla.edu/caap/generalized-anxiety-disorder-gad

Wagner, M. W., Kutash, K., Duchnowski, A. J., Epstein, M. H., & Sumi, W. C. (2005). The children and youth we serve: A national picture of the characteristics of students with emotional disturbances receiving special education. *Journal of Emotional and Behavioral Disorders, 13,* 79–96.

Walker, H. M., Horner, R. H., Sugai, G., Bullis, M., Sprague, J. R., Bricker, D., & Kauffman, M. J. (1996). Integrated approaches to preventing antisocial behavior patterns among school-age children and youth. *Journal of Emotional and Behavioral Disorders, 4,* 194–209.

Walker, H. M., Kavanagh, K., Stiller, B., Golly, A., Severson, H. H., & Feil, E. G. (1998). First step to success: An early intervention approach for preventing school antisocial behavior. *Journal of Emotional and Behavioral Disorders, 6,* 66–80.

Walker, H. M., Ramsey, E., & Gresham, F. M. (2004). *Antisocial behavior in school: Evidence-based practices.* Belmont, CA: Wadsworth.

Walker, H. M., & Severson, H. H. (1990). *Systematic screening for behavior disorders* (SSBD). Longmont, CA: Sopris West.

Walker, H. M., Severson, H. H., Nicholson, F., Kehle, T., Jensen, W. R., & Clark, E. (1994). Replication of the systematic screening for behavior disorders (SSBD) procedure for the identification of at-risk children. *Journal of Emotional and Behavioral Disorders, 2,* 66–77.

Walker, H. M., & Sprague, J. R. (1999). The path to school failure, delinquency, and violence: Causal factors and some potential solutions. *Intervention in School and Clinic, 35,* 67–73.

Walters, T. L., Barrett, P. M., & March, J. S. (2001). Cognitive-behavioral family treatment of childhood obsessive–compulsive disorder: Preliminary findings. *American Journal of Psychotherapy, 55,* 372–387.

Wehby, J. H., Symons, F. J., & Hollo, A. (1997). Promote appropriate assessment. *Journal of Emotional and Behavioral Disorders, 5,* 45–54.

Wenar, C., Kerig, P., & Ludlow, A. (2012). *Developmental psychopathology* (6th ed.). New York, NY: McGraw-Hill.

Woodcock, R., McGrew, K., & Mather, N. (2000). *Woodcock-Johnson III tests of achievement.* Itasca, IL: Riverside.

Zuckerman, M. (1999). *Vulnerability to psychopathology.* Washington, DC: American Psychological Association.

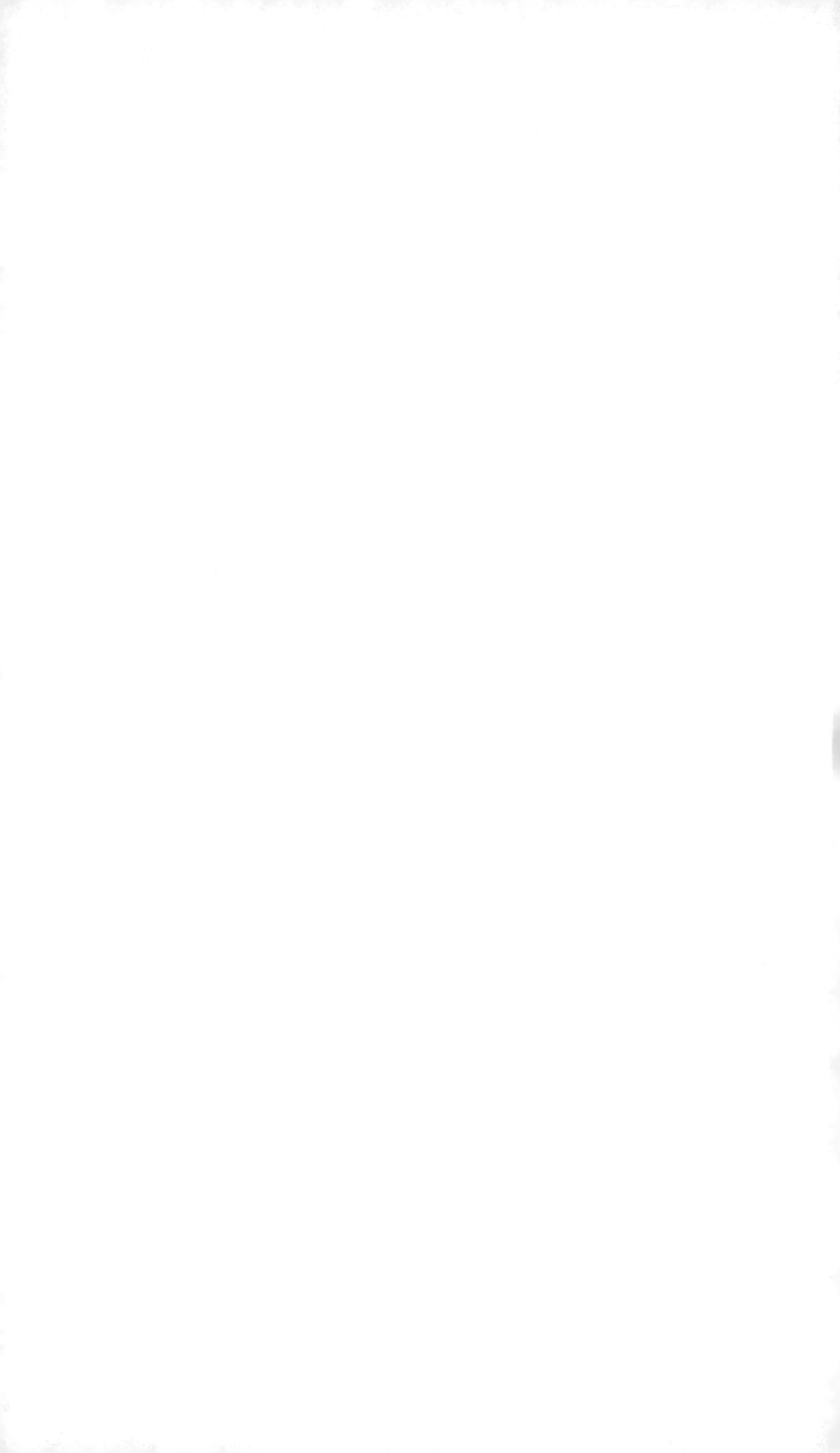

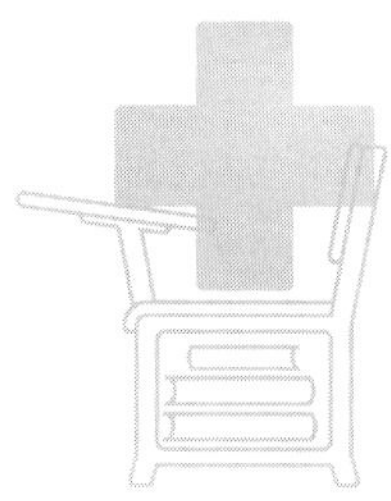

GLOSSARY

Abduct. To draw away from the median plane.

Abortifacient. An agent that causes abortion.

Abscess. A cavity filled with pus.

Acetone. A colorless liquid found in the urine of diabetic patients who are poorly controlled.

Achondroplasia. A type of dwarfism characterized by short limbs.

Acquired. Nongenetic, produced by external forces or influences.

Acuity. Keenness of vision or hearing.

Acute pancreatitis. Acute inflammation of the pancreas.

Adduct. To draw toward the median plane.

Adipose. Of or relating to fat.

Adrenaline (epinephrine). Secreted by the adrenal medulla and a powerful stimulant of the sympathetic nervous system.

Aerosolize. The process of dispersing in a fine mist.

Air studies. The introduction of air into the cerebrospinal fluid spaces for evaluation of brain anatomy.

Alexia. Loss of the ability to understand written language as the result of a cerebral lesion.

Allele. One or more contrasting characters transmitted by alternative genes.

Alpha-fetoprotein. A protein produced by the fetal liver that is markedly elevated in the amniotic fluid when the fetus has spina bifida or an open defect of the central nervous system.

Amblyopia. Decreased vision without apparent change in the eye structures.

Ambulation. The act of walking or moving about.

Amenorrhea. Absence or abnormal stoppage of the menses.

Amnesia. Loss of memory.

Amniocentesis. Surgical transabdominal perforation of the uterus to obtain amniotic fluid.

Amphetamine. A drug that acts as a central nervous system stimulant.

Amplification. Increase of auditory stimulus by the use of hearing aids.

Analgesic. A class of drugs used for the relief of pain.

Ancillary. Supplementary, additional.

Anemia. A condition in which blood is deficient in the quantity of hemoglobin or the number of red blood cells or both.

Anencephaly. Absence of the cerebral hemispheres and cranial vault in the brain.

Anomaly. A variance from the normal.

Anorexia. Loss of appetite for food.

Anorexia nervosa. Severe and prolonged inability or refusal to eat, sometimes associated with vomiting.

Anoxia. A severe reduction in the normal concentration of oxygen within the body.

Antacid. A drug that counteracts or relieves gastric (stomach) acidity.

Antenatal. Occurring before birth.

Anterior. Situated before or toward the front.

Anthropometric. Relating to the study of human body measurements, especially on a comparative basis.

Antibiotic. A chemical that inhibits the growth of or kills microorganisms.

Anticholinergic. An agent that blocks the parasympathetic nerves.

Anticonvulsant. A drug used to treat and prevent convulsions.

Antidepressant. A drug used to elevate the mood of a depressed individual.

Anxiolytic. A drug that inhibits anxiety.

Aortic stenosis. Obstruction of the aortic artery.

Aphasia. Defect or loss of the power to use words in speech or writing due to disease or injury of the brain.

Apnea. Transient attacks of failure of automatic control of breathing.

Arnold Chiari malformation. A congenital malformation of the brain in which the cerebellum and medulla protrude downward into the spinal cord.

Arteriosclerosis. Thickening and loss of elasticity of the arterial walls.

Arteriovenous malformation. An abnormal relationship between arteries and veins.

Arthritis. Inflammation of the joints due to infectious, metabolic, or constitutional causes.

Articular. Joint surface.

Articulator. A device for effecting a jointlike union.

Asphyxia. Lack of oxygen leading to cessation of life.

Asperger syndrome. High functioning autistic student.

Aspiration. The taking of foreign matter into the lungs when breathing or inhaling.

Assay. A biologic analysis to measure the quantity or purity of a substance.

Assistive technology. An umbrella term that includes assistive, adaptive, and rehabilitative devices for people with disabilities and includes the process used in selecting, locating, and using them. AT promotes greater independence by enabling people to perform tasks they were formerly unable to accomplish or had great difficulty accomplishing.

Astigmatism. Unequal curvature of the eye resulting in a distorted image on the retina.

Asymptomatic. Presenting no subjective evidence of disease.

Ataxia. Incoordination of movement.

Atonia. Deficient muscular tone often associated with chorea.

Atherosclerotic. A form of arteriosclerosis with yellow plaques containing cholesterol and lipids deposited within the walls of the arteries.

Attributional style. To explain by indicating a cause.

Auditory nerve. Eighth cranial nerve, the hearing nerve.

Augmentative communication device. An umbrella term that encompasses methods of communication for those with impairments or restrictions on the production or comprehension of spoken or written language. AAC systems are extremely diverse and depend on the capabilities of the user. They may be as basic as pictures on a board that the user indicates by pointing or can be advanced speech-generating devices based on speech synthesis technology capable of storing hundreds of phrases and words.

Aura. A subjective sensation or phenomenon that precedes a seizure.

Autistic. A severe disorder of communication and behavior characterized by self-absorption, withdrawal from contact with people, and preoccupation with inanimate objects.

Autoimmune. Directed against the body's own tissue.

Automatism. The performance of nonreflex acts without conscious volition.

Axon. That process of a neuron by which nerve impulses travel away from the cell body.

Bacteremia. The presence of bacteria in the blood.

Barbiturate. A drug that depresses the function of the central nervous system; a useful anticonvulsant.

Basal ganglia. These include the caudate nucleus, putamen, and globus pallidus and serve to coordinate movement.

Belladonna. A plant containing various anticholinergic alkaloids, including atropine.

Benign. Nonmalignant, nonrecurrent.

Benzodiazepine. Anticonvulsant drugs including diazepam (Valium) and Klonopin.

Bilateral. Affecting both sides.

Bilirubin. Bile pigment formed by the disintegration of red blood cells.

Binge. An unrestrained indulgence.

Binocular. Relating to the use of both eyes.

Bone mineral density. Assessment of the compactness of bone.

Bradycardia. Slowness of the heart rate.

Braille. A system of writing and printing for the blind by means of tangible points or dots.

Brain morphometry. Measuring the volume and size of the brain by neuroimaging techniques.

Brain stem. That section of the brain that includes the vital centers for heart and respiratory rate as well as the control of consciousness.

Bronchial. Any of the larger air passages of the lung.

Bronchitis. An inflammation of the larger air passages of the lung.

Bronchodilators. An agent that causes dilation of the lumina of the air passages of the lungs.

Café-au-lait spots. Coffee-colored skin spots associated with neurofibromatosis.

Carbohydrate. Sugar, starch, or cellulose.

Carcinoma. A malignant new growth or cancer.

Cardiomyopathy. Disease of the heart muscle.

Caries. Tooth cavities.

Catabolism. Destructive process by which complex substances are converted by living cells into more simple compounds.

Cataract. An opacity or density of the eye lens.

Cellulitis. Infection of the skin.

Cerebellum. Lies in the posterior portion of the cranial cavity and is concerned with coordination of movement.

Cerebral cortex. The main part of the brain, occupying the upper part of the cranial cavity.

Cerebrospinal fluid (CSF). The fluid that surrounds and bathes the brain and spinal cord.

Cervix. The lower and narrow end of the uterus.

Charcot-Marie-Tooth disease. Congenital weakness and wasting of the extremities, particularly the legs.

Chemotherapy. The treatment of a disease by chemicals or drugs.

Choreoathetosis. Movement characterized by chorea and athetosis.

Chorionic gonadotrophin. A substance formed in the placenta that stimulates the gonads.

Choriovillus. Fetal tissue that can be biopsied for a genetic diagnosis.

Chromosome. A rod-shaped body within the cell nucleus that contains the DNA that transmits hereditary characteristics.

Chronic. Marked by long duration or frequent recurrence.

Chronological age. The actual age of the individual.

Circumscribed. Restricted to a limited space.

Climacteric. Menopause.

Clitoris. A small, erectile body situated in the anterior angle of the external genitalia in the female.

Coarctation. A localized stricture.

Cognition. The act or process of knowing, including both awareness and judgment.

Coitus. Sexual intercourse.

Colostomy. Surgical opening between the colon (large bowel) and the surface of the body.

Comatose. A state of unconsciousness.

Comorbid. The presence of one or more diseases co-occurring with the primary disorder.

Compliance. The act or process of following a drug treatment or weight reduction program.

Conception. The act of becoming pregnant; the state of being conceived.

Concordance. The occurrence of a given trait in both members of a twin pair.

Condom. A sheath or cover for the penis used as a prophylactic.

Congenital. Existing at or dating from birth.

Congestive heart failure. The heart cannot produce the output required to sustain the metabolic needs of the body.

Conical. Cone shaped.

Conjunctiva. The delicate membrane that lines the eyelids and covers the surface of the eye.

Consanguinity. Relationship by blood.

Constitutional. Relating to the entire body rather than a particular organ.

Contracture. Fixation of a joint due to fibrosis of a muscle.

Cornea. The transparent structure forming the anterior part of the eye.

Corpus callosum. Neural pathways that connect the cerebral hemispheres.

Cortex. The outer or external layer of the brain; gray matter.

Cortical sulcal enlargement. An increase in the size of the depressions (i.e., a groove, trench, or furrow) on the outer layer of the brain.

Cortisol. A natural hydrocortisone product produced by the human adrenal gland.

Craniosynostosis. Premature closure of the sutures of the skull.

C-reactive protein. A blood test that measures the degree of inflammation.

Cyanosis. A bluish discoloration of the skin resulting from poor oxygenation.

Cycloplegia. The loss of the eye's ability to constrict the pupil.

Cystic fibrosis. An inherited disease characterized by fibrosis of the lungs and absence of digestive enzymes in the pancreas gland.

Cytoplasm. The protoplasm of a cell exclusive of that of the nucleus.

Decibel. A unit for expressing relative intensity of sound; zero is the average least perceptible sound and 130 is the average pain level.

Decongestant. An agent that reduces congestion or swelling.

Degradation. The act of reducing a chemical or compound to smaller units.

Dehydration. The condition that results from excessive loss of body water and electrolytes.

Delirium tremens. Alcoholic withdrawal characterized by anxiety, trembling, hallucinations, and excessive agitation.

Demyelination. Loss or destruction of myelin.

Dermatologic. Affecting the skin.

Detoxification. Treatment designed to free an addict from his or her drug habit.

Diffusion tensor MRI. An imaging method that is sensitive to the molecular movement of water, which indicates cellular integrity and pathology; this technique can provide a structural analysis of specific tracts within the central nervous system.

Dilantin. A drug used to control seizures.

Dilatation. The condition of being dilated or stretched beyond normal dimensions.

Diplegia. Weakness or paralysis of the legs.

Diploid. Double in appearance or arrangement, especially of the basic chromosome number.

Diplopia. Double vision due to weakness or paralysis of the eye muscles.

Distal. At the end of an extremity or organ.

Diuretic. An agent that promotes the excretion of urine.

Dopamine. An intermediate product in the synthesis of norepinephrine; acts as a neurotransmitter in the central nervous system.

Dorsiflexion. Backward flexion or bending of the hand or foot.

Dura. Thick, membranous protective covering of the brain.

Dwarfism. A condition characterized by short stature, less than average height.

Dysarthria. Imperfect articulation of speech due to a disturbance of motor control.

Dyscalculia. Impairment of the ability to do mathematical problems.

Dysesthesia. Impairment of any sense, especially touch.

Dysgraphia. Inability to write properly, sometimes as a part of a language disorder.

Dyskinesia. Fragmentary incomplete movements.

Dyslexia. An inability to read with understanding at age and grade level.

Dysmorphic. An abnormality in development.

Dysphagia. Difficulty in swallowing.

Dysplastic. Referring to abnormal development or growth.

Dyspraxia. Partial loss of ability to perform coordinated tasks.

Dystonia. Disordered tonicity of muscle.

Echolalia. The repetition of words or sentences by an individual, often without understanding.

Ectopic. Out of place or position.

Eczema. A skin disorder affecting the face, scalp, arms, and legs.

Edema. Swelling; collection of abnormally excessive amounts of fluid.

Ejaculation. Sudden expulsion of semen.

Electroencephalogram (EEG). The recording of electrical currents originating in the brain by means of electrodes placed on the scalp.

Electrolytes. Ions in the blood, including chloride, potassium, and sodium.

Electrophoresis. The movement of charged particles suspended in a liquid under the influence of an applied electric field.

Emaciation. A wasted or malnourished state.

Embryo. The developing organism from 2 weeks following fertilization to the end of the 8th week.

Embryogenesis. The development of a new organism by means of sexual reproduction.

Encephalitis. Infection of the brain.

Encephalocele. Hernia of the brain through a congenital or traumatic opening of the skull.

Encephalopathy. A process that damages or interferes with brain function.

Endometrium. The inner mucous membrane of the uterus.

End organ. The organ responsible for a particular function.

Enteritis. Inflammation of the small intestine.

Enucleation. The surgical removal of an organ (e.g., the eye).

Enzyme. A substance that accelerates or catalyzes specific chemical reactions within the organism.

Epicanthus. A vertical fold of skin on either side of the nose that covers the innermost portion of the eye.

Epidemic. A disease affecting many people in any region at the same time.

Epidemiologic. Pertaining to the incidence, distribution, and control of disease.

Epidermis. The outermost and nonvascular layer of skin.

Epididymis. An elongated cordlike structure lying along the testes which provides storage, transport, and maturation of spermatozoa.

Epigenetics. The study of changes in the expression of genes caused by certain base pairs in DNA or RNA being "turned off" or "turned on" again through certain chemicals.

Epiglottitis. A serious life-threatening infection of tissue covering the entrance to the larynx.

Epiphyseal. The end of a long bone.

Epiphysis. The end of a bone where the majority of growth takes place.

Ergot. A drug used for the treatment of migraine headaches.

Esophagus. The musculomembranous passage extending from the mouth to the stomach.

Esotropia. Deviation of the eye toward the nose.

Etiology. The cause of a disorder or condition.

Euphoric. A feeling of well-being or elation.

Eversion. The foot turned outward.

Evoked response potential. An electrical response (averaged on a computer) that follows stimulation of the central nervous system by a specific stimulus of the visual, auditory, or sensory system.

Exchange system. A diabetic diet that allows the trading of one item of food for another (e.g., a slice of bread for a serving of potatoes).

Executive brain function. Refers/defines complex cognitive functioning.

Exogenous. Outside the body or organ.

Exophoria. Outward deviation of the eye.

Exophthalmos. Abnormal protrusion of the eyeball.

Extension. Straightening out of a joint.

External rotation. Turned (rotated) away from the midline of the body.

Extrapyramidal. Outside the pyramidal tracts.

Fallopian tubes. Pair of tubes connecting the ovary to the uterus.

Femur. The bone that extends from the pelvis to the knee.

Fertilization. The act of rendering gametes fertile or capable of further development.

Fetus. A developing vertebrate organism; in the human, the period after the third month of intrauterine development.

Flaccid. Weak, soft, or loose.

Flexion. Bending or shortening of a joint.

Flora. Bacteria normally residing in the mouth and intestine.

Flux. An abnormal flow or discharge.

Focal neurologic signs. Neurologic abnormalities restricted to one portion of the body.

Footcandle. The amount of illumination produced by a standard candle at a distance of 1 ft.

Fovea (of the retina). A small pit in the retina that provides the clearest vision because of the concentration of a group of nerve cells called cones.

Fricatives. The sounds produced by a voiceless breath escaping through the larynx or vocal tract.

Friedreich's ataxia. An inherited disease that begins in childhood, is characterized by progressive loss of gait and speech impairment, and often results in sudden death because of cardiac arrhythmias.

Frontal lobe. The most anterior portion of the brain that controls many activities, including executive function.

Gangrene. Death of tissue usually associated with a loss of blood supply and followed by bacterial invasion.

Gastric. Relating to the stomach.

Gastroenteritis. Inflammation of stomach and intestines.

Gastroesophageal reflux (GER). Also known as acid reflux, a chronic symptom or damage caused by stomach acid coming up from the stomach into the esophagus.

Generic. Characteristic of an entire group or class.

Germ cell. The cell of origin that develops into the primitive embryo.

Gestation. The period of pregnancy.

Glaucoma. An eye disease characterized by increased pressure within the eye.

Global. Universal, comprehensive.

Glucose. A sugar.

Goiter. A visibly enlarged thyroid gland.

Gonad. The ovary or testes.

Gonadal dysgenesis. Defective development of the testes or ovary.

Gray matter. Neural tissue, especially of the brain and spinal cord, that contains cell bodies as well as nerve fibers, and forms most of the cortex and nuclei of the brain, the columns of the spinal cord, and the bodies of ganglia.

Gustatory. Pertaining to the sense of taste.

Guttural. Articulated in the throat.

Habilitation. The process of enhancing an individual's capabilities to the greatest potential.

Halitosis. Offensive breath.

Half-life. The time required to metabolize half of a drug or isotope.

Hallucination. A sense perception not founded upon objective reality.

Hallucinogen. A drug or chemical that produces hallucinations.

Hamstring. Muscle at the back of the thigh.

Heart murmur. A sound produced due to the abnormal flow of blood, usually the result of a heart defect.

Helical. Having the form of a helix.

Hematocrit. A measure of the volume of red blood cells.

Hematologic disturbances. Disturbances in the blood.

Hemiplegia. Paralysis on one side of the body.

Hemoglobin. The oxygen-carrying component in the red blood cells.

Hepatitis. Inflammation of the liver.

Hereditary. Genetically transmitted from parent to offspring.

Heterosexual. One who is sexually attracted to persons of the opposite sex.

Hormone. A chemical substance formed in one part of the body that has a specific action on an organ located in another site.

Huntington chorea. A rare hereditary disease characterized by progressive uncontrolled movements of the extremities and mental deterioration.

Hydrocephalus. An enlargement of the head due to an abnormal collection of cerebrospinal fluid.

Hyperkinesia. Abnormally increased activity.

Hyperopia. Farsightedness.

Hypertelorism. Abnormally increased distance between the eyes.

Hypertension. High arterial blood pressure.

Hyperthyroidism. Excessive activity of the thyroid gland.

Hypertrophy. The enlargement of an organ.

Hyperventilation. Deep breathing.

Hypochondriasis. Overconcern about one's health.

Hypoglycemia. An abnormally low blood glucose level.

Hypogonadal. Pertaining to the decreased function of the sex glands.

Hyposensitization. The process of decreasing sensitivity, usually by providing the patient with gradually increasing quantities of the offending substance.

Hypothalamic–pituitary axis. The anterior pituitary lobe secretes several important hormones that regulate the functioning of the thyroids, gonads, adrenal cortex, and other endocrine organs; the cells of the posterior lobe serve as a reservoir for hormones having antidiuretic and oxytocic action.

Hypothalamus. The portion of the brain that includes the optic chiasm, mamillary bodies, infundibulum, and hypophysis, which integrate peripheral autonomic mechanisms, endocrine activity, and many somatic functions.

Hypothyroidism. Deficiency of thyroid activity.

Hypotonia. Decreased muscle tone.

Hypoxia. Reduction of oxygen supply to tissues.

Hysterectomy. Surgical removal of the uterus (womb).

Iatrogenic. Induced by the physician or caregiver.

Individualized Education Program (IEP). A written document created by a team of professionals and parents that states the goals and objectives and services for a child with a disability.

Individual Family Service Plan (IFSP). A written document created by a team of professionals and the parents that states the outcomes, supports, and services for a child with a disability and his or her family.

Individuals With Disabilities Education Act (IDEA). A U.S. federal law ensuring children with disabilities a free and appropriate public education.

Ileostomy. Surgical creation of an opening from the surface of the abdominal wall into the small bowel.

Immunity. The ability to resist a certain disease or infection.

Immunoglobulin. A protein synthesized by lymphocyte and plasma cells that are responsible for the humoral aspects of immunity.

Impotence. Lack of ability to initiate an erection or to maintain an erection until ejaculation.

Incest. Sexual activity between close relatives (e.g., father and daughter; brother and sister).

Incidence. An expression of the rate at which a certain event occurs (e.g., number of new cases of a specific disease occurring during a certain period).

Incisors. Any of the four front teeth.

Infarction. Tissue destruction resulting from obstruction of circulation to the area.

Insomnia. Inability to sleep.

Insulin-dependent diabetes mellitus. A disease in which the body's cells cannot use glucose (sugar) properly for lack of or resistance to the hormone insulin, produced by the pancreas.

Intestinal motility. The ability of the intestine to move spontaneously.

Intracranial. Situated within the skull.

Intramuscular. Within the substance of a muscle.

In utero. Within the uterus.

Inversion. The foot turns inward.

Ipecac. A medication used to induce vomiting.

Ischemia. Deficiency of blood flow to a region of the body.

Jaundice. Abnormal deposition of bile pigment in the skin, resulting in a yellowish appearance.

Karyotype. The chromosome number and composition.

Keratoconus. A conical protrusion of the cornea.

Kernicterus. Excessive serum levels of bilirubin, resulting in brain damage.

Ketone. The substances acetone, acetoacetic acid, and b-hydroxybutyric acid.

Kinesthesia. The sense by which movement, weight, and position are perceived.

Labia. An elongated fold running downward and backward from the mons pubis of the female.

Lacrimation. The secretion of tears.

Lactation. The secretion of milk.

Larynx. The portion of the trachea that contains the vocal cords.

Lesion. A pathologic disruption of tissue or a loss of a part.

Lethal. Deadly, fatal.

Leukomalacia. Softening or destruction of the white matter.

Leukopenia. Decrease in white blood cells in the blood.

Lexicon. The vocabulary of language.

Likert scale. Rating scale designed to measure attitudes or opinions.

Limbic system. A highly complex, phylogenetically old portion of the brain that is thought to be involved with control of emotion.

Lingual. Pertaining to or toward the tongue.

Lissencephaly. Malformations of the brain due to abnormal convolutions of the cerebral cortex.

Locomotor. Pertaining to movement or locomotion.

Logogram. A letter, symbol, or sign used to represent an entire word.

Lupus erythematosis. A generalized connective tissue disorder.

Macroglossia. Excessive size of the tongue.

Macro-orchidism. Enlarged testes.

Macula. The anatomic area of the retina that provides the clearest vision.

Marfan syndrome. Tall stature, dilation of the aorta, displaced lenses in the eye, hypotonia, and normal intelligence.

Malabsorption. Impaired intestinal absorption of nutrients.

Malady. An illness, usually of a chronic type.

Malaise. A vague sensation of discomfort.

Malar. Relating to the cheek or the side of the head.

Malignancy. Cancer, a tumor with invasive properties.

Malingerer. One who feigns an illness.

Mallory-Weiss tears. Mucosal tears and bleeding at the junction of the stomach and esophagus caused by violent vomiting.

Malocclusion. Improper closure of the teeth.

Mastoid. The bony prominence located behind each ear.

Maturation. The process of becoming fully developed.

Maxilla. The upper jaw.

Mb. Megabyte.

Medial. Toward the middle.

Megavitamins. Extremely high doses of vitamins, sometimes used to treat autism and a wide range of developmental disorders.

Meiosis. The cellular process that results in the number of chromosomes in gamete-producing cells being reduced to one half.

Menarche. The onset of menstruation.

Meningitis. Infection of the brain and its covering membranes.

Meningomyelocele. Hernial protrusion of a part of the meninges and substance of the spinal cord through a defect in the bony spinal column.

Menses. The monthly flow of blood from the female genital tract.

Meta-analysis. Statistical methods for contrasting and combining results from different studies in the hope of identifying patterns among study groups.

Metabolic rate. The rate at which food is transformed into energy, which is then used for the maintenance of respiration, circulation, peristalsis, muscle tonus, body temperature, glandular activity, and other vegetative functions of the body.

Metabolism. The sum of chemical and physical activity that creates and destroys cells.

Metalinguistics. A branch of linguistics that deals with the relation between language and other cultural factors in a society.

Methylphenidate. Trade name Ritalin, the most commonly used stimulant medication for the treatment of attention-deficit/hyperactivity disorder.

Microcephaly. Abnormal smallness of the head, usually associated with cognitive impairment.

Milestone. A significant point or event in development.

Mites. Minute animals related to the spider.

Mitochondrial. Organelles in the cell cytoplasm that generate energy in the form of ATP (adenosine triphosphate).

Mitotic cell. A method of indirect division of a cell in which two daughter nuclei receive identical complements of the number of chromosomes characteristic of the somatic cells of the species.

Mitral valve. A bicuspid valve in the heart between the ventricle and the atrium.

Mitral valve prolapse. The downward displacement of the mitral valve, which is found between the two left chambers of the heart.

Monoarticular. Limited to one joint.

Monogamy. The practice of marrying only once during a lifetime.

Monozygotic twin. Derived from one fertilized ovum—an identical twin.

Morbidity. The condition of being diseased or unwell.

Morphogenesis. The development and establishment of form.

Mortality rate. The ratio of deaths to a total population in a given time or place.

Mucosa. A mucous membrane (e.g., vaginal, urethral).

Multidisciplinary. Pertaining to the cooperative participation by several professional groups.

Multifactorial. Arising through the interaction of many factors.

Musculoskeletal. Referring to muscles and the bony skeleton.

Mutagen. A chemical or physical agent that induces genetic mutations.

Myasthenia gravis. Muscle weakness due to a disorder of acetylcholine receptors at the neuromuscular junction.

Myelin. A fatlike substance that envelops certain nerve fibers or tracts.

Myopia. Nearsightedness.

Myotonic dystrophy. An inherited form of muscular dystrophy characterized by progressive weakness, baldness, cataracts, and a peculiar stiffness of certain muscles.

Nares. The nostrils.

Nasogastric tube. A soft tube inserted through a nostril into the stomach.

Neonatal. Pertaining to the initial month of life.

Neoplasm. Any new and abnormal growth of any tissue in the body.

Nephrosis. A disease of the kidneys characterized by loss of protein in the urine and generalized edema.

Neural tube. The primitive nervous system.

Neuromuscular. Pertaining to the peripheral nerves and muscles.

Neuron. Any of the conducting cells of the nervous system.

Neurotic. Pertaining to a functional nervous disorder without demonstrable physical lesion; pertaining to an emotionally unstable individual.

Neurulation. Formation of the neural plate in the embryo.

Neurotransmitter. A substance that is released from an axon and that inhibits or excites a target cell.

Nidus. The point of origin or focus of a morbid process.

Noonan syndrome. A child with short stature, shield chest, low hairline in neck, congenital heart disease, and a short webbed neck.

Noradrenaline. A catecholamine that is the principal neurotransmitter of adrenergic neurons.

Nystagmus. Abnormal, jerky eye movements.

Obesity. An excessive accumulation of body fat.

Occipital. Pertaining to the back or posterior part of the head.

Ocular. Pertaining to the eye.

Odds ratio. A method to quantify how strongly the presence or absence of property A is associated with the presence or absence of property B in a given population.

Olfactory. Pertaining to the sense of smell.

Ontogeny. The development of the individual organism.

Omphalocele. Protrusion of part of the intestine at birth through a large defect in the abdominal wall at the umbilicus.

Optic chiasm. The crossing of the optic nerves.

Optic nerve. The visual nerve.

Oral motor dysfunction. An inability to use the oral mechanism for functional speech or feeding, including chewing, blowing, swallowing, or making specific sounds.

Organ. A part of the body with specialized function (e.g., digestion, respiration).

Organic. Originating within the body and affecting the function of the individual.

Orgasm. The apex and culmination of sexual excitement.

Orthodontics. The dental specialty that is concerned with malocclusion of the teeth.

Orthographic. The representation of the sounds of a language by written or printed symbols.

Orthoptics. The prescription of eye movement exercises for the treatment of various visual defects, including muscular imbalance.

Orthotic. A supportive device to support, align, or correct deformities, or to improve the function of movable parts of the body.

Osmoregulation. Concerned with the regulation and maintenance of constant osmotic pressure.

Ossification. The formation of bone.

Osteoarthritis. Degenerative joint disease characterized by pain and stiffness, particularly after prolonged activity.

Osteogenesis imperfecta. An inherited condition in which the bones are abnormally brittle and subject to recurrent fractures.

Osteopenia. Decrease in bone mass.

Osteoporosis. Abnormal density of bones.

Osteotomy. The cutting of a bone by a surgeon.

Ototoxic. A drug that damages the hearing mechanism, resulting in deafness.

Ovulation. The discharge of an egg from a vesicular follicle of the ovary.

Ovum. The female reproductive cell, the egg.

Pallor. Paleness.

Palpebral. Eyelid.

Palpitations. A subjective sensation of an unduly rapid or irregular heartbeat.

Pancreas. A gland that lies behind the stomach; it produces digestive enzymes and insulin.

Parkinson disease. A neurological disease characterized by tremor, muscle rigidity, and decreased muscle movements due to a deficiency of dopamine in the central nervous system.

Parotid gland. Salivary gland, located in front of the ear.

Parturition. The act or process of giving birth to a child.

Pathogen. A disease-producing microorganism.

Pathogenesis. The sequence of events leading to the development of a disease.

Pathognomonic. Specifically distinctive or characteristic of a disease or pathologic condition.

Pathology. The study of structural changes within the body caused by disease.

Patterning. A system of physical therapy for the treatment of cerebral palsy, learning disorders, and a variety of other neurological disorders. Proponents have made controversial claims that this approach is an effective therapy for these disorders.

Pedodontics. The branch of dentistry concerned with conditions of the teeth and mouth in children.

Pedophilia. Sexual activity between adults and children.

Peptic. Related to the action of gastric juices.

Peptide. The constituent part of a protein; some peptides act as hormones.

Pericardial. A sac that surrounds the heart.

Perinatal. The period beginning the 28th week of gestation and ending 7–28 days after birth.

Periodontal. Situated or occurring around a tooth.

Periventricular. The area surrounding the ventricles of the brain.

Phallus. The penis or clitoris.

Pharyngitis. Inflammation with pain on swallowing at the back of the throat.

Phenotype. The visible properties of an individual that are produced by the interaction of the genotype and the environment.

Phenytoin. An anticonvulsant (Dilantin) effective in the management of generalized seizures.

Philtrum. The vertical groove in the median portion of the upper lip.

Phobia. Excessive fear.

Phoneme. A member of the set of the smallest units of speech that serve to distinguish one utterance from another.

Phonological. The science of speech sounds.

Photophobia. Abnormal intolerance of light.

Physiology. The study of body and organ function.

Pituitary. A gland situated in the base of the skull that secretes several important hormones.

Placebo. An inactive substance or preparation used in controlled studies to determine the efficacy of medicinal substances.

Placenta. The organ that unites the fetus to the uterus for the provision of various nutrients.

Plantar flexion. The foot pointed downward.

Plaque. A mass adhering to the enamel surface of the tooth.

Poliomyelitis. An acute viral disease that may involve the motor cells in the spinal cord; it can be prevented by a specific vaccine.

Polygenic. Pertaining to or determined by the action of several different genes.

Polymorphism. The quality or character of occurring in several different forms.

Posterior. Situated in back of or behind.

Postnatal. Pertaining to the time following birth.

Postural drainage. The process by which the patient is assisted in clearing sputum and secretions from the lungs by positioning first on one side and then the other.

Prader-Willi syndrome. Confined to males and is associated with low muscle tone, short stature, incomplete sexual development, cognitive disabilities, and behavioral problems. These boys have an insatiable appetite that leads to obesity unless vigorously treated. The syndrome results from a microdeletion of paternal chromosome 15. This phenomenon is referred to as imprinting.

Pragmatics. The relation between signs or linguistic expressions and their users.

Premorbid. The state of appearance prior to the onset of disease.

Prenatal. Pertaining to the period before birth.

Prepubertal. Preceding puberty.

Presbyopia. Farsightedness.

Prevalence. The total number of cases of a disease in existence at a certain time in a designated area.

Primordial. Original or primitive.

Progeny. Offspring, children.

Prognathism. Marked protrusion of the jaw.

Prognosis. A forecast as to the eventual outcome of a disease.

Prone. On the stomach or lying face down.

Prophylactic. Pertaining to the prevention of or warding off of a disorder.

Prosody. Accent of a syllable.

Prostaglandins. A group of naturally occurring fatty acids that have the ability to lower blood pressure, regulate acid secretion of the stomach, regulate body temperature, and control inflammation and vascular permeability.

Prostate. A gland in the male that surrounds the neck of the bladder and the urethra. The prostate contributes fluid to the seminal secretion.

Prosthesis. An artificial device to replace an absent portion of the body.

Proximal. Nearest to the center.

Psychoactive. A stimulant of the central nervous system.

Psychometric. The measurement of intelligence.

Psychopathology. The branch of medicine that deals with the causes and nature of mental disorders.

Psychopharmacologic agents. The use of drugs to modify psychological functions and states.

Psychosis. Mental illness.

Psychosomatic. Involving both mind and body.

Psychotropic. Drugs that modify the intensity of feelings or alter certain behaviors or experiences.

Ptosis. Drooping of the upper eyelid.

Pubescence. Arriving at the age of puberty.

Purging. To cause evacuation from the bowels by the use of a laxative.

Purulent. Pus.

Quadriceps. The groups of muscles on the upper or anterior surface of the thigh.

Quadriplegia. Paralysis of all four extremities.

Radiologic. Relating to the use of X-rays for diagnosis or use of radiation in treatment.

Recombinant DNA. DNA that has been artificially introduced into a cell so that it alters the genotype and phenotype of the cell and is replicated along with the natural DNA.

Refractive errors. The imperfect deviation of light by the eye so that the image is distorted by the time it reaches the retina.

Regional enteritis. A localized area of inflammation within the small intestine.

Regression. Progressive decline or loss of skills.

Related services. Services dedicated to helping children with disabilities benefit from special education. Related services can include, but are not limited to, speech-language pathology, audiology, interpreting services, psychology, physical therapy, occupational therapy, recreation, including therapeutic recreation, early identification and assessment of disabilities, counseling, including rehabilitation counseling, medical services for diagnostic or evaluation purposes, school health and school nurse services, social work, and parent counseling and training.

Renal. Pertaining to the kidney.

Replicate. Repeat.

Restless legs syndrome. A neurological disorder characterized by throbbing, pulling, creeping, or other unpleasant sensations in the legs and an uncontrollable and sometimes overwhelming urge to move them, particularly during sleep.

Reticular activating system. The portion of the brain that is concerned with the level of consciousness.

Retina. The innermost membrane of the eye; it is the perceptive structure of the eye and is connected to the brain by the optic nerve.

Rhinitis (allergic). Inflammation of the nose caused by an allergy.

Rhinorrhea. Discharge from the nose.

Rhizotomy. Surgical interruption of the roots of spinal nerves within the spinal canal.

Rickets. A bone-deforming disease of children caused by a deficiency of Vitamin D.

Rooting reflex. The infant's primitive instinct to seek a nipple or food source.

Rote. Memorization with little comprehension.

Rubella. German measles.

Rumination. The regurgitation of food following a meal.

Russell-Silver syndrome. Low birth weight, poor growth, short stature, delayed bone age, and various kidney problems.

Salicylates. Aspirin.

Salivation. Excessive flow or production of saliva.

Savant. A person with detailed knowledge in a specialized field.

Schizencephaly. A congenital malformation of the brain with abnormal clefts.

Schizophrenia. A psychotic disorder characterized by flights of ideas, disordered thought processes, and a loss of reality reasoning.

Sclera. The tough white outer coat of the eyeball.

Scoliosis. Curvature of the spine.

Scotopic. Pertaining to an eye that has adapted to the dark.

Scurvy. Vitamin C deficiency resulting in weakness, anemia, bleeding tendency, and spongy gums.

Sebaceous glands. Glands that secrete a greasy, lubricating substance called sebum.

Secondary amenorrhea. Cessation of menstruation after it has been established at puberty.

Secondary sexual characteristics. Sexual features unrelated to the genitalia, such as the beard in a male.

Semantics. The study of changes in the signification of words.

Sensorineural hearing loss. Hearing loss caused by injury to the auditory nerve.

Sensorium. The level or state of alertness or consciousness.

Sensory. Conveying nerve impulses from the sense organs to the brain.

Sequelae. The permanent consequences of an injury or disease.

Serotonin. Released by blood platelets and acts as a neurotransmitter in the central nervous system.

Serotonin reuptake inhibitors. These medicines are used mainly in the treatment of depression. They also are used to treat obsessive–compulsive disorder, panic disorder, and bulimia nervosa. These medicines affect the chemicals that nerves in the brain use to send messages to one another. These chemical messengers, called neurotransmitters, are released by one nerve and taken up by other nerves. These medicines work by inhibiting the reuptake of serotonin, an action that allows more serotonin to be available to be taken up by other nerves.

Shunt. The bypassing of an obstruction within the brain by redirecting the cerebrospinal fluid into the heart or peritoneal cavity through a plastic tube.

Sibilants. The *s, z, ch, zh,* or *j* sounds.

Sicca cell therapy. Implantation by injection of fetal sheep brain cells to promote brain growth and improve intelligence.

Sign. Objective evidence of a disease.

Sinusitis. An infection of the sinus, the air cavities within the cranial bones.

Skinfold thickness. A technique to measure the nutrition of an individual.

Slough. Shed or cast off.

Smokeless tobacco. "Snuff" or chewing tobacco.

Soft neurological signs. Abnormalities that are usually developmentally related, such as mirror movements of the hands (the opposite hand makes similar movements to the performing hand) and unusual posturing of the hands and arms when the upper extremities are extended. Soft signs do not contribute to the localization of central nervous system lesions, but rather reflect a more generalized immaturity of the brain such as occurs in learning disorders and cognitive impairment.

Somatic. Relating to the body.

Somatization. The conversion of mental experiences or states into bodily symptoms.

Spasticity. Increased tone and stiffness of the muscles.

Spermatogenesis. The first stage of formation of sperm cells.

Sphincter. A ring of muscle that serves to open and close an orifice.

Spina bifida. A developmental anomaly characterized by defective closure of the bony encasement of the spinal cord, through which the cord and meninges may protrude.

Squint. Crossing of the eyes.

Station. The position assumed while standing.

Stereopsis. The perception of objects in relief and not as all in one plane.

Stereotactic. Precise spatial positioning of a neurosurgical instrument within discrete areas of the brain that control specific functions.

Stimulant. An agent or remedy that produces stimulation.

Strabismus. Imbalance of the muscles of the eyeball, resulting in a squint.

Stupor. Partial loss of consciousness, near coma.

Subclinical. Pertaining to a condition not detectable by the usual tests.

Subcutaneous. Beneath the skin.

Subscapular. Under the scapula, the triangular bone in the back of the shoulder.

Substrate. A substance acted upon by an enzyme.

Sucrose. A disaccharide obtained from sugar cane.

Supine. On the back or lying face up.

Symptom. The patient's perception of a change from a normal condition, which may indicate the presence of disease.

Syndrome. A set of symptoms that occur together.

Synovitis. Inflammation of the synovial membrane, the lining of the joint cavities.

Syntax. The way that words are put together to form phrases, clauses, or sentences.

Synthesis. The production of a substance.

Systemic. Affecting the entire body.

Taxonomy. Classification.

Tay-Sachs disease. A lethal degenerative disease of the central nervous system, particularly among Ashkenazi Jewish children.

Teratogenic. Tending to produce anomalies of formation.

Tetanus. An acute disease that causes severe spasms and rigidity in certain muscles (lockjaw).

Thalamus. Main relay center for sensory impulses and cerebellar and basal ganglia projections to the cerebral cortex.

Thalidomide. A sedative drug that causes serious congenital anomalies in the fetus (amelia and phocomelia) when taken by a woman during early pregnancy.

Thermoregulation. Heat regulation.

Thrombocytopenia. Decreased platelets in the blood.

Tibial tubercle. Bony prominence on the tibia bone.

Tic. An involuntary, repetitive movement of a muscle(s).

Titer. The highest dilution of a serum that causes clumping of microorganisms or other particulate antigens.

Topical. Pertaining to a drug or substance that is applied to the skin.

Toxemia. Metabolic disturbances most frequently observed in pregnancy.

Toxin. A poison.

Tracheostomy. A surgical opening into the trachea.

Traumatic brain injury (TBI). An injury to the brain caused by an external (outside) force.

Transplantation. The transfer of an organ or tissue from one person (or place within the body) to another.

Tremor. Shaking, shivering, or trembling.

Triceps. The muscle along the back of the upper arm.

Trichobezoar. Hairball.

Trimester. A period of 3 months.

Turner syndrome. A form of abnormal development of the female gonads marked by short stature, undifferentiated (streak) gonads, and variable abnormalities, which may include webbing of the neck, low posterior hair line, increased carrying angle of elbow, cubitus valgus, and cardiac defects.

Ultrasound. The visualization of deep structures of the body by recording the reflections of pulses of ultrasonic waves directed into the tissues.

Umbilical. Relating to the navel.

Unilateral. One-sided.

Urethra. The canal conveying urine from the bladder to the exterior of the body.

Urinalysis. Physical, chemical, and microscopic examination of the urine.

Vasectomy. Sterilization in the male by surgical excision of the vas deferens (the tube connecting the testis and ejaculatory duct).

Vasopressin. A hormone that causes contraction of vascular tissue of capillaries.

Ventricular. A small cavity as in the brain or heart.

Ventricular arrhythmia. Variation from the normal rhythm of the heartbeat.

Virulent. The degree of pathogenicity of a microorganism as indicated by case fatality rates.

Virus. An infective agent responsible for a great number of diseases, including the common cold. The virus is smaller than most bacteria and is capable of multiplication only within a living cell.

Void. To urinate or empty the bladder.

Volatile. Tending to evaporate quickly.

Voluntary muscles. Muscle activity that is controlled by an individual.

Vulva. The region of the external genital organs of the female.

White matter. A neural tissue that consists largely of myelinated nerve fibers, has a whitish color, and underlies the gray matter of the brain and spinal cord or is gathered into nerves. White matter carries information between the nerve cells in the brain and the spinal cord.

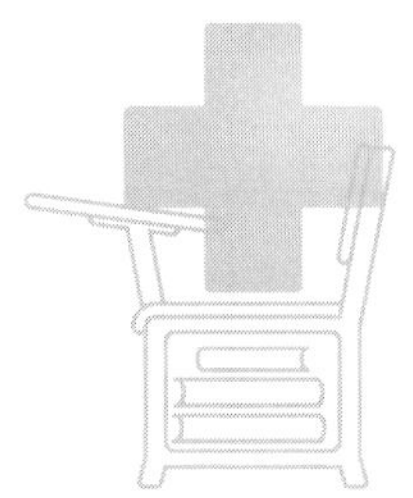

SUBJECT INDEX

A

B

C

D

E

F

G

H

J

K

L

M

O

P

Q

R

S

T

W

X

Y

Z

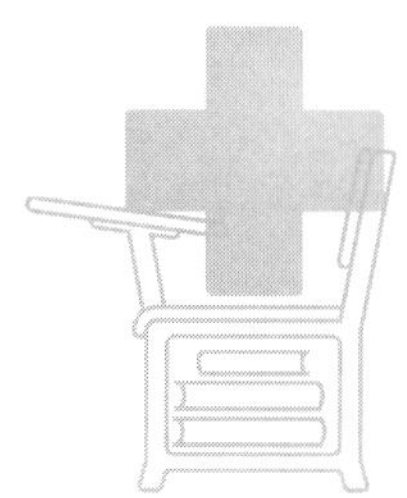

CONTRIBUTORS

Jennifer Accardo, MD, MSCE

Assistant Professor of Neurology and Pediatrics, Johns Hopkins University School of Medicine
Faculty, Kennedy Krieger Institute
Baltimore, Maryland

Pasquale J. Accardo, MD

James H. Franklin Professor of Developmental Pediatrics, Virginia Commonwealth University
Virginia Commonwealth University School of Medicine LEND Director
Richmond, Virginia

Heidi Andersen, MD

Infectious Diseases Fellow, Cincinnati Children's Hospital Medical Center
Cincinnati, Ohio

Christina M. L. Beeson, PhD Candidate

School of Psychology, Faculty of Social Sciences, University of Ottawa
Ottawa, Ontario

Kate Berz, DO

Assistant Professor of Pediatrics, Division of Sports Medicine, Department of Pediatrics, Cincinnati Children's Hospital
Cincinnati, Ohio

Patricia M. Blasco, PhD

Associate Professor, Department of Education, Portland State University
Portland, Oregon

Peter A. Blasco, MD

Associate Professor, Department of Pediatrics, Oregon Health and Science University, Director of Neurodevelopment Programs, Child Development and Rehabilitation Center, Portland, Oregon

Susan Bobbitt MD FRCPC (Pediatrics)

Subspecialty Resident, Developmental Pediatrics, University of Alberta
Edmonton, Alberta

Antonio F. Cianflone

Undergraduate Student, University of Manitoba
Winnipeg, Manitoba

Denis Daneman, MBBCh, FRCPC, DSc(Med)

Professor and Chairman, Department of Pediatrics, University of Toronto, Pediatrician-in-Chief, The Hospital for Sick Children
Toronto, Ontario

Caroline N. DeBenedictis, MD

Wills Eye Hospital
Philadelphia, Pennsylvania

Sarah Fotti, MD, FRCPC

Section of Child and Adolescent Psychiatry, Department of Psychiatry, College of Medicine, Faculty of Health Sciences, University of Manitoba
Winnipeg, Manitoba

Laurie Gaboury, PhD

Psychologist, Pediatric Center for Weight Loss and Health, Stollery Children's Hospital
Edmonton, Alberta

Jesse Godwin, MD

Division of Emergency Medicine, University of Toronto
Toronto, Ontario

Jorge E. Gonzalez, PhD

Associate Professor, Department of Educational Psychology, Texas A&M University
College Station, Texas

David B. Haslam, MD

Associate Professor, Clinical Director, Division of Infectious Diseases, and Director, Antimicrobial Stewardship Program, Cincinnati Children's Hospital
Cincinnati, Ohio

Robert H. A. Haslam, CM, MD, FAAP, FRCPC

Emeritus Professor of Pediatrics and Chairman, Department of Pediatrics and
Professor of Neurology, University of Toronto, Emeritus Pediatrician-in-Chief, The Hospital for Sick Children
Toronto, Ontario

Lana Dépatie, PhD, C.Psych

Psychologist, The Hospital for Sick Children
Toronto, Ontario

Dimitrios Ioannou, PhD

Assistant Professor, Department of Human and Molecular Genetics, Herbert Wertheim College of Medicine, Florida International University
Miami, Florida

Dilip J. Karnik, MD

Medical Director, Department of Pediatric Neurology at the Dell Children's Medical Center of Central Texas; Adjunct Professor, University of Texas at Austin, Austin, Texas

Laurence Y. Katz, MD, FRCPC

Professor of Psychiatry, Child and Adolescent Psychiatrist, Department of Psychiatry, College of Medicine, Faculty of Health Sciences, University of Manitoba
Winnipeg, Manitoba

Debra K. Katzman, MD, FRCPC

Professor of Pediatrics, Division of Adolescent Medicine, Department of Pediatrics, Senior Associate Scientist, Research Institute, The Hospital for Sick Children and the University of Toronto
Toronto, Ontario

Thaddeus E. Kelly (deceased)

Professor of Pediatrics, Division of Medical Genetics, University of Virginia School of Medicine
Charlottesville, Virginia

Alex V. Levin, MD, MHSc, FRCSC

Wills Eye Hospital
Philadelphia, Pennsylvania

Constance Mackenzie, MD, MSc, FRCPC

Assistant Professor, Department of Medicine, Divisions of Respirology and Pharmacology, Western University, London, Ontario and Assistant Medical Director, Ontario/Manitoba Poison Center, The Hospital for Sick Children
Toronto, Ontario

Laila Nurmohamed, MD, FRCPC

Child Maltreatment Fellow, University of Toronto, The Hospital for Sick Children
Toronto, Ontario

J. Ron Nelson, PhD

Professor of Special Education and Communication Disorders, University of Nebraska
Lincoln, Nebraska

Regina M. Oliver, PhD

Assistant Research Professor, Department of Special Education and Communication Disorders, University of Nebraska
Lincoln, Nebraska

Christine Orosz, PhD

Psychologist, Pediatric Center for Weight and Health, Child Health Center, Misericordia Community Hospital
Edmonton, Alberta

Vicky Papaioannou, MClSc, AUD(C), Reg.CASLPO

Assistant Professor and Head, Division of Audiology, Department of Otolaryngology, Head and Neck Surgery, University of Toronto and Department of Communication Disorders, The Hospital for Sick Children
Toronto, Ontario

Jitender Sareen, BSc, MD, FRCPC

Professor of Psychiatry, Psychology and Community Health Sciences, University of Manitoba, Group Leader of Manitoba Population Mental Health Research Group
Winnipeg, Manitoba

Herbert H. Severson, PhD

Senior Research Scientist, Oregon Research Institute, College of Education, University of Oregon
Eugene, Oregon

Bennett A. Shaywitz, MD

The Charles and Helen Schwab Professor in Dyslexia and Learning Development
Co-Director, Yale Center for Dyslexia & Creativity
Yale University School of Medicine
New Haven, Connecticut

Sally E. Shaywitz, MD

The Audrey G. Ratner Professor in Learning Development
Co-Director, Yale Center for Dyslexia & Creativity
Yale University School of Medicine
New Haven, Connecticut

Michelle Shouldice, MEd, MD, FRCPC

Associate Professor of Pediatrics, University of Toronto
Head, Division of Pediatric Medicine
The Hospital for Sick Children
Toronto, Ontario

Jeffrey R. Sprague, PhD

Professor, Special Education, Departments of Special Education and Clinical Sciences, University of Oregon
Eugene, Oregon

Helen G. Tempest, PhD

Assistant Professor, Department of Human and Molecular Genetics, Herbert Wertheim College of Medicine, Florida International University
Miami, Florida

Margaret Thompson, MD, FRCPC, FACMT, dABEM, dABEM(MedTox)

Assistant Professor, Departments of Pediatrics and Medicine, University of Toronto, Training Program Director, Clinical Pharmacology and Toxicology, Medical Director, Ontario/Manitoba Poison Center, The Hospital for Sick Children
Toronto, Ontario

Tracy Vaillancourt, PhD

Professor and Canada Research Chair, Faculty of Education, School of Psychology, Faculty of Social Sciences, University of Ottawa
Ottawa, Ontario

Ashley Vandermorris, MD, FRCPC

Subspecialty Resident, Adolescent Medicine, Division of Adolescent Medicine, Department of Pediatrics, The Hospital for Sick Children and University of Toronto
Toronto, Ontario

Hill M. Walker, PhD

Center on Human Development, UCEDD-University Center for Excellence in Developmental Disabilities, University of Oregon
Eugene, Oregon

Mary Anne Witzel, PhD (Retired)

Former Speech Pathologist, The Hospital for Sick Children
Toronto, Ontario

Lonnie Zwaigenbaum, MD

Associate Professor of Pediatrics, Department of Pediatrics, University of Alberta, Director, Autism Research, Glenrose Rehabilitation Hospital
Edmonton, Alberta

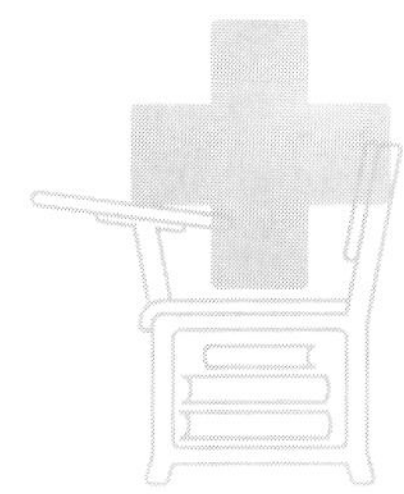

ABOUT THE EDITORS

Robert H. A. Haslam, CM, MD, FAAP, FRCPC, is a graduate of the University of Saskatchewan School of Medicine. Following an internship and a year of family medicine, he completed pediatric training at the Johns Hopkins University School of Medicine, followed by child neurology training at the University of Kentucky. In 1970, Haslam was appointed director of the John F. Kennedy Institute in Baltimore, MD, and assistant and then associate professor of pediatrics and neurology at the Johns Hopkins University School of Medicine. Haslam was named professor and chairman of the Department of Pediatrics at the University of Calgary, and director of research at the Alberta Children's Hospital in 1975. In 1986, he became professor and chairman of the Department of Pediatrics, as well as professor of medicine (neurology) at the University of Toronto and pediatrician-in-chief of pediatrics at the Hospital for Sick Children in Toronto. He has published more than 200 papers and book chapters and is a frequent invited speaker and visiting professor at national and international meetings. Currently, Haslam is a child neurologist at the Alberta Children's Hospital. His many awards and honors include the Arnold J. Capute Award by the American Academy of Pediatrics, in recognition of his notable contributions to the health and well-being of children with disabilities, and the Queen's Golden and Diamond Jubilee Medals, as well as the Order of Canada (CM), the highest civilian award in Canada, for notable contributions in pediatric research, education, child health, and advocacy.

Peter J. Valletutti, EdD, earned a doctorate in special education from the Teachers College, Columbia University. He has been a teacher and principal in the schools of New York State, as well as a professor and chairperson of special education at Coppin State College, in Baltimore, and Virginia State University, in Petersburg. He was an assistant professor in pediatrics at the Johns Hopkins University School of Medicine. He is former dean of education and graduate studies at Coppin State College. He has served as a consultant in special education and in the medical problems of children at the local, national, and international levels. The author of 24 texts in special education and rehabilitation, he is currently enjoying his retirement while working on several new writing projects.